普通高等教育"十一五"国家级规划教材
医学英文原版改编双语教材

供临床、基础、预防、口腔、药学、检验、护理等专业使用

TEXTBOOK OF PATHOLOGY

病 理 学

Original Editors
Parakrama Chandrasoma   Clive R. Taylor

Chief Editors of Adaptation Edition
Zhou Gengyin（周庚寅）
Jiang Xucheng（姜叙诚）

科学出版社
北京

· 版权所有　侵权必究 ·

举报电话:010-64030229;010-64034315;13501151303(打假办)

图字:01-2005-6067

Parakrama Chandrasoma, Clive R. Taylor
Concise Pathology, Third Edition
ISBN:0-8385-1499-5
Copyright © 1998 by Appleton & Lange

Original language published by the McGraw-Hill Companies, Inc. All rights reserved. No part of this publication may be reproduced or transmitted in any form or by any means, electronic or mechanical, including photocopying, recording, taping, or any information and retrieval system, without the written permission of the publisher.

This authorized English language reprint adapted edition is jointly published by McGraw-Hill Education (Asia) Co. and Science Press. This edition is authorized for sale in the People's Republic of China only, excluding Hong Kong SAR, Macao SAR and Taiwan province. Unauthorized export of this edition is a violation of the Copyright Act. Violation of this Law is subject to Civil and Criminal Penalties.

本书英文影印改编版由科学出版社和美国麦格劳-希尔教育(亚洲)出版公司合作出版。未经出版者预先书面许可,不得以任何方式复制或抄袭本书的任何内容。此版本仅限在中华人民共和国境内(不包括香港特别行政区、澳门特别行政区及台湾省)销售。未经许可之出口,视为违反著作权法,将受法律之制裁。

图书在版编目(CIP)数据

病理学 = TEXTBOOK OF PATHOLOGY/周庚寅,姜叙诚主编.—北京:科学出版社,2006.3
（普通高等教育"十一五"国家级规划教材,医学英文原版改编双语教材）
ISBN 978-7-03-016541-1

Ⅰ.病… Ⅱ.①周…②姜… Ⅲ.病理学－医学院校－教材　Ⅳ.R36

中国版本图书馆 CIP 数据核字（2006）第 141453 号

责任编辑:裴中惠　李国红　胡治国/责任校对:包志虹
责任印制:赵　博/封面设计:黄　超

版权所有,违者必究。未经本社许可,数字图书馆不得使用

科 学 出 版 社 出版
北京东黄城根北街 16 号
邮政编码:100717
http://www.sciencep.com
新科印刷有限公司 印刷
科学出版社发行　各地新华书店经销
*
2006 年 3 月第 一 版　　开本:787×1092 1/16
2017 年 1 月第九次印刷　印张:30 1/2
　　　　　　　　　　字数:1 011 000
定价:65.00 元
(如有印装质量问题,我社负责调换)

Contributors of Adaptation Edition

Chief Editors   Zhou Gengyin   Jiang Xucheng
Vice Chief Editors   Cui Jin   Wang Liantang
Secretary   Meng Bin
Contributors

Cui Jin	Kunming Medical College
Deng Hong	Zhejiang University School of Medicine
Dong Jianguo	Shanghai Jiaotong University School of Medicine
Gan Runliang	Nanhua University School of Medicine
Han Yuchen	China Medical University
Jiang Xucheng	Shanghai Jiaotong University School of Medicine
Li Lianhong	Dalian Medical University
Luo Dianzhong	Guangxi Medical University
Ma Yun	Guangxi Medical College
Meng Bin	Shandong University School of Medicine
Peng Tingsheng	Sun Yat-sen University, Faculty of Medicine
Qiu Xueshan	China Medical University
Shen Hong	Southern Medical University
Song Bo	Dalian Medical University
Song Jingyu	Yanbian University College of Basic Medicine
Song Wenjing	Tianjin Medical University
Wang Liantang	Sun Yat-sen University, Faculty of Medicine
Wang Yalan	Chongqing University of Medical Sciences
Yao Junxia	Yunyang Medical College
Zhang Jianzhong	Ningxia Medical College
Zhang Qinghui	Shandong University School of Medicine
Zhang Shuhua	Binzhou Medical College
Zhang Xianghong	Hebei Medical University
Zhang Zongji	Kunming Medical College
Zhou Gengyin	Shandong University School of Medicine

《病理学》改编委员会名单

主　　编　周庚寅　姜叙诚
副 主 编　崔　进　王连唐
秘　　书　孟　斌
编　　者（按拼音排序）
　　　　　　崔　进（昆明医学院）
　　　　　　邓　红（浙江大学医学院）
　　　　　　董建国（上海交通大学医学院）
　　　　　　甘润良（南华大学医学院）
　　　　　　韩昱晨（中国医科大学）
　　　　　　姜叙诚（上海交通大学医学院）
　　　　　　李连宏（大连医科大学）
　　　　　　罗殿中（广西医科大学）
　　　　　　马　韵（广西医科大学）
　　　　　　孟　斌（山东大学医学院）
　　　　　　彭挺生（中山大学中山医学院）
　　　　　　宋京郁（延边大学医学部基础医学院）
　　　　　　申　洪（南方医科大学）
　　　　　　邱雪杉（中国医科大学）
　　　　　　宋　波（大连医科大学）
　　　　　　宋文静（天津医科大学）
　　　　　　王连唐（中山大学中山医学院）
　　　　　　王娅兰（重庆医科大学）
　　　　　　姚俊霞（郧阳医学院）
　　　　　　张建中（宁夏医学院）
　　　　　　张庆慧（山东大学医学院）
　　　　　　张树华（滨州医学院）
　　　　　　张祥宏（河北医科大学）
　　　　　　章宗籍（昆明医学院）
　　　　　　周庚寅（山东大学医学院）

Preface for Adaptation Edition

Bilingual teaching, for example, in both Chinese and English, has been long promoted in China. However, we still lack a satisfactory textbook of pathology. Original editions of textbooks in English from abroad are not only too expensive for students but also somewhat unsuitable for teaching. Therefore there is a great demand for a suitable textbook. For this purpose, Science Press was authorized by McGraw-Hill Companies to have the copyright of **Concise Pathology** to be adapted for use in China.

The goal to adapt this textbook is to teach pathology according to the content, category and catalogue of textbook used in China based upon the style of the original book. The basic content of the book remains largely unchanged although the catalogue was rearranged to be consistent with pathologic textbook in China. Some chapters have been updated and largely rewritten.

Actually for Chinese authors to rewrite the original textbook of pathology in English is not easy because we have not yet had such experience before. We are deeply indebted to all the authors who have done their great endeavors to adapt and review the chapters in their areas of expertise. A lot of extra time with short notice was used to complete this edition accurately as well as quickly. We are especially grateful to the secretary for this book, Dr. Meng Bin, who organized this book so efficiently. We are particularly thankful to Professor Anders Zetterberg and his wife, from the Department of Oncology and Pathology, Karolinska Institute, Sweden, for helping in reviewing and correcting the English for some chapters during his academic visiting to the Department of Pathology, Shandong University School of Medicine.

There could be some errors in spelling or grammar in English, even in the basic knowledge of pathology. There is still room for improvement in future if it is republished. Hopefully the medical faculties and students will use this book and provide helpful suggestions and critiques in the future.

Zhou Gengyin, Jiang Xucheng
August, 2005

前 言

为使医学教育逐渐同世界接轨，双语教学在我们国家已倡导和推行多年，但至今仍然缺乏令人满意的病理学教科书。英语原版教材价格较高，且与中国目前的教学内容不甚吻合。基于对英语双语病理学教材的广泛需求，科学出版社获得了麦格劳-希尔公司《Concise Pathology》的合作改编权。其目的是在不改变原书风格和基本内容的前提下，通过改编使其内容及编排顺序比较符合中国的教学习惯。

由于缺乏经验和英语水平所限，虽是改编，实属不易。各位编委在担任繁重的医教研工作的同时，夜以继日、辛勤劳作，在较短的时间内完成了初稿和互审。本书编委会秘书孟斌博士在沟通信息和组织改编的过程中做了大量卓有成效的工作。在最后定稿期间，我们又特邀了瑞典卡罗琳斯卡医学院肿瘤病理科 Zetterberg 教授和他的夫人对某些章节的英语修辞和语法提出了建议和修改，在此表示衷心的感谢。

在改编过程中，对原书内容和目录进行了删节、调整和适当补充，个别章节有较大的更新和改动。在章节内容衔接上，尤其是英语语言的表达上，疏漏和错误之处在所难免。恳请同道和学生在实际使用过程中，不断提出意见，以期再版时进一步完善。

周庚寅　姜叙诚
2005 年 8 月

CONTENTS

Introduction   The Discipline of Pathology ·· (1)
Part A   **General Pathology** ··· (5)
   Chapter 1   Adaptation and Injury of Cell and Tissue ·· (5)
   Chapter 2   Tissue Repair ··· (33)
   Chapter 3   Hemodynamic Disorders and Abnormalities of Blood Supply ················ (47)
   Chapter 4   Inflammation ·· (75)
   Chapter 5   Neoplasia ·· (99)
Part B   **Systemic Pathology** ·· (145)
   Chapter 6   Diseases of the Cardiovascular System ·· (145)
   Chapter 7   Diseases of the Respiratory System ··· (183)
   Chapter 8   Diseases of the DigestiveSystem ·· (214)
   Chapter 9   The Diseases of Hematopoietic and Lymphoid Systems ······················ (271)
   Chapter 10   Diseases of Immunity ·· (289)
   Chapter 11   Diseases of the Urinary System ·· (315)
   Chapter 12   Diseases of the Genital System and Breast ······································· (347)
   Chapter 13   Diseases of the Endocrine System ··· (376)
   Chapter 14   Diseases of the Nervous System ·· (408)
   Chapter 15   Infectious Deseases ·· (433)
   Chapter 16   Parasitosis ··· (470)

Introduction The Discipline of Pathology

Cui Jin

WHAT IS PATHOLOGY?

Pathology is the study of disease. In its broadest sense, it is the study of how the organs and tissues of a healthy body - the basis of normal anatomy and physiology - change to those of a sick person. The study of pathology therefore provides an understanding of the disease processes encountered (*pathogenesis*), their causes (*etiology*), their structural and functional changes (*pathological change*), and their clinical effects (*clinical pathological correlation* and *prognosis*). In this way, pathology constitutes a logical and scientific basis of medicine. Pathology in this broad sense is what we aim to teach medical students.

Pathology is a bridge between basic science and clinical medicine. Before beginning the study of pathology, the normal structure and function of the body have been provided by basic medical courses of anatomy, embryology, histology, cellular biology, physiology and biochemistry. The basic science of pathology is that branch of medicine which is concerned with the response of the host to injury through a series of mechanisms or processes. For the student, this knowledge of the processes of disease provides a foundation for clinical medicine; for the pathologist these processes provide an unlimited area for basic research. The second task of pathology is to introduce the student to clinical medicine, which is concerned with the diagnosis and treatment of the disease entities. It must be emphasized that the student, before undertaking the study of the diseases themselves, should have correlative knowledge of the chemical, physical, and biologic agents that produce injury and of the fundamental pathologic processes through which the host responds. On the other hand, the pathologic diagnosis, which is an authoritative diagnosis based on pathologic features of organs and tissues observed grossly and microscopy, is more objective and precise than other clinical diagnosis such as iconography.

Pathology is not only basic scientific medicine but also practical clinic medicine; it is also named *Diagnostic Pathology or Surgical Pathology*. According to the different entity studied, pathology can be divided into *Human Pathology* and *Experimental Pathology*.

Human Pathology

The principal aim of human pathology considers structural abnormalities of cells and tissues grossly and microscopically examined from the patient's tissues. The surgical pathology laboratory in a hospital includes subdivisions such as autopsy, biopsy and cytology.

Autopsy means "see for yourself", this is one of the basic pathologic methods. Autopsy is a special surgical operation, performed by specially-trained physicians (usually a pathologist), on a dead body. Its purpose is to identify the cause of death, but also has several other functions:
- Clarify the causes of death in cases without clinical diagnosis or in those in which the patient's death was unexpected. Learn the patient's health status while alive.
- Diagnosis and treatment quality control. Autopsy findings may reveal flaws in diagnosis, treatment and therapy prevent future errors.
- Recognizing of negligence. Autopsies can also be ordered in every state when there is suspicion of foul play.
- Recognition of new diseases and new disease patterns.
- Source of information for the Secretary of Health, statistical analysis of the most frequent diseases, influence health policies and State and Municipal districts.
- Provide material for the residents, students and staff education. The clinical-pathological correlation done during all stages of the autopsy is an excellent exercise in pathology.
- Material for scientific research.
- Recognition of treatment effectiveness.

Biopsy is the removal of a sample of tissue from the body for examination. The tissue will be examined under a microscope to assist in diagnosis. Therefore, only very small samples are needed. Sometimes, it is enough just to scrape over an area. This is the case with cell examinations of the cervix. During examination of the large intestine, a biopsy can be taken with forceps through a tube known as an endoscope. In other cases, for instance, a liver or kidney biopsy, the biopsy is taken using a large hypodermic needle.

Cytology is responsible for preparation, staining and microscopic examination of patient samples. The cytological samples may be used for screening (cervical-vaginal), diagnosis (FNA) and improving overall diagnostic accuracy (brushes, washes). Pathologists perform Fine Needle Aspiration Biopsy (FNAB) using cytology to diagnose palpable masses. The pathologists in conjunction with Radiologists perform FNA of non-palpable thoracic, abdominal and soft tissue masses.

Experimental Pathology

Experimental pathology researches cellular processes incorporate animal experiment and tissue and cell cultures. **Animal Experimentation** is a pathological method using animal model to study disease and effects of disease within the body. We can become knowledgeable about diseases on all levels, from the molecular to the cellular and more. Animals are very different from human being in genus, so we must be careful when apply the results of experiments to explain human disease. Tissue and Cell culture is another major method in academic research. A viable culture from a human or animal tissue sample is obtained and maintained in vitro for experimental, diagnostic or therapeutic purposes.

WHO IS A PATHOLOGIST?

In western countries, a pathologist may be a physician (MD) or a person with a doctorate (PhD) in pathology who has been trained in the proper performance and interpretation of laboratory procedures. Training as a physician pathologist takes many years. In the United States, a five-year pathology residency follows the MD degree and covers all aspects of clinical and anatomic pathology. In England, pathology training also lasts for five years, being general in the first two years and more specialized in the last three. Pathologists in small hospitals maintain a basic knowledge of all areas of pathology. In large academic medical centers, an individual pathologist may specialize in surgical pathology, hematopathology, chemical pathology, microbiology, immunology, and so forth. The PhD program in pathology provides training in the scientific methods of pathology. PhD pathologists play a vital role in basic scientific research and function in many hospital laboratories in their spheres of expertise. Pathologists serve as consultants to their clinical colleagues, make diagnoses on biopsy material, run laboratories and interpret tests. They serve as educators for the hospital staff and have been termed "the doctor's doctor".

Training in clinical pathology includes learning the methodology of chemical, microbiologic, and immunologic procedures and learning how to operate the various instruments so as to produce accurate results. Training in anatomic pathology deals with microscopic diagnosis of disease by recognizing deviations from normal of cells and tissues by light and electron microscopic study.

The end product of a pathologic procedure is a **pathology report** that contains the result of the procedure. This may be a number (in chemical tests), the name of a microorganism (in microbiology), or a diagnosis based no the microscopic features of a tissue section (in surgical pathology). Interaction with the laboratory in terms of ordering the most appropriate laboratory procedures and being able to interpret the pathology report correctly is a vital part of the training of all physicians.

BASIC EXAMINATION METHOD FOR PATHOLOGY

The study methods of pathology include autopsy, biopsy, cytology, animal experiment, and tissue and cell culture as previous described. Main routine methods are:

A. Gross Examination

It is the basic method for pathologic examination. The morphological feature of a lesion – such as size, form, weight, color, circumscription, surface appearance, cut and position – can be observed by eye or assisted by using a ruler, steelyard, magnifying glass or other tools.

B. Histological and Cytological Examination

The specimens from patients are prepared as a section or smear, then stained, and examined by using microcopy. The diagnosis can be made via analysis the morphologic characteristics. The most common and basic stain method of a section is Haematoxylin and Eosin technique (H. E stain). However, other special stain methods or new techniques are necessary for assistance the diagnosis when it cannot be made by H. E stain. Special lesions on section must be examined grossly first noting density, color. Afterward, whole tissue can be examined carefully under low magnification, which is very important for making the diagnosis. High magnification examination is only used to observe cellular features.

C. Histochemistry and Cytochemistry Examination

Also called special stain method, some tissue structures and substances (e. g. protein, enzyme, nucleic acid, glycogen and lipid) are colored when a chemical group (e. g. carboxyl, phosphoric or aldehyde) reacts with the stain. For example, fat remains in the cytoplasm can be demonstrated by Sudan black B stains, and the glycogen in the cytoplasm, by PAS stains.

Other examination methods, such as *immunohistochemistry*, *electron microscopy*, *in situ hybridization*, *polymerase chain reaction* (*PCR*), chromosome analysis by fluorescence in situ hybridization (*FISH*), *flow cytometry* and *confocal laser scanning microscopy* are also now wildly used in clinical practice if necessary.

A BRIEF HISTORY OF PATHOLOGY

In 1761, **Dr. John Morgagni**, an Italian, wrote the great book "**The Seats and Causes of Disease, Investigated by Anatomy**" based on his series of 700 autopsies. This book summed up his lifetime's experience and is still a great read. Dr. Morgagni was among the most beloved people of his era. Thanks to his work, all disease was now recognized as **disease of organs** (*Organ Pathology*), and disease "sat" in different organs in different patients. Dr. Morgagni meticulously related his patients' symptoms to their diseased organs, making the first clinic-pathologic correlations. This was real progress, but Dr. Morgagni had no real idea of how disease in one organ caused malfunction in another organ, or even what disease is.

Dr. Rudolf Virchow (1821–1902), a German, is the greatest pathologist of all time. He liked to cut thin sections of diseased tissues with a razor, and look at them using the latest technology, the *microscope*. Dr. Virchow first achieved renown by discovering leukemia and myelin. In 1858, he wrote the famous book "**Cell Pathology**" which is the basis for all modern pathology. He established the principle that **all cells come from pre-existing cells** and he emphasized that **all disease is disease of cells** (*Cellular Pathology*). Dr. Virchow's ideas were introduced within months of two great unifying principles of today's science, the periodic table of the elements and the common origin of living things.

In the twentieth century, as the new techniques and methods developed and a new branches pathology can into be: *Ultrastructural Pathology*–Electron microscopy (EM) has contributed extensively to the understanding of cell structure and function as well as provided insight into pathologic processes. *Immunopathology* utilizes immunohistochemical methods to detect cell or tissue antigens on tissue section based on immunoenzimatic reactions using antibodies (mono or polyclonal). *Molecular Pathology* and *Genetic Pathology* are the subspecialties in which the principles, theories, and technologies of molecular biology and molecular genetics are used to make or confirm clinical diagnosis in neoplasia, infectious disease, tissue typing/identity testing, Mendelian genetic disorders and non-Mendelian genetic diseases. *Quantitative Pathology* is a branch of pathology concerned with the application of morphometry and image analysis technique.

Today there is a new emphasis on disease as it involves gene, molecules, cells, organs, whole persons and groups of people. Pathology deals with abnormal gross and microscopic anatomy, abnormal biochemistry, and abnormal physiology.

ORGANIZATION AND APPROACH OF THIS BOOK

The study of pathology is traditionally divided into general and systemic pathology, and we preserve this distinction.

In the *general pathology* chapters, the pathologic changes occurring in a hypothetic tissue are considered. This idealized tissue is composed of parenchymal cells and interstitial connective tissue and is the prototype of every tissue in the body. General pathology explores and explains the development of basic pathologic mechanisms without detailing the additional specific changes occurring in different organs.

In the *systemic pathology* chapters, the pathologic mechanisms discussed in the general pathology section are related to the various organ systems. In each system, normal structure, function, and the symptoms and signs that arise from pathologic changes are discussed briefly first. The diseases in each organ system are then considered, with emphasis given to those that are more common, so that the student can become familiar with most of the important diseases encountered in clinical practice.

Part A General Pathology

Chapter 1 Adaptation and Injury of Cell and Tissue

Zhang Zongji

CHAPTER CONTENTS
- Adaptation of Cell and Tissue
  - Atrophy
  - Hypertrophy and Hyperplasia
  - Metaplasia
- Mechanisms of Injury of Cell and Tissue
  - Causes of Cell Injury
  - Mechanisms of Cellular Injury
- Reversible Injury of Cell and Tissue
  - Hydropic Degeneration
  - Fatty Change
  - Hyaline Degeneration
  - Accumulation of Mucopolysaccharides
  - Deposition of Amyloid
  - Intracellular Accumulation of Glycogen
  - Deposition of Pathological Pigments
- Irreversible Cell Injury: Cell Death
  - Necrosis
  - Apoptosis
- Aging

The normal cell is a highly complex unit in which the various organelles and enzyme systems continuously carry out the metabolic activities that maintain cell viability and support its normal functions. Normal function is dependent on (1) the immediate environment of the cell; (2) a continuous supply of nutrients such as oxygen, glucose, and amino acids; and (3) constant removal of the products of metabolism, including CO_2. When cells encounter physiologic stress or pathologic stimuli, they can alter their structure and/or biochemical processes in order to achieve a new "steady state" and maintain near-normal physiologic functions; this is referred to as *adaptation*. If stressed cells cannot adequately adapt, critical cell functions may be impaired and the cell is said to be injured. Injury is defined as an alteration in cell structure or function resulting from some stress that exceeds the ability of the cell to compensate through normal physiologic adaptive mechanisms. Injury to a cell may be nonlethal (regeneration) or lethal (necrosis and apoptosis).

ADAPTATION OF CELL AND TISSUE

Within limits, most cells can adapt to environmental stresses by modifying their size/shape, pattern of growth, and/or metabolic activity. This process is referred to as *adaptation*. The adaptive changes in cell growth and differentiation that are particularly important in pathologic conditions include *atrophy*, *hypertrophy*, *hyperplasia* and *metaplasia* (see Figure 1-1).

ATROPHY

Atrophy is a decrease in the size of a tissue or organ, resulting from a decrease either in the size of individual cells or in the number of cells composing the tissue. Note that atrophy, which is a decrease in size of a normally formed organ, is distinct from agenesis, aplasia, and hypoplasia, which are abnormalities of organ development.

Atrophy is classified as two patterns: physiologic and pathologic atrophy.

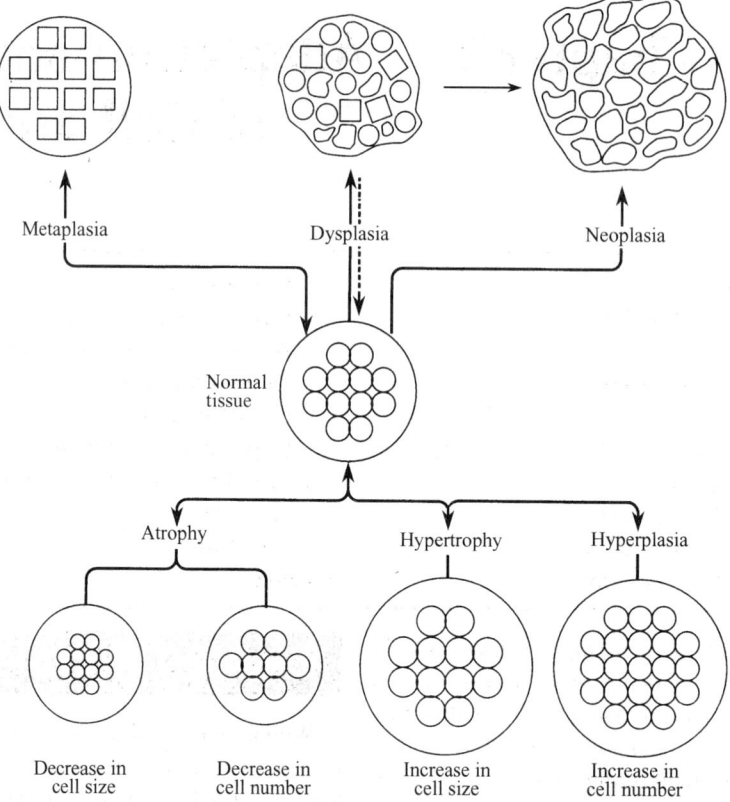

Figure 1-1 Adaptation and dysplasia of cell and tissue. Note that more than one abnormality may be present in a given case, e.g. the respiratory mucosa may show squamous metaplasia associated with dysplasia

Physiologic Atrophy

Physiologic atrophy is often seen when structures that are well developed and required at certain stages of development, later wither. A good example is that of endometrium, vaginal epithelium, and breast which occurs with menopause and the loss of estrogen stimulation. In the aging process, atrophy can be a normal morphologic change. It is most apparent in tissues populated by permanent cells, e.g. the brain and heart.

Pathologic Atrophy

A. Atrophy of Disuse

Atrophy of disuse occurs in immobilized skeletal muscle and bone, as when a fractured limb is put in a cast or when a patient is restricted to complete bed rest. Skeletal muscle atrophies rapidly with disuse. Initially, there is a rapid decrease in cell size that is readily reversible when activity is resumed. With more prolonged immobilization, muscle fibers decrease in number as well as in size. Because skeletal muscle can regenerate only to a very limited extent, restoration of muscle size after loss of muscle fibers can only occur through compensatory hypertrophy of the surviving fibers, which often requires a long rehabilitation period. Bone atrophy results when bone resorption occurs more rapidly than bone formation; it is characterized by decreased size of the trabeculae (decreased mass), leading to osteoporosis of disuse.

B. Denervation Atrophy

Skeletal muscle is dependent on its nerve supply for normal function and structure. Damage to the lower motor neuron at any point between the cell body in the spinal cord and the motor end plate leads to rapid atrophy of the muscle fibers supplied by that nerve. When denervation is temporary, physical therapy and electrical stimulation of the muscle are important to prevent muscle fiber loss and ensure that normal function can be restored when nerve function is reestablished. Many primary muscle diseases (e.g. the genetically determined **dystrophies**) also show irregular atrophy of muscle fibers.

C. Atrophy Due to Loss of Trophic Hormones

Many endocrine glands are dependent on trophic hormones for normal cellular growth, and withdrawal of these hormones leads to atrophy. Pituitary disease associated with decreased secretion of pituitary trophic hormones results in atrophy of the thyroid, adrenals, and gonads. High-dose adrenal corticosteroid therapy, which is sometimes used for immunosuppression, causes atrophy of the adrenal glands because it suppresses pituitary corticotrophin (ACTH) secretion. Such patients soon lose the ability to secrete cortisol and become dependent on exogenous steroids. Withdrawal of steroid therapy in such patients must be gradual enough to permit regeneration of the atrophied adrenal.

D. Atrophy Due to Lack of Nutrients

Severe protein-calorie malnutrition (marasmus) results in the utilization of body tissues such as skeletal muscle as a source of energy and protein after other sources such as adipose stores have been exhausted. Marked muscle atrophy is seen in marasmus.

A decrease in blood supply (ischemia) to a tissue as a result of arterial disease result in atrophy of the tissue due to progressive cell loses. Cerebrovascular disease, for example, is associated with cerebral atrophy, including neuronal loss.

E. Pressure Atrophy

Prolonged compression of tissue causes atrophy. A large, encapsulated benign neoplasm in the spinal canal may produce atrophy in both the spinal cord it compresses and the surrounding vertebrae. It is likely that such atrophy results from compression of small blood vessels, resulting in ischemia, and not from the direct effect of pressure on cells.

Morphology

In atrophic organs, there is a decreasing size and weight, the color is always darker than normal, consistency becomes hard or firm, and the margins of the organs is shrunken. On the surface of organs the arteries may be tortuous (Figure 1-2). Histologically, the size and/or the number of the parenchyma cells are decreased. Pigment deposition can be seen in the atrophic cytoplasm. At the same time, the interstitial connective tissue and the adipose tissue can proliferate. Under electron microscopy, decrease in the size of a cell results from a reduction in the amount of cytoplasm and the number of cytoplasmic organelles; it is usually associated with diminished metabolism. Degenerating organelles are taken up in lysosomal vacuoles for enzymatic degradation (autophagy). Residual organelle membranes often accumulate in the cytoplasm as brown lipofuscin pigment.

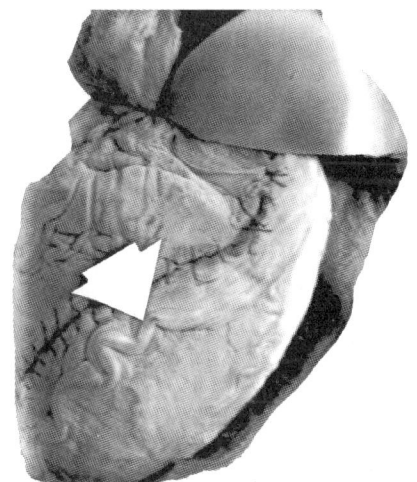

Figure 1-2 Atrophic heart, showing the decrease of size, and the coronary on the surface is tortuous (**arrow**)

HYPERTROPHY AND HYPERPLASIA

Hypertrophy is an increase in the size of a tissue due to increased size of individual cells (Table 1-1). It occurs in tissues made up of permanent cells, in which a demand for increased metabolic activity cannot be met through cell multiplication.

Hyperplasia is an increase in the size of a tissue as a result of increased numbers of component cells (Table 1-1). It is the principal mechanism accounting for increased size in tissues composed of labile and stable cells.

Table 1-1 Hypertrophy and hyperplasia of organs

Tissue	Cause of Increased Demand
Skeletal muscle hypertrophy	Physical activity, weight lifting
Cardiac muscle hypertrophy	Increased pressure load (high blood pressure, valve stenosis) or increased volume load (valve incompetence causing regurgitation of blood)
Smooth muscle (wall of intestine, urinary bladder) hypertrophy	Obstructive lesions
Renal hypertrophy	Unilateral disease of one kidney; removal of one kidney
Uterine myometrial hypertrophy	Pregnancy (hormone-induced)
Bone marrow hyperplasia erythroid hyperplasia	Increased destruction of erythrocytes (hemolytic process); prolonged hypoxia (living at high altitudes)
Megakaryocytic hyperplasia	Increased destruction of platelets in the periphery
Myeloid hyperplasia	Increased demand for neutrophils (as in inflammation)
Lymph node hyperplasia	Antigenic stimulation (proliferative immune response)
Breast hyperplasia	Pregnancy and lactation (hormone-induced)

Not uncommonly, increased size of a tissue is due to a combination of hypertrophy and hyperplasia.

Causes of Hypertrophy and Hyperplasia

Hypertrophy results from increased amounts of cytoplasm and cytoplasmic organelles in cells. In secretory cells, the synthetic apparatus – including the endoplasmic reticulum, ribosome, and the Golgi zone – becomes prominent. In contractile cells such as muscle fibers, there is an increase in size of cytoplasmic myofibrils. Hyperplasia results when cells of a tissue are stimulated to undergo mitotic division, thereby increasing the number of cells.

A. Physiologic Hypertrophy and Hyperplasia

Hypertrophy and hyperplasia may occur as an adaptation to increased demand (Table 1-1, Figures 1-3, and 1-4). Hypertrophy and hyperplasia are controlled responses reflecting increased demand; if the demand is removed, the tissues revert toward normal.

B. Pathologic Hypertrophy and Hyperplasia

Abnormal hypertrophy and hyperplasia occur in an appropriate stimulus of increased functional demand.

Myocardial hypertrophy, if it occurs without recognizable cause (e.g. in the absence of hypertension or valvular or congenital heart disease), is considered an example of pathologic hypertrophy. Such hypertrophy is frequently associated with abnormal cardiac function producing **cardiomyopathy.**

Endometrial hyperplasia is an important result of increased estrogen stimulation, particularly when estrogens are not opposed by progesterone secretion, as typically occurs near menopause. It is associated with irregular, often excessive uterine bleeding. The presence of excessive trophic hormones causes hyperplasia of the target organs, e.g. excessive secretion of ACTH causes bilateral adrenal hyperplasia. The hyperplasic target organs frequently show increased function. In the case of the adrenal gland, there is increased cortisol secretion (Cushing's syndrome).

Thyroid hyperplasia (**goiter; Graves' disease**) results from increased TSH stimulation of the thyroid or from the action of autoantibodies that are able to bind to TSH receptors in thyroid cell membranes.

Hyperplasia of the prostate gland is common in older men and is due to hyperplasia of the glandular and the stromal elements. The cause is not known, although it is believed that waning androgen levels may be responsible.

METAPLASIA

Metaplasia is an abnormality of cellular differentiation in which one type of mature cell is replaced by a different type of mature cell — and the latter is not normal for the tissue involved (Table 1-2). Metaplasia results from abnormal differentiation of stem cells (Figures 1-1, 1-5, and 1-6). The new, metaplastic tissue is structurally normal, however, so the regular cellular organization is maintained. Metaplasia is reversible.

Chapter 1 Adaptation and Injury of Cell and Tissue

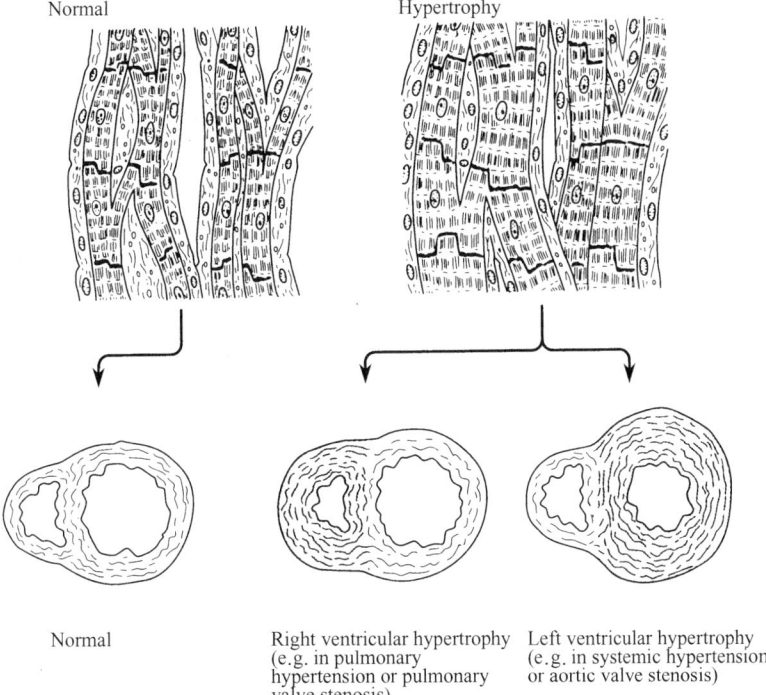

Figure 1-3 Cardiac muscle hypertrophy, showing the increase in size of cardiac muscle fibers. Hypertrophy may involve any of the cardiac chambers if they are subjected to an increased pressure or volume load (**right and left ventricular hypertrophy and a few of their common causes are shown**)

Table 1-2 Metaplasia[1]

Type of Metaplasia	Site	Causative Factors
Epithelial metaplasia		
Squamous metaplasia	Multiple sites Bronchus Endocervix Urinary bladder	Vitamin A deficiency Cigarette smoking, chronic inflammation Chronic inflammation Chronic inflammation, schistosomiasis
Intestinal metaplasia	Esophagus Stomach	Acid reflux Alkaline reflux, chronic inflammation
Gastric metaplasia	Esophagus Intestine	Acid reflux Unknown
Serous or mucinous metaplasia	Germinal epithelium of ovary	Trauma of multiple ovulation
Mesenchymal metaplasia		
Osseous metaplasia	Fibrous scars Areas of calcification	Unknown Unknown
Myeloid metaplasia[2]	Spleen, liver	Unknown

[1] See test for details of cell types involved.

[2] Myeloid metaplasia is the appearance of myeloid (bone marrow) elements outside the bone marrow and is not metaplasia in the strict sense because it is usually the result of extreme hyperplasia of bone marrow with extension of hematopoiesis into extramedullary sites such as the spleen and liver. (The last-named sites are normal sites of hematopoiesis in the fetus).

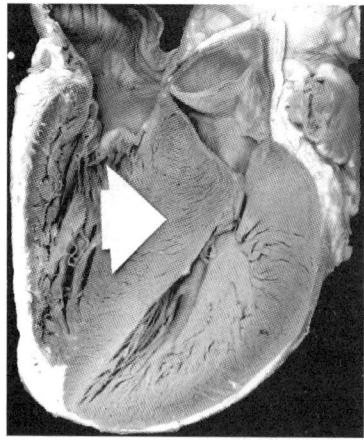

Figure 1-4 Hypertrophic heart, showing the size of the heart is as large as a normal heart, but the weight is increased. On the cut surface, the musculature of the left ventricle and septum is clearly enlarged, and the papillary muscles and trabeculae carneae are thickened. Without dilatation of the left ventricle, concentric hypertrophy results

manner that is abnormal for that location, resulting in epithelium of a type different from that usually present. Epithelial metaplasia is thus a manifestation of the varied potential for differentiation in stem cells and typically occurs following chronic physical or chemical irritation.

In **squamous metaplasia** - the most common type of epithelial metaplasia - nonsquamous pseudostratified columnar or cuboidal epithelium is replaced by a normal-appearing stratified squamous epithelium. Squamous metaplasia is common in the endocervix and the bronchial mucosa (Figure 1-5), it occurs less frequently in the endometrium and urinary bladder.

Glandular metaplasia occurs in the esophagus, where the normal squamous epithelium is replaced by glandular, mucus-secreting epithelium (either gastric or intestinal in type), usually as a result of acid reflux into the esophagus (see Barrett's esophagus). Metaplasia may also occur in the stomach and intestine, where the mucosa of one part is replaced by that of another, e.g. replacement of gastric mucosa with intestinal mucosa (intestinal metaplasia) or vice versa (gastric metaplasia). It may also affect the germinal epithelium of the ovary, as in the formation of serous and mucinous cysts.

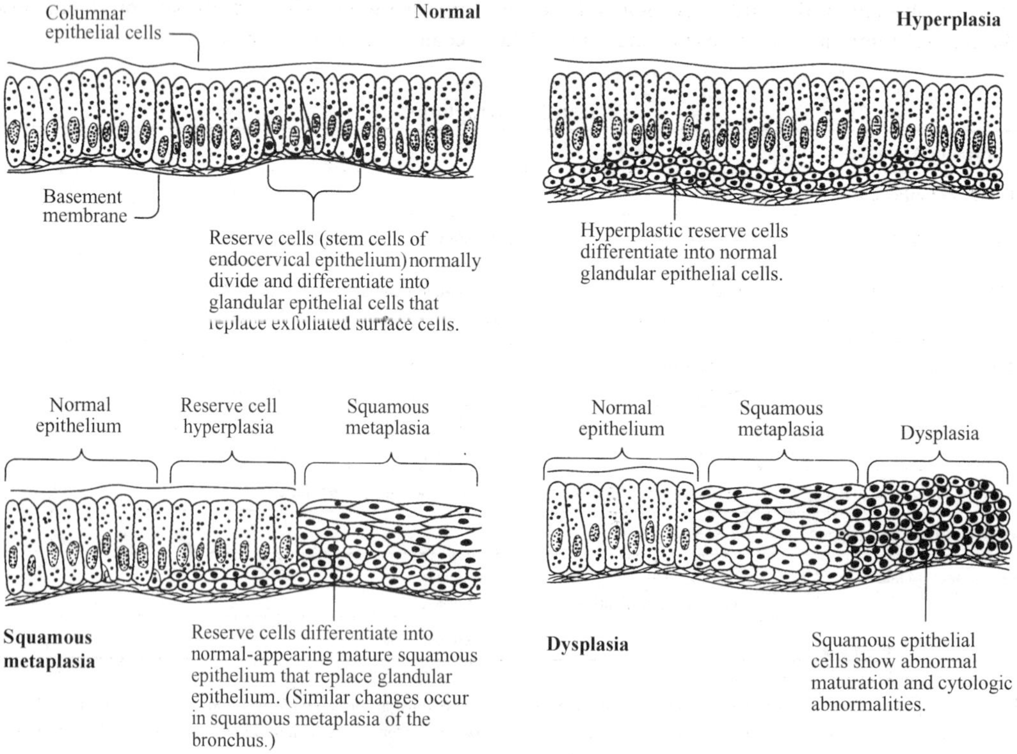

Metaplasia most commonly involves epithelium. As the germinative stem cells multiply to replace cells shed at the surface, they differentiate in a

Figure 1-5 Hyperplasia, squamous metaplasia, and dysplasia occurring in the uterine endocervical epithelium. Similar changes may occur in the bronchial epithelium

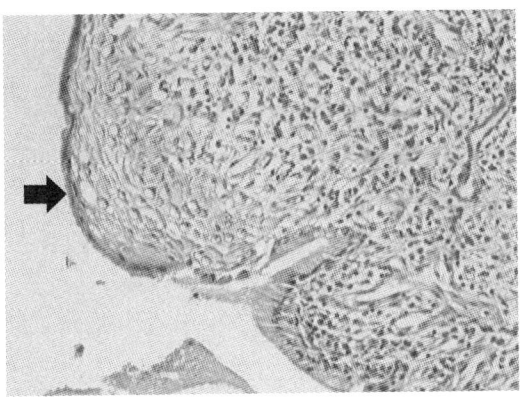

Figure 1-6 Endocervix, showing squamous metaplasia. The normal columnar epithelium (below) has been replaced by a squamous epithelium (arrow)

Metaplasia can occurs in mesenchymal tissue and is best exemplified by osseous metaplasia in scars and other fibroblastic proliferations. Metaplasia in mesenchymal tissue is the same as epithelial metaplasia in representing the potential for diverse differentiation of mesenchymal stem cells.

Most metaplasia is of little clinical significance, although important functional deficits may result in some areas; loss of cilia and of mucus production in the bronchi may predispose to development of infection. Metaplastic tissue is structurally normal and itself carries no increased risk of development of cancer.

MECHANISMS OF INJURY OF CELL AND TISSUE

CAUSES OF CELL INJURY

A variety of injurious agents act on human tissues (Figure 1-7) to produce tissue damage either directly or indirectly. A noxious agent may act directly on the tissue and interfere with its structure or biochemical function. An example is a burn, in which heat causes immediate direct destruction of cell membranes, tissue components, and coagulation of intracellular proteins. However, an injurious agent may act at some site other than the tissue in question to produce an abnormality in the immediate environment of the cell or cause accumulation of some toxic substance, which in turn causes cell damage. Representative causes of indirect injury include accumulation of toxic products seen in kidney and liver failure or a change in extracellular pH, electrolyte concentrations, or core body temperature. These indirect injuries may result in cell damage to many different tissues throughout the body, e. g. structural and functional abnormalities in the brain from liver failure (hepatic encephalopathy).

1. Oxygen deprivation

Hypoxia is an extremely important and common cause of cell injury. Oxygen reaches the cells via arterial blood but is ultimately derived from the atmosphere. Most of the oxygen carried in blood is bound to hemoglobin. Lack of oxygen in the cells (hypoxia) may result from (1) **respiratory obstruction or disease**, preventing oxygenation of blood in the lungs; (2) **ischemia**, or failure of blood flow in the tissue, due either to generalized circulatory failure or to local vessel obstruction; (3) **anemia** (e. g. decreased hemoglobin in the blood), resulting in decreased oxygen carriage by the blood; or (4) **alteration of hemoglobin** (as occurs in carbon monoxide poisoning), making it unavailable for oxygen transport and leading to the same result as anemia.

2. Physical agents

Many forms of physical injury can be harmful to cells and tissues. For example, extremes of heat or cold (burns, heat stroke, heat exhaustion, frostbite, and hypothermia), mechanical injury (crush injury, fractures, lacerations, and hemorrhage), electric shock, radiation and sudden changes in atmospheric pressure all have direct effects on cells and tissues.

3. Chemical agents

A very large number of drugs and environmental chemical agents are capable of causing cell injury. The list includes inorganic compounds, ions, and organic molecules – including byproducts of normal metabolism and toxins synthesized by microorganisms. Two basic mechanisms of chemical injury are recognized: (1) a compound can react directly with some critical molecular component of the cell interfering with its function. For example, cyanide inactivates the enzyme cytochrome oxidase in mitochondria required for aerobic respiration. (2) A compound that is itself harmless to cells can be rendered toxic when it is metabolized and converted to a toxic substance (such as a free radical). This is the way in which acetaminophen overdose is toxic to the liver.

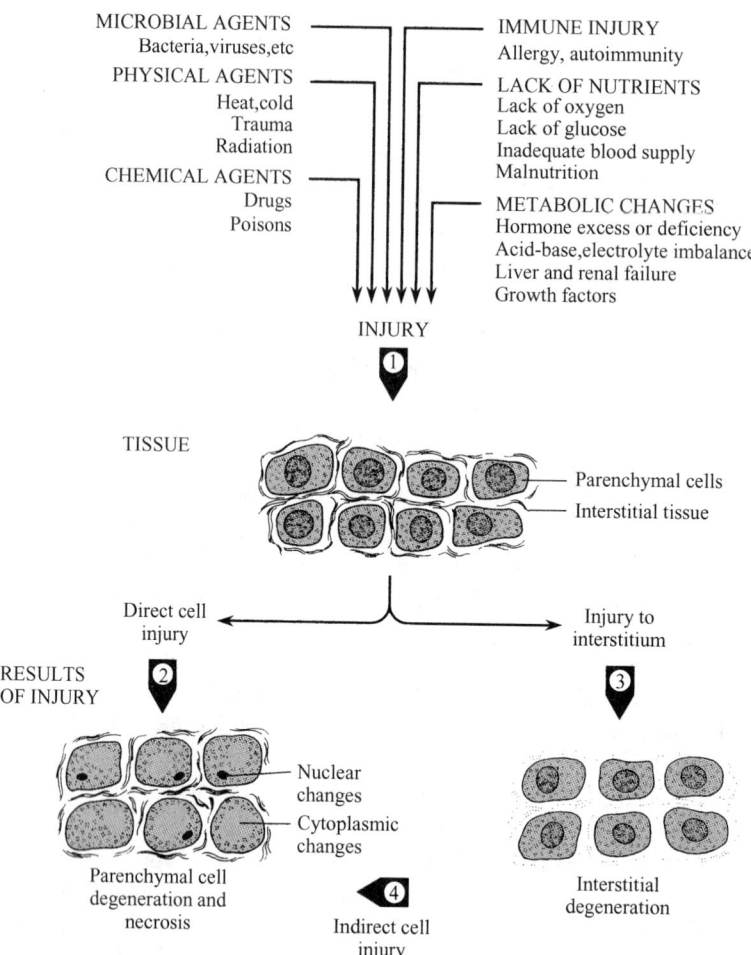

Figure 1-7 General causes and effects of tissue injury. Many different types of injuries act on tissues ① to cause direct parenchymal cell injury ② or interstitial injury ③ Interstitial abnormalities may cause indirect parenchymal cell injury④

4. Infectious agents

This very common category of cell injury results from the parasitization of the body by pathogenic viruses, bacteria, fungi, protozoa, or helminths. Pathogenic organisms produce disease by either: (1) replicating inside host cells and disrupting the structural integrity of the cell, (2) producing a toxin that is harmful to host cells, or by (3) triggering an inflammatory or immune response that inadvertently injures host cells.

5. Immunologic agents

Although the immune system defends our body against foreign materials, exaggerated immune reactions (anaphylaxis, allergy) or the inappropriate targeting of the body's own cells by the immune system (autoimmunity) can result in acute or chronic inflammation and cell injury. Abnormal suppression of the immune system can increase vulnerability to microbial invasion.

6. Genetic defects

Inherited or acquired mutations in important genes can alter the synthesis of crucial cellular proteins leading to developmental defects or abnormal metabolic functioning. Acquired mutations to somatic cells during life can affect cell differentiation and replication leading to diseases such as cancer.

7. Nutritional Imbalances

Deficiencies or excesses in normal cellular substrates (e. g. calories, proteins, carbohydrates, minerals and vitamins) can produce problems such as obesity, malnutrition, scurvy, iron deficiency anemia, etc.

MECHANISMS OF CELLULAR INJURY

Cell injury is associated with damage to the structural and functional molecules of the cell. Injury to a cell may be nonlethal or lethal (Figure 1-8).

Nonlethal injury to a cell may produce cell degeneration, which is manifested as some abnormality of biochemical function, a recognizable structural change, or a combined biochemical and structural abnormality. Degeneration is reversible but may progress to necrosis if injury persists. When it is associated with abnormal cell function, cell degeneration may also cause clinical disease.

Lethal injuries to the cell of a living individual cause cell death, including necrosis and apoptosis. Necrosis is accompanied by biochemical and structural changes (see below) and is irreversible. The

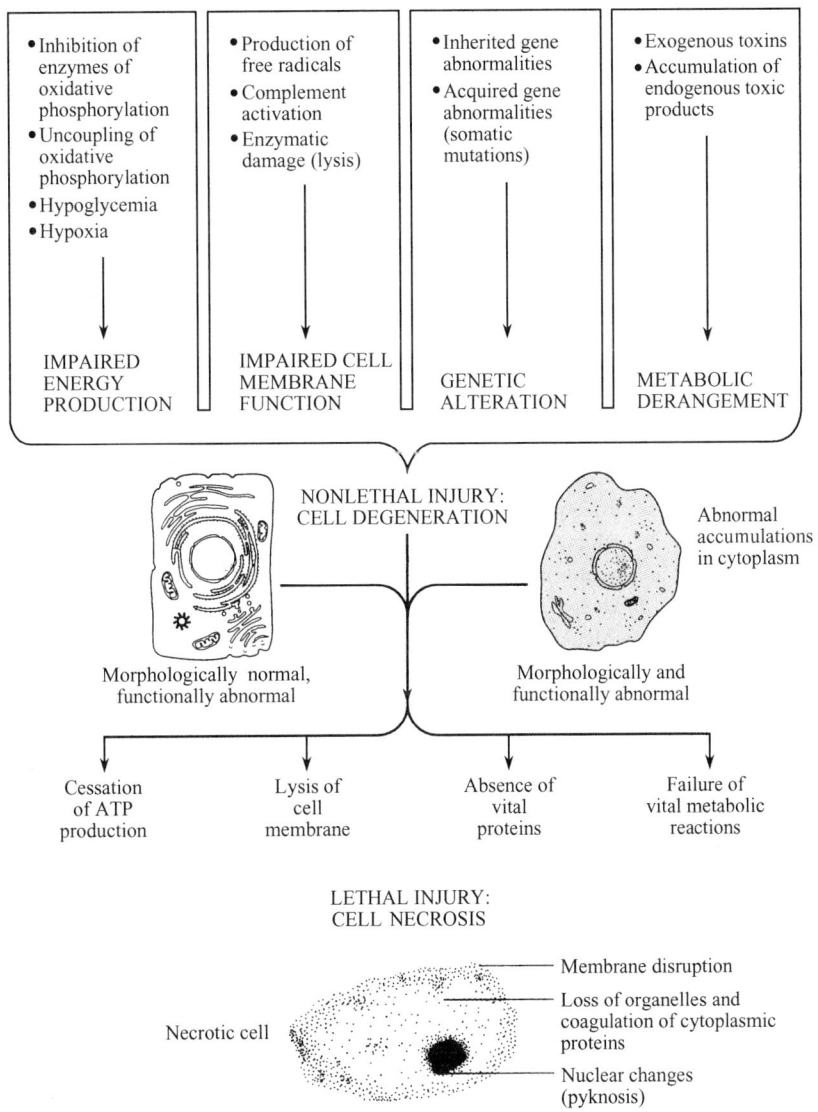

Figure 1-8 Mechanisms of injury leading to cell degeneration and necrosis

necrotic cells cease to function; if necrosis is sufficiently extensive, clinical disease results. Necrosis should be distinguished from apoptosis - genetically programmed cell death. In apoptosis, there is an orderly disassembly of cellular proteins and DNA with minimal disruption to normal tissue. Apoptosis is a normal physiologic process designed to eliminate unwanted, functionally abnormal, or senescent (old and worn out) cells. It plays an important role in the developing embryo, certain hormone-dependent tissues, and in aging. However, in some instances, apoptosis may be a pathologic process induced by cell injury (e.g. viral infection, radiation injury, etc.). The details of apoptosis are discussed later.

Mechanical Trauma

Mechanical trauma may cause subtle but significant dislocations of the intracellular organization of organelles or may destroy the cell by completely disrupting it. For example, a surgical incision or accidents can destroy the cells and tissues directly. Ice crystals which occur in freezing can mechanically injury the structure of the cell membrane.

Impaired Cell Membrane Function

Selectively permeable lipid membranes are essential for maintaining the internal environment of cells. By controlling what molecules enter and leave the cell, the plasma membrane helps conserve important resources, and keeps the cell in osmotic equilibrium with extracellular fluid. Energy-dependent protein "pumps" embedded in the plasma membrane establish differences in ion concentrations and electrical charge between the inside and outside of the cell (resting membrane potential).

Cell membranes can be disrupted by degrading phospholipids - the primary molecular component of biologic membranes. Damage to the plasma membrane increases the cell permeability to sodium and water. This causes the cell to swell, and may even lead to disruption of the cell (lysis). Potassium may leak out of the cell affecting its ability to maintain resting membrane potential. Injury to the membrane of mitochondria impairs energy metabolism. Lysosomal injury releases hydrolytic enzymes into the cytoplasm leading to auto-digestion of cellular proteins. Damage to the endoplasmic reticulum interferes with protein synthesis and the intracellular transport of biologically important compounds.

Impaired Energy Production

A. Normal Energy Production

High-energy phosphate bonds of adenosine triphosphate (ATP) represent the most efficient energy source for the cell. ATP is produced by phosphorylation of ADP, a reaction that is linked to the oxidation of reduced substances in the respiratory chain of enzymes. Oxygen is required (oxidative phosphorylation). Cells require a constant energy supply, mainly in the form of ATP, to drive metabolism and biosynthetic reactions.

B. Causes of Defective Energy (ATP) Production

1. Hypoglycemia

Glucose is the main substrate for energy production in most tissues and is the sole energy source in brain cells. Low glucose levels in blood (hypoglycemia) therefore result in deficient ATP production that is most profound in the brain.

2. Hypoxia

Depriving the cell of oxygen (hypoxia), or disturbing mitochondrial function, interferes with the cell's ability to utilize oxygen in generating adequate amounts of ATP. This, in turn, impairs the ability of the cell to utilize nutrients in synthesizing structural and functional proteins necessary for maintaining the cell. Depletion of ATP also shifts energy metabolism towards anaerobic glycolysis.

3. Enzyme Inhibition

Cyanide poisoning is a good example of a chemical interfering with a vital enzyme. Cyanide inhibits cytochrome oxidase, the final enzyme in the respiratory chain, causing acute ATP deficiency in all cells of the body and rapid death.

4. Uncoupling of oxidative phosphorylation

Uncoupling of oxidation and phosphorylation occurs either through chemical reactions or through physical detachment of enzymes from the mitochondrial membrane. Mitochondrial swelling, which is a common change associated with many types of injury, causes uncoupling of oxidative phosphorylation.

C. Effects of Defective Energy Production

Generalized failure of energy production will first affect those cells with the highest demand for oxygen because of their high basal metabolic rate. Brain cells are maximally affected. The earliest clinical signs of hypoxia and hypoglycemia are disturbances of the normal level of consciousness.

Genetic Alteration

Damage to cellular DNA interferes with cell replication, and impairs the synthesis of important structural and functional proteins.

Inherited genetic abnormalities are passed from generation to generation, frequently in predictable fashion according to Mendelian laws. **Acquired genetic abnormalities** are somatic mutations resulting from damage to genetic material by any of several agents, including ionizing radiation, viruses, and mutagenic drugs and chemicals. The clinical and pathologic effects of genetic abnormalities depend on (1) the severity of damage, (2) the precise gene or genes damaged, and (3) when the damage was sustained. When genetic damage is inherited or occurs during gametogenesis or early fetal development, clinical effects may be present at birth (congenital genetic disease). Acquired genetic disease results when genetic damage occurs postnatally.

The Role of Oxygen-derived Free Radicals

When mitochondria generate energy by reducing molecular oxygen to water, small amounts of partially reduced forms of oxygen (superoxide, hydrogen peroxide, and hydroxyl radicals) are produced in the process. These "free radicals" are short-lived molecules containing an unpaired electron in an outer orbital – an electron that is not contributing to normal intramolecular bonding. These are essentially "free chemical bonds" which are energetically unstable and highly reactive. Free radicals are generally transient products of oxidation-reduction reactions or result when a covalent bond is broken and one electron from each pair remains with each atom. Although free radicals play an important physiologic role in intracellular oxidation-reduction reactions and the bacteria killing function of white blood cells, they can also interact with biologically important molecules-removing electrons or hydrogen atoms and disrupting covalent bonds. Fortunately, cells normally produce only very small amounts of oxygen-derived free radicals, and they also have molecular scavengers (anti-oxidants) to neutralize them before they can do any harm.

When cells are injured, large amounts of free radicals can accumulate-rapidly depleting anti-oxidants and allowing free radicals to react with critical biochemical components of the cell. Free radicals can attack the double bonds of unsaturated phospholipids in cell membranes which eventually degrade the structural integrity of cell membranes. Free radicals also impair the functions of enzymes by causing fragmentation of polypeptide chains or the cross-linking of sulfhydryl (-SH) groups in proteins. Free radicals also cause strand breaks or abnormal cross-linking in DNA.

Denaturation of Cellular Enzymes or Structural Proteins

Almost all vital cellular processes are dependent on enzymes-protein catalysts that facilitate biochemical reactions inside the cell. Without enzymes, synthesis and metabolic reactions would occur too slowly to be useful to the cell.

Damage to structural proteins can impair the intracellular transport system of cells and disrupt the supportive protein cytoskeleton of cells.

REVERSIBLE INJURY OF CELL AND TISSUE

Under some conditions, many normal or abnormal amounts of various substances may be accumulated either in the cytoplasm or in the interstitial tissues. These may be harmless or may cause varied degree of injury. This is also named as degeneration.

Degeneration and accumulation of endogenous substances are seen Table 1-3.

HYDROPIC DEGENERATION

Hydropic degeneration, or **clouding swelling**, is an early and reversible effect of cell injury, including hypoxia, toxins and so on. These injurious agents can cause dysfunction of the energy-dependent sodium pump in the plasma membrane, and resulting influx of sodium and water into cell.

Table 1-3 Endogenous substances accumulating in tissues as a result of deranged metabolism

Accumulated Substance	Effects in Parenchymal Cells	Effects in Interstitial Tissues
Water	Cloudy swelling Hydropic change	Edema
Lipid		
Triglyceride	Fatty change	
Cholesterol		Atherosclerosis Xanthoma
Complex lipids (phospholipids)	Lipid storage disease	
protein	Ubiquitin/protein Complexes Heat shock proteins	Amyloidosis
Glycogen	Glycogen storage diseases	
Mucopolysaccharide	Mucopolysaccharidoses	Myxoid degeneration
Minerals		
Iron	Hemochromatosis	Localized hemosiderosis
Calcium	Contributes to necrosis	Calcification
Copper	Wilson's disease	Wilson's disease
Pigments		
Bilirubin	Kernicterus	Jaundice
Lipofuscin	Brown atrophy	
Urate		Gout
Homogentisic acid		Alkaptonuria

Morphologically, in the hydropic swelling of the organs or tissues there is an increasing weight and turgor. The parenchyma cells are enlarged in various degrees and crowded together, and the cytoplasm is translucent and stains more lightly. Sometimes these large round cells are called balloon like enlarged cells. The nucleus is usually in the center of the cell. Some small, clear vacuoles may be seen within the cytoplasm on microscopy (Figure 1-9). The vacuoles represent distended cisternae of the endoplasmic reticulum or sequestered remnants of it.

FATTY CHANGE (Fatty Degeneration)

Fatty change is the accumulation of triglyceride in the cytoplasm of parenchymal cells. It is common in the liver and rare in the kidney and myocardium and occurs as a nonspecific response to many types of injury.

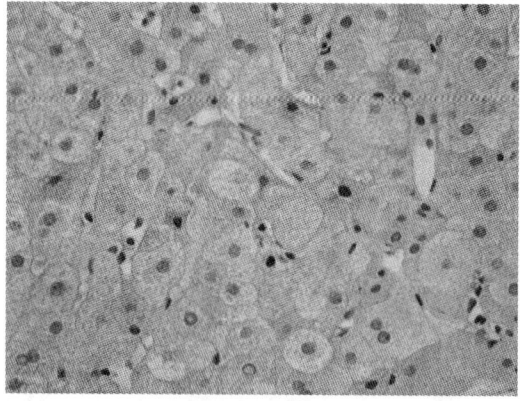

Figure 1-9 Hydropic swelling of hepatocytes. The cytoplasm of the liver cells is lucent. Some of the liver cells are enlarged with translucent cytoplasm that appears as a vacuole, also called balloon-like enlarged cells

Normal Triglyceride Metabolism in the Liver

The liver plays a central role in triglyceride metabolism. Free fatty acids are carried in the blood to the liver, where they are converted to triglycerides, phospholipids, and cholesteryl esters. After these lipids form complexes with specific lipid acceptor proteins (apoproteins), which are also synthesized in the liver cell, they are secreted into the plasma as lipoproteins. When triglycerides are metabolized normally, there are so little triglycerides in the liver cell that it cannot be seen in routine microscopic sections.

Causes of Fatty Liver

Accumulation of triglycerides in the cytoplasm of liver cells (fatty liver) represents an abnormality of the metabolic pathway and occurs in the following conditions: (1) When there is increased mobilization of adipose tissue, resulting in an increase in the amount of fatty acids reaching the liver, e. g. in starvation and diabetes mellitus. (2) When the rate of conversion of fatty acids to triglycerides in the liver cell is increased because of overactivity of the involved enzyme systems. This is the main mechanism by which alcohol, a powerful enzyme inducer, causes fatty liver. (3) When oxidation of triglycerides to acetyl-CoA and ketone bodies is decreased, e. g. in anemia and hypoxia. (4) When synthesis of lipid acceptor proteins is deficient. Protein malnutrition and several hepatotoxins, e. g. carbon tetrachloride and phosphorus, cause fatty liver in this way.

Types of Fatty Liver

A. Acute Fatty Liver

Acute fatty liver is a rare but serious condition associated with acute liver failure. In acute fatty liver, triglyceride accumulates as small, membrane-bound droplets in the cytoplasm (microvacuolar fatty change, Figure 1-10).

B. Chronic Fatty Liver

Chronic fatty liver is much more common. It is associated with chronic alcoholism, malnutrition, and several hepatotoxins. Fat droplets in the cytoplasm fuse to form progressively larger globules

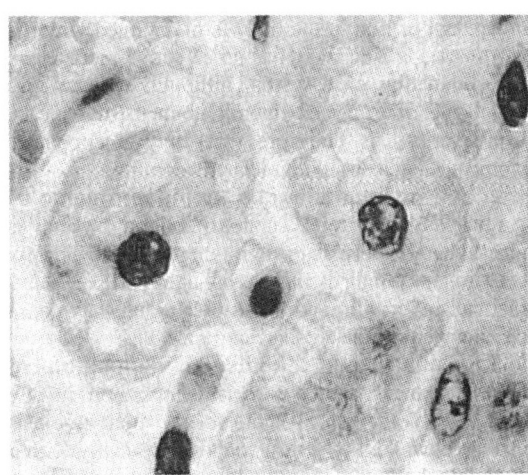

Figure 1-10 Acute microvacuolar fatty change of the liver in Reye's syndrome. The cytoplasm of the liver cells is filled with numerous small vacuoles representing the lipid that has been dissolved out of the tissue during processing. The nuclei are centrally located

(macrovacuolar fatty change, Figure 1-11). The distribution of fatty change in the liver lobule varies with different causes (Figure 1-12). Grossly, the fatty liver is enlarged and yellow, with a greasy appearance when cut. Even when severe, chronic fatty liver is rarely associated with clinically detectable liver dysfunction.

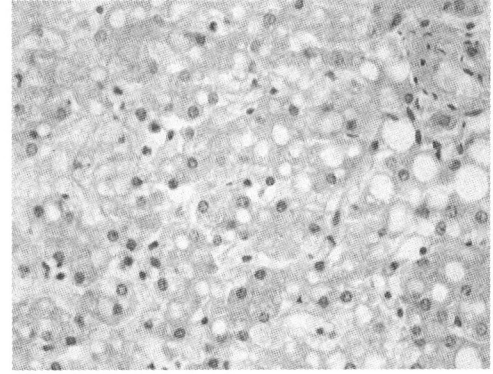

Figure 1-11 Macrovacuolar fatty change of the liver in chronic alcoholism. The large fat globules in the cytoplasm appear as empty spaces that have displaced the nucleus to the side

Fatty Change of the Myocardium

Triglyceride deposition in myocardial fibers occurs

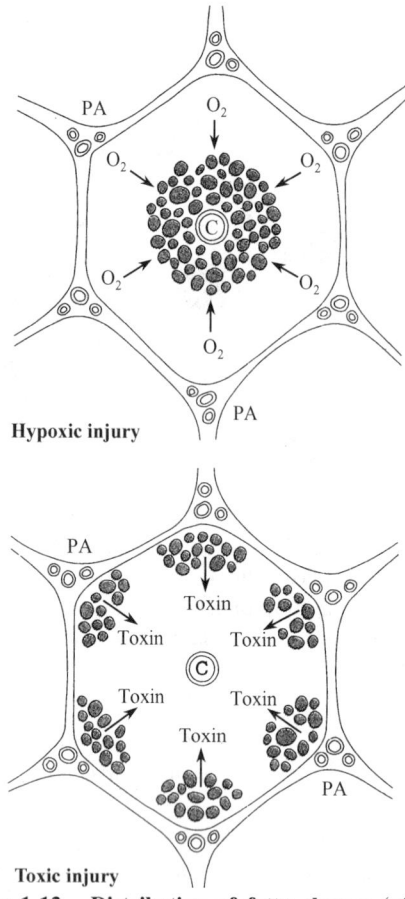

Figure 1-12 Distribution of fatty change (tinted circles) in the liver in hypoxic and toxic liver injuries. In hypoxic injury, fatty change occurs centrizonalling; in toxic injury, fatty change occurs around the portal areas, The rules relating to this distribution, which are dependent on the mode of entry of oxygen and toxins into the liver lobule, are not without exception. Carbon tetrachloride, for example, causes centrizonal fatty change

in chronic hypoxic states, notably severe anemia. In chronic fatty change, bands of yellow streaks alternate with red-brown muscle ("thrush breast" or "tiger skin" appearance); this usually causes no clinical symptoms. Toxic diseases such as diphtheritic myocarditis and Reye's syndrome produce acute fatty change. The heart is flabby and shows diffuse yellow discoloration; myocardial failure commonly follows.

Microscopic Features of Fatty Change

Any fat present in tissues dissolves in the solvents that are used to process tissue samples for microscopic sections. In routine tissue sections, therefore, cells in the earliest stages of fatty change have pale and foamy cytoplasm. As fat accumulation increases, cytoplasmic vacuoles appear. Positive demonstration of fat requires the use of frozen sections made from fresh tissue. Fat remains in the cytoplasm in frozen sections, where it can be demonstrated by fat stains such as oil red O and Sudan black B.

HYALINE DEGENERATION

Hyaline degeneration is applied to material of homogeneous, glassy, usually eosinophilic appearance seen on microscopy of hematoxylin and eosin stain. It is a purely descriptive adjective, and many different formed tissue elements, as well as cell cytoplasm or interstitial tissue, may assume a hyaline appearance.

A. Hyaline of Connective Tissue

It commonly occurs in dense collagenous fibrous scar which may assume a homogeneous pink hyaline appearance grossly. Microscopic examination shows excessive collagen as thick, hyalinized bands.

B. Hyaline of the Arterial Wall

In the kidney, brain, spleen, retina and other organs, the walls of arterioles usually become thickened. Hyalinization in arteries occurs in longstanding hypertension. The hyaline material arises by intramural deposition of plasma protein and lipids and reduplication of the intimal basement membrane. The narrowing of the lumens usually result in the ischemia of organs (Figure 1-13).

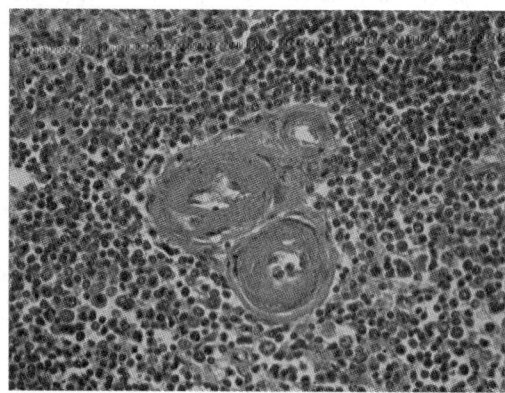

Figure 1-13 Hyaline degeneration of the central artery of the spleen, showing numerous homogenous eosinophilic material deposit under the intima, which results in thickened of the parts of the central artery as well as narrowing of the lumen

C. Intracellular Accumulation of Protein

In many injuries, overabundant proteins deposition in cell cytoplasm results in morphological changes of tissue. On microscopy the round, eosinophil droplets usually can be seen in cytoplasm. These droplets can appear as homogeneous, filament-like and crystalloid by electron microscopy. For example: (1) In many conditions such as glomerulonephritis, abnormal amounts of plasma proteins leak into the glomerolar filtrate, part of the protein is resorbed by the tubular epithelium where it is seen as hyaline droplets. (2) Russell bodies in plasma cells constitute spherical hyaline immunoglobulin deposits, it usually occurs in some chronic inflammation. (3) Mallory hyaline appears in the hepatocyte cytoplasm in alcoholics, particularly when it has led to cirrhosis of the liver, and certain other forms of liver cell injury (Figure 1-14). And (4) Lewy bodies appears in neurons of Parkinson's disease.

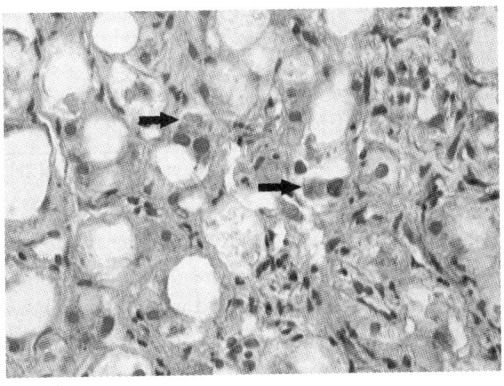

Figure 1-14 Mallory body, so called "alcoholic hyaline" in the cirrhosis associated with alcohol abuse. The irregular dark configuration within the liver cells (arrow)

ACCUMULATION OF MUCOPOLYSACCHARIDES (Myxoid Degeneration)

An increase in the amount of mucopolysaccharides (glycosaminoglycans) in the ground substance of the interstitium is termed myxoid (myxomatous) degeneration. Special stains (e.g. alcian blue, colloidal iron) are necessary to demonstrate mucopolysaccharides; myxoid degeneration appears on microscopic examination of hematoxylin and eosin-stained sections as loose, weakly basophilic material.

Myxoid degeneration of the interstitium occurs in hypothyroidism (myxedema) through an unknown mechanism. Myxoid degeneration is common in joint capsules, where it may lead to formation of a cystic tumor (ganglion) on a tendon or aponeurosis. Myxoid degeneration also occurs in the stroma of neoplasms such as neurofibromas.

A form of myxoid degeneration may occur in the aorta and cardiac valves, especially the mitral valve. This change is common in Marfan's syndrome (see above) and may be associated with valvular incompetence and aortic rupture. A similar form of myxoid degeneration - largely confined to the mitral valve leaflets - occurs in otherwise normal individuals and is the most common cause of mitral valve incompetence (floppy valve syndrome).

DEPOSITION OF AMYLOID (Amyloidosis)

The term amyloid denotes a variety of fibrillary proteins deposited in interstitial tissues in certain pathologic conditions. All types of amyloid have the following physicochemical characteristics:
a. In histologic sections, amyloid stains as follows:
• With Congo red stain, amyloid appears red with apple-green birefringence when viewed under polarized light.
• With H and E, it stains homogeneous pink.
• Amyloid may also be stained immunohistochemically using antibodies specific to the various subtypes of fibrils.
b. On electron microscopy, amyloid appears as non-branching fibrils 7.5 - 10 nm wide.
c. On x-ray diffraction, amyloid exhibits a pleated β-sheet structure that renders the protein very resistant to enzymatic degradation, contributing to its accumulation in tissues.

Chemical Composition

The chemical structure of amyloid protein is quite variable (see Table 1-4, where AL, AA, etc are explained).

A. Amyloid of Immunoglobulin Origin

In AL amyloid, the protein is composed of fragments of the light chains of immunoglobulin molecules. AL is produced by neoplastic plasma cells

Table 1-4 Amyloidosis

Amyioid Protein	Principal Constituent	Associated Diseases	Distribution
AL	Lmmunoglobulin light chain	Primary amyloidosis Plasma cell myeloma B cell malignant lymphoma	Tongue, heart, gastrointestinal tract liver, spleen, kidney (primary distribution)
AA	Serum A protein (α_1-globulin)	Rheumatoid arthritis	Tongue, heart, gastrointestinal tract (primary distribution)
AA	Serum A protein (α_1-globulin)	Chronic infections (tuberculosis, leprosy bronchiectasis, osteomyelitis) Hodgkin's disease Inflammatory bowie disease	Liver, kidney, spleen (secondary distribution)
AA	Serum A protein (α_1-globulin)	Familial Mediterranean fever	Liver, kidney spleen
AF	Prealbumin	Familial amyloidosis (Portuguese, Swedish, etc)	Peripheral nerves, kidney
AS	Prealbumin	Senile amyloidosis Cardiac amyloidosis Cerebral amyloid angiopathy	Heart, spleen, pancreas Heart Cerebral vessels
AE	Peptide hormone precursors (e.g. calcitonin)	Medullary carcinoma of thyroid Pancreatic islet cell adenomas	Locally within the neoplasm
AD	Unknown	Lichen amyloidosis	Skin (dermis)
Alzheimer	A_4 peptide[1] or beta amyloid precursor protein	Alzheimer's disease Down's syndrome	Neurofibrillary tangles, plaques, and angiopathy

[1] A_4 peptide = Alzheimer 4000-MW peptide (derived from a 40,000-MW precursor protein found in serum and cerebrospinal fluid; encoded in chromosome 21).

(myeloma) and B lymphocytes (B cell lymphomas). Amyloid light chains resemble the free light chains (Bence Jones proteins) or light chain fragments that are produced by the neoplastic plasma cells or B lymphocytes.

B. Amyloid of Other Origin

Other amyloid fibrils are composed of (1) serum amyloid-associated protein, an acute phase protein (MW 18,000) produced by the liver during any inflammatory process; (2) prealbumin; and (3) other peptide fragments (Table 1-4). In addition, all amyloids contain small amounts of amyloid P protein and, usually, heparan sulfate.

Classification

The clinical classification of amyloidosis is based on protein type and tissue distribution.

A. Systemic Amyloidosis

1. Primary pattern of distribution

In systemic amyloidosis with a primary distribution, amyloid is found in the heart, gastrointestinal tract, tongue, skin, and nerves. This distribution is seen in primary amyloidosis and neoplasms of B lymphocytes (plasma cell myeloma and B cell malignant lymphomas). An underlying plasma cell neoplastic process with a monoclonal immunoglobulin is detectable in serum in more than 90% of patients with primary amyloidosis. In these cases, amyloid is AL. In rheumatoid arthritis, a nonimmunoglobulin amyloid (AA) is deposited in this primary pattern.

2. Secondary pattern of distribution

In systemic amyloidosis with a secondary distribution, amyloid is found in the liver, spleen, kidney, adrenals, gastrointestinal tract, and skin. It occurs secondarily to chronic inflammatory diseases such as tuberculosis, leprosy, chronic osteomyelitis, chronic pyelonephritis, and inflammatory bowel disease (reactive systemic amyloidosis, secondary amyloidosis). The amyloid protein is AA and is derived from plasma α_1-globulins.

B. Localized Amyloidosis

Localized amyloidosis may take the form of nodular, tumor-like masses that occur rarely in the tongue, bladder, lung or skin. These amyloid tumors are commonly associated with localized plasma cell neoplasms. In Alzheimer's disease, deposits of a special form of amyloid occur in the extracellular brain substance (plaques).

C. Amyloid in Neoplasms

Amyloid is present in the stroma of many endocrine neoplasms, e.g. medullary carcinoma of the thyroid. The amyloid protein is AE, usually derived from precursor molecules of certain peptide hormones (e.g. calcitonin).

D. Heredofamilial Amyloidosis

Familial amyloidosis has been reported in only a few families. The amyloid type is AF or AA. Familial amyloidosis is classified as neuropathic, nephropathic, or cardiac, depending on the site of maximal involvement. Familial Mediterranean fever, a disease transmitted by autosomal recessive inheritance, is characterized by fever and inflammation of joints and serosal membranes.

E. Senile Amyloidosis

Small amounts of amyloid (AS type) are frequently found in the heart, pancreas, and spleen in the elderly. In the late stages of diabetes mellitus, amyloidosis occurs in the abnormal pancreatic islets. This may be a distinct type of amyloid composed of islet amyloid polypeptide, which has been shown to have hormonal activity, affecting glucose uptake in muscle.

Effects of Amyloid Deposition

Amyloid is deposited in interstitial tissue, commonly in relation to the basement membrane of cells and small blood vessels. Tissues affected by amyloidosis are often enlarged (hepatosplenomegaly, cardiomegaly, thickened peripheral nerves, macroglossia). Affected tissues are also firmer and less flexible or distensible than normal tissues. Therefore, blood vessels affected by amyloidosis do not constrict normally and tend to bleed after injury; diagnostic biopsy may be followed by hemorrhage for this reason. The gross appearance of involved tissue appears pale gray and waxy. Pathologic and clinical effects of amyloidosis are illustrated in Figures 1-15 and 1-16.

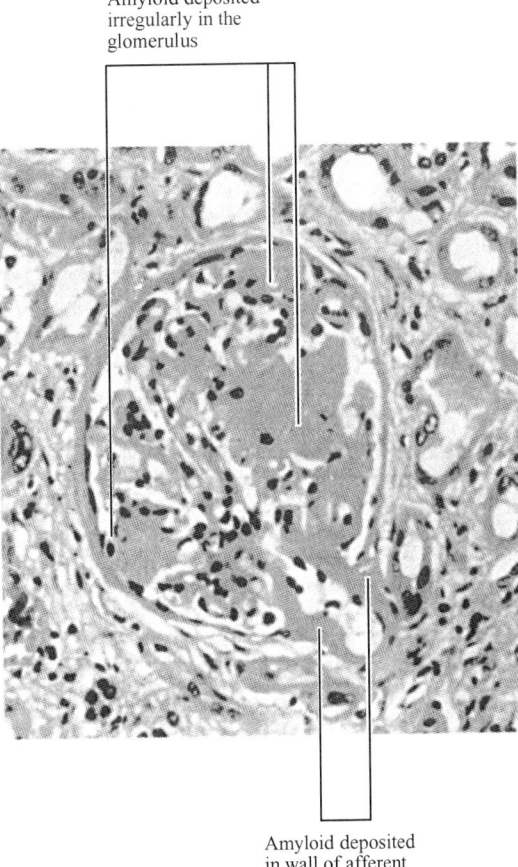

Figure 1-15 Amyloidosis involving a glomerulus. Amyloid appears as a homogeneous acellular material that stains pink with hematoxylin and eosin

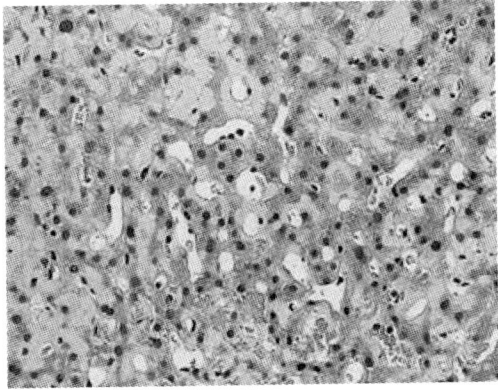

Figure 1-16 Amyloidosis of the liver. Amyloid is deposited in the space of Disse and compresses the liver cell plates

INTRACELLULAR ACCUMULATION OF GLYCOGEN

Glycogen accumulation is encountered in patients having deranged carbohydrate or glycogen metabolism. Intracellular accumulation of glycogen usually occurs in **diabetes mellitus** or **glycogen storage disease.** In diabetes mellitus, increased glucose is reabsorbed by the renal tubular epithelial cells, especially affecting the terminal straight portion of the proximal convoluted tubules and the loop of Henle. Glycogen accumulates and causes clear vacuolation of the cytoplasm of the cell in these tubules on H. E section. On PAS stained sections, glycogen appears rose-red color. Glycogen accumulation in the diabetic is also encountered in hepotocytes, myocardium and β-cell of pancreatic islets. In the glycogen storage disease, there is a genetic lack of one or more of the enzymes involved in either the mobilization of glycogen or the synthesis of normal glycogen, and glycogen also accumulates intracellularly.

DEPOSITION OF PATHOLOGICAL PIGMENTS

Pigments are the colored substances in tissues. Some pigments exist in normal tissues such as melanin in skin, but other's occur in abnormal conditions such as hemosiderin in lung. They are either exogenous, coming from outside the body (example as carbon), or endogenous, synthesized within body itself (example as lipofuscin, melanin and hemosiderin).

Coal Dust

Coal dust is the most common exogenous pigment; usually occurring in the coal miner and the urban dweller. When inhaled into alveoli and deposited, some black pigment can be seen in lung grossly. Then the dusts are phagocytosed by alveolar macrophages and transported through lymphatic channels to the tracheobronchial lymph nodes. Aggregates of the dust blacken the draining lymph nodes and pulmonary parenchyma. Heavy accumulations may induce emphysema or pulmonary sclerosis that can result in serious lung disease.

Melanin

Melanin, which is normally present in skin, hair follicles, iris, choroids and other sites, is synthesized in melanocytes by the tyrosinase-mediated oxidation of tyrosine to dihydroxyphenylalanine (DOPA). It is an endogenous dark brown granular cytoplasmic pigment. Melanin synthesis is under adrenal and pituitary control. Adrenal steroids suppress and pituitary adrenocorticotropic hormone (ACTH) stimulates its synthesis. Aggregates of these melanophores create freckles which darken after exposure to sunlight because of the actinic stimulation of melanin synthesis in melanocytes. The local aggregate of melanin can occur in melanotic nevus, melanoma and other diseases.

Lipofuscin

With light microscopy, lipofucin appears as yellow-brown, fine cytoplasmic granules which present in certain normal cells, such as the epithelial cells of the epididymis, the interstitial cells of the testis and the ganglion cells of the hippocampus. However, larger amounts of lipofucins are found in cells undergoing slow regressive changes, such as that which occurs in the atrophy accompanying advanced age and in chronic injury (Figure 1-17). Lipofucin granules represent residual bodies containing depolymerized indigestible residues of organellar membranes.

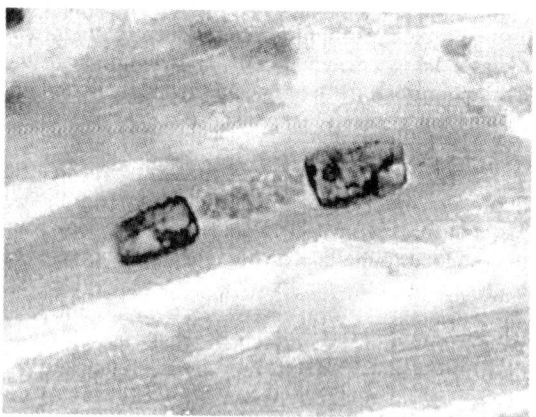

Figure 1-17 Myocardial fiber with lipofuscin pigment in the perinuclear region. On sections stained with hematoxylin and eosin, lipofuscin has a golden brown color (arrow)

Deposition of Iron (Hemosiderosis and Hemochromatosis)

A. Normal Iron Metabolism

Iron metabolism is normally regulated so that the total amount of iron in the body is maintained within a narrow range. The body has no effective mechanism for eliminating excess iron, although women lose 20 – 30 mg of iron each month in menstrual blood. Iron overload is therefore rare in premenopausal women, whereas iron deficiency is common.

B. Hemosiderosis and Hemochromatosis

An increase in the total amount of iron in the body is termed hemosiderosis or hemochromatosis. The excess iron accumulates in macrophages and parenchymal cells as ferritin and hemosiderin and may cause parenchymal cell necrosis (Figure 1-18).

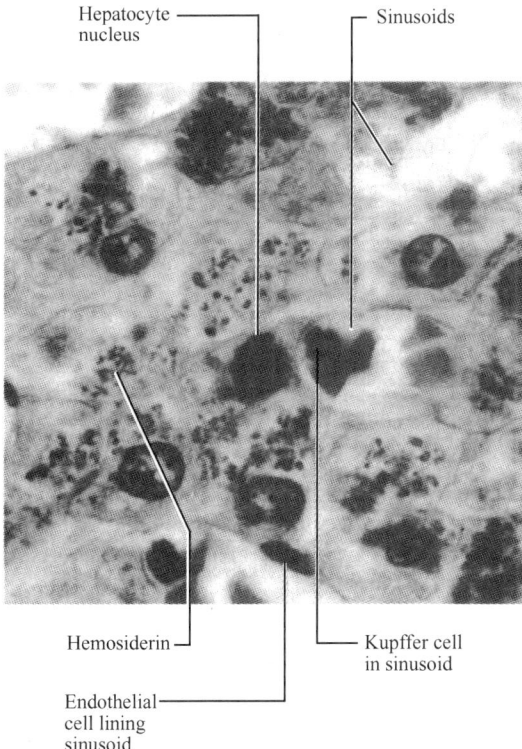

Figure 1-18 Hemochromatosis of the liver, showing hemosiderin pigment deposited in hepatocytes and Kupffer cells. Hemosiderin stains golden brown with hematoxylin and eosin and deep blue with Prussian blue stain

C. Causes and Effects of Deposition of Iron

Localized hemosiderosis is common, in any tissue that is the site of hemorrhage. Hemoglobin is broken down and its iron is deposited locally; either in macrophages or in the connective tissue, in the form of hemosiderin (as in a bruise). Localized hemosiderosis has no clinical significance.

Generalized hemosiderosis is less common, occurring with relatively minor iron excess following multiple transfusions, excessive dietary iron, or excess absorption of iron in some hemolytic anemias. The excess iron is deposited as hemosiderin in macrophages throughout the body, notably in bone marrow, liver, and spleen. Generalized hemosiderosis can be diagnosed in bone marrow and liver biopsies and, apart from indicating the presence of iron overload of minor degree, has no clinical significance.

Hemorrhage is the presence of blood in interstitial tissue outside the blood vessels. Hemorrhage results from escape of erythrocytes across intact vessels (diapedesis) or from vascular rupture.

Erythrocytes are rapidly broken down in interstitial tissue, and the iron in hemoglobin molecules is ingested by macrophages in the interstitium and converted to **hemosiderin**, which appears as a brown, granular pigment in the cytoplasm of macrophages. Hemosiderin may spill over from macrophages to be deposited in interstitial connective tissue (localized hemosiderosis). The porphyrin in the hemoglobin molecule is broken down by local macrophages to form bilirubin, which may be absorbed in the blood or deposited in interstitial connective tissue as a golden-yellow, crystalline pigment called **hematoidin**. Neither hemosiderin nor hematoidin deposited in interstitial tissues cause cellular dysfunction.

Deposition of Calcium (Calcification)

Deposition of calcium in the interstitium is common and takes one of two forms.

A. Metastatic Calcification

Metastatic calcification is due to an increase in serum calcium or phosphorus levels. Calcification occurs in previously normal tissues, most commonly the arterial walls, alveolar septa of the lung, and kidneys.

Calcification affecting the renal interstitium (nephrocalcinosis) may cause chronic renal failure. Extensive calcification of blood vessels may result in ischemia, particularly in the skin. Rarely, extensive involvement of pulmonary alveoli causes abnormalities in diffusion of gases. Apart from these instances, calcification does not impair function of parenchymal cells in tissues.

Deposition of calcium in tissues is visible radiologically. Microscopically, calcium is intensely basophilic (stains blue with hematoxylin). Deposits of calcium appear granular in the early stages of calcification; larger deposits are amorphous.

B. Dystrophic Calcification

In dystrophic calcification, calcium and phosphorus metabolism and serum levels are normal, and calcification occurs as a result of local abnormality in tissues. Functional impairment is uncommon. Dystrophic calcification may provide radiologic markers; e. g. a calcified pineal gland accurately points to the midline of the brain.

IRREVERSIBLE CELL INJURY: CELL DEATH

Cell death may be caused by various severe injuries. Cell death appears as necrosis and apoptosis.

NECROSIS

Necrosis refers to a sequence of morphologic changes that follow cell death in living tissue. The morphologic structural changes that accompany necrosis result from two processes: (1) Enzymatic digestion of the cell by its own hydrolytic lysosomal enzymes (sometimes called **liquefaction necrosis**) (2) Denaturation and precipitation of cellular proteins (**coagulation necrosis**).

Necrosis may occur directly or may follow cell degeneration.

Morphological Evidence of Necrosis

A. Early Changes

In early necrosis, the cell is morphologically normal. There is a delay of 1 – 3 hours before changes of necrosis are recognizable on electron microscopy and at least 6 – 8 hours before changes are apparent on light microscopy. For example, if a patient has a heart attack (myocardial necrosis caused by anoxia due to occlusion of a coronary artery) and dies within minutes, autopsy will reveal no structural evidence of necrosis; if, on the other hand, death occurs 2 days after the heart attack, changes due to necrosis are obvious.

B. Nuclear Changes

Nuclear changes are the best evidence of cell necrosis. The chromatin of the dead cell clumps into coarse strands, and the nucleus becomes a shrunken, dense, and deeply basophilic mass (i. e. it stains dark blue with hematoxylin). This process is called **pyknosis** (Figure 1-19). The pyknotic nucleus may then break up into numerous small basophilic particles (**karyorrhexis**) or undergo lysis as a result of the action of lysosomal deoxyribonucleases (**karyolysis**). In rapidly occurring necrosis, the nucleus undergoes lysis without a pyknotic stage.

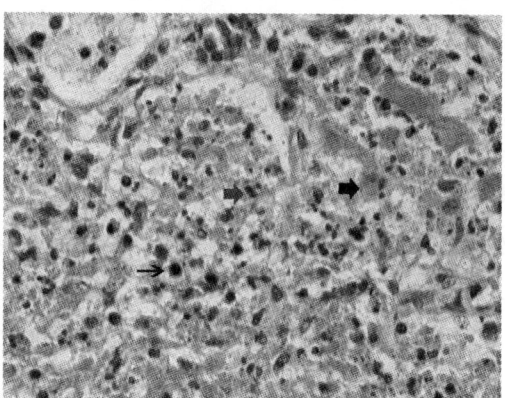

Figure 1-19 Morphologic features of necotic cells, showing the nuclear pyknosis (thin arrow), karyorrhexis (grey thick arrow) and karyolysis (blank thick arrow)

C. Cytoplasmic Changes

About 6 hours after the cell undergoes necrosis, its cytoplasm becomes homogeneous and deeply acidophilic – i. e. it stains pink with an acidic stain such as eosin. This is the first change detectable by light microscopy, and it is due to denaturation of cytoplasmic proteins and loss of ribosomes. The RNA of the ribosomes is responsible for the basophilic tinge in normal cytoplasm. When specialized organelles are present in the cell, such as myofibrils in myocardial cells, these are lost early. Swelling of mitochondria and disruption of organelle membranes causes cytoplasmic vacuolation. Finally, enzymatic digestion of the cell by enzymes released by the cell's own lysosomes causes lysis (**autolysis**).

D. Biochemical Changes

The influx of Ca^{2+} into the cell is closely related to irreversible injury and the appearance of morphologic changes of necrosis. In the normal cell, the intracellular calcium concentration is about 0.001 that of extracellular fluid. This gradient is maintained by the cell membrane, which actively transports Ca^{2+} out of the cell. In experimental systems in which cell injury is induced by ischemia and/or toxic agents, intracellular calcium accumulation occurs only when the cell is irreversibly damaged. Calcium ions activate endonucleases (hydrolyze DNA), phospholipases (disrupt membranes), and proteases (digest the cytoskeleton).

Types of Necrosis

Different cells show different morphologic changes after they undergo necrosis; the differences reflect variations in cell composition, speed of necrosis, and type of injury (Figure 1-20).

A. Coagulative Necrosis

In this type of necrosis, the necrotic cell retains its cellular outline, often for several days. The cell, devoid of its nucleus, appears as a mass of coagulated, pink-staining, homogeneous cytoplasm.

Coagulative necrosis typically occurs in solid organs, such as the kidney, heart (myocardium), and adrenal gland, usually as a result of deficient blood supply and anoxia. It is also seen with other types of injury, e.g. coagulative necrosis of liver cells due to viruses or toxic chemicals, and coagulative necrosis of skin in burns.

B. Liquefactive Necrosis

Liquefaction of necrotic cells results when lysosomal enzymes released by the necrotic cells cause rapid liquefaction. Lysis of a cell as a result of the action of its own enzymes is autolysis. Liquefactive necrosis is typically seen in the brain following ischemia (Figures 1-21 and 1-22).

Liquefactive necrosis also occurs during pus formation (suppurative inflammation) as a result of the action of proteolytic enzymes released by neutrophils. Cellular lysis by enzymes derived from a source other than the cell itself is heterolysis.

C. Fat Necrosis

1. Enzymatic fat necrosis

Fat necrosis most characteristically occurs in acute pancreatitis when pancreatic enzymes are liberated from the ducts into surrounding tissue. Pancreatic lipase acts on the triglycerides in fat cells, breaking these down into glycerol and fatty acids, which complex with plasma calcium ions to form calcium soaps. The gross appearance is one of opaque chalky white plaques and nodules in the adipose tissue surrounding the pancreas.

Rarely, pancreatic disease may be associated with entry of lipase into the bloodstream and subsequent widespread fat necrosis throughout the body; the subcutaneous fat and bone marrow are most affected.

2. Nonenzymatic fat necrosis

Nonenzymatic fat necrosis occurs in the breast, subcutaneous tissue, and abdomen. Many patients have a history of trauma. Nonenzymatic fat necrosis is also termed traumatic fat necrosis even though trauma is not established as the definitive cause. Nonenzymatic fat necrosis evokes an inflammatory response characterized by numerous foamy macrophages, neutrophils, and lymphocytes. Fibrosis follows, producing a mass that may be difficult to distinguish from a cancer.

D. Caseous and Gummatous Necrosis

Caseous (cheese-like) and gummatous (gum- or rubber-like) necrosis occur in infectious granulomas (localized chronic inflammatory lesions such as tuberculosis and syphilis). Histologically, the necrotic focus appears as amorphous granular debris seemingly composed of fragmented, coagulated cells with a granulomatous reaction.

E. Fibrinoid Necrosis

Fibrinoid necrosis is a type of connective tissue necrosis seen particularly in autoimmune diseases (e.g. rheumatic fever, polyarteritis nodosa, and systemic lupus erythematosus). Collagen and smooth muscle in the media of blood vessels are especially involved. Fibrinoid necrosis of arterioles also occurs in accelerated (malignant) hypertension.

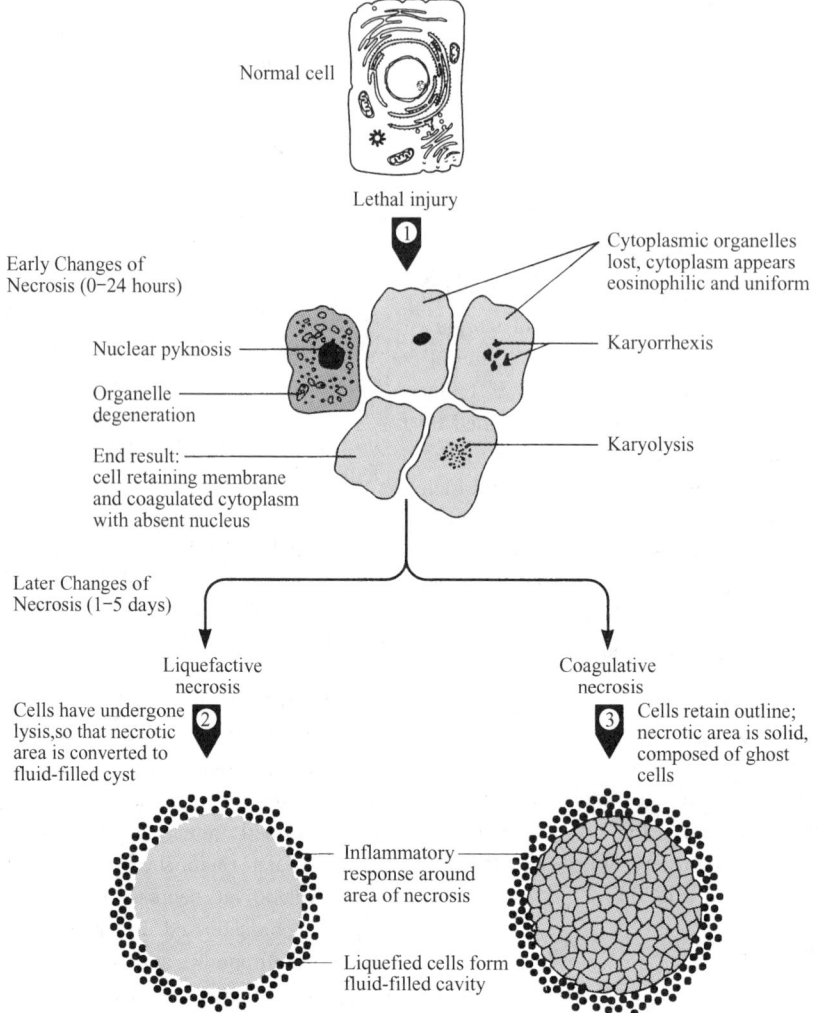

Figure 1-20 Necrosis of cells caused by lethal injury①, showing early changes and the difference between liquefactive necrosis ② and coagulative necrosis ③

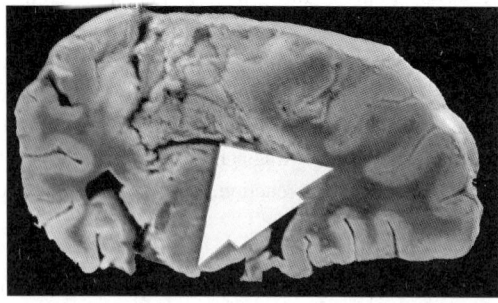

Figure 1-21 Cerebral infarct, showing liquefactive necrosis of the cerebral hemisphere. The involved area has been converted to a fluid-filled cyst that collapsed when the brain was cut and the fluid drained out (arrow)

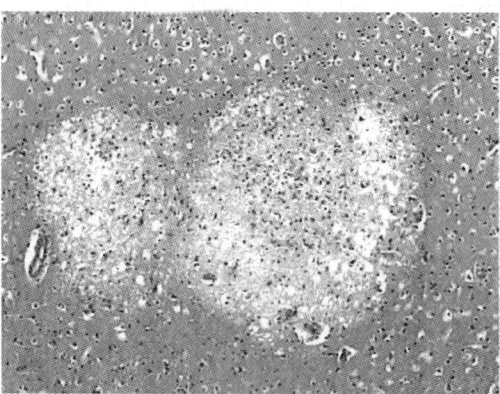

Figure 1-22 Liquefactive necrosis of the cerebral tissue, showing some pink, loose and rete-liked areas in the tissue. Areas of encephalomalacia are the characteristic feature of Epidemic encephalitis B

Frinoid necrosis is characterized by loss of normal structure and replacement by a homogeneous, bright pink-staining necrotic material that resembles fibrin microscopically (Figure 1-23). Note, however, that fibrinoid is not the same as fibrinous, which denotes deposition of fibrin as occurs in inflammation and blood coagulation. Areas of fibrinoid necrosis contain various amounts of immunoglobulins, complement, albumin, breakdown products of collagen, and fibrin.

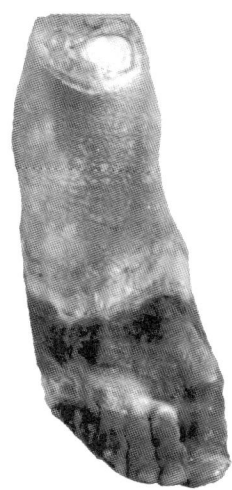

Figure 1-24 Dry gangrene of the feet, showing necrosis of the distal parts of feet. Note the black, dry, shriveled appearance

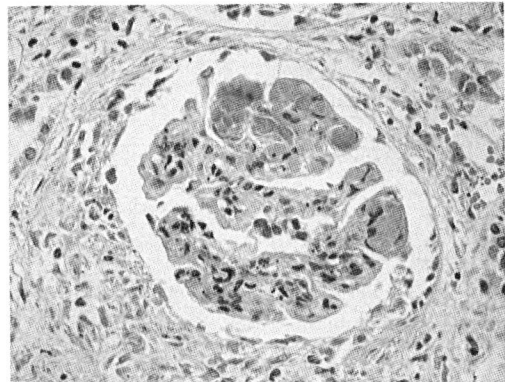

Figure 1-23 Fibrinoid necrosis of glomerulus arteriole. In hematoxylin-and eosin-stained section, the necrotic area stains bright pink, resembling fibrin

F. Gangrene

The term gangrene is widely used to denote a clinical situation in which extensive tissue necrosis is complicated to a variable degree by secondary bacterial infection.

1. Dry gangrenes (Figure 1-24)

Dry gangrene most commonly occurs in the extremities as a result of ischemic necrosis of tissues due to arterial obstruction. The necrotic area appears black, dry, and shriveled and is sharply demarcated from adjacent viable tissue. Secondary bacterial infection is usually insignificant. Treatments consist of surgical removal of dead tissue (debridement).

2. Wet gangrene

Wet gangrene results from severe bacterial infection superimposed on necrosis. It occurs in the extremities as well as in internal organs such as the intestine. Acute inflammation and growth of invading bacteria cause the necrotic area to become swollen and reddish-black, with extensive liquefaction of dead tissue. Wet gangrene is a spreading necrotizing inflammation that is not clearly demarcated from adjacent healthy tissue and is thus difficult to treat surgically. Bacterial fermentation produces a typical foul odor. The type of bacteria involved varies with the site. The mortality rate is high.

3. Gas gangrene

Gas gangrene is a wound infection caused by *Clostridium perfringens* and other clostridial species. It is characterized by extensive necrosis of tissue and production of gas by the fermentative action of the bacteria. The gross appearance is similar to that of wet gangrene, with the additional presence of gas in the tissues. Crepitus (a crackling sensation on palpation over the site) can often be detected clinically, and gas may be seen on soft tissue x-rays. Again, the mortality rate is high.

Clinical Effects of Necrosis

A. Abnormal Function

Necrosis of cells leads to functional loss that frequently causes clinical disease, as in heart failure resulting from extensive myocardial necrosis. The severity of clinical disease depends on the type of tissue involved and the extent of tissue destruction in relation to the amount and continued function of surviving tissue. Necrosis in the kidney, for example, does not cause renal failure even when an entire kidney is lost because the other kidney can compensate. Necrosis of a small area of the motor cortex in the brain, however, results in muscle paralysis.

The clinical manifestations of necrosis vary. Abnormal electrical activity originating in areas of cerebral or myocardial necrosis may result in seizures or cardiac arrhythmias. Failure of peristalsis in an area of intestinal wall necrosis may cause functional intestinal obstruction. Bleeding into necrotic tissue often produces symptoms, e.g. expectoration of blood (hemoptysis) with pulmonary necrosis.

B. Bacterial Infection

Bacteria grow readily in necrotic tissue and may disseminate throughout the body via the lymphatics or bloodstream. This potentially fatal development makes gangrene a serious condition that often requires surgical removal of the affected tissue.

C. Release of Contents of Necrotic Cells

Necrotic cells release their cytoplasmic contents (e.g. enzymes) into the bloodstream, where their presence signifies that cell death has occurred. These enzymes may be detected by various tests whose specificity depends on distribution of the enzyme in different cells of the body, e.g. elevation of the MB isoenzyme of creatine kinase is specific for myocardial necrosis because this enzyme is found only in myocardial cells. Elevation of aspartate amino-transferase levels (AST, formerly called glutamic-oxaloacetic transaminase [SGOT] is less specific because this enzyme is present not only in myocardium but also in liver and other cells.

D. Systemic Effects

Cell necrosis is commonly associated with fever (due to release of pyrogens from the necrotic cells) and neutrophil leukocytosis (increased number of neutrophils in the peripheral blood due to the associated acute inflammatory reaction).

E. Local Effects

Ulceration of epithelial surfaces may produce local hemorrhage (e.g. a bleeding peptic ulcer). Swelling of tissues due to edema may lead to severe pressure effects in a confined space (e.g. the cranial cavity). Obviously, the exact effect depends upon the site of necrosis and its extent.

Evolution of Necrosis

In the living patient, most necrotic cells and their debris disappear by a combined process of extracellular enzyme digestion and leukocyte phagocytosis, or absorb by through lymphatic and capillary, or isolated and ejected from peripheral tissue (resolution). If necrotic cells and tissues are not promptly eliminated, they can be replaced with granulation tissue and collagen (organization) or encapsulated by collagen (encapsulation), furthermore, they also tend to attract calcium salt and other minerals (dystrophic calcification).

APOPTOSIS

Introduction

The word "apoptosis" is derived from Greek word meaning "falling leaves" and was first used to describe a new form of cell death distinct from necrosis. Apoptosis is the morphologic appearance of **programmed cell death** which is an important mechanism in both development and homeostasis in adult tissues for the removal of either superfluous, infected, transformed or damaged cells by activation of an intrinsic suicide program. It is characterized by specific morphologic and biochemical properties.

The normal metazoan development and health require the precise regulation of cell death. Apoptosis plays a critical role in important biological processes. Although apoptosis is important for the normal development and health of an animal, its aberrant activation may contribute to a number of diseases, for example, AIDS, neurogenerative disorders, and ischemic injury. In contrast, impaired apoptosis may be a significant factor in the etiology of such diseases as cancer, autoimmune disorders, and viral infections.

Morphological Evidence

On light and electron microscopy, some of the essential features of an apoptotic cell include (Figure 1-25):

A. Cell Shrinkage

An apoptotic cell shrinks, forms blebs, detaches from its neighbors and has loss of the specialized membrane structures e.g. microvilli and desmosomes. Organelles become tightly packed making the cytoplasm appear dense but the plasma membrane and cellular organelles remain intact.

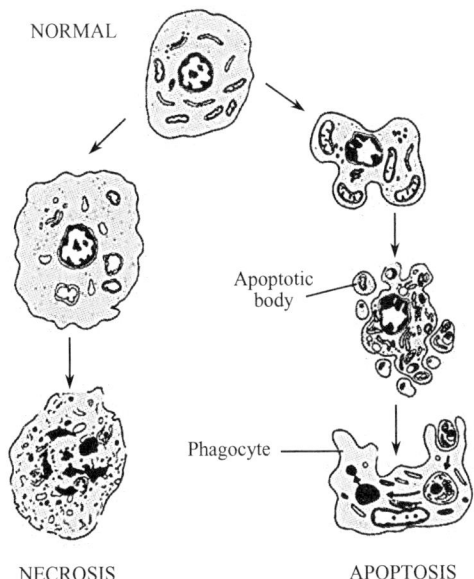

Figure 1-25 The sequential ultrastructural changes seen in necrosis (left) and apoptosis (right). Necrosis is characterized by cellular swelling, chromatin clumping and membrane damage. In apoptosis, the morphological changes consist of nuclear chromatin condensation and fragmentation, cytoplasmic budding and phagocytosis of the extruded apoptotic bodies

B. Chromatin Condensation

Chromatin condenses to the periphery of the nucleus forming crescents. The nucleus has loss of pores and become fragmented (karyorrhexis).

C. Apoptotic Bodies Formation

Cytoplasmic membrane blebbing formed and apoptotic bodies composed cytoplasm, organelles and nuclear fragments.

D. Phagocytosis of Apoptotic Bodies by Neighbouring Cells or Macrophages

On H and E stained sections, apoptosis usually involves a single cell or clusters of cells which appear as round masses with intensely eosinophilic cytoplasm. Chromatin condenses to the periphery of the nucleus and aggregates into well-delineated masses of various shape sand sizes. Then the cell shrinks, forms blebs and cytoplasmic buds and fragment as apoptosis bodies (Figure 1-26). During the process of apoptosis the plasma membrane and cellular organelles remain intact, and the cells don't release their cytoplasmic contents, so apoptosis does not elicit an inflammatory response. These fragments are quickly extruded and phagocytosed or degraded, even substantial apoptosis may be histologically inapparent.

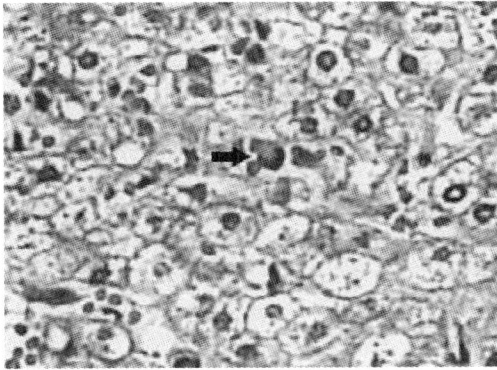

Figure 1-26 Apoptosis of hepatocyte, showing the cells have increased eosinophilia staining, their nucleus is deep staining and the chromatin condenses to the periphery of the nucleus forming crescents (arrow)

Mechanisms of Apoptosis

Apoptosis is currently the subject of considerable research activity. The basic processes of apoptosis include four components (Figure 1-27):

A. Triggered by Signals

3 different mechanisms trigger the apoptosis program: (1) Signals arising within the cell. In many cases, absence of survival factors, e.g. growth factor etc, is enough to drive a cell into apoptosis. (2) Death activators binding to receptors at the cell surface. For example, tumor necrosis factor (TNF-α) and Fas ligand (FasL) binds to a cell-surface receptor named Fas (also called CD95). (3) Dangerous reactive oxygen species also cause cell death.

B. Control and Regulation

There are some specific proteins in cytoplasm and cell membrane connection the original death signals to the final execution program. These proteins are important because their actions play a key rule in the process of apoptosis. There are two main apoptotic pathways:

1. The mitochondrial pathway

The protein Bcl-2 appears localized or associated with intracellular membranes of mitochondria, endoplasmic reticulum, and nuclei. Ecotopic expression of *bcl-2* suppresses cell death induced by oxidizing agents and appears to affect glutathione levels. Genetic evidence indicates that *ced-9/bcl-2* belongs to an emerging family. Some of the members of this family can suppress apoptosis like *bcl-2*, e. g. bcl-xL. Other members make cells more susceptible to apoptotic stimuli, e. g. *bax* and *bcl-xS*. Bcl-2 which is bound to a molecule of the protein Apaf-1 (apoptotic protease activating factor-1), and Bax penetrate mitochondrial membranes causing cytochrome to leak out. The released cytochrome c and Apaf-1 bind to molecules of caspase 9, triggering execution caspase activation.

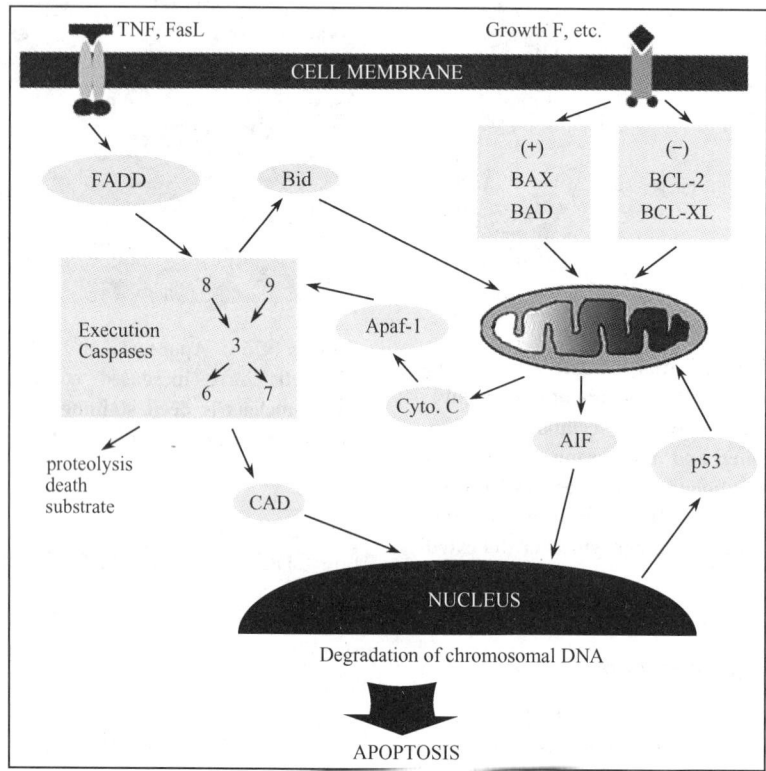

Figure 1-27 Overview of the mechanisms of apoptosis

2. The death receptor pathway

TNF and Fas receptor bind the complementary death activator (TNF and FasL respectively), and transmits a signal to the cytoplasm that leads to activation of caspase 8 which initiates a cascade of caspase activation.

C. Execution

The final pathway of apoptosis is characterized by a distinctive constellation of biochemical events that result from the synthesis and/or activation of a number of cytosolic catabolic enzymes. One set of mediators implicated in apoptosis belong to the asparate-specific cysteinyl proteases or **caspases.** More than 10 caspases have been identified. Some of them (e. g. caspase 8 and 10) are involved in the initiation of apoptosis, others (caspase 3, 6, and 7) execute the death order by destroying essential proteins in the cell. Activation of one or more such caspase enzymes may lead to a cascade of activation of other proteases, such as down-stream endonuclease. Activation results in the characteristic DNA fragmentation – DNA breakdown into 180-to 200-base pair fragments which may be visualized as a distinctive "laddering" of DNA into discrete-sized pieces on agarose gel electrophoresis. While cell volume and shape changes may in part result from cleavage of components of the cytoskeleton.

Neurons, and perhaps other cells, have another way to self-destruct that - unlike the two paths described above - does not use caspases. Apoptosis-inducing factor (**AIF**) is a protein that is normally located in the intermembrane space of mitochondria. When the cell receives a signal, AIF is released from the mitochondria (like the release of cytochromec), migrates into the nucleus and binds to DNA, which triggers the destruction of the DNA and cell death.

D. Removal of Dead Cells

There are some marker molecules on the surfaces of apoptotic cells. It facilitates uptake and disposal by adjacent cells or phagocytes. And then the apoptotic cell is recognized and engulfed by phagocytes without release of proinflammatory mediators. This process is so efficient that dead cells disappear without leaving a trace, and inflammation is virtually absent.

Difference Between Necrosis And Apoptosis

The execution of apoptosis minimizes the leakage of cellular constituents from dying cells. For example, proteases could damage adjacent cells or stimulate an inflammatory response. This cardinal feature of apoptosis distinguishes it from necrosis, which usually results from trauma that causes injured cells to swell and lyse, releasing the cytoplasmic material that stimulates an inflammatory response (Figure 1-25, Table 1-5)

Table 1-5 General characteristics of necrosis and apoptosis

	Necrosis	Apoptosis
Stimuli	Toxins, severe hypoxia, massive insult, ATP depletion	Physiological and pathological conditions without ATP depletion
Patterns of death	Groups of neighboring cells	Single cells
Histologic appearance	Cell swells; organelles swell; disruption of organelles occurs Plasma membrane is lysed	Cell contracts; chromatin condenses; apoptotic bodies form Plasma membrane remains intact and blebbed
DNA breakdown	Diffuse and Random	Internucleosomal cleavage

Cellular processes	No protein synthesis
	No RNA transcription
	Energy independent
	ATP depletion
		Programmed cascade of reactions
		  Caspase activation
		  Internucleosomal endonucleases
		  Transglutaminase activation
		Requires
		  New RNA transcription
		  Protein synthesis
		  ATP

Tissue reaction	Inflammation occurs	No inflammation occurs Apoptotic bodies are phagocytized

AGING

Aging is the final phase of human development and may be defined as the aggregate of structural changes that occur with the passage of time; it is characterized by progressive inability to sustain vital functions, with death the eventual result.

Several different hypotheses have been proposed to explain aging, but no one of them is entirely satisfactory, and it is probable that aging is due to a combination of several processes. For example, according to programmed aging hypothesis, the genome of every cell is programmed at conception to cease mitotic division after a certain time. This has been demonstrated by normal fibroblasts and other cells in tissue culture, which undergo a finite number (40 - 60) of divisions. Two mechanisms are proposed: (1) Incomplete replication of chromosome ends, and (2) the regulation of clock gene. However, DNA damage hypothesis hold that aging is the result of DNA damage, due either to somatic mutations or to failure of DNA repair mechanisms in aging cells. DNA changes lead to errors in RNA transcription and in that way cause defects in cellular synthesis of protein. Although these changes undoubtedly occur in aging cells, they could just as easily be the result of the aging process rather than the cause.

As life expectancy increases, the study of aging (gerontology) becomes increasingly important. It is crucial to distinguish changes that are part of the aging process from diseases that are common in older individuals. Changes of cellular structures and function are inevitable with aging. The morphologic alterations include decreased cell size and number and to atrophy of organs, irregular nuclei, pleomorphic vacuolated mitochondria, diminished endoplasmic reticulum, and distorted Golgi apparatuses. The decline of cellular function appears as the reducing of mitochondria oxidative phosphorylation, decreasing synthesis of enzymatic and receptor proteins, and diminishing capacity for nutrient uptake and for repair of chromosomal damage.

Abnormal immune function in the elderly predisposes to development of infections. Older individuals frequently develop autoantibodies and show an increased incidence of autoimmune diseases such as pernicious anemia, Hashimoto's thyroiditis, and Addison's disease. Cancer is predominantly a disease of older individuals and may in part be related to the decreased ability of the immune system to rid the body of cancer cells.

Chapter 2 Tissue Repair

Cui Jin

CHAPTER CONTENTS
- Cell Regeneration
    - Types of Regeneration
    - The Proliferative Potential of Different Cell Types
    - Regeneration Process of Variety Tissue
- Repair by Scar Formation
    - Preparation
    - Ingrowth of Granulation tissue
    - Production of Fibronectin
    - Collagenization
- Healing of Skin Wound
    - Types of Skin Injury
    - Healing Processes
- Mechanisms of Cellular Regeneration
    - Growth Factors
    - Chalon and Contact Inhibition
    - Extracellular Matrix
- Fracture Healing

Tissue injuries associated with inflammation are eventually followed by some form of repair (**healing**). Removal of inflammatory and necrotic cellular debris must precede any such healing. Healing occurs rapidly after transitory injury such as a single minor traumatic episode. Healing is also rapid if the injurious agent is quickly inactivated by the host response, whether inflammatory or immune. With persistent low-grade injury, healing occurs concurrently with ongoing chronic inflammation.

The ideal result of healing is to restore the tissue to its normal (preinjury) state, a process termed **resolution**. Removal of debris associated with the inflammatory response is sufficient to restore a tissue to its normal state if injury has been minor (e.g. if minimal parenchymal cell necrosis has occurred). After removal of cellular debris, any necrotic parenchymal cells may be replaced by new parenchymal cells of the same type in a process known as **regeneration**.

When resolution and regeneration are not possible, necrotic cells are replaced with collagen; this is termed **organization** or repair by scar formation. In many instances, a combination of healing processes occurs.

The mechanism of healing depends on the type of inflammation, the extent of tissue necrosis, the types of cells involved, and the regenerative ability of damaged parenchymal cells.

CELL REGENERATION

Replacement of lost parenchymal cells by division of adjacent surviving parenchymal cells (regeneration) can also restore injured tissue to normal. Whether regeneration occurs depends on (1) the regenerative capacity of involved cells (e.g. their ability to divide), (2) the number of surviving viable cells, and (3) the presence of a connective tissue framework that will provide a base for restoration of normal tissue structure.

Before regeneration can occur, the necrotic cells must be removed. This involves an acute inflammatory response, liquefaction of cells by neutrophil enzymes, and removal of debris by lymphatics and macrophages as described in the preceding section.

TYPES OF REGENERATION

Physiological Regeneration

Physiological regeneration is a normal process going on continuously, e.g. in gut epithelium, or continually, e.g. in hair follicle epithelium, involving cell division for the replacement of cells lost naturally. Blood, epithelial, bone and connective tissue cells show this phenomenon.

Pathological Regeneration

In pathological conditions, e.g cell and tissue injury, the regeneration of adjacent surviving parenchymal cells restore the injured tissue. This process is referred to as pathological regeneration.

THE PROLIFERATIVE POTENTIAL OF DIFFERENT CELL TYPES

The cells of the body can be divided into three groups - **labile**, **stable**, and **permanent** - on the basis of their regenerative capacity (Table 2-1).

Labile Cells (Intermitotic Cells)

Labile cells normally divide actively throughout life to replace cells that are being continually, lost from the body. Labile cells have a short G_0 (resting, or intermitotic) phase. Continued loss of mature cells of a given tissue is a continuous stimulus for resting cells to enter the mitotic cell cycle. Examples of labile cells include basal epithelial stem cells of all epithelial linings and hematopoietic stem cells in bone marrow (Table 2-1). Mature differentiated cells in these particular tissues cannot divide; their numbers are maintained by division of their parent labile cells.

Table 2-1 Classification of cells on the basis of their regenerative capacity

Cell Types	Mitotic Capacity	Examples
Labile (intermitotic)	Short G_0 phase: almost always in mitotic cell cycle	Hematopoietic stem cells Basal cells of epithelia Hair follicle cells Germ cells

Stable (reversibly postmitotic)	Long G_0 phase: can divide actively when stimulated	Parenchymal cells
		   Liver
		   Kidney
		   Lung, etc
		Mesenchymal cells
		   Osteodlast
		   Chondrocyte
		   Fibroblast
		   Endothelial cell

Permanent (irreversibly postmitotic)	None (can not divide)	Neurons Ganglion cells Cardiac muscle[1] Skeletal muscle[1]

[1] Cardiac and skeletal muscle cells demonstrate limited mitotic capability in experimental settings. In humans, they are functionally permanent cells.

Stable Cell (Reversibly Postmitotic or Quiescent Cells)

Stable cells typically have a long life span and are therefore characterized by a low rate of division. They remain in the G_0 phase for long periods (often years) but retain the capacity to enter the mitotic cell cycle if the need arises. The parenchymal cells of most solid glandular organs (liver, pancreas) and mesenchymal cells (fibroblasts, endothelial cells) are examples of stable cells. Unlike labile cells, which are undifferentiated cells that divide frequently and must undergo maturation before becoming functional, stable cells are differentiated functional cells that only revert to a dividing mode at need. Although stable cells have a long resting phase, they can divide rapidly upon demand, e.g. parenchymal cells of the liver swiftly regenerate after necrosis of hepatocytes.

Permanent Cell (Irreversibly Postmitotic Cells)

Permanent cells have no capacity for mitotic division in postnatal life. Examples of permanent cells include neurons in the central and peripheral nervous system and cardiac muscle cells.

REGENERATION PROCESS OF VARIETY TISSUE

After injury, the regeneration process requires (1) the regenerative ability of the cells, and (2) the intact of tissue framework.

Epithelial Regeneration

As discussed above, the epithelial cell is a kind of labile cells. Injury to epithelial cells is followed by rapid regeneration. The cells at the cut margins start to regenerate by division and migrate out as a thin layer over the denuded surface. While the epithelial surface is being restored as a thin sheet, its cells start to multiply and differentiate, restoring the original thickness and variety of specialized cells to the epithelium. For example, surgical removal of the endometrium through curettage or physiologic loss of endometrium during menstruation is followed by complete regeneration of cells from the basal germinative layer within a few days. Regeneration in tissues with labile cells occurs only when enough labile cells have been spared by injury (Figure 2-1). In the example cited above, overly zealous surgical curettage of the endometrium that removes the entire endometrial lining, including the basal layer, precludes regeneration. Healing then occurs by scar formation, which leads to failure of menstruation and infertility.

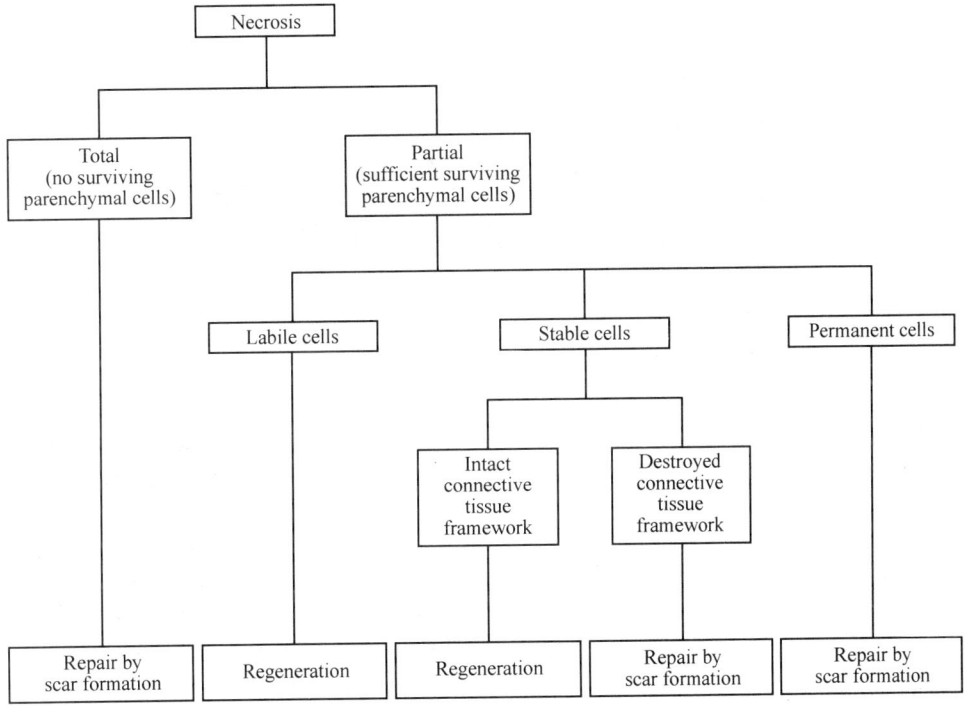

Figure 2-1 Factors influencing regeneration and repair by scar formation after injury to tissues containing labile and stable cells

Because glands are composed of epithelial cells, regeneration of these tissues requires (1) enough viable tissue remaining to provide a source of parenchymal cells for regeneration and (2) an intact connective tissue framework (Figure 2-1). If the basement membrane is not destroyed, epithelial cells from the glands lining the basal layer can regenerate and restore glands to the origin structure. Otherwise, the injuring glands will be replaced by granulation tissues. For example, injuries to the kidney illustrate the need for an adequate connective tissue framework. Selective necrosis of renal tubular cells (acute renal tubular necrosis) with sparing of the renal tubular framework is rapidly followed by regeneration, and the lost cells are replaced by division of surviving tubular cells. On the other hand, when necrosis of

Regeneration of Connective Tissue

Injury to permanent cells is always followed by connective tissues/scar formation. No regeneration is possible. There are three stages to this process: (1) migration and proliferation of fibroblast, (2) deposition of extracellular matrix (ECM), (3) maturation and reorganization of the fibrous tissue. The details of this process will be discuses later (see *REPAIR BY SCAR FORMATION*).

Angiogenesis

Damage to blood vessel often occurs during injury. Angiogenesis refers to the process of blood vessel healing at the sites of injury. Angiogenesis begins with the degradation of the basement membrane by proteases secreted by activated endothelial cells that migrate and proliferate. This leads to the formation of solid endothelial cell sprouts in the stromal space. Vascular loops are formed and capillary tubes develop with formation of tight junctions and deposition of a new basement membrane (Figure 2-2).

both the parenchyma and the connective tissue framework occurs (renal infarct), no regeneration is possible, and healing occurs by scar formation.

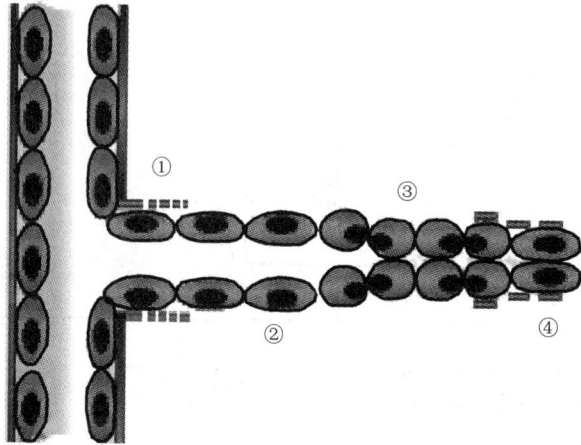

Figure 2-2 The process of angiogenesis. ① Proteolysis of ECM; ② Migration of endothelial cells; ③ Endothelial cells proliferation; ④ Lumen formation, maturation, and inhibition of growth

Regeneration of Peripheral Nerves

Once a peripheral nerve has been transected, the axon distal to the site of injury rapidly degenerate and ultimately disappears, a process termed Wallerian degeneration. The myelin sheath and axon of the remaining intact nerve degenerate back to the next node of Ranvier. Then macrophages enter the area to remove the myelin and axonal debris. During this process, the basement membrane which surrounds the axon and Schwann cell remain intact. Schwann cells line up on the basement membrane tube and synthesize growth factors, which attract axonal sprouts formed at the terminal end of the proximal segment of the severed axon. The basement membrane tubes provide pathways for the regenerating axons to follow to muscles and skin. The Schwann cells then remyelinate the newly formed axons; however, the newly formed myelin is thinner than normal and the newly formed internodes are shorter than normal. Axonal regeneration may be accompanied by recovery of function in the denervated area, but this is incomplete. If there has been severe trauma to nerve and disruption of its fascicular architecture, a fibrous scar can form and obstruct regenerated axons. These then form a tangled, often painful mass of intertwined nerve fibers termed a traumatic neuroma.

Regeneration of Other Tissues

A. Bone

Injury to bone tissue is followed by rapid regeneration. We will discuss details later in *FRACTURE*

HEALING.

B. Cartilage

In mature cartilage, the injury defects are likely to be filled with fibrous tissues, or the lesion may precipitate a degeneration of adjacent cartilage. Restitution of tissue is performed by the perichondrium, in which the chondroblasts proliferate and then transform to chondrocytes.

C. Tendon

Fibroblasts from the cut tendon's sheath and other sources proliferate, become active, and lay down orderly collagen fibers, which can restore most of the original strength of the tendon.

D. Skeletal Muscle

If the cut is small, myotubes regenerating from each side may fuse and restore the fibers. Just outside the sarcolemma of intact muscle fibers lie satellite cells that act as residual, peripheral myoblasts which are able to respond to injury by becoming active myoblasts. But in many conditions, the injured skeletal muscle is usually replaced by scar.

E. Smooth and Cardiac Muscle

In general, muscle lesion will be filled with granulation tissue. Only small amounts of new muscle tissue will form to replace what was lost. Surviving muscle fibers may hypertrophy in an attempt to restore the strength of the muscle as a whole.

REPAIR BY SCAR FORMATION

A scar is a mass of collagen that is the end result of repair by organization and fibrosis. Repair by scar formation occurs (1) when resolution fails to occur in an acute inflammatory process; (2) when there is ongoing tissue necrosis in chronic inflammation; and (3) when parenchymal cell necrosis cannot be repaired by regeneration.

As discussed above, regeneration fails when necrotic cells are permanent cells, when the connective tissue framework of a tissue composed of stable cells has been destroyed, or when necrosis is so extensive that no cells are available for regeneration.

The process of repair by scar formation can be divided into several overlapping phases (Figure 2-3).

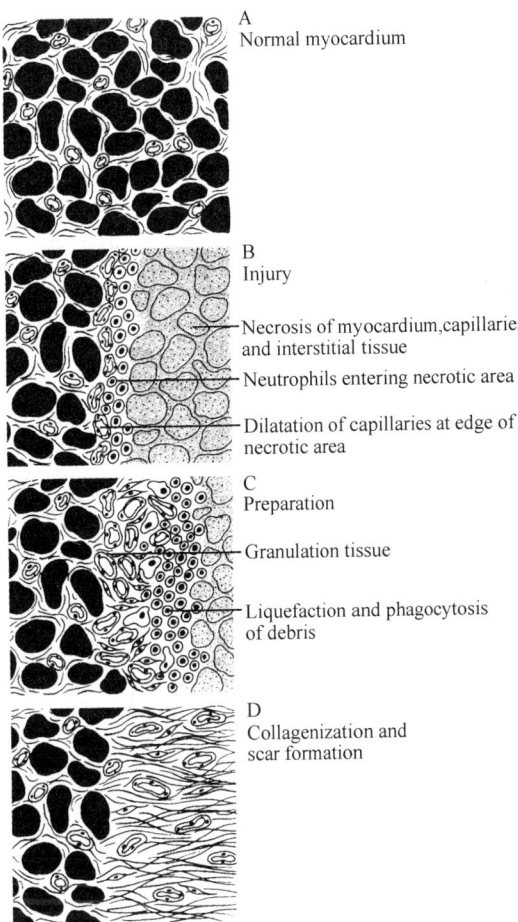

Figure 2-3 Repair of a myocardial infarct by scar formation. A normal myocardium is shown in A. The infarct evokes an acute inflammatory response and is invaded from the periphery by neutrophils (B), which liquefy the necrotic tissue. This is followed by entry of macrophages and granulation tissue (C), which removes the necrotic debris and leads to replacement of the necrotic zone by scar (D)

PREPARATION

The area of injury is prepared for scar formation by removal of the inflammatory exudate, including fibrin, blood, and any necrotic tissue. This debris is liquefied by lysosomal enzymes derived from neutrophils that have migrated to the area. Liquefied material is removed by lymphatics; any particulate residue is removed by macrophage phagocytosis.

This preparatory process is similar to that occurring in resolution and regeneration.

INGROWTH OF GRANULATION TISSUE

Granulation tissue forms and fills the injured area while necrotic debris is being removed. **Granulation tissue** is highly vascularized connective tissue composed of newly formed capillaries, proliferating fibroblasts, and residual inflammatory cells. (Note: Granulation tissue must be distinguished from granuloma, which is an aggregate of macrophages associated with chronic inflammation.) Capillaries are derived by vascular proliferation in healthy tissue at the periphery of the involved area. Fibroblasts migrate with capillaries to the injured area. The proliferation of capillaries, fibroblasts, and other cells in the healing process is controlled by a variety of growth-stimulatory or growth-inhibitory factors.

On gross examination, granulation tissue is soft and fleshy (it appears pink and granular) because of the numerous capillaries. Microscopic examination shows the thin-walled capillaries lined by endothelium and surrounded by fibroblasts (Figures 2-4A and 2-4B). Both endothelial cells and fibroblasts are metabolically very active, with large nuclei and prominent nucleoli; mitotic figures may be seen. Electron microscopy demonstrates prominent rough endoplasmic reticulum in the cytoplasm of fibroblasts, an indicator of active protein synthesis.

Over time — the duration depends on the extent of injury — the entire area of repair is replaced by ingrowing granulation tissue (organization).

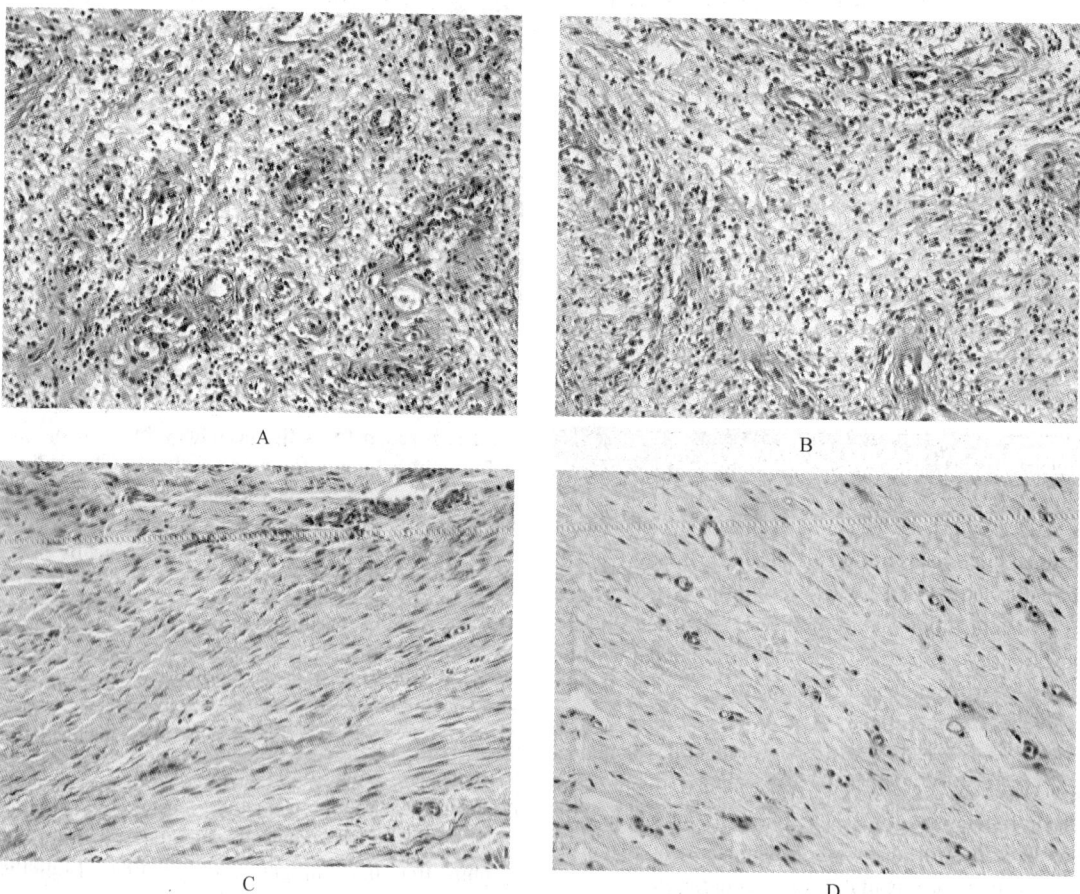

Figure 2-4 Scar formation from granulation tissue. Early granulation tissue (A) is composed of capillaries, fibroblasts, and inflammatory cells. Progressive collagenization (B, C) results in a dense cellular scar (D)

PRODUCTION OF FIBRONECTIN

Fibronectin is a glycoprotein (MW 44,000) that plays a key role in the formation of granulation tissue and is present in large amounts during wound healing. In the early phases, it is derived from plasma, but later it is synthesized by fibroblasts, macrophages, and endothelial cells in granulation tissue. Fibronectin is chemotactic for fibroblasts and promotes organization of endothelial cells into capillary vessels.

COLLAGENIZATION

Collagen is the major fibrillary protein of connective tissue. It is synthesized by fibroblasts in the form of a precursor, tropocollagen (procollagen), which has a molecular weight of 285,000 and a long, rod-like shape. During or shortly after secretion, final removal of the terminal part of the peptide chain by an enzyme leads to formation of an insoluble molecule of fibrillary collagen. Under the light microscope, collagen appears as a fibrillary mass that stains pink with routine H and E stain and green or blue with trichrome stains. Collagen fibers are flexible but inelastic and are responsible for much of the tensile strength of scar tissue. The terms fibrous tissue and scar tissue are synonymous with collagen. (*Note*: Fibrin is a molecule derived from plasma fibrinogen and is entirely distinct from collagen; fibrinous and fibrous are therefore adjectives characterizing unrelated entities.)

Synthesis of tropocollagen by fibroblasts requires hydroxylation of proline by an enzyme whose activity requires ascorbic acid (vitamin C); and hydroxylation and oxidation of lysine, which permit crosslink-age between adjacent polypeptide tropocollagen chains. The detection of hydroxyproline released into the serum or urine by injury to collagen serves as a useful laboratory test in certain diseases of connective tissue.

A. Types of Collagen

Several types of collagen (types I-V) are recognized on the basis of biochemical variations in the structure of their polypeptide chains. Young fibroblasts in granulation tissue form type III collagen that is later replaced by stronger, cross-linked type I collagen.

B. Turnover of Collagen

Scar tissue is not inactive; continuous slow removal of collagen in the scar by the enzyme collagenase is balanced by synthesis of new collagen by fibroblasts. Even long-established scars may weaken if the normal activity of fibroblasts is impaired, as occurs in vitamin C deficiency or administration of corticosteroids.

Maturation

The collagen content of granulation tissue progressively increases with time. A young scar consists of granulation tissue and abundant collagen together with a moderate number of capillaries and fibroblasts (Figure 2-4C). It appears pink on gross examination because of the vascularity. As the scar matures, the amount of collagen increases and the scar becomes less cellular and vascular. The mature scar is composed of an avascular, poorly cellular mass of collagen (Figure 2-4D) and is white on gross examination.

Contraction And Strengthening

Contraction and strengthening constitute the final phase of repair by scar formation. Contraction decreases the size of the scar and enables the surviving cells of the organ to function with maximal effectiveness; e.g. the conversion of a large myocardial infarct to a small scar permits optimal function of the remaining myocardium.

Contraction begins early in the repair process and continues as the scar matures. Early contraction is due to active contraction of actomyosin filaments in certain specialized myofibril-containing fibroblasts (also called myofibroblasts). Later contraction is a property of the collagen molecule itself.

The tensile strength of a scar is dependent on the amount of collagen and progressively increases, from about 10% of normal at the end of the first week to about 80% of normal over several months. The increasing tensile strength is due to an increase in the amount of collagen, change in the type of collagen (from type III to type I), and an increase in covalent linkages between collagen molecules. The fully formed scar is a firm, inelastic, flexible structure.

HEALING OF SKIN WOUND

Understanding the mechanisms involved in the healing of skin wounds provides insight into healing in general. The skin is composed of epidermis, which is made up of stratified squamous epithelium – the basal germinative layer of which is composed of labile (stem) cells – and dermis, which is composed of collagen, blood vessels, and skin appendages (adnexa) such as hair follicles, sweat glands, sebaceous glands, and apocrine glands. Stable cells make up the dermal connective tissue and adnexa.

TYPES OF SKIN INJURY

Skin injuries are classified on the basis of the severity and nature of involvement.

A. Abrasion (Scrape)

The mildest form of skin injury is characterized by removal of the superficial part of the epidermis. Because the underlying basal germinative layer of labile cells is intact, the epithelium regenerates from below, and the integrity of the epithelium is restored with no scarring.

B. Incision (Cut) and Laceration (Tear)

Incisions and lacerations involve the full thickness of the skin (both epidermis and dermis) but with minimal loss of germinative cells. If the skin edges are carefully apposed, as in a sutured surgical incision, only a small gap remains to be repaired. Simple incisions constitute ideal skin wounds with regard to the healing process because they do not contain foreign material and are not infected. They therefore heal quickly and without incident. This process, in which necrosis and inflammation are minimal, is known as healing by first intention (see below).

C. Wounds with Epidermal Defects

Severe injuries (e.g. crush injuries, extensive lacerations, burns) are characterized by denudation of large areas of the complete epidermis, including the basal germinative cells, with variable necrosis of underlying dermis. In contrast with an abrasion, the absence of labile epidermal cells at the base of the wound necessitates epidermal regeneration from surviving basal germinative cells around the margins. The extensive necrosis that is present in such wounds is accompanied by a phase of inflammation prior to the repair process (healing by second intention; see below).

HEALING PROCESSES

A. Healing by First Intention (Primary Union)

1. Simple repair

Clean incised wounds and lacerations in which the edges of the wound are in close apposition heal by first intention (Figure 2-5). The small gap in the epidermis and dermis fills with clotted blood, which forms a scab and seals the skin opening within 24 hours to prevent the entry of infectious agents into the wound. The epidermis regenerates by rapid division of basal cells at the edges of the wound. These cells grow under the scab and reestablish continuity of the epidermis within 48 hours. As the epidermal cells mature and start shedding the superficial keratinized layers, the scab separates, usually at the end of the first week.

In the subjacent dermis, the wound fills with clotted blood and heals by scar formation. The small amount of clot and tissue debris is liquefied by neutrophilic enzymes and removed by macrophage phagocytosis. Neutrophils appear in the wound within 24 hours, rapidly complete the liquefaction process, and are usually replaced by macrophages by day 3. The growth of fibroblasts and new vessels (granulation tissue) into the prepared dermal gap begins within 48 hours, and collagen can be demonstrated there within 72 hours after injury. By day 5, the dermal gap is filled with a small amount of collagenizing granulation tissue (Figure 2-5). The amount of collagen increases for about 4-6 weeks.

2. The scar

The young scar that becomes visible when the scab separates from the skin is initially pink because of the vascularity of the dermal granulation tissue. Over the next few weeks the scar turns white as a result of a decrease in the number of blood vessels and an increased amount of collagen in the maturing scar. Eventually, the scar assumes normal skin color as the epidermis matures.

3. Tensile strength

In the first postoperative week, a surgical incision is artificially held together by sutures, clips, or tape.

B. Healing by Second Intention (*Secondary Union*)

Wounds that fail to heal by first intention heal by second intention (secondary union [Figure 2-6]).

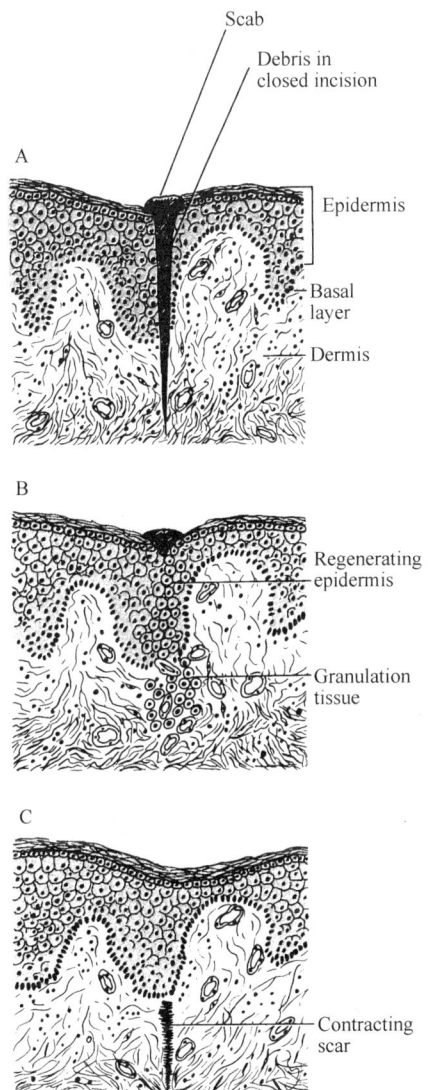

Figure 2-5 Healing of a surgical incision by first intention. A: Debris in the narrow gap between apposed skin edges is removed by neutrophils and macrophages. B: The epidermis regenerates rapidly, and granulation tissue in the dermal gap becomes collagenized to form a thin dermal scar (C)

When the sutures are removed at the end of the first week (leaving them in place longer increases the risk of wound infection), the tensile strength of the young scar is only about 10% that of normal skin. Scar strength increases to about 30%–50% of normal skin by 4 weeks and to 80% after several months.

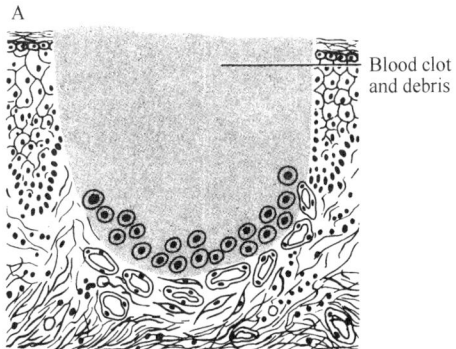
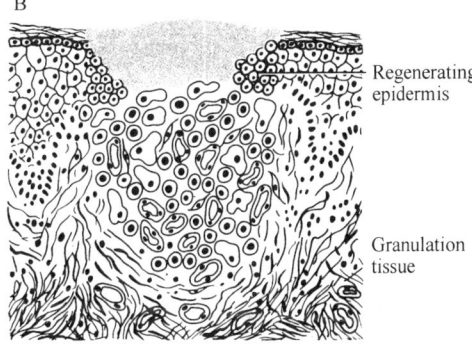
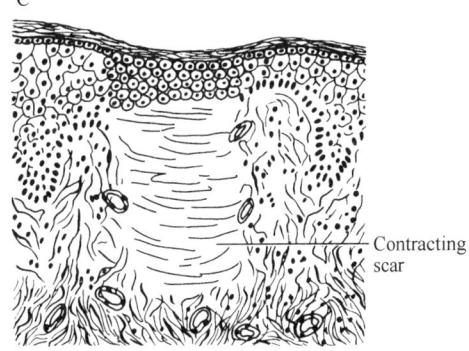

Figure 2-6 Healing by second intention of a large wound with extensive necrosis. A: The large area of tissue necrosis evokes acute inflammation with entry of neutrophils from the periphery. Slow liquefaction of debris and ingrowth of granulation tissue from the base (B) leads to scar formation (C). The epidermis regencrates slowly from the edges.

1. Reasons for failure of the primary healing process

Primary union fails to occur in the following circumstances: (1) in lacerations characterized by inability to achieve apposition of wound margins; (2) when foreign material is present; (3) when necrosis is extensive; and (4) when infection occurs. If infection develops after the skin edges are apposed, acute inflammation with suppuration leads to rupture of the wound and drainage of pus.

2. Process of secondary healing

The processes involved are essentially the same as those in healing by first intention but take much longer because of the more extensive damage. Infection is controlled by acute inflammation. The fluid exudate and necrotic tissue are then removed by enzymatic liquefaction, lymphatic drainage, and macrophage phagocytosis. Surgical removal of dead tissue and foreign material from the wound (debridement) greatly aids this clearing process. Granulation tissue then grows from the healthy tissue at the base of the wound and displaces the necrotic tissue toward the surface of the skin.

The epidermis regenerates from basal cells at the edges of the wound. In large wounds, reepithelialization may take several weeks. In these situations, surgical transplantation of skin (skin grafting) can help to speed healing.

When complete epithelialization of the surface of the wound has occurred, collagenization transforms the underlying granulation tissue to scar tissue. The eventual size of the mature scar is much smaller than that of the original wound as a result of contraction.

Skin appendages such as hair follicles and glands are regenerated if enough residual cells remain to provide a source of proliferating cells. In extensive skin wounds with total destruction of skin appendages, the resulting dermal scar is typically devoid of these structures.

C. Causes of Defective Wound Healing (Table 2-2.)

Surgeons must recognize the presence of any factors that impair healing because such adverse factors increase the overall risk of surgery and may even contraindicate surgery. If surgery is performed, recovery may take longer, and the risk of wound breakdown (which may be life-threatening) is also increased.

Table 2-2 Factor that adversely affect wound healing

Local	Systemic
Infection	Advanced age
Poor blood supply(ischemia)	Protein malnutrition
Presence of foreign material	Vitamin C deficiency
Presence of necrotic tissue	Zinc deficiency
Movement in injured area	Corticosteroid excess
Irradiation	Decreased number of
Tension in injured area	Neutrophils
	Macrophages
	Diabetes mellitus
	Cytotoxic (anticancer) drugs
	Severe anemia
	Bleeding disorders
	Ehlers-Danlos syndrome

1. Failure of collagen synthesis

Lack of collagen synthesis is one of the most common causes of defective wound healing and may result from vitamin C, protein, or zinc deficiency. Preoperative correction of negative protein balance with nutritional supplementation in malnourished patients improves the chances for uneventful healing.

Ehlers-Danlos syndrome is a group of rare inherited disorders characterized by defective collagen formation, hyperextensible joints, fragile tissues, and impaired wound healing. The basic defect appears to involve failure of cross-linkage of collagen chains.

2. Excessive collagen production

Synthesis of excessive amounts of collagen in wound healing results in formation of abnormal nodular masses of collagen (keloids) at the sites of skin injury (Figure 2-7A). Keloids often result from minor skin wounds and cause extensive disfigurement. Microscopic examination shows excessive collagen as thick, hyalinized bands (Figure 2-7B). Keloid formation tends to occur more frequently in blacks and demonstrates a familial tendency but with no recognizable single-gene inheritance pattern. The cause is not known. Excision of a keloid for cosmetic reasons is generally followed by formation of a new keloid.

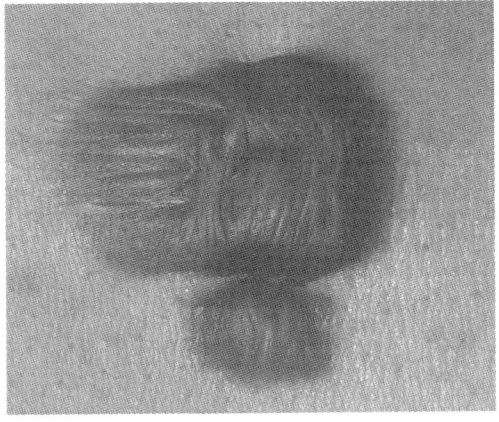
A

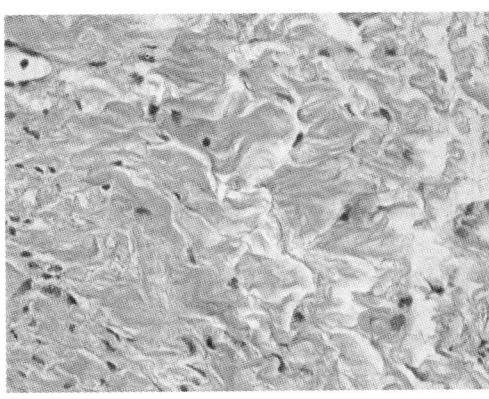
B

Figure 2-7　Keloid formation. The keloid is an irregularly contracted skin nodule (A) composed of thick hyalinized bands of collagen (B)

3. Local factors

Important local factors that cause defective wound healing include the following:
a. Foreign or necrotic tissue or blood: The presence of foreign bodies, necrotic tissue, or excessive blood in the wound impairs healing. At surgery, foreign material and necrotic tissue should be removed and hemostasis ensured before the incision is closed.
b. Infection: Infection in the wound will result in acute inflammation and (commonly) abscess formation, with breakdown of the wound and delayed healing.
c. Abnormal blood supply: Ischemia due to arterial disease and impaired venous drainage both hinder wound healing.
d. Decreased viability of cells: Irradiation of a tissue or administration of antimitotic drugs in cancer chemotherapy is associated with poor wound healing. These facts have important implications for the management of cancer patients because the timing of surgery in relation to radiotherapy must be adjusted to minimize the risks associated with defective healing.

4. Diabetes mellitus

Diabetes mellitus is associated with impaired wound healing, probably as a result of deficient microcirculation and increased incidence of infection.

5. Excessive levels of adrenal corticosteroids

Corticosteroid excess, whether due to administration of exogenous corticosteroids or to endogenous adrenal hyperactivity (Cushing's syndrome), is associated with impaired wound healing. Corticosteroids interfere with neutrophil and macrophage function.

MECHANISMS OF CELLULAR REGENERATION

The repair and regeneration of injured tissues are not only dependent on the regenerative abilities of surviving cells, but also on many other factors, e.g. cytokines.

GROWTH FACTORS

Growth factors are proteins that bind to receptors

on the cell surface with the primary result of activating cellular proliferation and/or differentiation. Many growth factors are quite versatile, stimulating cellular division in numerous different cell types; others are specific to a particular cell-type. Table 2-3 summarizes the most important factors released at sites of injury.

Table 2-3 Major growth factors in wound healing

Factor	Principal Source	Primary Activity	Comments
Platelet-derived growth factor (PDGF)	Platelets, endothelial cells, placenta	Promotes proliferation of connective tissue, glial and smooth muscle cells	Two different protein chains form 3 distinct dimer forms; AA, AB and BB
Fibroblast growth factors (FGF)	Wide range of cells; protein is associated with the ECM	Promotes proliferation of many cells; inhibits some stem cells	At least 19 family members, 4 distinct receptors
Epidermal growth factor (EGF)	Submaxillary gland, Brunners gland	Promotes proliferation of mesenchymal, glial and epithelial cells	
Transforming growth factors-β (TGF-β)	Common in transformed cells	May be important for normal wound healing	Related to EGF
Vascular epidermal growth factor (VEGF)	Original from tumor, protein is associated with the endothelial cells	Promotes angiogenesis and proliferation of epithelial cells	
Cytokines (e.g. IL-1, TNF)	Wide range of cells	Chemotactic for fibroblasts, stimulate synthesis of collagen and collagenase	Detailed in Chapter 4 as mediators of inflammation

CHALON AND CONTACT INHIBITION

Not much is known about chalon compared to growth factors. Chalon may be secreted by many tissues to inhibit cell growth, and only affects the same type of tissue. For example, differentiated epithelial cells can secrete epidermal chalon which can inhibit the proliferation of basal cells.

Normal cells will stop growing when they begin touching other cells while filling in an area. This is called "contact inhibition" of cells. Although the precise mechanism is unknown, research has shown that contact inhibition has been implicated as an important antiproliferative mechanism in the development and maturation of tissues. For example, Exogenous TGF-beta2 in aqueous humor suppresses Sphase entry in cultured rat corneal endothelial cells. It is not known whether TGF-beta2 contributes to the mitotic inhibition that occurs during in vivo endothelial development.

EXTRACELLULAR MATRIX (ECM)

The extracellular matrix (ECM) is a complex structural entity surrounding and supporting cells that are found within mammalian tissues. The ECM is often referred to as the **connective tissue.** The ECM is composed of 3 major classes of biomolecules: (1) **Structural proteins**: e.g. collagen and elastin, (2) **Specialized proteins**: e.g. fibrillin, fibronectin, and laminin, (3) **Proteoglycans.** These proteins are important because they are responsible for tissue strength and resilience. They also play a dynamic role in injury healing, promoting cell growth and differentiation by signal transduction pathways, scaffolding for tissue renewal, establishment of tissue microenvironments and storage, and presentation of regulatory molecules.

FRACTURE HEALING

Fracture, the most common bone lesion, is defined as a break in the continuity of a bone or a part of its mineralized structure caused by a traumatic physical force. Fracture is divided as two types: **Traumatic fracture** may be the result of an excessive impact, rotation, bending, or other mechanical force acting on previously normal bone. **Pathologic or spontaneous fracture** may be the consequence of an unnoticed or trivial injury of previously diseased bone. A fracture is described as complete or incomplete, simple (closed) or compound open if contiguous to an open external or internal wound, and comminuted if the bone is grossly splintered. A stress fracture is one that is caused by the cumulative effect of repeated episodes of physical stress on previously normal bone.

The basic process of fracture healing (Figure 2-8) include in:

A. Hematoma

The immediate effects of a simple fracture are to break the bone cortex and trabeculae, lift up or tear the periosteum, and sever the periosteal, endosteal, and Haversian blood vessels. This injury result in the extravasations and pooling of blood and blood clots filled between the bone fragments, as well as any space created by tearing of adjacent tissue, such as beneath the elevated periosteum, in the adjacent muscle and other soft tissues. Many bone cells and other cells at the fracture site undergo necrosis as a result of physical injury and ischemia. An acute inflammatory response occurs in regions of tissue injury and necrosis.

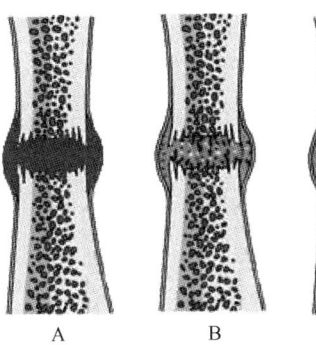
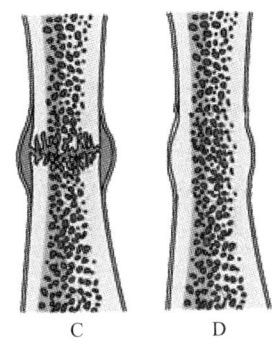

Figure 2-8 Process of fracture healing including bleed and hematoma formation (A), provisional callus (B), bony callus (C) and Bone remodeling (D)

B. Provisional Callus

By the second or third day, hematoma and exudate organized by granulation tissue develops from the periosteum and endosteum. And then the rapidly proliferating chondroblasts and osteoblasts appear in the areas proximate to the injured periosteum and endosteum. By the fifth or sixth day, the formation of primitive or woven bone begins around the fracture (called callus) which bridges the gap between the bone fragments and immobilizes them. When this has completed, pluripotent cells migrate into the granulation tissue. These cells become chondrocytes and later osteocytes, which produce cartilage and bone respectively. The structure surrounding the fracture site is slightly harder, this is a provisional callus.

C. Bony Callus

As time goes on, some calcium is deposited in the cartilaginous matrix further hardening the provisional callus and splinting the fractured ends of the bone. More and more woven bone is made by the osteoblasts. This woven bone is initially remodelled into lamellar bone. In this manner, the provisional callus is replaced by bony callus.

D. Bone Remodeling

At the last stage, the bulky external and internal callus of woven bone is slowly decreased in size and replaced by strong lamellar bone, and firm bony union is established. The process of bone remodeling by osteoclastic resorption and osteoblastic reformation takes place over subsequent weeks or months. The final result of fracture healing in a setting of good alignment, close positioning, and firm immobilization of bone fragments is to attain a normal anatomical and functional reconstitution of the bone cortex and medulla.

Many factors are important in the fracture healing process. The rate of healing and the ability to remodel a fractured bone vary tremendously for each person and depend on your age, your health, the kind of fracture, and the bone involved (Table 2-4).

Table 2-4 Variables that influence fracture healing

Influencing Type	Influencing Factor
Injury	Type Intensity Duration
Patient	Age Metabolic state Disease and motion
Treatment	Apposition Stabilization Loading and motion
Tissue type	Bone Dense fibrous tissue Cartilage Muscle

Chapter 3 Hemodynamic Disorders and Abnormalities of Blood Supply

Wang Liantang, Peng Tingsheng, Yang Shicong

CHAPTER CONTENTS
- Edema
- Hyperemia and Congestion
    - Morphology
    - Venous Congestion in Heart Failure
- Hemostasis and Thrombosis
    - Normal Hemostasis
    - Abnormal Hemostasis
    - Factors in Thrombosis
    - Types of Thrombi
    - Sites of Thrombosis
    - Evolution of Thrombi
- Disseminated Intravascular Coagulation (DIC)
    - Causes
    - Effects
    - Treatment
- Embolism
    - Origin of Emboli
    - Types and Sites of Embolism
- Infarction
    - Classification of Infarcts
    - Morphology of Infarcts
    - Venous Infarction
    - Factors That Influence Development of an Infarct
    - Evolution of Infarcts
- Shock

The health of cells and tissue depends not only on an intact circulation to deliver oxygen and remove wastes but also on normal fluid homeostasis; the major causes of morbidity and mortality in developed countries are associated, in some way, with failure to maintain normal fluid status. The maintenance of adequate blood circulation is a highly complex process that depends on proper function of the heart, the integrity of the vasculature, and the maintenance of a delicate balance between the coagulation and fibrinolytic systems. Failure of blood supply to a tissue (ischemia) may be localized, due to arterial obstruction or deficient venous drainage, leading to infarction (ischemic necrosis of tissue); orgeneralized, due to severe decrease in cardiac out put, leading to a generalized decrease in tissue perfusion (shock). Normal homeostasis encompasses maintenance of vessel wall integrity as well as intravascular pressure and, osmolarity within certain physiologic ranges. Changes in vascular volume, pressure, or protein content or alternation in endothelial function affect the net movement or water across the vascular wall. Such water extravasation into the interstitial spaces is called edema and has importance on its locations.

EDEMA

Approximately 60% of lean body weight is water, with 2/3 intracellular and the rest extracellular, most of which is interstitial fluids (merely 5% of the total body water is blood plasma). Depending on its location, the term edema can be designated as hydrothorax, hydropericardium, or hydroperitoneum (i. e. ascites). Anasarca is a severe and generalized edema, subcutaneous.

In general, the opposing effects of vascular hydrostatic pressure and plasma colloid osmotic pressure are the major factors that govern fluid movement between vascular and interstitial spaces. Either increased capillary pressure or diminished colloid osmotic pressure can result in increased interstitial fluid. As extravascular fluid accumulates in either case, the increased tissue hydrostatic and plasma colloid osmotic eventually achieve a new equilibrium, or water reenter the venues. Excess interstitial fluid can be removed via lymphatic drainage, ultimately returning to bloodstream by thoracic duct; thus obstruction of lymphatic tissue can cause edema through damaging the draining route. Lastly, retention of sodium in renal disease also results in edema.

Causes

A. Increase Hydrostatic Pressure

Localized increase in intravascular pressure may result from impaired venous return e. g. secondary to deep venous thrombosis in the lower extremities, with a restricted edema in the affected leg. Generalized increment of venous pressure often occur in congestive heart failure, which affects the right ventricular function with reduced cardiac output and hence reduced renal hyperfusion, resulting in systemic edema. In brief, if the failing heart cannot increase cardiac output, the extra fluid in increased pressure and eventually edema, which would be worsen unless cardiac output is restored or renal water retention reduced.

B. Reduces Plasma Osmotic Pressure

This can result from excessive loss (nephritic syndrome, characterized by a leaky glomerular capillary wall) or reduced synthesis (liver disease e. g. cirrhosis or protein malnutrition) of albumin, the serum protein most responsible for maintaining colloid osmotic pressure. In both cases, reduced plasma osmotic pressure leads to a net movement of fluid into the interstitial tissues The mechanism of compensation cannot work if the defect of serum protein persists.

C. Lymphatic Obstruction

Impaired lymphatic drainage and consequent lymph edema is usually localized; it can result from inflammatory or neoplastic obstruction. For example, the parasitic infection filariasis often causes massive lymphatic and lymph node fibrosis in the inguinal region (elephantiasis). In breast cancer, resection of the lymphatic channels as well as scarring related to surgery and radiation can result in severe edema of the arm Also, infiltration and obstruction of the superficial lymphatic can cause edema of the overlying skin, giving rise to the so-called peau d'orange (orange peel) appearance resulting from an accentuation of depressions in the skin at the site of hair follicles.

D. Sodium and Water Retention

These are clearly contributory factors in several forms of edema. Increased salt, with the obligate accompanying water, causes increased hydrostatic pressure (due to expansion of the intravascular colloid osmotic pressure), e. g. poststreptococcal glomerulonephritis and acute renal failure.

Clinical Correlation

The effects of edema may range from merely annoying to fatal. Subcutaneous tissue edema in cardiac or renal failure is vital primarily because it indicates underlying diseases; and if severe it can impair wound healing or the clearance of the infection. Pulmonary edema can cause death by interfering with normal ventilator function, at the same time creating a favorable environment for bacterial infection. Brain edema is serious and can be rapidly fatal, if severe, brain can be pushed out through e. g. the foramen magnum (herniate), or the brain stem vascular supply can be compressed. Either condition can injure the medullary and cause death.

Morphology

Edema is most easily recognized grossly; microscopically, edema fluid generally is manifested only as subtle cell swelling, with clearing and separation of the extracellular matrix elements. Although any organ or tissue in the body may be involved, edema is most commonly seen in subcutaneous tissues, lungs, and brain. Severe, generalized edema is also called anasarca.

Subcutaneous edema may have different distributions depending on the cause. It can be diffuse, or it may be more prominent in the regions with the highest hydrostatic pressures. Edema of the dependent parts of the body (e. g. The legs when standing, the sacrum the recumbent) is a prominent feature of cardiac failure, particularly of the right ventricle. Edema due to renal dysfunction or nephritic syndrome is generally more severe and affects all parts of the body. It may be initially manifested in tissue with a loose connective tissue matrix, such as the eyelids, causing periorbital edema. Finger pressure over significantly edematous subcutaneous tissue displaces the interstitial fluid and leaves a finger-shaped depression, so-called pitting edema.

Pulmonary edema is a common clinical problem most frequently seen in the setting of left ventricular failure and other diseases. The lungs are typically 2-3 times their normal weight, and sectioning reveals frothy, sometimes blood-tinged fluid representing a mixture of air, edema fluid, and extravasated red cells.

Edema of the brain may be localized (e. g. abscesses or neoplasm) or generalized, (encephalitis or hypertensive crises), depending on the nature and extent of the injury. With generalized edema, the brain is grossly swollen with narrowed sulci and distended gyri showing signs of flattening against unyielding skull.

HYPEREMIA AND CONGESTION

A local increased volume of blood in a particular tissue may cause hyperemia or congestion.

Hyperemia is an active process, after arteriolar dilation the blood flow is augmented at local sites, such as sites of inflammation, or in skeletal muscle during exercise, or in stomach replete with food. The affected tissue is redder because of engorgement with oxygenated blood.

Congestion is a passive process, resulting from impaired venous return from a tissue. It may occur systemically, as in cardiac failure, or it may be local, resulting from an isolated venous obstruction. The tissue has a blue-red color (cyanosis), especially as worsening congestion leads to accumulation of deoxygenated hemoglobin in the affected tissues. Congestion of capillary beds is closely related to the development of edema, so that congestion and edema commonly occur together. In long standing congestion, called chronic passive congestion, the stasis of poorly oxygenated blood causes chronic hypoxia, which can result in parenchymal cell degeneration or death, sometimes with microscopic scarring. Capillary rupture at these sites of chronic congestion may also cause small foci of hemorrhage; breakdown and phagocytosis of the red cell debris can eventually result in small clusters of hemosiderin-laden macrophages.

MORPHOLOGY

In situations where collateral drainage is inadequate, congestion of the tissue occurs in addition to edema, as is seen in the face when the superior vena cava is occluded. So the cut surfaces of hyperemia or congestion tissues are wet and darkly red color. In acute severe venous congestion, hydrostatic pressure may rise enough to cause capillary rupture and hemorrhage, e.g. orbital congestion and hemorrhage in cavernoussinus occlusion. In extreme cases, venous infarction may result.

VENOUS CONGESTION IN HEART FAILURE

Specific types of venous congestion occur in heart failure when venous blood backs up in the circulatory system because of failure of the heart to pump all of the venous return.

A. Pulmonary Venous Congestion

Left heart failure causes congestion of the pulmonary circulation. **Acute pulmonary congestion** causes dilation of alveolar capillaries with transudation of fluid into the alveoli (pulmonary edema) (Figure 3-1A). Intra-alveolar hemorrhage may also result. **In chronic pulmonary congestion**, the long-standing increase in pulmonary venous pressure stimulates development of fibrosis in alveolar walls (Figure 3-1B). The septa become thickened and fibrotic, the escape of erythrocytes into alveoli over a long period causes accumulation of hemosiderin-laden macrophages ("**heart failure cells**") in the alveoli (Figure 3-1C).

B. Hepatic Venous Congestion

Right heart failure causes congestion of the systemic circulation. In addition to peripheral (ankle) edema, there is also hepatic venous congestion. In acute hepatic congestion, because the central portion of the hepatic lobule is the last to receive blood, dilation of the central hepatic veins and congestion of the sinusoids in the central part of the hepatic lobule appears firstly. In chronic hepatic congestion, the central regions of the hepatic lobules are grossly red-brown and slightly depressed (owing to a loss of cells), while the peripheral zones are uncongested tan or paler tissue, which sometimes fatty, then create a mottled effect (so-called nutmeg liver because of its resemblance to the cut surface of a nutmeg) (Figure 3-2). Microscopically, there is evidence of centrilobular necrosis with hepatocyte drop-out and hemorrhage, including hemosiderin-laden macrophages. As congestion increases, hypoxia due to reduced blood flow occurs, with fatty change of liver cells that enhances the mottled appearance. The cells of the central zone of the liver lobule may eventually undergo necrosis; they are then replaced by fibrous tissue; Contraction of the centrizonal fibrous tissue alternating with

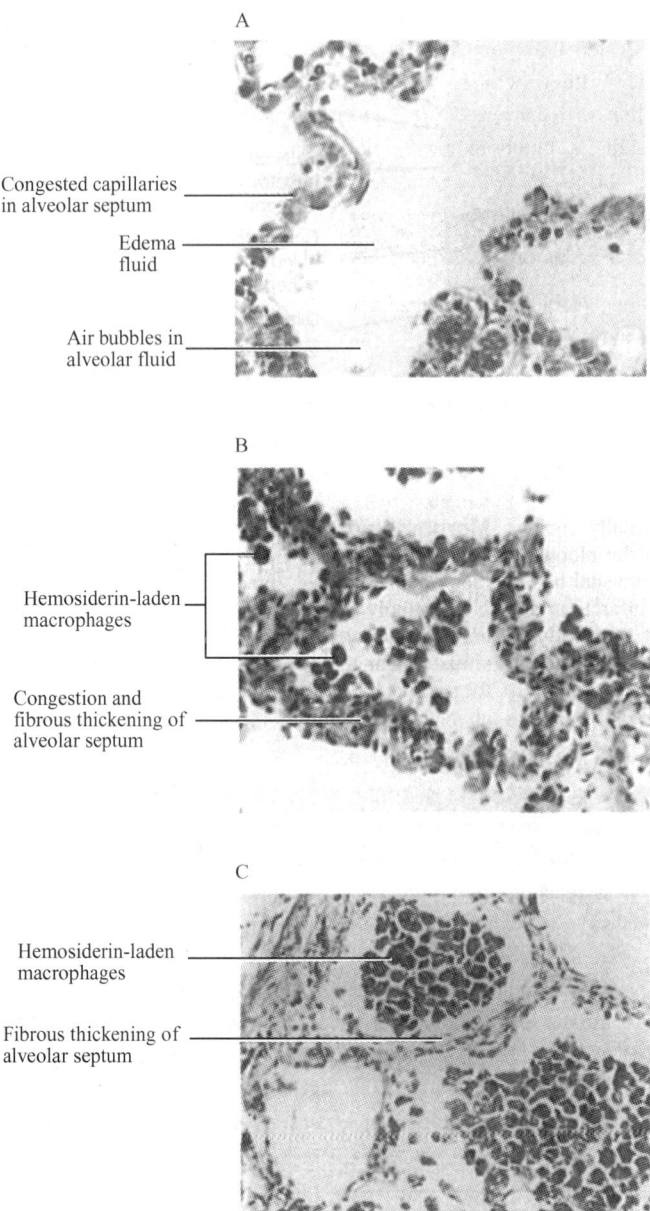

Figure 3-1 A: Acute congestion and edema of the lung in a patient with acute left ventricular failure. The alveolar septa show congestion, and the alveoli are filled with edema fluid. B: Chronic venous congestion of the lung. The alveolar septa are thickened by fibrosis, and the alveoli contain scattered hemosiderin-laden macrophages. C: Chronic venous congestion of the lung, later stage. The alveolar septa show fibrosis, and there are numerous hemosiderin-laden macrophages in the alveoli

the surviving peripheral zonal cells may result in a nodular liver (cardiac cirrhosis).

HEMOSTASIS AND THROMBOSIS

Normal hemostasis results from well-regulated processes that maintain blood in a fluid, clot-free state in normal vessels while inducing the rapid formation of a localized hemostatic plug at the site of vascular injury. The pathologic converse to hemostasis is thrombosis. Thrombosis is the formation of a solid mass from the constituents of blood (platelets, fibrin, and entrapped red and white blood cells) within the heart or vascular system in a living orga-

Chapter 3 Hemodynamic Disorders and Abnormalities of Blood Supply

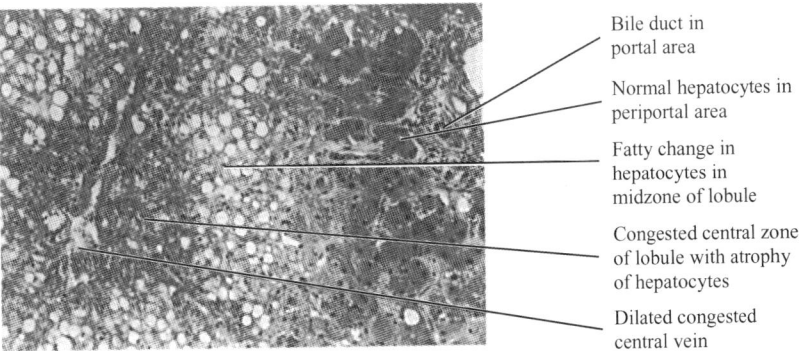

Figure 3-2 Chronic venous congestion of the liver. The central vein is distended with blood, and the central zone shows congestion and atrophy of liver cells. The midzonal hepatocytes show fatty change

nism. Thrombosis is usually distinguished from blood clotting, although the distinction is somewhat arbitrary and both invoke the coagulation cascade. Clotting occurs in tissues when blood escapes from an injured vessel (hematoma formation). It also occurs in vessels after death (postmortem clotting of blood) and in vitro (in a test tube outside the body). In one word, Both hemostasis and thrombosis are dependent on three general components: the vascular wall, platelets, and the coagulation cascade.

Thrombosis can be thought as the formation of a blood clot (thrombus) in uninjured vessels, or thrombotic occlusion of a vessel after relatively minor injury. A thrombus is generally attached to the endothelium and is composed of layers of aggregated platelets and fibrin, whereas a blood clot contains randomly oriented fibrin with entrapped platelets and red cells. We begin our discussion with the process of normal hemostasis and a description of how it is regulated.

NORMAL HEMOSTASIS (Figure 3-3)

Thrombosis is a normal hemostatic mechanism that acts to stop bleeding when a vessel is injured. Under normal conditions, there is a delicate and dynamic balance between thrombus formation and dissolution of thrombus (fibrinolysis).

The role of the important factors in normal Hemostasis process:

a. Endothelium: (1) antithrombotic properties including antiplatelet effects, anticoagulant properties, and fibrinolytic properties. (2) prothrombotic properties. In summary, intact endothelial cells serve primarily to inhibit platelet adherence and blood clotting. However, injury or activation of endothelial cells results in a procoagulant phenotype that contributes to localized clot formation.

b. Platelets: Platelets play a central role in normal hemostasis, The series of platelet events can be summarized as follows: (1) Platelets adhere to the ECM at sites of endothelial injury and become activated. (2) Upon activation, platelets secrete granule products (e.g. ADP) and synthesize TXA2. (3) Platelets also expose phospholipid complexes important in the intrinsic coagulation pathway. (4) Injured or activated endothelial cells release tissue factor to activate the extrinsic coagulation cascade. (5) Injured or activated endothial cells released ADP stimulates formation of a primary hemostatic plug, which is eventually converted (via ADP, thrombin, and TXA2) into a larger definitive secondary plug. f. Fibrin deposition stabilizes and anchors the aggregated platelets.

c. Coagulation cascade: The coagulation cascade is essentially a series of enzymatic conversions, turning inactive proenzymes into activated enzymes and culminating in the formation of thrombin. Thrombin then converts the soluble plasma protein fibrinogen into the insoluble fibrous protein fibrin.

Following trauma, the usual initiating factor in thrombus formation is endothelial injury, which leads to formation of a hemostatic platelet plug and activation of the coagulation and fibrinolytic systems.

A. Formation of Hemostatic Platelet Plug (Figure 3-4.)

Injury to the vascular endothelium exposes subendothelial collagen, which has a strong thrombogenic

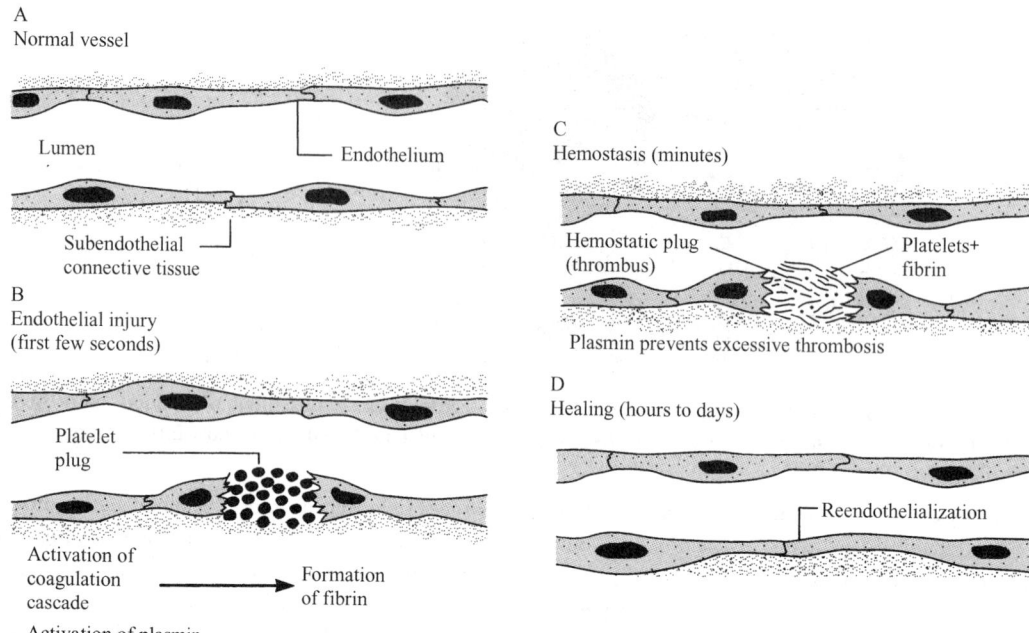

Figure 3-3 Mechanisms of normal Hemostasis. A: In normal uninjured vessels, subendothelial connective tissue, especially collagen and elastin, is not exposed to the circulating blood. B: In the first few seconds after injury, exposure of subendothelial tissue attracts platelets, which adhere and aggregate at the site of injury. Endothelial injury also activates Hageman factor (factor XII), which in turn activates the intrinsic pathway of the coagulation cascade. Release of tissue thromboplastins activates the extrinsic pathway. C: Hemostasis is achieved in minutes. Platelet degranulation stimulates further platelet aggregation. Fibrin formed by activation of the coagulation cascade combines with the mass of aggregated platelets to form the definitive hemostatic plug that seals the injury. Plasmin (fibrinolysin) formed by activation of the fibrinolytic pathway prevents excessive fibrin formation. D: During healing (hours to days), the thrombus retracts, and organization and fibrosis of the thrombus occur. Reendothelialization of the vessels is the final step

effect on platelets and results in the adherence of platelets at the site. The platelets adhering to the injured endothelium aggregate to form a hemostatic plug, which is the beginning of a thrombus. Platelet aggregation in turn leads to degranulation of platelets, which releases serotonin, ADP, ATP, and thromboplastic substances. ADP – itself a powerful platelet aggregator-causes further accumulation of platelets. The layers of platelets alternating with fibrin in a thrombus appear on microscopic examination as pale lines (lines of Zahn, Figure 3-6).

B. Coagulation of Blood (Figure 3-4.)

Activation of Hageman factor (factor XII in the coagulation cascade) results in the formation of fibrin by activation of the intrinsic coagulation pathway. (For further details, see Figure 3-5.) Tissue thromboplastins released by injury activate the extrinsic coagulation pathway, which contributes to fibrin formation. Factor XIII acts on fibrin to produce an insoluble fibrillary polymer that – with the platelet plug – makes up the definitive hemostatic plug: Fibrin appears on microscopic examination as a pink-staining fibrillary meshwork intermingled with amorphous pale platelet masses (Figure 3-6).

ABNORMAL HEMOSTASIS

The normal balance that exists between thrombus formation and fibrinolysis ensures that just the right amount of thrombus is formed in response to endothelial injury so that hemorrhage from the vessel is prevented. Fibrinolytic activity prevents the formation of excessive thrombus. A disturbance of this balance results in abnormal thrombosis or abnormal bleeding.

Excessive thrombus formation results in narrowing or occlusion of the vessel lumen. This usually occurs

Chapter 3 Hemodynamic Disorders and Abnormalities of Blood Supply

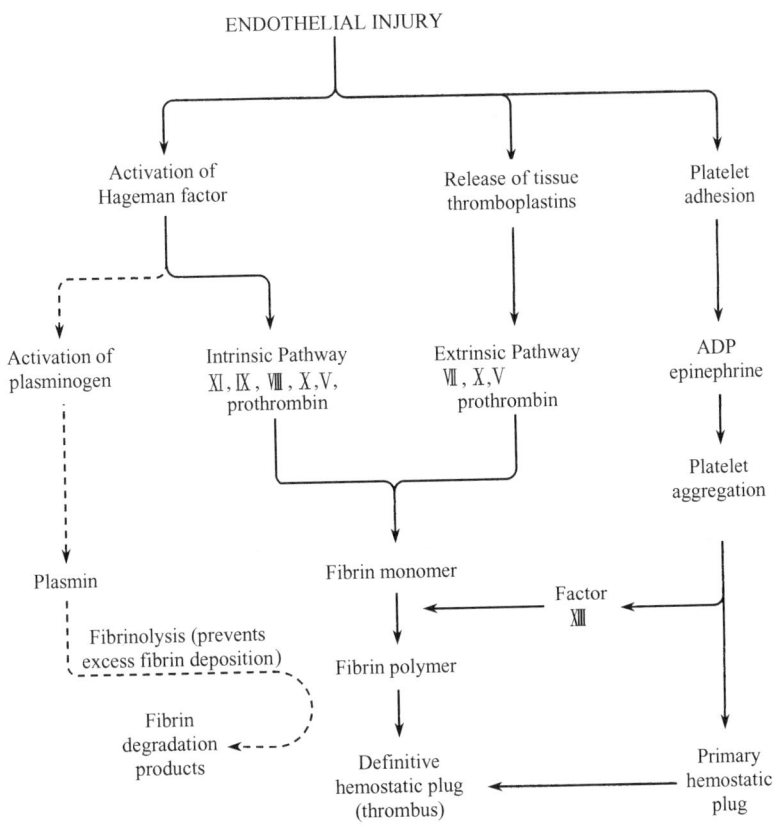

Figure 3-4 Effect of endothelial injury on the coagulation system and platelets, resulting in formation of the definitive Hemostasis plug, or thrombus. Note that simultaneous activation of the opposing fibrinolytic system provides a degree of control over the extent of thrombus formation

as a result of local factors at the site that overwhelm the ability of a normally functional fibrinolytic system to prevent excess thrombosis. Decreased fibrinolysis alone almost never produces excessive thrombosis.

In contrast, decreased ability to form thrombi results in excessive bleeding and occurs in a variety of bleeding disorders, including decreased platelets in the blood, deficiency of coagulation factors, and increased fibrinolytic activity. These disorders are considered in Bleeding disorders.

FACTORS IN THROMBOSIS

Having discussed the process of hemostasis, we can now turn our attention to the dysregulation that under-lies pathologic thrombus formation.

Pathogenesis. Three primary influences predispose to thrombus formation, the so-called Virchow triad: (1) endothelial injury, (2) stasis or turbulence of blood flow, and (3) blood hypercoagulability (Figure 3-7).

Endothelial damage is the dominant influence and by itself can lead to thrombosis. It is particularly important in thrombus formation in the heart and arterial circulation, for example, within the cardiac chambers when there has been endocardial injury (e.g. myocardial infarction or valvulitis), over ulcerated plaques in severely atherosclerotic arteries, or at sites of traumatic or inflammatory vascular injury. It is important to note that endothelium does not need to be denuded or physically disrupted to contribute to the development of thrombosis; any perturbation in the dynamic balance of prothrombotic and antithrombotic effects can influence local clotting events. Thus, significant endothelial dysfunction may occur from the hemodynamic stresses of hypertension, turbulent flow over scarred valves, or bacterial endotoxins. Even relatively subtle influences such as homocystinuria, hypercholesterolemia, radiation, or products absorbed from cigarette smoke may be sources of endothelial injury and dysregulation. Regardless of the cause, physical loss of endothelium leads to expo-

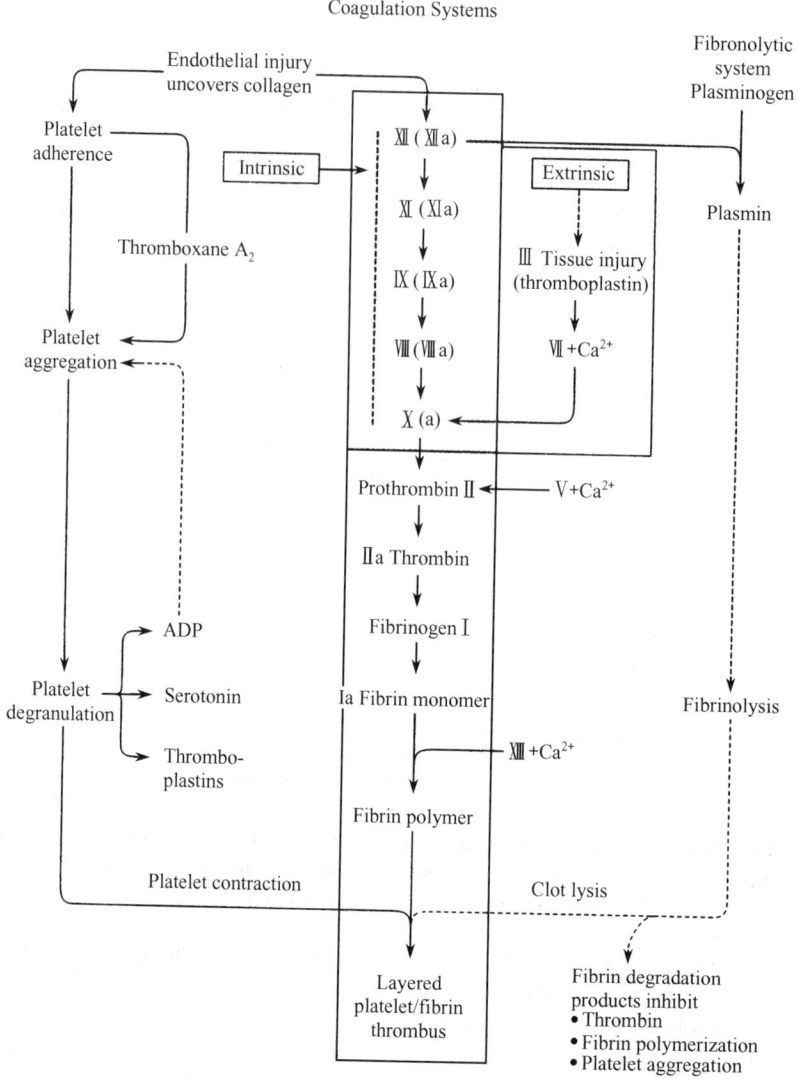

Figure 3-5 Coagulation and fibrinolytic systems. The balance between these two systems is very finely tuned. If this balance is disturbed, pathologic thrombosis or excessive bleeding may result. (a, actived factor.)

sure of subendothelial collagen (and other platelet activators), adherence of platelets, release of tissue factor, and local depletion of PG12 and PA such as tissue plasminogen activator (tPA) or urokinase (uPA). Dysfunctional endothelium may elaborate greater amounts of procoagulant factors (e.g. adhesion molecules to bind platelets, tissue factor, PAL etc.) and smaller amounts of anticoagulant effectors (e.g. thrombomodulin, PGI2, t-PA).

Alterations in normal blood flow. Turbulence contributes to arterial and cardiac thrombosis by causing endothelial injury or dysfunction, as well as by forming countercur-rents and local pockets of stasis; stasis is a major factor in the development of venous thrombi. Normal blood flow is laminar such that the platelet elements flow centrally in the vessel lumen, separated from the endothelium by a slower-moving clear zone of plasma. Stasis and turbulence therefore (1) disrupt laminar flow and bring platelets into contact with the endothelium, (2) prevent dilution of activated clotting factors by fresh-flowing blood, (3) retard the inflow of clotting factor inhibitors and permit the build-up of thrombi, and (4) promote endothelial cell activation, predisposing to local thrombosis, leukocyte adhesion, and a variety of other endothelial cell effects.

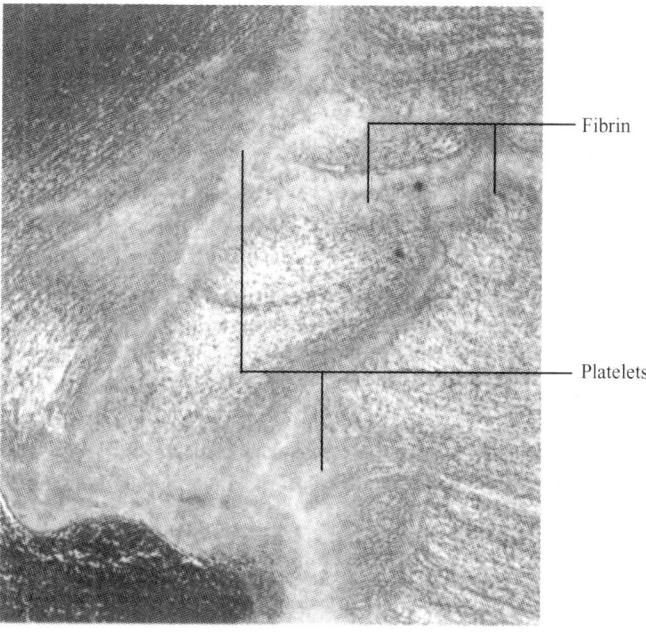

Figure 3-6　Thrombus, showing alternating zones of amorphous platelets (lines of Zahn) and fibrillary fibrin

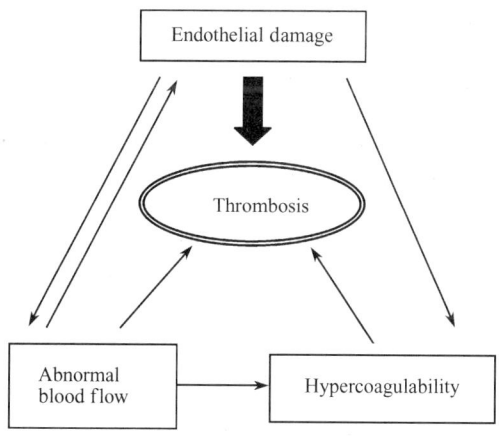

Figure 3-7　The factors influenced thrombosis and the relationship among them

Turbulence and stasis contribute to thrombosis in a number of clinical settings. Ulcerated atherosclerotic plaques not only expose subendothelial ECM but also generate local turbulence. Abnormal aortic and arterial dilations called aneurysms cause local stasis and are favored sites of thrombosis. Myocardial infarctions not only have associated endothelial injury but also have regions of noncontractile myocardium, adding an element of stasis in the formation of mural thrombi. Mitral valve stenosis (e. g. after rheumatic heart di-sease) results in left atria dilation.

Hypercoagulability generally contributes less frequently to thrombotic states but is nevertheless an important (and interesting) component in the equation. It is loosely defined as any alteration of the coagulation pathways that predisposes to thrombosis, and it can be divided into primary (genetic) and secondary (acquired) disorders.

Of the inherited causes of hypercoagulability, mutations in the factor V gene and prothrombin gene are the most common. The characteristic alteration is a mutant factor Va that cannot be inactivated by protein C; as a result, an important antithrombotic counter-regulatory pathway is lost. Less common primary hyper-coagulable states include inherited deficiencies of antico-agulants such as antithrombin Ⅲ, protein C, or protein S; affected patients typically present with venous thrombosis and recurrent thromboembolism in adolescence or early adult life. Congenitally elevated levels of homocys-teine contribute to arterial and venous thromboses (and indeed to the development of atherosclerosis), likely via inhibitory effects on antithrombin Ⅲ and endothelial thrombomodulin.

Although these hereditary disorders are uncommon, the basis of the thrombotic tendencies is reasonably well understood. However, the pathogenesis of acquired thrombotic diatheses in a number of common clinical settings is more complicated and multifactorial. In some of the acquired conditions (e. g. cardiac failure or trauma), factors such as stasis or vascular injury may be most important. Among acquired causes (oral contraceptive use and the hyperestrogenic state of pregnancy), hypercoagulability may be related to increased hepatic synthesis of coagulation factors and reduced synthesis of antithrombin III. In disseminated cancers, release of procoagulant tumor products predisposes to thrombosis. The hypercoagulability seen with advancingage may be due to increasing platelet aggregation and reduced PGIZ release by endothelium. Smoking and obesity promote hypercoagulability by unknown mechanisms.

TYPES OF THROMBI

thrombi can be divided into four types described as follows:

Pale thrombus is the thrombus often in the fast-flowing arterial circulation such as coronary, cerebral, and femoral arteries, which are composed predominantly of fibrin and platelets, with few entrapped erythrocytes (Figure 3-6). The thrombi typically are firmly adherent to the injured arterial wall and are gray-white and friable.

Red thrombi are composed of platelets, fibrin, and large numbers of erythrocytes trapped in the fibrin mesh. Red thrombi typically occur in the venous system, where the slower blood flow encourages entrapment of red cells.

Mixed thrombus often arise in the slowly moving venous blood, containing an original part as pale thrombus. The blood flow move slowly after the original part, and then amount of erythrocytes coagulate, forming the body of the thrombus with pale layers of platelets and fibrin that alternate with darker layers containing more red cells. Mixed thrombus in aortic lumen are termed mural thrombus, abnormal myocardial contraction or injury to the endomyocardial surface leads to the formation of cardiac mural thrombus (Figure 3-9).

Hyaline thrombus or microthrombus usually appears in DIC, which will be discussed following. Numerous microthrombi are seen in micro-circulation ie. glomerular capillaries (Figure 3-13).

SITES OF THROMBOSIS

A. Arterial Thrombosis (Figure 3-8 and Figure 3-9)

Arterial thrombosis is common and typically occurs after endothelial damage and local turbulence has been caused by atherosclerosis. Large- and medium-sized arteries such as the aorta, carotid arteries, arteries of the circle of Willis, coronary arteries, and arteries of the intestine and limbs are mainly affected.

Less commonly, arterial thrombosis is a complication of arteritis, as occurs in polyarteritis nodosa, giant cell arteritis, thromboangiitis obliterans, and Henoch-Schölein purpura. Medium - and small-sized arteries are commonly affected.

B. Cardiac Thrombosis

Thrombi form within the chambers of the heart in the following circum-stances.

1. Inflammation of cardiac valves

Endocardial damage occurring in association with inflammation of the cardiac valves (endocarditis, valvulitis) leads to local turbulence and deposition of platelets and fibrin on the valves. These thrombi are called, vegetations (Figure 3-10). Vegetations may be large and friable (as occurs in infective endocarditis), and fragments of thrombus often break off and are carried in the circulation as emboli (see below).

2. Damage to mural endocardium

Myocardial infarction and ventricular aneurysms are associated with damage to the mural endocardium. Thrombi forming on the walls are often large and may also give rise to emboli.

3. Turbulence and stasis in atrial chambers

Thrombi often form in chambers of the atrium when turbulence and stasis of blood occur, typically in patients with mitral valve stenosis or atrial fibrillation. Thrombi may be so large (ball thrombus) that they obstruct the mitral valve orifice. Fragments of atrial thrombi may become detached and form emboli.

C. Venous Thrombosis

1. Thrombophlebitis

Thrombophlebitis denotes venous thrombosis occurring secondary to acute inflammation of the vein.

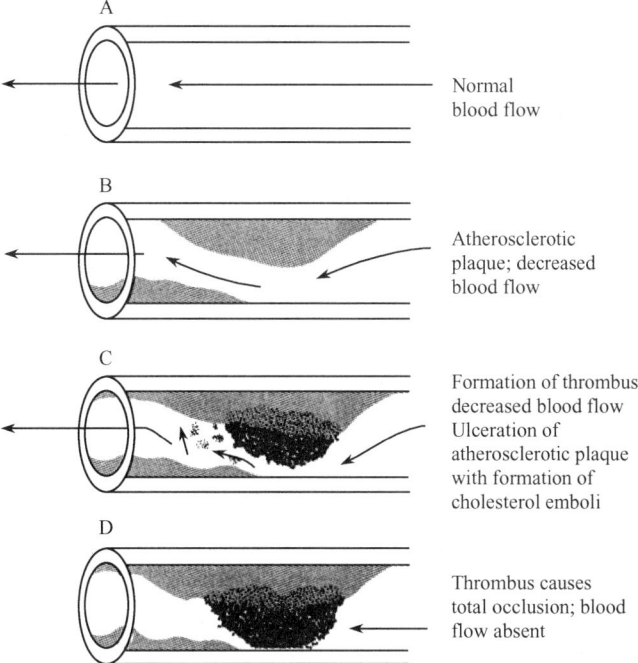

Figure 3-8 Thrombosis in an atherosclerotic artery. A: Normal artery, showing typical laminar blood flow. B: Atherosclerotic artery, showing atherosclerotic plaques. The endothelium is intact, but the vessel lumen is narrowed. Decreased blood flow and increased turbulence are present. C: Ulcerated atherosclerotic plaque from which fragments of the plaque have become detached and passed distally as cholesterol emboli (see Figure 9-28). Blood flow is further decreased and turbulence increased. Thrombosis has occurred over the ulcerated area. D: Extension of thrombosis has caused total occlusion of the artery, and there is no blood flow in the vessel

Thrombophlebitis is a common phenomenon in infected wounds or ulcers and characteristically involves the superficial veins of the extremities. The affected vein is firm and cord-like and shows signs of acute inflammation (pain, redness, warmth, swelling). This type of thrombus tends to be firmly attached to the vessel wall; they rarely form emboli.

Rarely, thrombophlebitis occurs in multiple superficial leg veins (thrombophlebitis migrans) in patients with visceral cancers, most commonly pancreatic and gastric cancer (Trousseau's syndrome).

2. Phlebothrombosis

Phlebothrombosis denotes venous thrombosis occurring in the absence of obvious inflammation. Phlebothrombosis occurs mostly in the deep veins of the leg (deep vein thrombosis). Less commonly, veins of the pelvic venous plexus are involved. Deep vein thrombosis is common and has important medical implications because the large thrombi that form in these veins are only loosely attached to the vessel wall and are often easily detached. They travel in the circulation to the heart and lung and lodge in the pulmonary arteries (pulmonary embolism \[Figure 3-17\ ]).

a. Causes: Up to 50% of patients with deep vein thrombosis show a mutation of the factor V gene, with the result that factor V is less readily degraded by activated protein C. The mutation is known as the Leiden or Q506 mutation (producing a substitution of glycine for arginine at position 506); heterozygous individuals have a tenfold increase in risk for thrombosis, and homozygous individuals a hundredfold increase.

Otherwise, factors causing deep vein thrombosis are those typical of thrombosis in general, although endothelial injury is usually minimal. Sluggish blood flow is an important factor. In the venous plexus of the calf muscles, blood flow is normally maintained by calf muscle contraction (the muscle pump). Prolonged immobilization in bed favors stasis of blood and thrombosis. The routine use of physical thera-

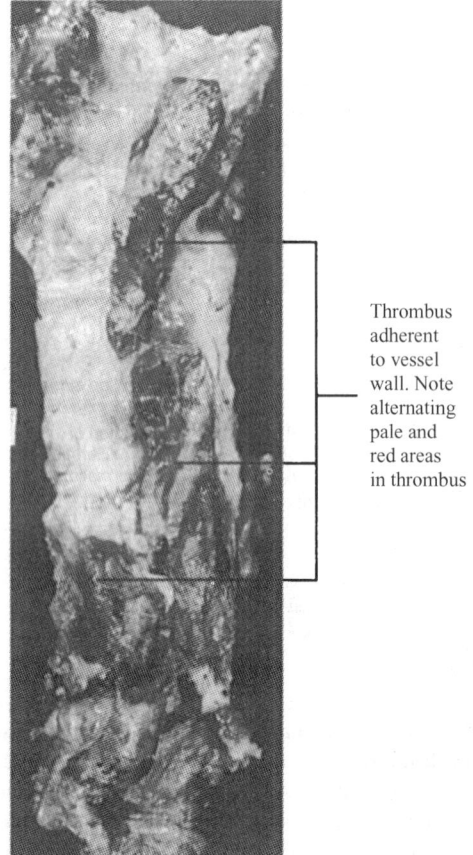

Thrombus adherent to vessel wall. Note alternating pale and red areas in thrombus

Figure 3-9 Abdominal aorta, showing multiple large thrombi attached to the endothelial surface. The thrombi have alternating pale and red areas

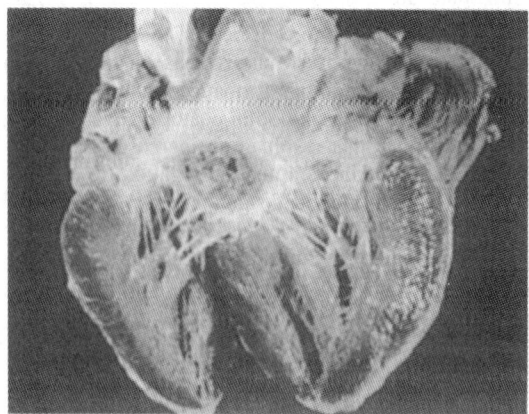

Figure 3-10 Vegetation (thrombus) on mitral valve in subacute infective endocarditis

py, compressive stockings, and early ambulation after surgery has considerably decreased the incidence of postoperative deep vein thrombosis. Other factors predisposing to thrombus formation include changes in the composition of blood in postoperative or postpartum patients that result in an increased tendency toward platelet adhesion and aggregation, as well as increased levels of some coagulation factors (fibrinogen and factors VII and VIII). Oral contraceptives-particularly those with high estrogen levels may cause increased blood coagulability. Cardiac failure also contributes to sluggish blood flow in the deep veins of the calf. In practice, several of these factors may act together.

b. Clinical findings: Deep vein thrombosis of the legs may cause few or no clinical symptoms. Mild edema of the ankles and calf pain when the ankle is dorsiflexed (Homans' sign) are helpful diagnostic features. In many patients, pulmonary embolism is the first clinical manifestation of phlebothrombosis. Deep vein thrombosis can be detected by venography, ultrasonography, and other radiologic techniques.

EVOLUTION OF THROMBI

Thrombus formation evokes a host of response that is designed to remove the thrombus and repair the injured blood vessel. Several outcomes are possible (Figure 3-11).

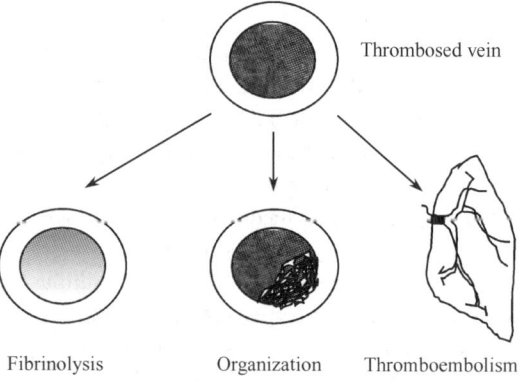

Figure 3-11 Potential evolution of thrombi

A. Fibrinolysis

Lysis of the thrombus (fibrinolysis) accompanied by reestablishment of the lumen is the ideal end result. The fibrin constituting the thrombus is dissolved by plasmin, which is activated by Hageman factor (factor XII) whenever the intrinsic coagulation pathway is activated (i.e. the fibrinolytic system is activated at the same time as the clotting sequence; this mechanism for clot lysis is a built-in control function that normally prevents excessive thrombosis, Figure 3-4). Fibrinolysis is effective in preventing excess fibrin formation and in dissolving small thrombi. Fibrinolysis is much less effective in dissolving large thrombi occurring in arteries, veins, or the heart itself. Drugs such as streptokinase and tissue plasminogen activator (alteplase, recombinant; t-PA), which activate the fibrinolytic system, are effective when used immediately after thrombosis in causing lysis of the thrombus and re-establishing perfusion. They have been used with some success in the treatment of acute myocardial infarction, deep vein thrombosis, and acute peripheral arterial thrombosis.

B. Organization and Recanalization

Organization and recanalization commonly occur in large thrombi. Slow liquefaction and phagocytosis of the thrombus are followed by in growth of granulation tissue and collagenization (organization). The vessels in the granulation tissue frequently enlarge, and may establish new channels across the thrombus (recanalization) (Figure 3-12) through which some blood flow maybe restored. Recanalization occurs slowly over several weeks, and although it does not prevent the acute effects of thrombosis, it may slightly improve tissue perfusion over the long term (Figure 3-12).

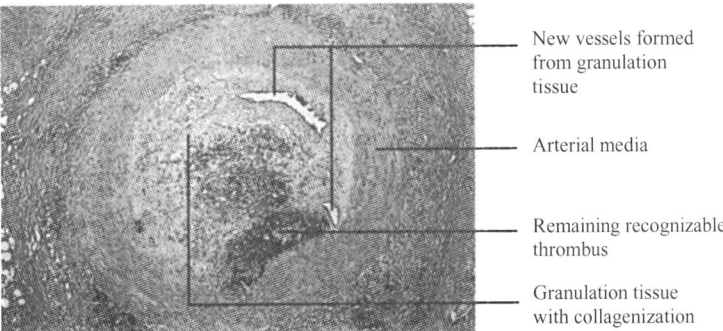

Figure 3-12 Early organization and recanalization of a thrombosed vessel. As the process progresses, the thrombus is completely replaced by collagen and the vascular channels in the granulation tissue dilate

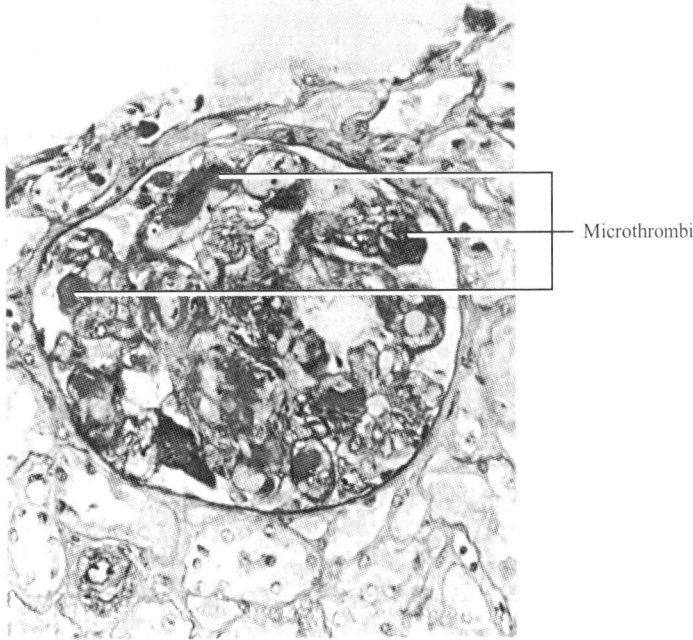

Figure 3-13 Disseminated intravascular coagulation(DIC). Numerous microthrombi are seen in glomerular capillaries

C. Thromboembolism

Sometimes a fragment of thrombus is detached and carried in the circulation to lodge at a distant site – a process termed thromboembolism (see below).

DISSEMINATED INTRAVASCULAR COAGULATION (DIC)

Disseminated intravascular coagulation is the widespread development of small thrombi in the microcirculation throughout the body (Figure 3-13). It is a serious and often fatal complication of numerous diseases and requires early recognition and treatment.

CAUSES (TABLE 3-1)

In many cases, the cause of disseminated intravascular coagulation is unknown. Diffuse endothelial injury, as occurs in infections due to gram-negative bacteria (gram-negative sepsis, endotoxic shock), is a common cause. Viral and rickettsial infections may result in direct infection and damage to endothelial cells. Immunologic injury to the endothelium, as occurs in type II and type III hypersensitivity, may also precipitate DIC. Disseminated intravascular coagulation may occur when thromboplastic substances enter the circulation, as occurs in amniotic fluid embolism (amniotic fluid contains thromboplastin, which has procoagulant activity), snakebite (particularly Russell's viper), promyelocytic leukemia (the promyelocytes contain thromboplastic substances), and any condition associated with extensive tissue necrosis.

EFFECTS (FIGURE 3-14)

A. Decreased Tissue Perfusion

The multiple occlusions of the microcirculation in disseminated intravascular coagulation result in widespread impaired tissue perfusion, leading to shock, accumulation of lactic acid, and micro infarction in many organs. Note that the disseminated thrombi may not be demonstrable at autopsy owing to concurrent fibrinolytic activity (see below).

B. Bleeding

Disseminated thrombosis also results in the consumption of coagulation factors in the blood (consumption coagulopathy). Paradoxically, thrombocytopenia develops and, together with depletion of fi-

Table 3-1 Disorders associated with disseminated intravascular coagulation (DIC)

Infectious diseases
Gram-negative bacteremia
Meningococcal sepsis
Gram-positive bacteremia
Disseminated fungal infections
Rickettsial infections
Severe viremias (e.g. hemorrhagic fevers)
Plasmodium falciparum malaria
Neonatal and intrauterine infections
Obstetric disorders
Aminotic fluid embolism
Retained dead fetus
Abruptio placentae
Liver diseases
Massive liver cell necrosis
Cirrhosis of the liver
Malignant diseases
Acute promyelocytic leukemia
Metastatic carcinoma, mainly adenocarcinoma
Miscellaneous disorders
Small vessel vasculitides
Massive trauma
Burns
Heat stroke
Surgery with extracorporeal circulation
Snakebite (Russell's viper)
Intravascular hemolysis

brinogen and other coagulation factors, leads to abnormal bleeding. This bleeding tendency is aggravated by excessive activation of the fibrinolytic system (activation of Hageman factor XII, which initiates the intrinsic coagulation pathway, also leads to conversion of plasminogen to plasmin). Fibrin degradation products resulting from the action of plasminon fibrin also have anticoagulant properties, further exacerbating the bleeding tendency. In many patients with disseminated intravascular coagulation, the predominant clinical effect is hemorrhage.

TREATMENT

Treatment includes heparin to inhibit the formation of thrombi as well as administration of platelets and plasma to restore the depleted coagulation factors. Monitoring the levels of fibrin degradation products, fibrinogen, and platelets aids diagnosis and assesses the effectiveness of therapy.

EMBOLISM

Embolism is the occlusion or obstruction of a vessel by an abnormal mass (solid, liquid, or gaseous)

Chapter 3 Hemodynamic Disorders and Abnormalities of Blood Supply

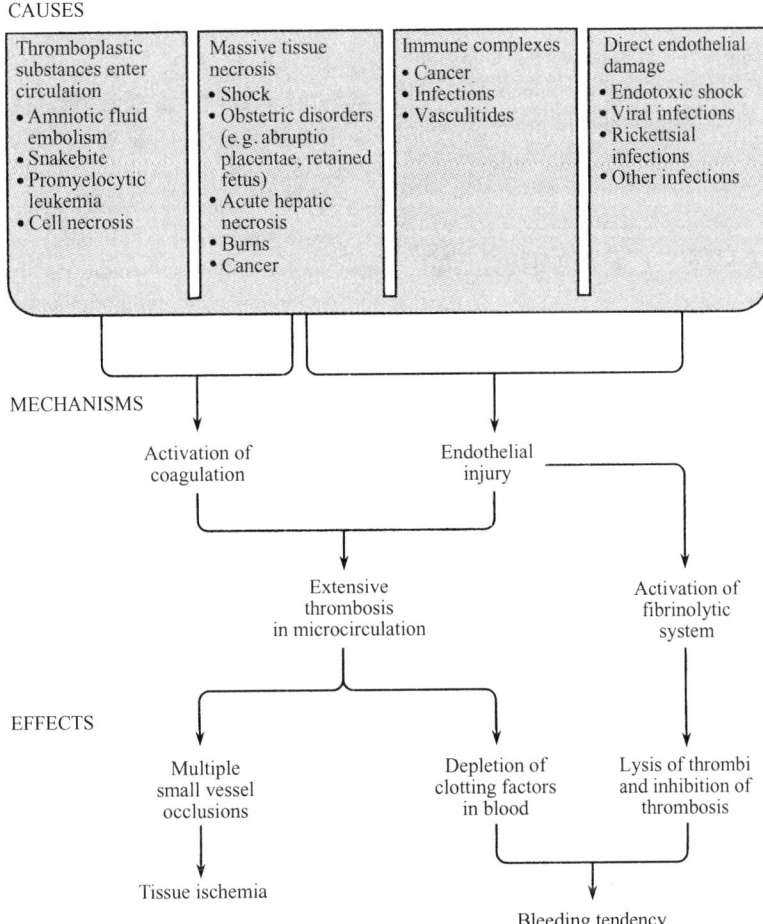

Figure 3-14 Initiating factors and mechanisms in disseminated intravascular coagulation (DIC). A key difference between DIC and normal thrombus formation is that in DIC both coagulation and fibrinolysis occur diffusely throughout the microcirculation – in contrast to the more localized nature of normal thrombosis. In some instances, thrombosis predominates, resulting in ischemic effects; in others, fibrinolysis predominates, resulting in hemorrhage

transported from a different site by the circulation. Most emboli are detached fragments of thrombi that are carried in the bloodstream to their sites of lodgment (thromboembolism). Numerous other substances serve as less common causes of embolism.

ORIGIN OF EMBOLI

The site of embolism is governed by the point of origin and size of the embolus.

A. Origin in Systemic Veins

Emboli that originate in systemic veins (as a result of venous thrombosis) or in the right side of the heart (e.g. infective endocarditis affecting the tricuspid valve) lodge in the pulmonary arterial system unless they are so small (e.g. fat globules, tumor cells) that they can pass through the pulmonary capillaries. The point of lodgment in the pulmonary arterial circulation depends on the size of the embolus (see below). Rarely, an embolus originating in a systemic vein passes across a defect in the cardiac interatrial or interventricular septum (thus bypassing the lungs) to lodge in a systemic artery (paradoxic embolism).

Emboli that originate in branches of the portal vein lodge in the liver, e.g. cancer cells from colonic or pancreatic cancer.

B. Origin in Heart and Systemic Arteries

Emboli originating in the left side of the heart and systemic arteries (as a result of cardiac or arterial thrombosis) lodge in a distal systemic artery in sites such as the brain, heart, kidney, extremity, intestine, etc.

TYPES AND SITES OF EMBOLISM (TABLE 3-2)

A. Thromboembolism

Detached fragments of thrombi are the most common cause of clinically significant embolism.

1. Pulmonary embolism

a. Causes and incidence: The most serious form of thromboembolism is pulmonary embolism, which may cause sudden death. Pulmonary embolism has an incidence of 20 to 25 per 100,000 hospitalized patients. Although the rate of fatal pulmonary emboli (as assessed at autopsy) has declined from 6% to 2% over the last quarter century, pulmonary embolism still causes about 200,000 deaths per year in the United States. Over 95% of pulmonary emboli originate in the deep veins of the leg (phlebothrombosis). More rarely, thrombi in pelvic venous plexuses are the source. Pulmonary embolism is common in the following conditions that predispose to the development of phlebothrombosis: (1) The immediate postoperative period. About 30%-50% of patients show evidence of deep vein thrombosis after major surgery. Only a small number of these patients develop clinically significant pulmonary embolism. (2) The immediate postpartum period. (3) Lengthy immobilization in bed. (4) Cardiac failure. (5) Use of oral contraceptives.

b. Clinical effects (Figure 3-15-1 and Figure 3-15-2): The size of the embolus is the factor most influencing the clinical effects of pulmonary embolism.

Table 3-2 Types of embolism

Origin and Type of Embolism	Circulatory System Involved	Clinical Effect

Thrombi in right side of heart and systemic veins
  Deep vein thrombosis
  Right-sided infective endocarditis
	Pulmonary	Circulatory arrest, lung infarction
		Pulmonary hypertension

Thrombi in left side of heart and systemic veins
  Cardiac valvular vegetations
  Cardiac mural thrombus
  Cardiac artrial thrombus
  Cardiac aneurysmal thrombus
  Aortic aneurysmal thrombus
	Systemic	Infarction in brain, kidney, intestine, peripheral arteries

Air embolism
  Puncture of jugular vein
  Childbirth of abortion
  Blood transfusion using positive pressure
  Pneumothorax
	Pulmonary (right ventricle)	Total obstruction of pulmonary flow causes sudden death

Nitrogen gas embolism Decompression sickness	Pulmonary and systemic	Ischemia in lung, brain, nerves
Fat embolism Trauma (i.e. serious fractures of large bones)	Mostly pulmonary; some fat globules pass to systemic	Microinfarcts and hemorrhages in lung, brain, skin
Bone marrow embolism Trauma	Pulmonary	No clinical significance
Atheromatous embolism Ulcerated atheromatous plaque	Systemic	Microinfarcts in lung, kidney
Amniotic fluid embolism Childbirth	Pulmonary	DIC
Tumor embolism	Depends on location of tumor	Metastasis

Chapter 3 Hemodynamic Disorders and Abnormalities of Blood Supply · 63 ·

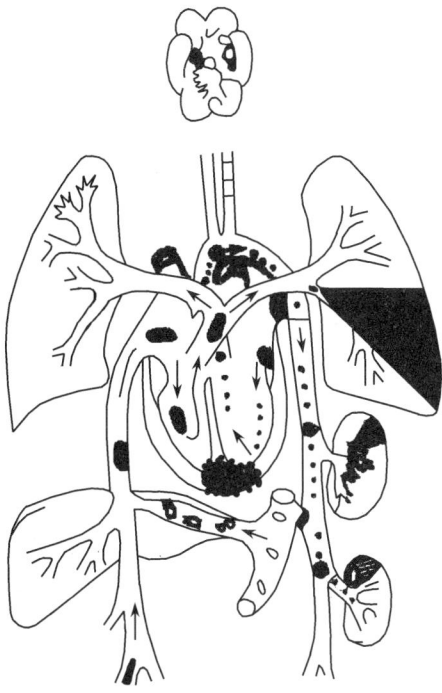

Figure 3-15-1 Embolus of different sites: Embolus in the vein can cause pulmonary infarction through the right ventricle; while those from the arteries can cause cardio infarcion and renal infarction. And according to the pattern of blood supply, each of these lesions have its unique shape

- **Massive emboli**: Large emboli (several centimeters long and of the same diameter as the femoral vein) may lodge in the outflow tract of the right ventricle or in the main pulmonary artery, where they cause circulatory obstruction and sudden death (Figure 3-16). Large emboli lodging in a large branch of the pulmonary artery may also cause sudden death, probably as a result of severe vasoconstriction of the entire pulmonary arterial circulation induced reflexly by lodgment of the embolus (Figure 3-17).
- **Medium-sized emboli**: Moderate-sized emboli often lodge in a major branch of the pulmonary artery. In healthy individuals, the bronchial artery supplies blood (and oxygen) to the lung, and the function of the pulmonary artery is mainly gas exchange (not local tissue oxygenation). In a normal person, therefore, a moderate-sized pulmonary embolus creates an area of lung that is ventilated but not perfused with regard to gas exchange. This results in abnormal gas exchange and hypoxemia, but infarction of the lung does not occur. In a patient with chronic left heart failure or pulmonary vascular disease, however, the bronchial arterial circulation is impaired, and the lung is therefore dependent on the pulmonary artery for perfusion of tissue as well as gas exchange. In these patients, obstruction of a pulmonary artery by a moderate-sized embolus results in **pulmonary infarction.**

- **Small emboli**: Small emboli lodge in minor branches of the pulmonary artery with no immediate effects (Figure 3-18). In many instances, the emboli either fragment soon after lodgment or dissolve during fibrinolysis, in which case clinical effects are minimal. If numerous small emboli occur over a long period, however, the pulmonary microcirculation may be so severely compromised that pulmonary hypertension results.

2. Systemic arterial embolism

a. Causes: Thromboembolism occurs in systemic arteries when the detached thrombus originates in the left side of the heart or a large artery. Systemic arterial thromboembolism commonly occurs (1) in patients who have infective endocarditis with vegetations on the mitral and aortic valves; (2) in patients who have suffered myocardial infarction in which mural thrombosis has occurred; (3) in patients with mitral stenosis and atrial fibrillation due to left atrial thrombosis; and (4) in patients with aortic and ventricular aneurysms, which often contain mural thrombi. Thromboemboli from any of these locations pass distally to lodge in an artery of some other organ. Because of the anatomy of the aorta, cardiac emboli tend to pass more frequently into the lower extremities or into the circulation derived from the right internal carotid artery than into other systemic arteries.

b. Clinical effects: The clinical effects of systemic thromboembolism are governed by the size of the obstructed vessel, the availability of collateral arterial circulation, and the susceptibility of the tissue to ischemia. Infarction is common when emboli lodge in the arteries of the brain, heart, kidney, and spleen. Infarction occurs in the intestine and lower extremities only when large arteries are occluded or when the collateral circulation in these tissues is compromised.

B. Air Embolism

Air embolism occurs when enough air bubbles enter the vascular system to produce clinical sympt-

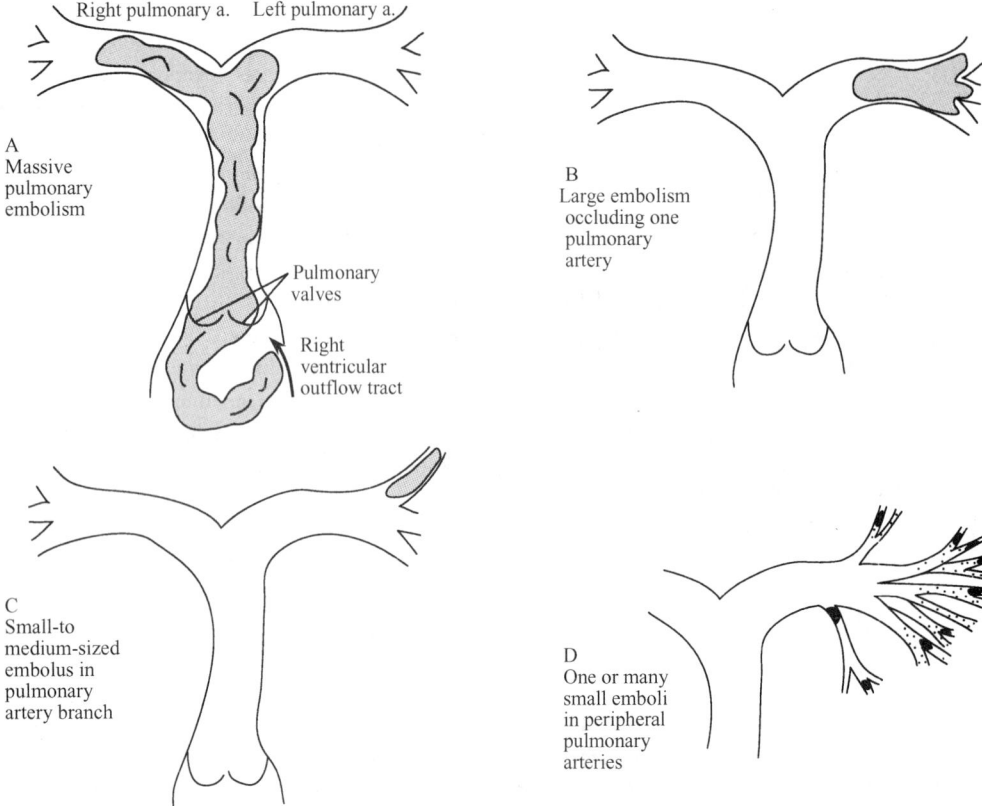

Figure 3-15-2   Clinical effects of pulmonary embolism. A: Massive pulmonary embolism causes circulatory arrest and sudden death (Figure 3-16). B: A large embolism occluding one pulmonary artery may cause pulmonary infarction or sudden death due to reflex vasoconstriction of the pulmonary circulation (See Figure 3-17). Some healthy indivduals may show no ill effects, but this is unusual with a large embolism. C: A small to medium-sized embolus in a pulmonary arterial branch typically has no effect in healthy individuals. Pulmonary infarction may occur if the bronchial circulation is compromised, as in patients with left heart failure and pulmonary hypertension. D: Small emboli have no effect unless they are numerous, in which case they may cause pulmonary hypertension

oms; about 150 mL of air causes death. The condition is rare.

1. Causes

• **Surgery of or trauma to internal jugular vein**: In injuries to the internal jugular vein, the negative pressure in the thorax tends to suck air into the jugular vein. This phenomenon does not occur in injuries to other systemic veins because they are separated by valves from the negative pressure in the chest.

• **Childbirth or abortion**: Air embolism may occur during childbirth or abortion, when air may be forced into ruptured placental venous sinuses by the forceful contractions of the uterus.

• **Blood transfusions**: Air embolism during blood transfusions occurs only if positive pressure is used to transfuse the blood and only if the transfusion is inadvertently not discontinued at its completion. The use of collapsible plastic packs for blood transfusion has greatly reduced the risk of this catastrophe.

2. Clinical effects

When air enters the blood-stream, it passes into the right ventricle, creating a frothy mixture that effectively obstructs the circulation and causes death. More rarely, the frothy air-blood mixture obstructs a pulmonary artery.

C. Nitrogen Gas Embolism (Decompression Sickness)

1. Cause

Decompression sickness is a form of embolism that

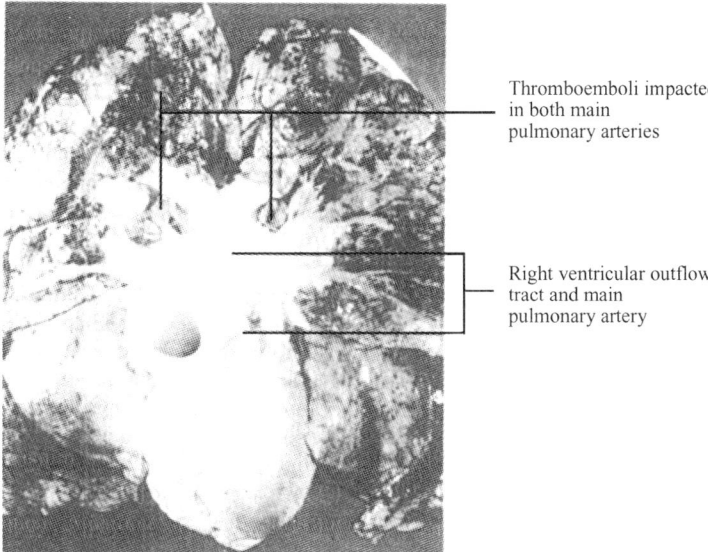

Figure 3-16 Massive pulmonary embolism. The main pulmonary artery has been opened and shows impacted thromboemboli at the orifices of both right and left main pulmonary arteries. This led to sudden death from circulatory obstruction. *Note*: When the pulmonary arteries were further opened, the emboli were seen to be very large. Only their tips are shown here

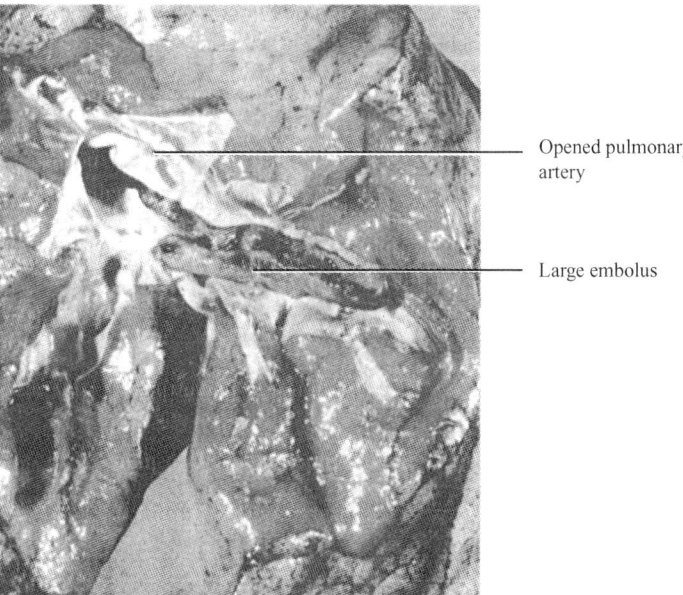

Figure 3-17 Pulmonary embolism. The pulmonary artery has been opened to reveal a large thromboembolus within it. Note the branching of the embolus, probably corresponding to the configuration of the vein in which it originated

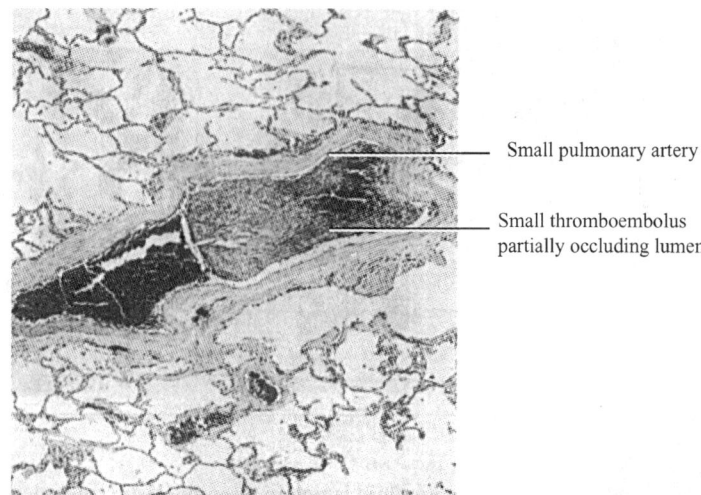

Figure 3-18 Pulmonary thromboembolism partially occluding a small branch of the pulmonary artery in the lung. This has no immediate effect, but pulmonary hypertension may result if recurrent and numerous emboli occur

occurs in caisson workers and under-sea divers if they ascend too rapidly after being submerged for long periods. The disorder is also called the bends or caisson disease (caissons are high-pressure underwater chambers used for deep water construction work). When air is breathed under high underwater pressure, an increased volume of air, mainly oxygen and nitrogen, goes into solution in the blood and equilibrates with the tissues.

If decompression to sea level is too rapid, the gases that have equilibrated in the tissues come out of solution. Oxygen is rapidly absorbed into the blood, but nitrogen gas coming out of solution cannot be absorbed rapidly enough and forms bubbles in the tissues and bloodstream that act as emboli.

Scuba divers breathing high-pressure compressed air who ascend rapidly from depths as shallow as 10m may also develop decompression sickness, and those who engage in this recreational activity should be taught and cautioned to ascend slowly.

Decompression sickness can also occur in unpressurized aircraft if they ascend too rapidly to high altitudes (above 2000 m). Mountain climbers who climb too rapidly to high altitudes are also at risk.

2. Clinical effects

Platelets adhere to nitrogen gas bubbles in the circulation and activate the coagulation cascade. The resulting disseminated intravascular thrombosis aggravates the ischemic state caused by impaction of gas bubbles in capillaries. Involvement of the brain in severe cases may cause extensive necrosis and death. In less severe cases, nerve and muscle involvement causes severe muscle contractions with Intense pain (the bends). Nitrogen gas emboli in the lungs cause severe difficulty in breathing (the chokes) that is associated with alveolar edema and hemorrhage.

D. Fat Embolism

1. Causes

Fat embolism occurs when globules of fat enter the bloodstream, typically after fractures of large bones (e.g. femur) have exposed the fatty bone marrow. Rarely, extensive injury to subcutaneous adipose tissue causes fat embolism. Although fat globules can be found in the circulation in as many as 90% of patients who have sustained serious fractures, few patients demonstrate clinically significant signs of fat embolism.

Although simple mechanical rupture of fat cells at trauma sites may explain how fat globules can enter the circulation, other factors are probably involved. It has been shown that fat globules enlarge once they are in the circulation, which explains why small globules that bypass lung capillaries may later become obstructed in systemic capillaries. It is thought that release of catecholamines due to the stress of trauma mobilizes free fatty acids, which coalesce to form progressively enlarging fat globules. Adhesion of platelets to fat globules further increases their size and causes thrombosis. When this process is extensive, it is equivalent to disseminated intravascular coagulation.

2. Clinical effects

Circulating fat globules first encounter the capillary network of the lung. Larger fat globules (> 20 μm) are arrested in the lung and cause respiratory distress (dyspnea and abnormal gas exchange). Smaller fat globules escape the lung capillaries and pass into the systemic circulation, where they may obstruct small systemic arteries. Typical clinical features of fat embolism include a hemorrhagic skin rash and brain involvement manifested as acute diffuse neurologic dysfunction.

The possibility of fat embolism must be considered if respiratory distress, cerebral dysfunction, and a hemorrhagic rash occurs 1 - 3 days after major trauma. The diagnosis can be confirmed by demonstrating fat globules in urine and sputum. About 10% of patients with clinical fat embolism die. At autopsy, fat globules can be demonstrated in many organs using frozen sections and special fat stains (e.g. oil red O).

E. Bone Marrow Embolism

Fragments of bone marrow containing fat and hematopoietic cells may enter the circulation after traumatic injury of bone marrow and may be found in the pulmonary arteries of patients who have suffered rib fractures during-cardiopulmonary resuscitative efforts. Bone marrow embolism is of no clinical significance.

F. Atheromatous (Cholesterol) Embolism

Large ulcerated atheromatous plaques often release cholesterol and other atheromatous material into the circulation (Figure 3-19). Emboli are carried distally to lodge in small systemic arteries. Such embolization in brain produces transient ischemic attacks, characterized by reversible acute episodes of neurologic dysfunction.

G. Amniotic Fluid Embolism

The contents of the amniotic sac may rarely (1:80,000 pregnancies) enter ruptured uterine venous sinuses during tumultuous labor in childbirth. Although rare, amniotic fluid embolism is associated with a mortality rate of about 80% and is a significant cause of maternal deaths. Amniotic fluid is rich in thromboplastic substances that induce disseminated intravascular coagulation, which is the main mechanism by which the disorder is manifested clinically.

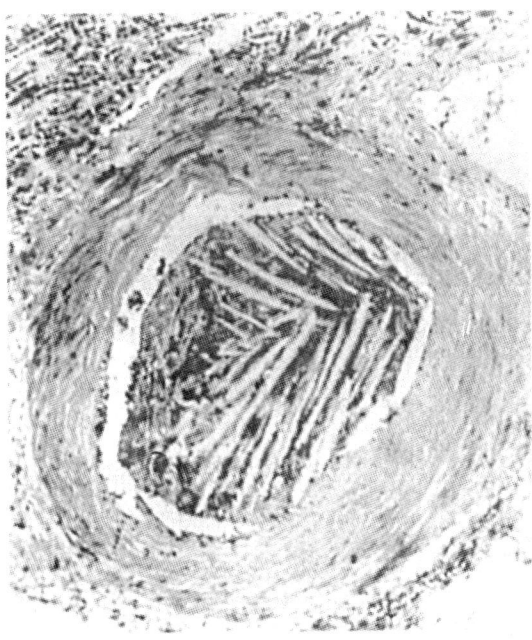

Figure 3-19 Cholesterol embolus derived from an ulcerated atheromatous plaque lodged in a branch of the renal artery

Amniotic fluid also contains fetal squamous epithelium (desquamated from the skin), fetal hair, fetal fat, mucin, and meconium, all of which may undergo embolization and become lodged in the pulmonary capillaries, a finding that is useful in makingan autopsy diagnosis of amniotic fluid embolism (Figure 3-20).

H. Tumor Embolism

Cancer cells often enter the circulation during metastasis of malignant tumors (see Chapter of Neoplasia). Typically, these solitary cells or small clumps of cells are too small to obstruct the vasculature. Occasionally, larger fragments of tumor constitute significant emboli-with renal carcinoma, especially in the inferior vena cava; and with hepatic carcinoma, especially in the hepatic veins.

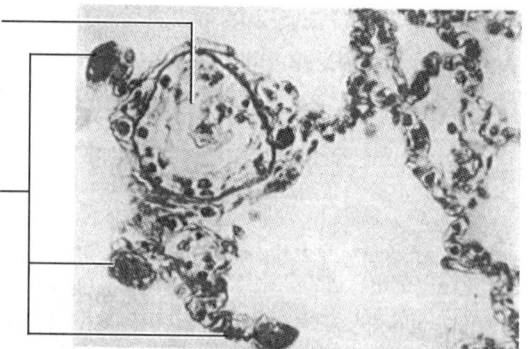

Figure 3-20 Amniotic fluid embolism of lung

INFARCTION

Infarction is the development of an area of localized necrosis in a tissue resulting from sudden reduction of its blood supply (Figure 3-21). Both parenchymal cells and interstitial tissue undergo necrosis. Infarction is most commonly due to arterial obstruction by thrombosis or embolism. More rarely, obstruction of venous drainage results in infarction.

CLASSIFICATION OF INFARCTS

The appearance of an infarct varies with the site. Various classification schemes are used.

A. Pale Versus Red

Pale (white, anemic) infarcts (Figure 3-21) occur as a result of arterial obstruction in solid organs such as the heart, kidney, spleen, and brain that lack significant collateral circulation. The continuing venous drainage of blood from the ischemic tissue accounts for the pallor of such infarcts.

Red (or hemorrhagic) infarcts are found in tissues that have a double blood supply - eg, lung and liver - or in tissues such as intestine that have collateral vessels permitting some continued flow into the area although the amount is not sufficient to prevent infarction. The infarct is red because of extravasation of blood in the infarcted area from necrotic small vessels.

Red infarcts may also occur in tissue if dissolution or fragmentation of the occluding thrombus permits reestablishment of arterial flow to the infarcted area. Venous infarcts are always associated with congestion and hemorrhage. They are red infarcts (Figure 3-22).

B. Solid Versus Liquefied

In all tissues other than brain, infarction usually produces coagulative necrosis of cells. leading to a solid infarct (see Chapter 1). In brain, on the other hand, liquefactive necrosis of cells leads to the formation of a fluid mass in the area of infarction. The end result is frequently a cystic cavity (Figure 3-23).

C. Sterile Versus Septic

Most infarcts are sterile. Septic infarcts are characterized by secondary bacterial infection of the necrotic tissue. Septic infarcts occur (1) when microorganisms are present in the occluding thrombus or embolus, e. g. emboli in acute infective endocarditis; or (2) when infarction occurs in a tissue (e. g. intestine) that normally contains bacteria; or (3) when bacteria from the blood-stream cause secondary infection (this is unusual because blood is normally sterile). Septic infarcts are characterized by acute inflammation that frequently converts the infarct to an abscess. Secondary bacterial infection of an infarct may also result in gangrene (e. g. in the intestine).

MORPHOLOGY OF INFARCTS

Infarction occurs in tissue supplied by an artery that, when occluded, leaves an insufficient collateral blood supply (Figure 3-24). Infarcts in kidney, spleen, and lung are wedge-shaped, with the occluded artery situated near the apex of the wedge and

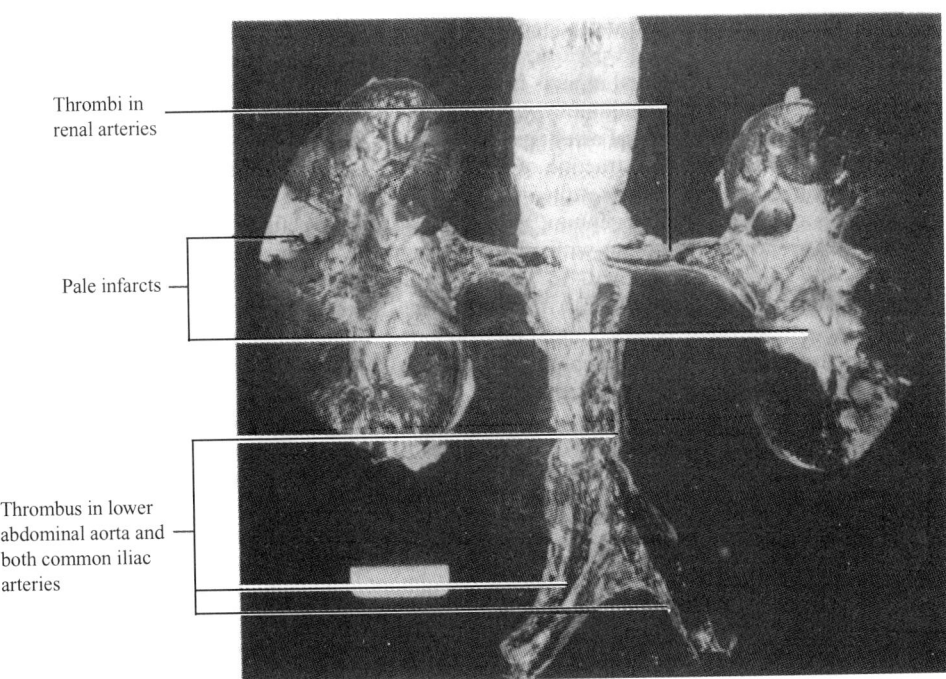

Figure 3-21 Bilateral renal infarction secondary to renal artery thrombosis. The infarcts are pale and wedge-shaped. Note the presence of extensive thrombosis at the bifurcation of the aorta

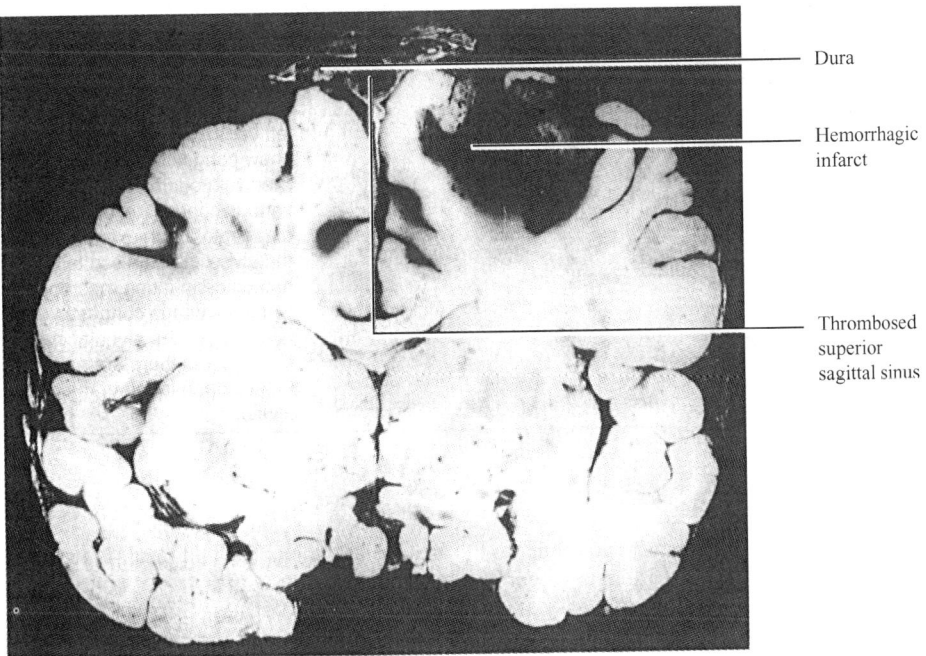

Figure 3-22 Hemorrhagic infarction of the parasagittal region of one cerebral hemisphere secondary to thrombotic occlusion of the superior sagittal sinus

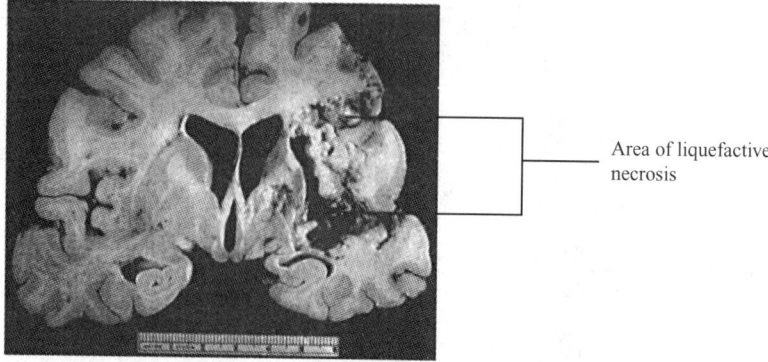

Figure 3-23 Cerebral infarct. The involved area has been converted to a fluid-filled cyst

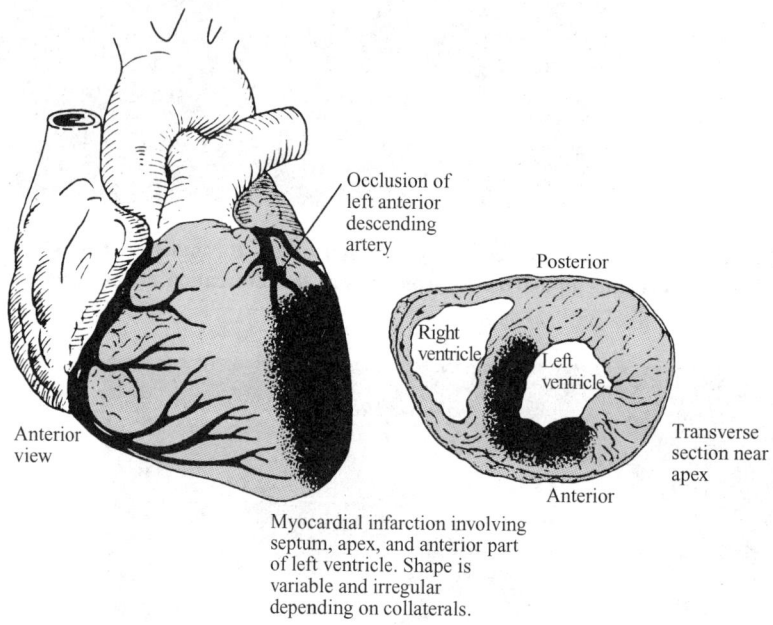

Figure 3-24 Distribution of infarction in the myocardium following acute occlusion of the left anterior descending artery. In cases where collaterals have developed, the infarcted area may be much smaller

the base of the infarct located on the surface of the organ. The characteristic shape of infarcts in these organs is due to the symmetric dichotomous branching pattern of the arteries supplying them.

The shape of cerebral and myocardial infarcts is irregular and determined by the distribution of the occluded artery and the limits of collateral arterial supply (Chapter 6). In some patients, obstruction of the left anterior descending coronary artery results in infarction of the anterior inter ventricular septum, apex, and anterolateral left ventricle; in patients with extensive collaterals, the infarcted area may be much smaller. The thickness of the infarct is similarly variable. Intestinal infarcts develop in loops of bowel in accordance with the pattern of arterial supply. The most common infarcts of the intestine occur in the small intestine as a result of occlusion of the superior mesenteric artery.

VENOUS INFARCTION

Venous infarction results when total occlusion of all venous drainage from a tissue occurs (e.g. superior sagittal sinus thrombosis (Figure 3-22), renal vein thrombosis, superior mesenteric vein thrombosis). The result is severe edema, congestion, hemorrhage, and a progressive increase in tissue hydrostatic pressure. When tissue hydrostatic pressure increases sufficiently, arterial blood flow into the tissue is obstructed, leading to ischemia and infarction. Venous infarcts are always hemorrhagic (see Classification of Infarcts, below). Special types of venous infarction occur in strangulation, in which constriction of the neck of a hernial sac results in infarction of the contents of the sac; and torsion, where twisting of the pedicle of an organ, most commonly the testis, results in venous obstruction and hemorrhagic infarction.

FACTORS THAT INFLUENCE DEVELOPMENT OF AN INFARCT

The consequences of a vascular occlusion can range from no or minimal effect, all the way up to death of a tissue or even the individual. The major determinants are as follows:

A. Nature of the Vascular Supply

The availability of an alternative blood supply is the most important factor in determining whether occlusion of a vessel will cause damage. For example, lungs have a dual pulmonary and bronchial artery blood supply; thus, obstruction of small pulmonary arterioles does not cause infarction in an otherwise healthy individual with an intact bronchial circulation. Similarly, the liver, with its dual hepatic artery and portal vein circulation, and the hand and forearm, with their dual radial and ulnar arterial supply, are all relatively resistant to infarction. In contrast, renal and splenic circulations are end-arterial, and obstruction of such vessels generally causes infarction.

B. Rate of Development of Occlusion

Slowly developing occlusions are less likely to cause infarction because they provide time for the development of alternative pathways of flow. For example, small interarteriolar anastomoses, normally with minimal functional flow, interconnect the three major coronary arteries in the heart. If one of the coronaries is only slowly occluded (e.g. by an encroaching atherosclerotic plaque), flow within this collateral circulation may increase sufficiently to prevent infarction, even though the major coronary artery is eventually occluded.

C. Vulnerability to Hypoxia

The susceptibility of a tissue to hypoxia influences the likelihood of infarction. Neurons undergo irreversible damage when deprived of their blood supply for only 3 to 4 minutes. Myocardial cells, although hardier than neurons, are also quite sensitive and die after only 20 to 30 minutes of ischemia. In contrast, fibroblasts within myocardium remain viable after many hours of ischemia.

D. Oxygen Content of Blood

The partial pressure of oxygen in blood also determines the outcome of vascular occlusion. Partial flow obstruction of a small vessel in an anemic or cyanotic patient might lead to tissue infarction, whereas it would be without effect under conditions of normal oxygen tension. In this way, congestive heart failure, with compromised flow and ventilation, could cause infarction in the setting of an otherwise inconsequential blockage.

EVOLUTION OF INFARCTS (FIGURE 3-25)

An infarct is an irreversible tissue injury characterized by necrosis of both parenchymal cells and the connective tissue framework. Necrosis induces an acute inflammatory response in the surrounding tissue, with congestion (forming a red rim around a pale infarct in the first few days) and neutrophil emigration (Figures 3-25 and 3-26). Lysosomal enzymes from neutrophils then cause lysis of the infarcted area (heterolysis), and macrophages phagocytose the liquefied debris. In growth of granulation tissue occurs. Acute inflammatory cells are replaced by lymphocytes and macrophages as active necrosis ceases. Lymphocytes and plasma cells probably represent an immune response to the release of endogenous cellular antigens.

Collagen production by fibroblasts in the granulation tissue ultimately leads to scar formation. Because of contraction, the resulting scar is much smaller than the area of the original infarct. Cytokines released by chronic inflammatory cells are partly responsible for stimulating fibrosis and neovascularization (Chapter 2).

Evolution of a **cerebral infarct** differs from the above (Chapter 14). Necrotic cells undergo liquefac-

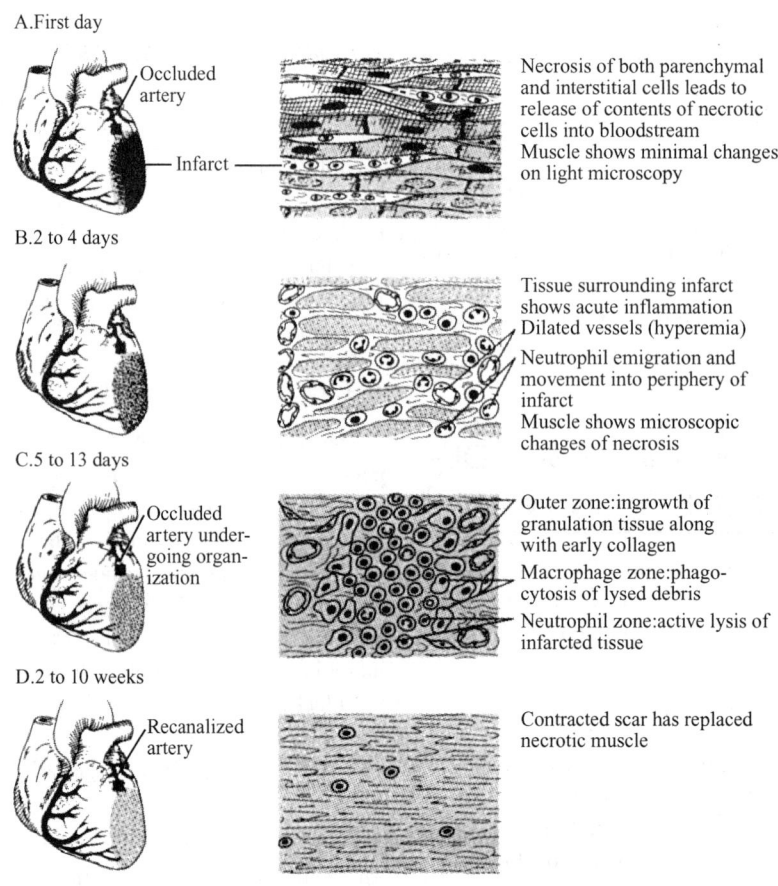

Figure 3-25 Evolution of a myocardial infarct

tion because of their enzyme content (autolysis). Neutrophils are less conspicuous than in infarcts of other tissues. Liquefied brain cells are phagocytosed by special macrophages (microglia), which become distended with foamy, pale cytoplasm (Figure 3-27). The infarcted area is converted into a fluid-filled cystic cavity that becomes walled off by proliferation of reactive astrocytes (a process termed gliosis, which represents the cerebral analogue of fibrosis). The rate of evolution of an infarct and the time required for complete healing vary with size. A small infarct may heal within 1 – 2 weeks, whereas healing of a larger one may take 6 – 8 weeks or longer. Evaluation of the gross and microscopic changes in an infarcted area enables the pathologist to assess the age of an infarct, which is an important consideration at autopsy in establishing the sequence of events that caused death.

SHOCK

Shock is a clinical state characterized by a generalized decrease in perfusion of tissues associated with decrease in effective cardiac output.

Causes

A. Hypovolemia (decrease blood volume)

Hypovolemia may be due to hemorrhage or excessive fluid loss, as occurs in diarrhea, vomiting, burns, dehydration, or excessive sweating.

B. Peripheral Vasodilatation

Widespread dilation of small vessels leads to excessive pooling of blood in peripheral capacitance vessels, due to the caution of metabolic, toxic, or neurotrogenic stimuli during anesthesia or spinal cord injury. The result is reduction of the effective blood volume and therefore a decreased cardiac output (peripheral circulatory failure).

C. Cardiogenic Shock

Cardiogenic shock results from a severe reduction in

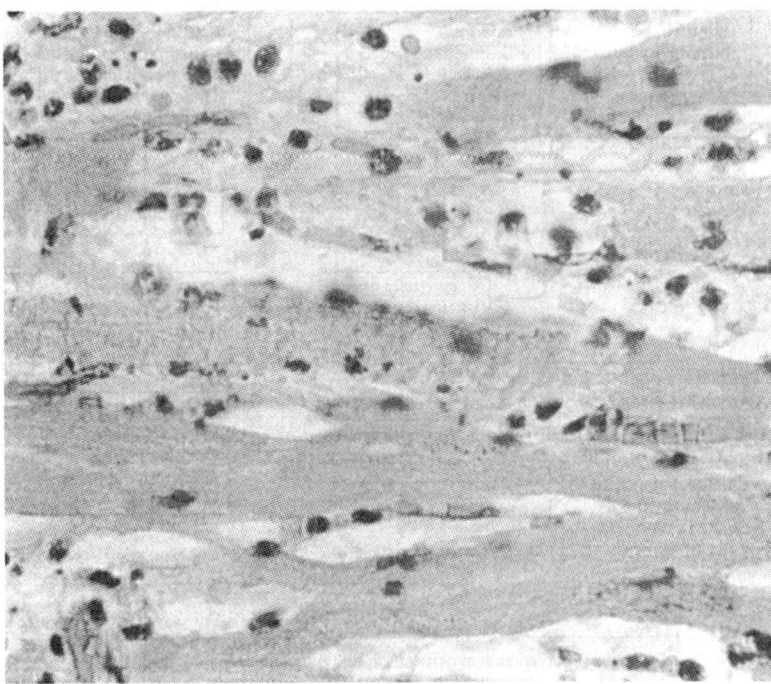

Figure 3-26 Myocardial infarct 2-4 days old, showing infiltration of the infarcted area by neutrophils. Note early of the muscle fibers

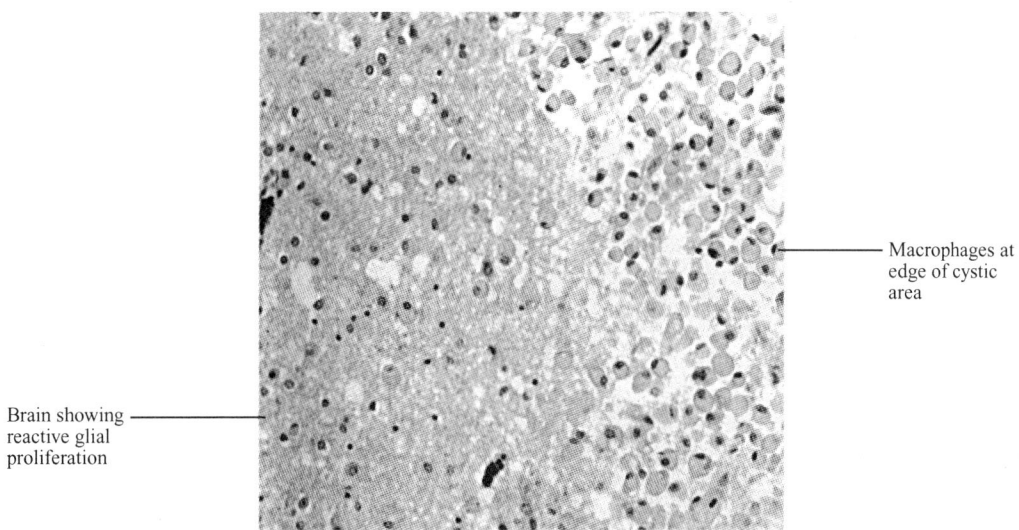

Figure 3-27 Edge of a cerebral infarct, showing the lining of the cystic cavity

cardiac output due to primary cardiac disease, e. g. acute myocardiac infarction, acute myocarditis, and certain arrhythmias.

D. Obstructive Shock

Obstruction to blood flow in the heart or main pulmonary artery, e. g. massive pulmonary embolism or a large left atrial thrombus impacting in the mitral valve orifice, causes obstructive shock. Severely impaired filling of the ventricles produces a significant fall in cardiac output.

Clinicopathologic Features

A. Stages of Compensation

Compensatory mechanisms activated by a decrease in cardiac output include reflex sympathetic stimulation, which increases the heart rate (tachycardia) and causes peripheral vasoconstriction to maintain blood pressure in vital organs (brain and myocardium). The earliest clinical evidence of shock is a rapid, low-volume pulse (thread).

Some less vital tissues e. g. skin, becomes cold and clammy. Vasoconstriction in renal arterioles decreases the pressure and rate of glomerular filtration, with resulting decreased urine output (oliguria). Both representing early stage of shock.

B. Stage of Impaired Tissue Perfusion

Prolonged excessive vasoconstriction is harmful because it impairs tissues perfusion, tissue fluid exchange and oxygenation, and leads to sludging, which further impedes capillary blood flow.

Impaired tissue perfusion has several adverse effects. It promotes anaerobic glycolysys, leading a production of lactic acid and lactic acidosis, which is almost always present in shock. Impaired tissue perfusion, if severe or sustained, produces cell necrosis, most apparent in the kidney – acute renal tubular necrosis (figure 9-11), and in the lung, acute alveolar damage (shock lung) (figure 9-12); in the liver, anoxic necrosis of the central region hepatic lobules. Ischemia necrosis of the intestine is important because it is frequently associated with hemorrhage or release of bacterial endotoxins that further aggravate the shock state.

C. Stage of Decompensation

As a result of increasing capillary hypoxia and acidosis, there is a progressive fall in blood pressure (hypotension). Cerebral hypoxia then causes acute brain dysfunction, (loss of consciousness, edema, neuronal degeneration). Myocardial hypoxia leads to further diminution of cardiac output, and death may occur rapidly.

Prognosis

The prognosis for a patient in shock depends on several factors. When this can be treated most patients survive even if they are in an advanced stage of shock when first seen. In the recovered patients, necrotic cells-renal tubular cells and alveolar epithelial cells usually regenerate, regaining normal function. Patients who die are those in whom the cause of shock cannot be ealily corrected.

Chapter 4 Inflammation

Jiang Xucheng

CHAPTER CONTENTS
- Introduction to Inflammation
   - Conception of Inflammation
   - Cardinal Clinical Signs
   - Systemic Clinical Signs
- Acute Inflammation
   - Morphologic and Functional Changes
   - Mediators of Acute Inflammation
   - Types of Acute Inflammation
   - Course of Acute Inflammation
   - Diagnosis of Acute Inflammation
- Chronic Inflammation
   - Chronic Inflammation in Response to Antigenic Injurious Agents
   - Chronic Inflammation in Response to Non-antigenic Injurious Agents
   - Function and Result of Chronic Inflammation
   - Mixed Acute and Chronic Inflammation
   - Chronic Suppurative Inflammation
   - Recurrent Acute Inflammation
   - Clinical and Pathologic Diagnosis

INTRODUCTION TO INFLAMMATION

CONCEPTION OF INFLAMMATION

Inflammation is a complex reaction to injurious agents that consists of vascular response, cellular reaction, and systemic reactions. Inflammation is fundamentally a defensive response.

Inflammation is divided into acute inflammation and chronic inflammation based on the process and duration of the response.

CARDINAL CLINICAL SIGNS

Clinically, acute inflammation is characterized by 5 cardinal signs: **rubor** (redness), **calor** (increased heat), **tumor** (swelling), **dolor** (pain) and **functio laesa** (loss of function) (Figure 4-1). The first four were described by Celsus (ca 30 BC-38 AD); the fifth was a later addition by Virchow in the nineteenth century. Redness and heat are due to increased blood flow to the inflamed area; swelling is due to accumulation of fluid; pain is due to release of chemicals that stimulate nerve endings; and loss of function is due to a combination of factors. These signs are manifested when acute inflammation occurs on the surface of the body, but not all of them will be apparent in acute inflammation of internal organs. Pain occurs only when there are appropriate sensory nerve endings in the inflamed site - for example, acute inflammation of the lung (pneumonia) does not cause pain unless the inflammation involves the parietal pleura, where there are pain-sensitive nerve endings. The increased heat of inflamed skin is due to the entry of a large amount of blood at body core temperature into the normally cooler skin. When inflammation occurs internally - where tissue is normally at body core temperature - no increase in heat is apparent.

SYSTEMIC CLINICAL SIGNS

Acute inflammation may be accompanied by systemic features in addition to the local cardinal signs described earlier.

A. Fever

Fever is one of the most prominent manifestations of the acute inflammation and may result following the entry of pyrogens and prostaglandins into the circulation at the site of inflammation. These act upon the brain stem to reset body temperature.

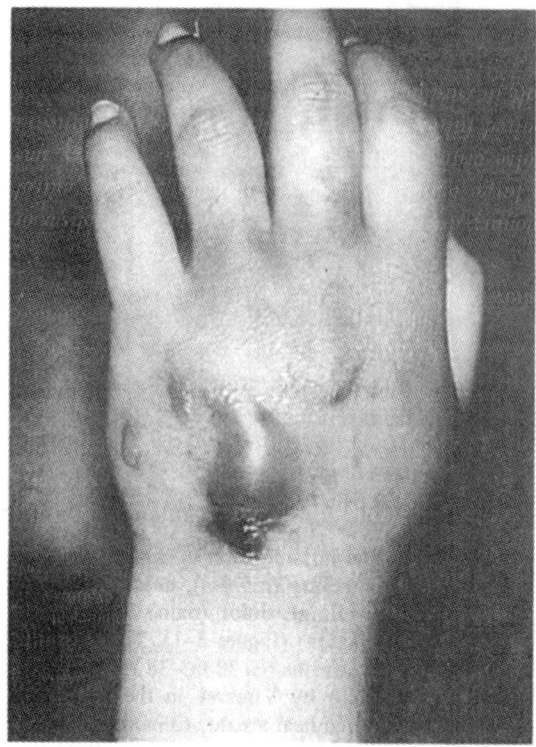

Figure 4-1 Cardinal signs of acute inflammation. Note swelling and redness of the skin around an infected burn. Marked tenderness, increased local temperature, and loss of function were also present

B. Changes in the Peripheral White Blood Cell Count (Figure 4-2)

The total number of neutrophils in the peripheral blood is increased (**neutrophil leukocytosis**). Leukocytosis is a common feature of inflammation, the leukocyte count could climbs to 15,000 or 20,000 cells/μL or even higher. Initially, this is due to accelerated release of neutrophils from bone marrow. Later, neutrohil production in the marrow is increased. Peripheral blood neutrophils tend to be the less mature forms, and they frequently contain large cytoplasmic granules (**toxic granulation**). A rise in the number of more immature neutrophils in the blood is referred as shift to the left. Viral infections tend to produce neutropenia (decreased number of neutrophils in the blood) and lymphocytosis (excess of normal lymphocytes in the blood). Acute inflammation resulting from viral infection therefore represents an exception in that the microcirculatory changes and fluid exudation are accompanied by a lymphocytic rather than a neutrophil response.

C. Changes in Plasma Protein Levels

The levels of certain plasma proteins typically increase when acute inflammation is present. These acute phase proteins are mostly synthesized in the liver, and include C-reactive protein (CRP), α1-antitrypsin, fibrinogen, serum amyloid A protein (SAA), haptoglobin, and ceruloplasmin. Increased levels of these substances in turn lead to an **increased erythrocyte sedimentation rate**, a simple and useful (though nonspecific) clue to the presence of inflammation.

ACUTE INFLAMMATION

Acute inflammation is the early (almost immediate) response of a tissue to injury. It is nonspecific and may be evoked by any injury short of one that is immediately lethal. Acute inflammation may be regarded as the first line of defense against injury and is characterized by changes in the microcirculation: exudation of fluid and emigration of leukocytes from blood vessels to the area of injury. Acute inflammation is typically of short duration, occurring before the immune response becomes established, and it is aimed primarily at removing the injurious agent.

The causative factors that could induce acute inflammation include: (1) infections and microbial toxins; (2) trauma; (3) physical and chemical agents; (4) tissue necrosis; (5) foreign bodies or materials, and (6) immune reactions.

Until the late 18th century, acute inflammation was regarded as a disease. John Hunter (1728 – 1793, London surgeon and anatomist) was the first to realized that acute inflammation was a response to injury that was generally beneficial to the host: "But if inflammation develops, regardless of the cause, still it is an effort whose purpose is to restore the parts to their natural functions."

MORPHOLOGIC AND FUNCTIONAL CHANGES

The morphologic and functional changes in acute inflammation were described in the late nineteenth century by Cohnheim, who demonstrated the vascular changes of injury in the vessels of a frog tongue. The two main components of the acute inflammatory response are the microcirculatory response and the cellular response.

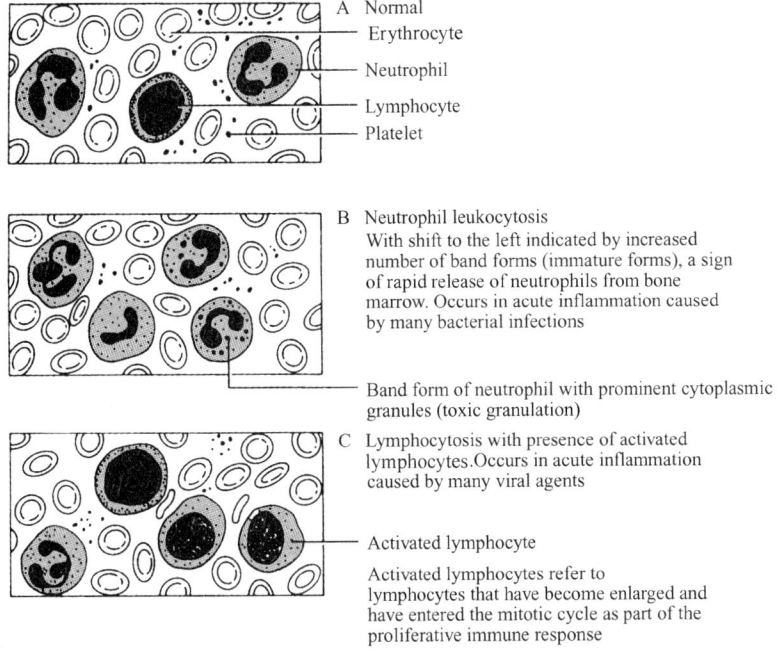

Figure 4-2 Changes in peripheral blood leukocytes in acute inflammation. The exact change observed varies with different agents and may give clues to the cause of the disease

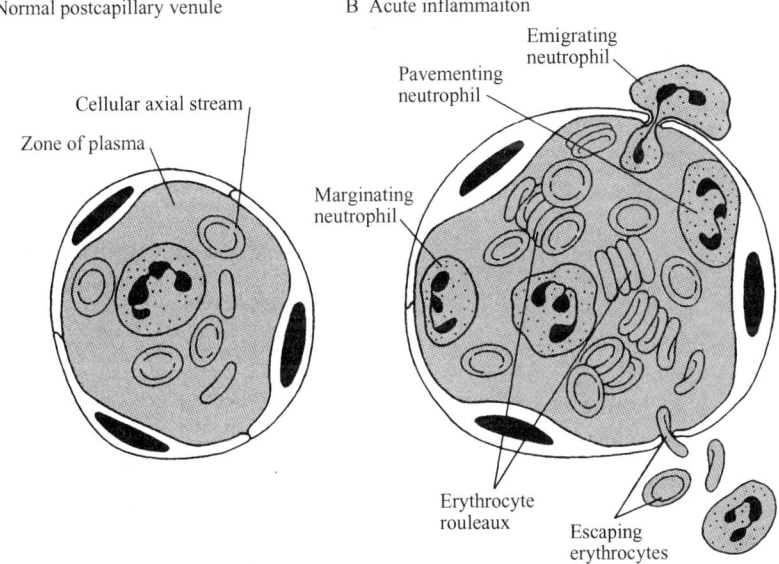

Figure 4-3 Microcirculatory changes in acute inflammation. The postcapillary venule is dilated and has swollen endothelial cells. Rouleau formation of erythrocytes and margination and emigration of leukocytes are also seen. Postcapillary venules generally show the greatest change

Microcirculatory Response

A. Vasodilation and Stasis

The first change in the microcirculation is a transient and insignificant vasoconstriction, which is then followed by marked, active dilation of arterioles, capillaries, and venules. Vasodilation is induced by action of mediators, e.g. histamine and nitric oxide, on vascular smooth muscle. This vasodilation causes an initial marked increase in blood in the area (**hyperemia**) (Figures 4-3 and 4-4). Subsequently, as fluid is lost into the exudates (see below), **stasis** may supervene, with very sluggish blood flow.

B. Increased Permeability

The permeability of capillaries and venules is a function of the intercellular junctions between vascular endothelial cells. These pores normally permit the passage of small molecules ($MW < 40,000$). Pinocytosis permits selective transfer of larger molecules across the capillary into the interstitium. In normal capillaries, fluid passes out of the microcirculation and into tissues under the influence of capillary hydrostatic pressure — and returns because of plasma colloid osmotic pressure. Normally, fluid that passes out of the microcirculation is an ultrafiltrate of plasma (Table 4-1).

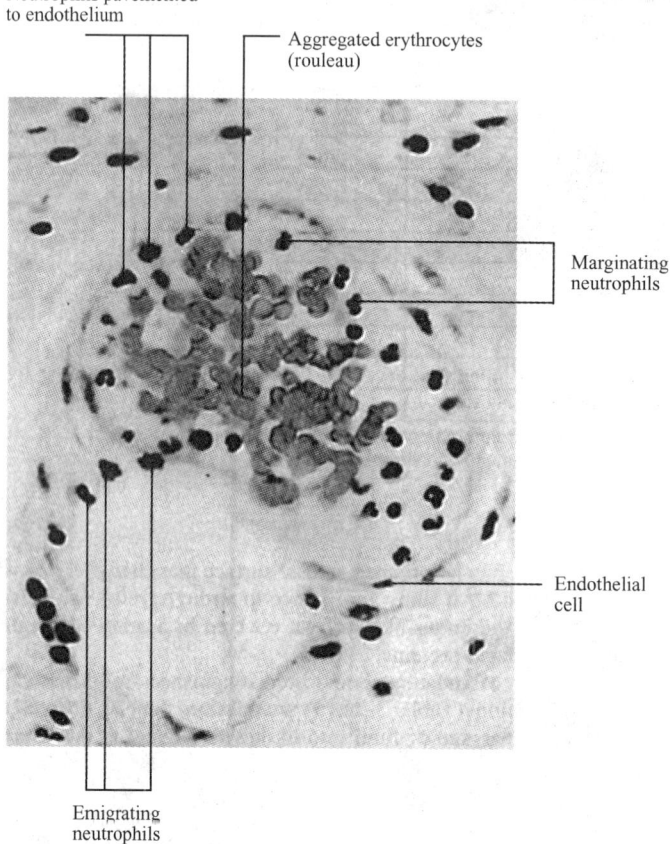

Figure 4-4 Marginating, pavementing, and emigrating neutrophils in a venule in an area of acute inflammation

Table 4-1 Differences between exudates and transudates

	Ultrafiltrate of Plasma	Transudate	Exudate	Plasma
Vascular permeability	Normal	Normal	Increased	—
Protein content	Trace	0 – 1.5 g/dL	1.5 – 6 g/dL	6 – 7 g/dL[1]
Protein types	Albumin	Albumin	All[2]	All[2]
Fibrin	No	No	Yes	No (fibrinogen)
Specific gravity	1.010	1.010 – 1.015	1.015 – 1.027	1.027
Cells	None	None	Inflammatory	Blood

[1] The protein content of an exudates depends on the plasma protein level. In patients with very low plasma protein levels, and exudate may have a lower protein content than 1.5g/dL.

[2] All = albumin, globulins, complement, immunoglobulins, proteins of the coagulation and fibrinolytic cascades.

Increased vascular permeability is a hallmark of acute inflammation. In acute inflammation, there is an immediate (but reversible) marked increase in the permeability of venules and capillaries due to active contraction of actin filaments in endothelial cells. The effect is separation of intercellular functions from one another (widening of the pores). Direct damage to the endothelial cells by the noxious agent may also contribute. Other mechanisms for increased leakage of the endothelium include leukocyte-mediated endothelial injury, increased transcytosis across the endothelial cytoplasm and leakage from new blood vessels formed in inflammation. Delayed prolonged leakage could be caused by mild to moderate thermal injury, x-radiation or ultraviolet radiation and certain bacterial toxins. The mechanism of such leakage is unknown. Increased amounts of fluid and high-molecular-weight proteins are able to pass through these abnormally permeable vessels (see Exudation of Fluid, below).

Increase in permeability in acute inflammation occurs in several phases: (1) an immediate phase mediated mainly by the actions of histamine and leukotrienes; (2) a delayed response mediated by kinins, complement etc. and (3) a prolonged response which occurs after direct endothelial injury. These permeability changes are effected by various chemical mediators (Table 4-2).

Table 4-2 Mediators of acute inflammation

Mediator	Vasodiltation	Increased Permeability		Chemotaxis	Opsonin	Pain
		Immediate	Sustained			
Histamine	+	+ + +	−	−	−	−
Serotonin (5-HT)	+	+	−	−	−	−
Bradykinin	+	+	−	−	−	+ +
Complement 3a	−	+	−	−	−	−
Complement 3b	−	−	−	−	+ + +	−
Complement 5a	−	+	−	+ + +	−	−
Prostaglandins	+ + +	+	+ ?	−	−	−
Leukotrienes	−	+ + +	+ ?	+ + +	−	−
Lysosomal proteases	−	−	+ +[1]	−	−	−
Oxygen radicals	−	−	+ +[1]	−	−	−

[1] Proteases and oxygen-based free radicals derived from neutrophils are believed to mediate a sustained increase in permeability by means of their damage to endothelial cells.

C. Exudation of Fluid

The passage of a large amount of fluid from the circulation into the interstitial tissue produces swelling (inflammatory edema), one of the major features of acute inflammation. Increased passage of fluid out of the microcirculation because of increased vascular permeability is termed **exudation.** The composition of an exudate approaches that of plasma (Table 4-1); it is rich in plasma proteins, including immunoglobulins, complement, and fibrinogen, because the abnormally permeable endothelium no longer prevents passage of these large molecules. Fibrinogen in an acute inflammation exudates is rapidly converted to fibrin by tissue thromboplastins. Fibrin can be recognized microscopically in an exudates as pink strands or clumps (Figure 4-4). Grossly, fibrin is most easily seen on an acute inflamed serosal surface that changes from its normal shiny appearance to a rough, yellowish bread and butter-like surface, covered by fibrin and coagulated proteins.

Exudation should be distinguished from transudation (Table 4-1). **Transudation** denotes increased passage of fluid into tissue through vessels of *normal* permeability. The force that causes outward passage of fluid from the microcirculation into the tissues is either increased hydrostatic pressure or decreased plasma colloid osmotic pressure. A transudate has a composition similar to that of an ultrafiltrate of plasma. In clinical practice, identification of edema fluid as a transudate or an exudates is of considerable

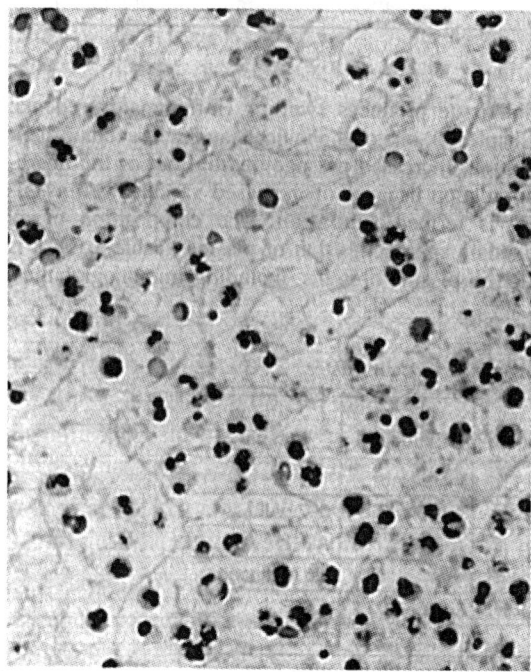

Figure 4-5 An acute inflammatory exudates, showing strands of fibrin and numerous neutrophils. Scattered macrophages are also present

diagnostic value because it provides clues to the cause of the disorder, e. g. examination of peritoneal (ascites) fluid (Table 4-3).

Table 4-3 Selected causes of transudative and exudative peritoneal effusion (ascites)

Transudate	Exudate
Cirrhosis of the liver	Bacterial peritonitis
Portal vain obstruction	Tuberculous peritonitis
Right heart failure	Metastatic neoplasms
Constrictive pericarditis	Mesothelioma (cancer of mesothelial cells)
Meigs' syndrome[1]	Connective tissue disease (e. g. systemic lupus erythematosus)
Malnutrition (kwashiorkor)	

[1] Meigs' syndrome is the occurrence of peritoneal and pleural effusion due to transudation of fluid from the surface of an ovarian tumor.

Exudation helps combat the offending agent (1) by diluting it; (2) by causing increased lymphatic flow; and (3) by flooding the area with plasma, which contain numerous defensive proteins such as immunoglobulins and complement. The increased lymphatic drainage conveys noxious agents to the draining lymph nodes, thereby facilitating a protective immune response. Occasionally, with virulent organisms, the lymphatics may inadvertently promote spread and may actually themselves become inflamed (lymphangitis), together with the lymph nodes.

Cellular Response

Leukocytes are recruited from the circulation during the process of acute inflammation. Leukocyte infiltration plays an important role in limiting the spread of injury and in defending the host tissue. In the inflamed area, leukocytes ingest offending agents, kill bacterial and other microbes, and get rid of necrotic tissue.

A. Types of Cells Involved

Acute inflammation is characterized by the active emigration of inflammatory cells from the blood into the area of injury. Neutrophils (polymorphonuclear leukocytes) (Figure 4-5) dominate the early phase (first 24 hours). After the first 24 – 48 hours, phagocytic cells of the macrophage (reticuloendothelial) system – and immunologically active cells such as lymphocytes and plasma cells – enter the area. Neutrophils remain predominant for several days, however.

B. Margination, Adhesion and Transmigration of Neutrophils

In a normal blood vessel, the cellular elements of blood are confined to a central axial stream, which is separated from the endothelial surface by a zone of plasma (Figure 4-3A). This separation is dependent on normal blood flow, which creates physical forces that tend to keep the heaviest cellular particles in the center of the vessel.

As the rate of blood flow in the dilated vessels decreases in acute inflammation, the orderly flow of blood is disturbed. Erythrocytes form heavy aggregates (**rouleaux**) in a phenomenon termed **sludging** (Figure 4-3B).

The process of the leukocytes from the vessel lumen to the interstitial tissue is called extravasation, which include several steps: (1) margination, rolling and adhesion to endothelium in the lumen; (2) transmigration across the endothelium (diapedesis); and (3) migration toward the site of injury.

As a result of disturbed blood flow, leukocytes move to the periphery in contact with the endothelium (margination), to which many then adhere (pavementing) (Figures 4-3B and 4-4). Pavementing is a normal process that is much exaggerated in inflammation as a result of increased expression of various cell adhesion molecules (CAMs) on both leukocytes and endothelial cells. For example, expression of beta 2 integrins (the CD 11-CD 18 complex), which include leukocyte function antigen-1 (LFA-1), is enhanced by the action of such chemotactic factors as C5a (complement anaphylatoxin) and leukotriene TB4. The complementary CAMs on endothelial cells are similarly upregulated by the action of interleukin-1 (IL-1) and TNF (tumor necrosis factor, which is not confined to tumors); these include ICAM 1, ICAM 2, and ELAM-1 (endothelial leukocyte adhesion molecule). LAM-1, which promotes the passage of lymphocytes across high endothelial vesicles into lymph nodes, also plays a role in neutrophil and lymphocyte emigration in inflammation.

Adhesion of leukocytes to endothelial cells are regulated by the binding of complementary adhesion molecules on the leukocyte and endothelial surface. Adhesion molecules involved in the inflammatory response include four molecular families: the selectins, the immunoglobulin superfamily, the integrins, and mucin-like glycoproteins.

C. Emigration of Neutrophils

The adherent neutrophils actively leave post capillary venules through intercellular junctions (Figure 4-3 and 4-4) and pass through the basement membrane to reach the interstitial space (**emigration**). Penetration through the wall takes 2 – 10 minutes; in interstitial tissue, neutrophils move at a rate of up to 20μm/min.

D. Chemotactic Factors (Table 4-2)

In the interstitial tissue, neutrophils move toward the site of injury, this movement oriented along a chemical gradient is termed **chemotaxis**. The active emigration of neutrophils and the direction in which they move are governed by **chemotactic factors**. Complement factors C3a and C5a (collectively know as anaphylatoxin) are potent chemotactic agents for neutrophils and macrophages, as is leukotriene LTB4. Interaction between neutrophil surface receptor and these chemotaxins increases neutrophil motility (via an influx of Ca^{2+} ions, which stimulates contraction of actin) and promotes degranulation. Various cytokines play an increasing role as the immune response develops.

Erythrocytes enter an inflamed area passively – in contrast to the active process of leukocyte emigration. Red blood cells are pushed out of the vessel by hydrostatic pressure through the widened intercellular junctions behind emigrating leukocytes (**diapedesis**). In severe injuries associated with disruption of the microcirculation, large numbers of erythrocytes enter the inflamed area (**hemorrhagic inflammation**).

E. Phagocytosis: (See Figure 4-6)

1. Recognition

The first step in phagocytosis is recognition of the injurious agent by the phagocytic cell, either directly

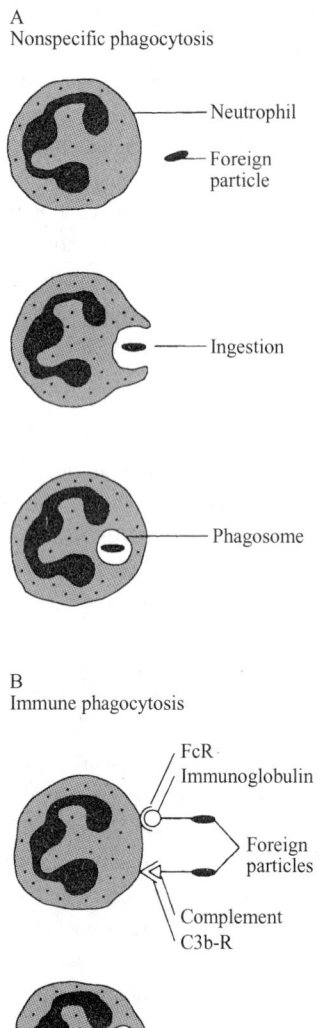

Figure 4-6 Phagocytosis by neutrophils immune phagocytosis (B) is much more efficient than nonspecific phagocytosis (A). The presence on the cell membrane of receptors to the Fc fragment of the immunoglobulin molecule (FcR) and C 3b component of complement (C 3b-R) are important in immune phagocytosis. Note that macrophages have similar phagocytic capability

(as occurs with large, inert particles) or after the agent has been coated with immunoglobulin or complement factor 3b (C3b) (**opsonization**). The coating agents are **opsonins**. Opsonin enhance the capability of phagocytosis through the complementary receptors on leukocytes. Opsonin-mediated phagocytosis is the mechanism operating in the immune phagocytosis of microorganisms. Both IgG and C3b are effective opsonins. Immunoglobulin that is specifically reactive with antigens on the injurious agent (specific antibody) is the most effective opsonin. C3b is generated locally by activation of the complement cascade. Early in acute inflammation - before the immune response has developed - nonimmune factors dominate, but as immunity develops, they are superseded by the more efficient immune phagocytosis.

2. Engulfment

On the surface of neutrophils and macrophages, there are receptors, one is the receptor for Fc fragment of IgG, and the other is the receptor for C3b. Once recognized by a neutrophil or macrophage, a foreign particle is engulfed by the phagocytic cell to form a membrane-bound vacuole called **phagosome**, which fuses with lysosomes to form a **phagolysosome**.

3. Microbial killing

When the offending agent is a microorganism, it must be killed before degradation can occur. The same factors that are instrumental in cell injury are also effective in killing microorganisms. The formation of the phagolysosome allows the enzymes to have access to the engulfed microorganism, and the killing takes place.

• **The hydrogen peroxide (H_2O_2) -myeloperoxidase-halide system** is the most important microbicidal mechanism in neutrophils whose cytoplasmic granules contain myeloperoxidase. Superoxide ions are formed by the action of an oxidase in the plasma membrane. Superoxide is spontaneously transformed to microbicidal H_2O_2 in the lysosome. In addition, myeloperoxidase, in combination with a halide ion (usually chloride), greatly potentiates the microbicidal effect of H_2O_2, probably by forming highly toxic ions such as HOCl.

• Toxic oxygen-based radicals, e.g., superoxide ($O_2^- \cdot$ hydroxyl \[OH · \]), and singlet oxygen, are produced in all phagocytic cells. Microbial killing resulting from the action of these oxygen-based radicals may be direct or may be mediated by ferric ions. Reaction of superoxide with ferric ion results in the formation of ferrous ion, which reacts with hydrogen peroxide to form hydroxyl radicals. Hydroxyl radicals react with bacterial cell wall phospholipids, causing loss of bacterial cell membrane integrity (lipid peroxidation).

● Other bactericidal agents released by neutrophil granules include hydrolases, proteases (cathepsin G), lactoferrin, and lysozyme. Lysosome was first discovered in tears by Alexander Fleming, who called it "tear antiseptic". It acts by attacking muramic acid linkages in bacterial cell walls.

● Immunologic mechanisms such as **macrophage-activating factor**, a lymphokine released by sensitized T lymphocytes, assist microbial killing by macrophages.

● As the immune response develops, a variety of other microbicidal mechanisms come into effect (Figure 4-7).

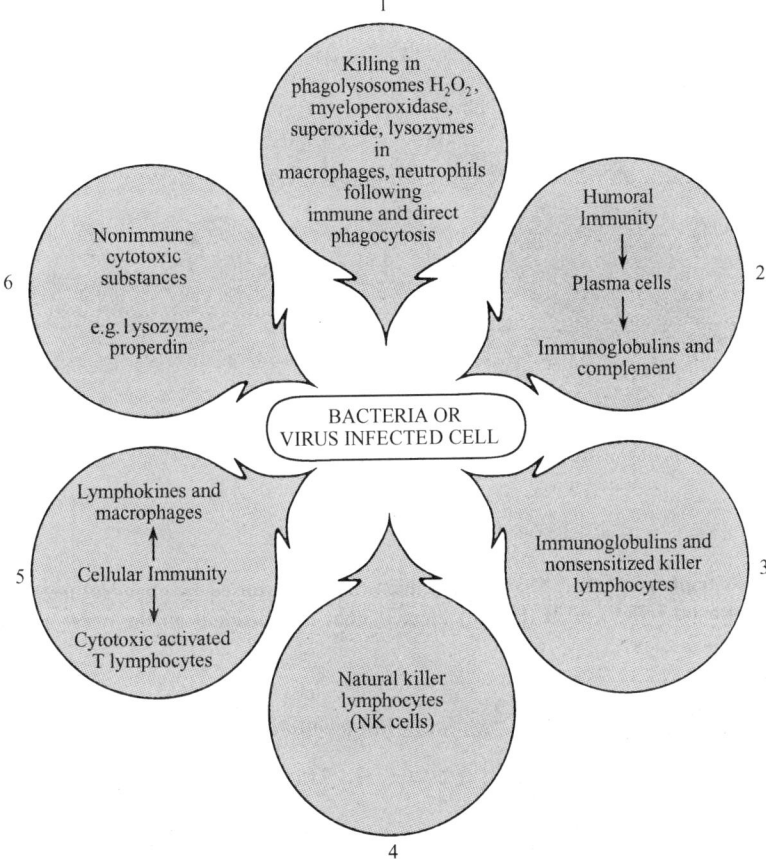

Figure 4-7 Mechanisms of microbial killing

MEDIATORS OF ACUTE INFLAMMATION

A variety of endogenous chemical mediators play some important roles in the modulation of inflammatory response. These mediators are divided into cell-derived mediators and plasma-derived mediators. Main cell-derived mediators include vasoactive amines (histamine and serotonin), postagladin (PG), leukotriene (LT), products of leukocytes and components of lysosomes, cytokine, chemokine and nitric oxide (NO). Complement system, kinin and clotting system are among plasma-derived mediators.

The Triple Response (Figure 4-8)

Sir Thomas Lewis, in a series of elegant and simple experiment in 1927, elucidated the basic factors that mediate acute inflammation. Firmly stroking the forearm with a blunt instrument such as a pencil evokes the **triple response**: (1) Within 1 minute, a red line appears along the line of stroke as a result of dilation of arterioles, capillaries, and venules at the site of injury. (2) simultaneously, a red flare develops as a result of vasodilation in the tissue surrounding the injury; and (3) a wheal forms because of exudation of fluid along the line of injury.

Lewis showed that vasodilation in tissue surrounding the injury - the flare, a minor part of the acute inflammatory response - is mediated by a local axon reflex (Figure 4-8). The major components of acute inflammation - the red line and the wheal - were shown to be independent of neural connections in the tissue. Lewis then demonstrated that local injection of histamine (Lewis's " H substance") produced a reaction equivalent to the red line and wheal. This discovery laid the foundation for understanding the role of chemical mediators in acute inflammation.

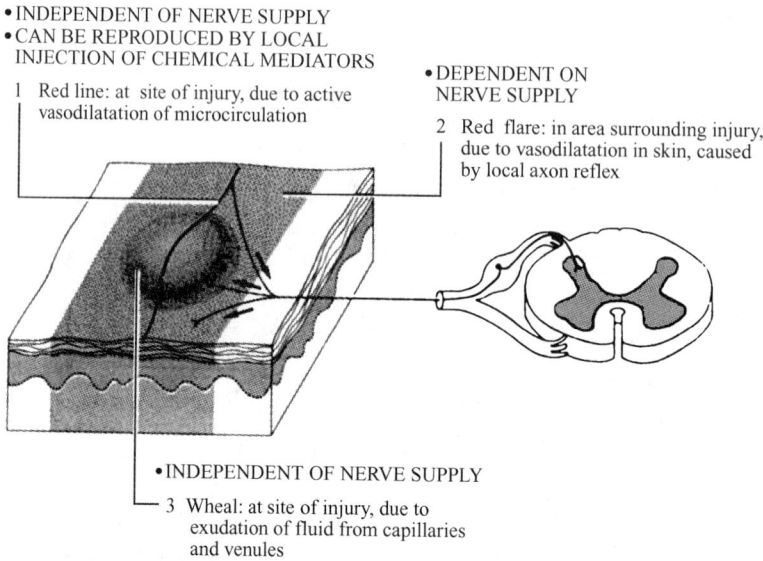

Figure 4-8 Lewis's triple response. The red line and wheal are caused by chemical mediators; the flare is mediated by a local axon reflex and is the only element that is dependent on the nerve supply

Specific Mediators (Table 4-2)

In the years since Lewis's experiments, it has become apparent that histamine can account for only a small part of the acute inflammatory response. Many other chemical mediators have been discovered, but the exact role of individual mediators in inflamed tissue is unknown; their actions in vivo can only be postulated on the basis of their demonstrated in vitro activity.

A. Vasoactive Amine

Histamine and **serotonin** are released from mast cells and platelets and can be identified early in the course of acute inflammation. Histamine is more important than serotonin in humans; it acts mainly on venules that have H_1-histamine receptors. Both of these amine cause vasodilation and increased permeability and are probably the main agents responsible for the immediate phase of the acute inflammatory response. Histamine levels decrease rapidly within an hour after the onset of inflammation.

B. The Kinin System

Bradykinin, the final product of the kinin system, is formed by the action of **kallikrein** on a precursor plasma protein (high-molecular-weight kininogen). Kallikrein is present in its inactive form prekallikren in plasma and is activated by activated factor XII (Hageman factor) of the coagulation cascade. Bradykinin causes increased vascular permeability and stimulates pain receptors.

C. The Coagulation Cascade

Note that the coagulation cascade, leading to production of fibrin, is also initiated by Hageman factor (activated factor XII). The fibrinopeptides that are also formed in the catabolism of fibrin (fibrinolysis) also cause increased vascular permeability and are chemotactic for neutrophils.

D. The Complement System

C5a and C3a, which are formed in the activation of complement, cause increased vascular permeability by stimulating release of histamine from mast cells. C5a is a powerful chemotactic agent for neutrophils and macrophages. C3b is an important opsonin. C5a activates the lipoxygenase pathway of arachidonic acid metabolism (see below).

E. Arachidonic Acid Metabolites

Arachidonic acid is a 20-carbon unsaturated fatty acid found in phospholipids in the cell membranes of neutrophils, mast cells, monocytes, and other cells. Release of arachidonic acid by phospholipases initiates a series of complex reactions that culminate in the production of prostaglandings, leukotrienes, and other mediators of inflammation (Figure 4-9).

F. Neutrophil Factors

Proteases and toxic oxygen-based free radicals generated by the neutrophil are believed to cause endothelial damage leading to increased vascular permeability.

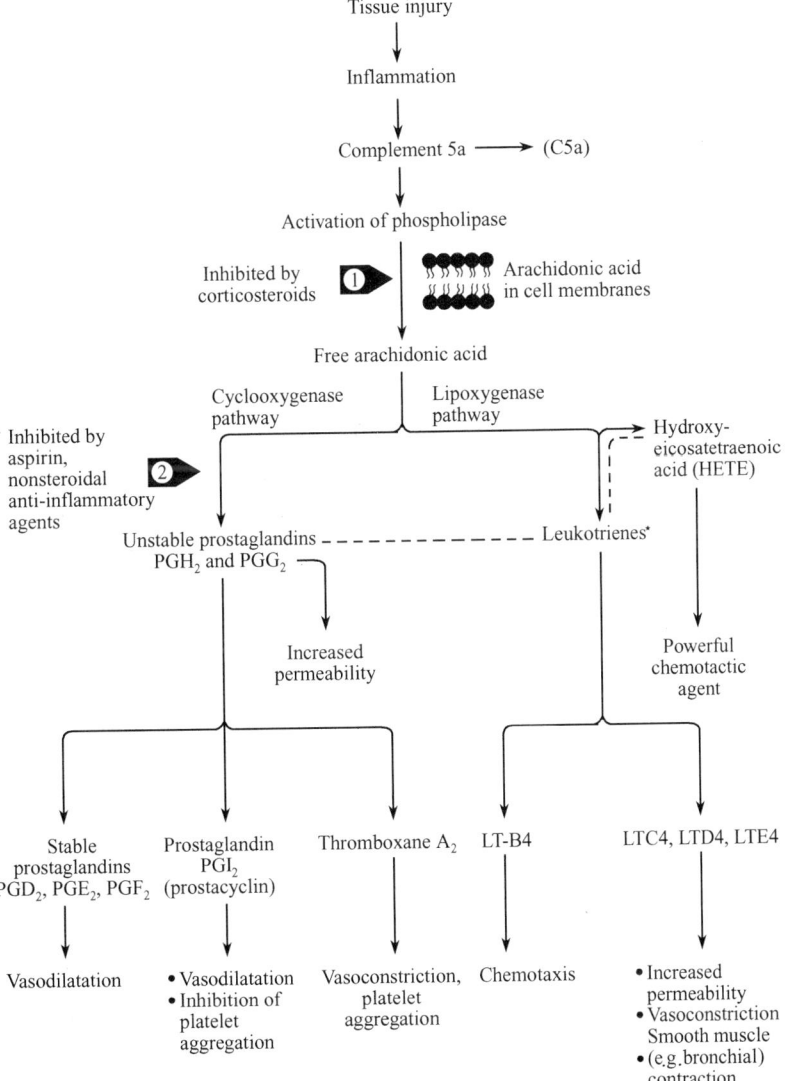

Figure 4-9 Metabolites of arachidonic acid and their influence on the acute inflammatory response.
★ Note that LTC4, LTD4 and LTE4 appear to equate with slow-reacting substance of anaphylaxis (SRS-A) of the older literature. These are key mediators of anaphylactic hypersensitivity reactions

G. Other Mediators and Inhibitors

Numerous other chemical mediators of acute inflammation have been described that are ignored here because they play either a minor or a dubious role. Negative feedback (inhibition) of inflammation also occurs but is not well understood; possible inhibitory factors include C1 esterase inhibitor (inhibits the complement cascade) and α_1-antitrypsin (inhibits proteases).

TYPES OF ACUTE INFLAMMATION

The preceding description of acute inflammation is that of the classic, most frequently occurring form. It is important to recognize variations from this common type because they provide clues to the causative agent (Table 4-4).

Table 4-4 Types of Acute Inflammation

Type	Features	Common Causes
Classic type	Hyperemia; exudation with fibrin and neutrophils; neutrophil leukocytosis in blood	Bacterial infections; response to cell necrosis
Acute inflammation without neutrophils	Paucity of neutrophils in exudates; lymphocytes and plasma cells predominant; neutrophils, lymphocytosis in blood	Viral and rickettsial infections (immune response contributes)
Allergic acute inflammation	Marked edema and numerous eosinophils, esosinophilia in blood	Certain hypersensitivity immune reactions
Serous inflammation	Marked fluid exudation	Burns; many bacterial infections
Catarrhal inflammation (inflammation of mucous membranes)	Marked secretion of mucus	Infections, e.g. common clod (rhinovirus); allergy (e.g. hay fever)
Fibrinous inflammation	Excess fibrin formation	Many virulent bacterial infections.
Necrotizing inflammation, hemorrhagic inflammation	Marked tissue necrosis and hemorrhage	Highly virulent organisms (bacterial, viral, fungal), e.g. plague (*Yersinia pestis*), anthrax (*Bacillus anthracis*) herpes simplex encephalitis, mucormycosis
(Pseudomembranous) inflammation	Necrotizing inflammation involving mucous membranes. The necrotic mucosa and inflammatory exudates from an adherent membrane on the mucosal surface	Toxigenic bacteria, e.g. diphtheria bacillus (*Corynebacterium diphtheriae*) and *Clostridium difficile*
Suppurative (purulent) inflammation	Exaggerated neutrophil response and liquefactive necrosis of parenchymal cells; pus formation. Marked neutrophil leukocytosis in blood	Pyogenic bacteria, e.g. staphylococci, streptococci, gram-negative bacilli, anaerobes

Morphologic Patterns of Acute Inflammation

Several types of acute inflammation are recognized, these types of acute inflammation have some morphologic features and might point to possible cause of the disease.

A. Serous Inflammation

Serous inflammation is characterized by accumulation of excessive clear watery fluid with a variable protein content, which implies increased vascular permeability. The inflammatory reaction occurs in skin (burn blisters), and in peritoneal, pleural and pericardial cavities.

- **Catarrhal inflammation**: "Catarrh" means "flow down", catarrhal inflammation is a mild exudative inflammation of a surface mucousmembrance without apparent tissue destruction. The example of serous catarrhal inflammation is the marked serous exudation in common clod.

B. Fibrinous Inflammation

Severe injuries cause greater increasing in vascular permeability. Large amounts of fibrinogen pass the vessel wall, and fibrins are formed in the extracellular spaces as a result of activation of the coagulation system. Examples of the fibrinous inflammation include fibrinous pericarditis or pleuritis. Excessive fibrinous exudation usually lead to organization and fibrosis in the affected area. **Pseudo-membranous inflammation** is the fibrinous inflammation occurred on a mucosal surface, and a membranous film consisting mainly of fibrin mixed with necrotic cells appears on the surface of the affected mucosa. The typical changes of diphtheria and bacillary dysentery are all belong to pseudo-membranous inflammation.

C. Suppurative (Purulent Inflammation)

The characteristics of suppurative inflammation is the formation of purulent exudates or pus. Pus is made up of neutrophils, necrotic cells and edema fluid. A localized collection of purulent inflammation accompanied by liquefactive necrosis is referred to abscess.

D. Hemorrhagic Inflammation

Obvious hemorrhage occurs when the blood vessels in the inflamed areas are severally injured. Marked hemorrhage is the predominant pathological change in some infections diseases, e. g. endemic hemorrhagic fever, leptospirosis and plague.

COURSE OF ACUTE INFLAMMATION

The acute inflammatory response is aimed at neutralizing or inactivating the agent causing the injury. There are several possible outcomes:

A. Resolution

In uncomplicated acute inflammation, tissue returns to normal in a process of resolution. In which the exudates and cellular debris are liquefied and removed by macrophages and lymphatic flow.

B. Repair

When tissue necrosis has occurred before the agent is neutralized, repair ensues, and dead cells are either replaced by regeneration or repaired by scar formation.

C. Suppuration

In virulent bacterial infections, exaggerated emigration of neutrophils with liquefactive necrosis occurs (suppurative inflammation). The liquefied mass of necrotic tissue and neutrophils is called **pus**. When an area of suppuration becomes walled off, an abscess results (Figure 4-10).

D. Chronic Inflammation

When the noxious agent is not neutralized by the acute inflammatory response, the body mounts an immune response, which leads to chronic inflammation.

DIAGNOSIS OF ACUTE INFLAMMATION (Table 4-5)

Local cardinal signs of inflammation permit diagnosis of acute inflammation when the process involves surface structures - skin, conjunctiva, mouth, etc. Acute inflammation in internal organs such as the lung and kidney may first manifest with systemic changes as fever and alterations in the blood (white cell count, proteins, etc). More rarely, it is necessary to examine a fluid exudates or tissue sample (biopsy) to establish the presence of acute inflammation.

Table 4-5 Summary of clinical and laboratory evaluation of acute inflammation

Systemic features
Fever (usually of acute onset and rapidly rising)
Changes in peripheral white blood cell count
Neutrophil leukocytosis with shift to the left
Lymphocytosis and neutropenia in acute viral infections
Local features I (cardinal clinical signs; seen at site of injury only)
Redness
Swelling
Heat
Pain
Loss of function

- **Laboratory evaluation**
  Examination of inflammatory exudates
  Characteristic high protein levels and high specific gravity
  Presence of acute inflammatory cells (neutrophils; lymphocytes in viral infections)
  Biopsy and microscopic examination of tissue
  Hyperemia
  Edema
  Neutrophils
  Fibrin
  Diagnostic tests
  Microbiologic (culture and Gram-stained smear)
  Immunologic: Serum antibody levels, complement levels etc

(Continued)

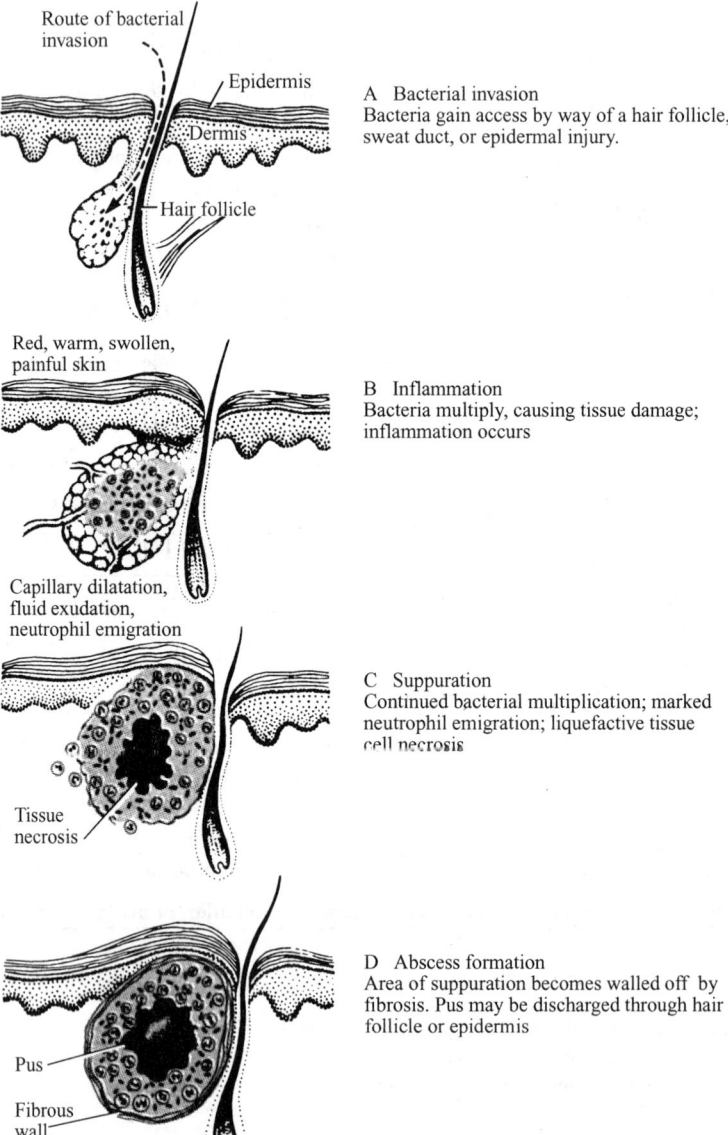

Figure 4-10 Bacterial infection (A) of a hair follicle of the skin, resulting in acute inflammation (B) followed by suppuration with liquefactive necrosis (C) and abscess formation (D)

CHRONIC INFLAMMATION

Chronic inflammation is the sum of the responses mounted by tissue against a persistent injurious agent: bacterial, viral, chemical, immunologic, etc. The tissue affected by chronic inflammation commonly show evidence of the following pathologic processes:

A. Immune Response

Manifestations of the immune response in injured tissue include the response of lymphocytes, plasma cells, and macrophages (Figure 4-11). Plasma immunoglobulin levels may be elevated.

B. Phagocytosis

Immune phagocytosis is mediated by macrophages that have been activated by T cell lymphokines, and it involves antigens that have opsonings (immunoglobulins and complement factors) attached to their surfaces. **Nonimmune phagocytosis** is directed against foreign nonantigenic particles.

C. Necrosis

Commonly there is some degree of necrosis that may affect only scattered individual cells or may be extensive.

D. Repair

Repair of tissues damaged by persistent injury is characterized by new blood vessel formation, fibroblastic proliferation, and collagen deposition (fibrosis).

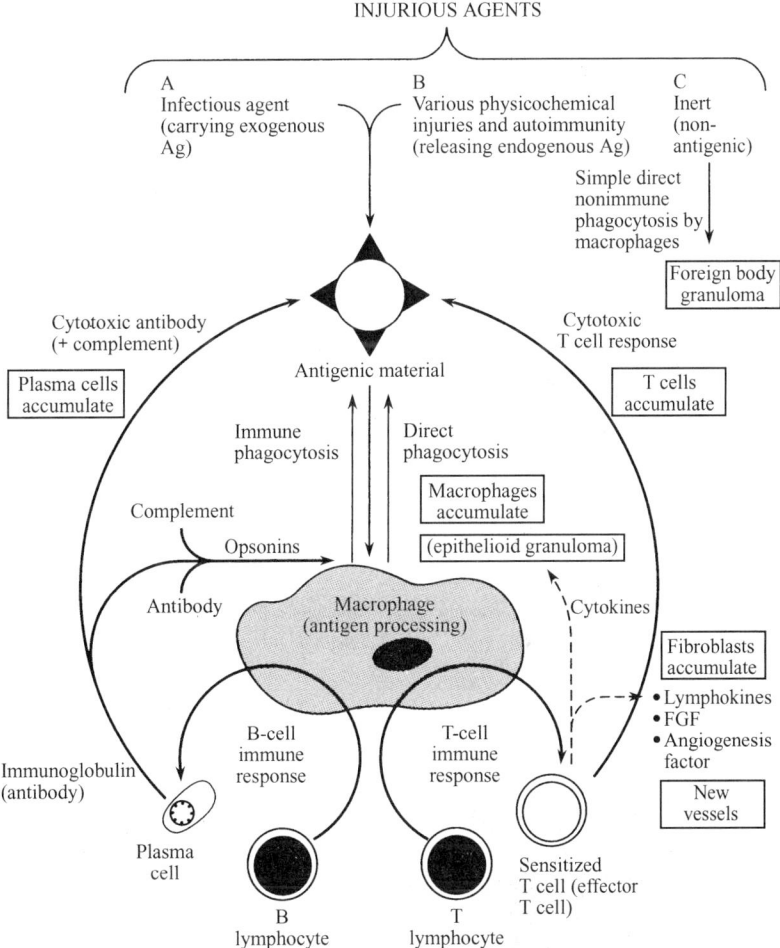

Figure 4-11 Chronic inflammation. Cellular components seen as part of the immune response. In most cases, the persistent injurious agent is antigenic and leads to an immune response involving T cells, B cells, and macrophages. Foreign body granuloma formation, on the other hand, appears to be a direct phagocytic response to inert (i.e. nonantigenic) material, and the immune response is not involved

Chronic inflammation is the inflammatory response of prolonged duration, and it lasts for several weeks or months, or even years. Chronic inflammation may follow an acute inflammatory response that fails to vanquish the agent, or may occur without a clinically apparent acute phase. Chronic inflammation is recognized and defined by its morphologic features (Table 4-6). The main features of chronic inflammation include: (1) Mononuclear cell infiltration. Inflammatory cells predominant in chronic inflammation include macrophages, lymphocytes and plasma cells. Macrophages play dominant rolls in chronic inflammation; (2) tissue destruction; (3) granulation issue formation and fibrosis. Chronic inflammation is distinguished from acute inflammation by the absence of cardinal signs such as redness, swelling, pain and increased temperature. Active hyperemia, fluid exudation and neutrophil emigration are absent in chronic inflammation. It is distinguished pathologically from acute inflammation by being of a duration that is long enough to permit the tissue manifestations of the immune response and repair. Most agents associate with chronic inflammation cause insidious but progressive and often extensive **tissue necrosis** accompanied by ongoing **repair by fibrosis.** The amount of fibrosis in the tissues is a function of the duration of chronic inflammation.

Table 4-6 Differences between acute and chronic inflammation

	Acute	Chronic
Duration	Short (days)	Long (weeks to months)
Onset	Acute	Insidious
Specificity	Nonspecific	Specific (where immune response is activated)
Inflammatory cells	Neutrophils, macrophages	Lymphcytes, plasma cells, macrophages, fibroblasts
Vascular changes	Active vasodilation, increased permeability	New vessel formation (granulation tissue)
Fluid exudation and edima	+	-
Cardinal clinical signs (redness, heat, swelling, pain)	+	-
Tissue necrosis	- (Usually) + (Suppurative and necrotizing inflammation)	+ (ongoing)
Fibrosis (collagen deposition)	-	+
Operative host responses	Plasma factors: complement, immunoglobulins, properdin, etc; neutrophils, nonimmune phagocytosis	Immune response, phagocytosis, repair
Systemic manifestations	Fever, often high	Low-grade fever, weight loss, anemia
Changes in peripheral blood	Neutrophil leukocytosis; lymphocytosis (in viral infections)	Frequently none, variable leukocyte changes, increased plasma immunoglobulin

The specific feature of chronic inflammation occurring in response to different noxious stimuli depend on the relative magnitude of each of the processes described above. For example, an agent that induces extensive release of cytokines will produce chronic inflammation characterized by numerous macrophages. This would differ from chronic inflammation against an agent that evokes a cytotoxic T lymphocyte response, which is characterized by the presence of T lymphocyte alone. Chronic inflammation, therefore, displays a range of tissue changes. Study of these processes is often rewarded by insights about the agent causing the disease. It is from this perspective that we approach the study of chronic inflammation.

CHRONIC INFLAMMATION IN RESPONSE TO ANTIGENIC INJURIOUS AGENTS

Mechanisms

Chronic inflammation usually occurs in response to an injurious agent that is antigenic, e. g. a microorganism, but may also develop in response to self antigens released from damaged tissues. The immune response is triggered by the first contact with the antigen but takes some days to become apparent in the tissue. Local persistence of the antigen leads to accumulation of activated T lymphocytes, plasma cells, and macrophages at the site of injury (Figure 4-11). Because these cells are the prominent cell types in chronic inflammation, effector cells of the immune response are also called **chronic inflammatory cells**.

Although it is triggered at the time of injury, the immune response takes several days to develop because the nonsensitized lymphocytes that initially respond to antigens must pass through several division cycles before increased numbers of effector lymphocytes become manifest in the tissues. Simple uncomplicated acute inflammation usually resolves upon removal of antigen prior to any apparent tissue manifestation of the immune response.

Macrophages (monocytes) are recruited to the lesion from the blood by such chemotactic factors as C5a and TGFβ. Local activation occurs under the influence of multiple cytokines (Table 4-3), particularly γ interferon and IL-4. Macrophages in turn release a variety of factors that perpetuate the developing immune response, including cytokines (IL-1, IL-6, and TNF-α), complement components, prostaglandin (Figure 4-9), and various growth factors such as FGF (fibroblast growth factor), PDGF (platelet-derived growth factor), and TGFβ (transforming growth factor). Multiple proteases and hydrolases contribute to the phagocytic and microbicidal effect.

Morphologic Types

Differentiation of the various types of chronic inflammation is based both on the nature of the inciting agent and the subsequent immune response against it.

A. Granulomatous Chronic Inflammation

Granulomatous inflammation is a special type of chronic inflammation, and is characterized by the formation of granuloma. A granuloma is defined as an aggregate of macrophages. Two types of granuloma are recognized: (1) epithelioid cell granuloma, which represents an immune response in which the macrophages are activated by lymphokine of specifically stimulated T cells; and (2) foreign body granuloma, which represents nonimmune phagocytosis of foreign nonantigenic material by macrophages.

1. Characteristic features

Chronic granulomatous inflammation is characterized by the formation of **epithelioid cell granulomas. Epithilioid cells** are activated macrophages that appear on microscopic examination as large cells with abundant pale, foamy cytoplasm; they are called epithelioid cells because of a superficial resemblance to epithelial cells (Figure 4-12A). Epithelioid cells appear to have enhanced ability to secrete lysozyme and a variety of enzymes but decreased phagocytic potential. An epithelioid cell granuloma is an aggregate of these activated macrophages. Macrophage aggregation is induced by lymphokines produced by activated lymphocytes. Granulomas are usually surrounded by lymphocytes, plasma cells, fibroblasts, and collagen. A typical feature of epiehtlioid cell granulomas is the formation of **Langhans-type giant cells** that are derived from fusion of macrophages and characterized by 10 – 50 nuclei around the periphery of the cell (Figures 4-12 and 4-13).

2. Causes

Epithelioid cell granulomas form when two conditions are satisfied: (1) When macrophages have successfully pahgocytosed the injurious agent but it survives inside them. The abundant pale, foamy cytoplasm reflects the presence of extensive rough reticulum (secretory function). (2) When an active T lymphocyte-mediated cellular immune response occurs. Lymphokines produced by activated T lymphocytes (Table 4-3) inhibit migration of macrophages and cause them to aggregate in the area of injury and form granulomas (Figure 4-14).

Epithelioid granulomas occur in several different types of disease states (Table 4-7).

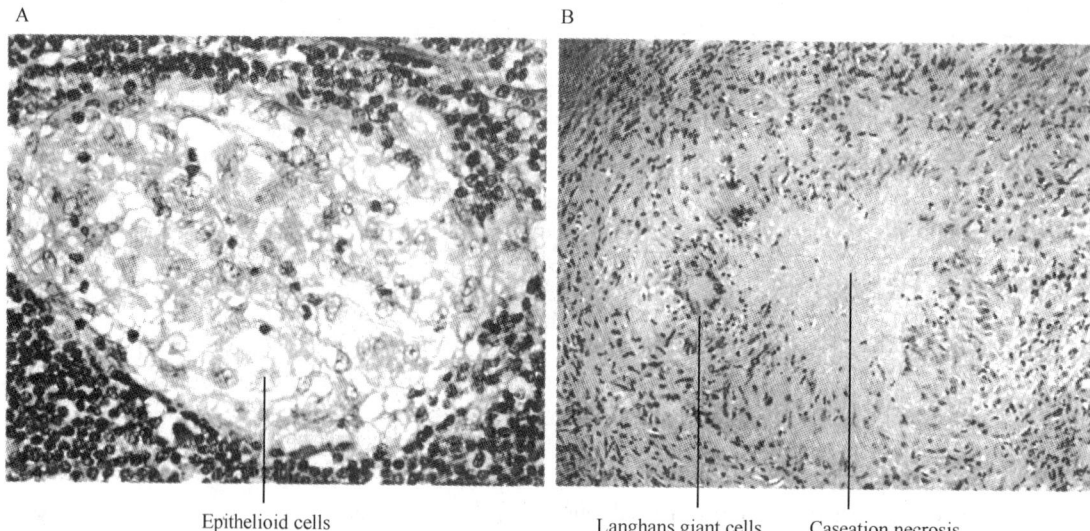

Epithelioid cells   Langhans giant cells   Caseation necrosis

Figure 4-12 Epithelioid cell granuloma (composite) A: Early granuloma composed of an aggregate of epithelioid cells with vesicular nuclei, abundant cytoplasm, and indistinct borders. This is surrounded by lymphocytes. B. Granuloma with central caseation. Note the presence of Langhans giant cells

Table 4-7 Common causes of epithelioid cell granulomas

Disease	Antigen	Caseous Necrosis
Immunologic response		
Tuberculosis	*Mycobacterium tuberculosis*	+ +
Leprosy (tuberculoid type)	*Mycobacterium leprae*	−
Histoplasmosis	*Histoplasma capsulatum*	+ +
Coccidio do mycosis	*Coccidioides immitis*	+ +
Q fever	*Coxiella burnetii* (rickettsial organism)	−
Brucellosis	*Brucella* species	−
Syphilis	*Treponema pallidum*	+ +[1]
Sarcoidosis[2]	Unknown	−
Crohn's disease[2]	Unknown	−
Berylliosis[3]	Beryllium (? + protein)	−
Nonimmunologic response		
Foreign body (e.g. in intravenous drug abuse)	Talc, fibers (? + protein)	−

[1] Granuloma formation occurs in late syphilis. The necrosis in syphilitic granulomas resembles caseous necrosis in its pathogenesis and microscopic appearance but differs in its gross appearance, being firm and rubbery rather than cheesy. This is called gummatous necrosis, and the syphilitic granuloma is called a gumma.

[2] Strongly suspected to be of infectious origin, but agent unknown.

[3] Contact hypersensitivity to beryllium.

3. Changes in affected tissues

Initially microscopic, granulomas expand and fuse with adjacent granulomas over time to form large masses that sometimes resemble malignant tumors. Parenchymal tissue around the granuloma is lost as a result of necrosis and is replaced by scar tissue when healing occurs.

In many infectious granulomas (e.g. those due to a specific microorganism), central **caseous necrosis** is a common feature. On gross examination, caseous mate-

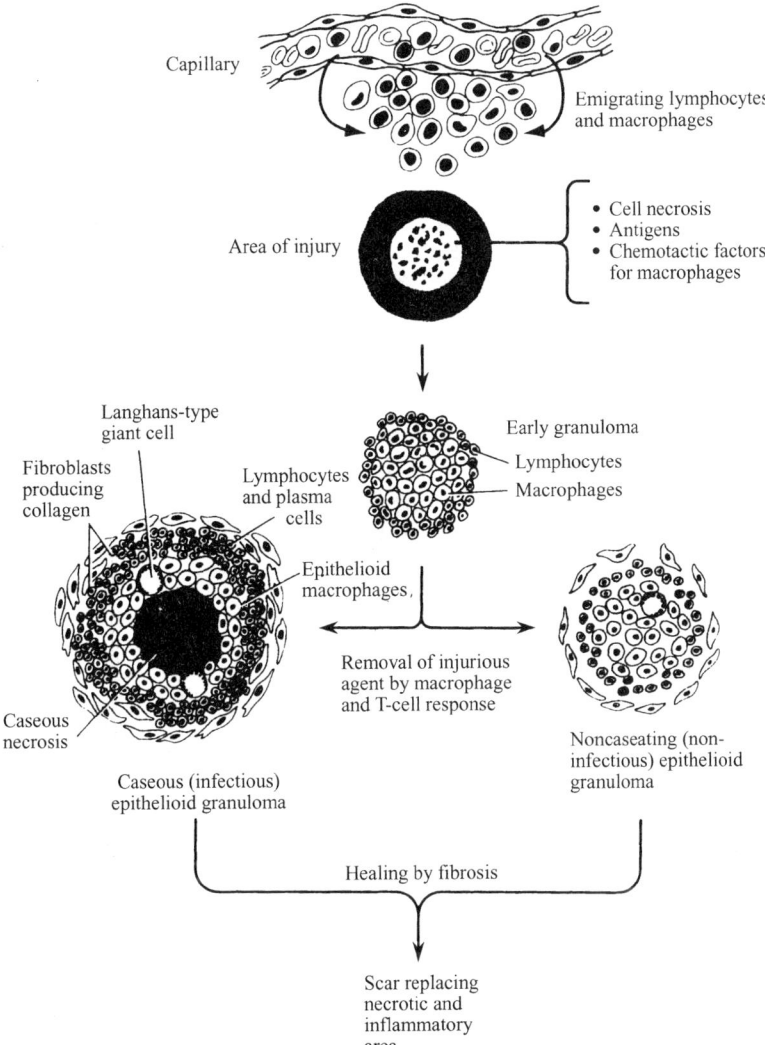

Figure 4-13 Phases in formation of epithelioid granulomas during chronic inflammation. Caseous necrosis occurs especially in those cases in which an infectious agent is responsible for the injury (e. g. tuberculosis)

rial appears yellowish-white and resembles crumbly cheese; on microscopic examination, the center of the granuloma is finely granular, pink, and amorphous (Figure 4-12B). A similar form of necrosis called **gummatous necrosis** occurs in syphilis except that gross characteristics display a more rubbery consistency (hence the term gummatous). Caseous or gummatous necrosis results from a T lymphocyte-mediated hypersensitivity reaction (type IV hypersensitivity). Caseation does not occur in noninfectious epithelioid granulomas.

B. Nongranulomatous Chronic Inflammation

1. Characteristic features

Nongranulomatous chronic inflammation is characterized by the accumulation of sensitized lymphocytes (specifically activated by antigen), plasma cells, and macrophages in the injured area. These cells are scattered diffusely throughout the tissue, however, and do not form granulomas. Scattered tissue necrosis and fibrosis are common.

2. Causes and changes in affected tissue

Nongranulomatous chronic inflammation represents a composite of several different types of immune response due to different antigenic agents (Table 4-8).

a. Chronic viral infections: Persistent infection of parenchymal cells by viruses evokes an immune

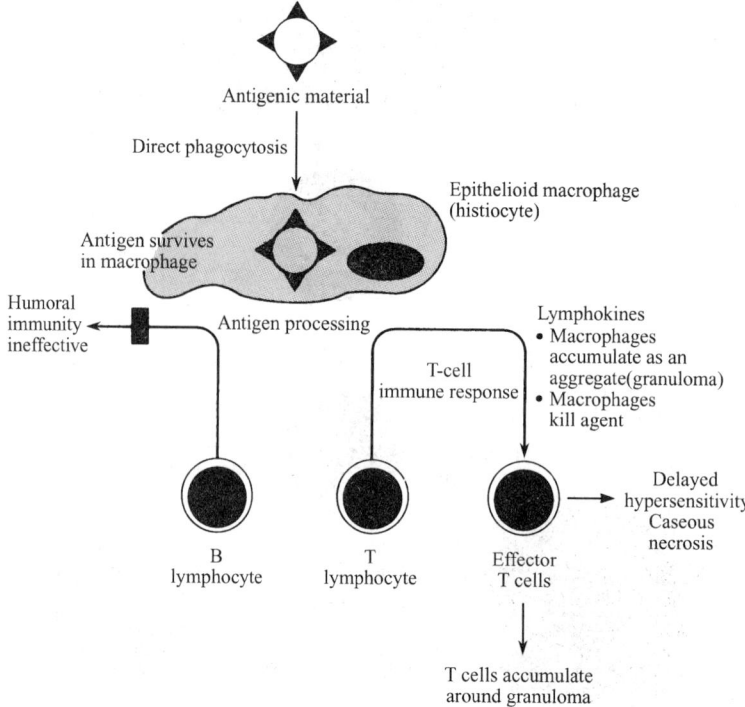

Figure 4-14 Immune mechanism of epithelioid granuloma

Table 4-8 Common causes of nongranulomatous chronic inflammation

Characterized by lymphocytic and plasma cell infiltration of tissue associated with cell necrosis and fibrosis

    Chronic viral infections (cytotoxic B and T cell responses)
    Chronic viral hepatitis
    Chronic viral infections of the central nervous system
  Autoimmune diseases (cytotoxic B and T cell responses)
    Hashimoto's autoimmune thyroiditis
    Chronic autoimmune atrophic gastritis
    Rheumatoid arthritis
    Chronic ulcerative colitis
  Chronic toxic diseases (cell necrosis caused by the toxin results in conversion of cell molecules to antigens)
    Chronic alcoholic pancreatitis
    Chronic alcoholic liver disease

Characterized by diffuse accumulation of macrophges with numerous intracytoplasmic microorganisms:

Deficient T cell response
Lepromatous leprosy
Mycobacterium avium-intracellulare infection in patients with AIDS
Rhinoscleroma (*Klebsiella rhinoscleromatis*)
Leishmaniasis

Characterized by the presence of numerous eosinophils in conjunction with other inflammatory cells

Infections with metazoan parasites
Recurrent type I hypersensitivity reactions, e.g. bronchial ashma, allergic nasal polyps, atopic dermatitis

response whose main components are a B cell response and a T cell cytotoxic response (Figure 4-15). The affected tissue shows accumulation of lymphocytes and plasma cells that produce cytotoxic effects on the cell containing the viral antigen, causing cell necrosis (Figure 4-16). This cytotoxic effect is mediated either by killer T lymphocytes or by cytotoxic antibody acting with complement. Ongoing parenchymal cell necrosis is associated with repair characterized by fibroblast proliferation and deposition of collagen.

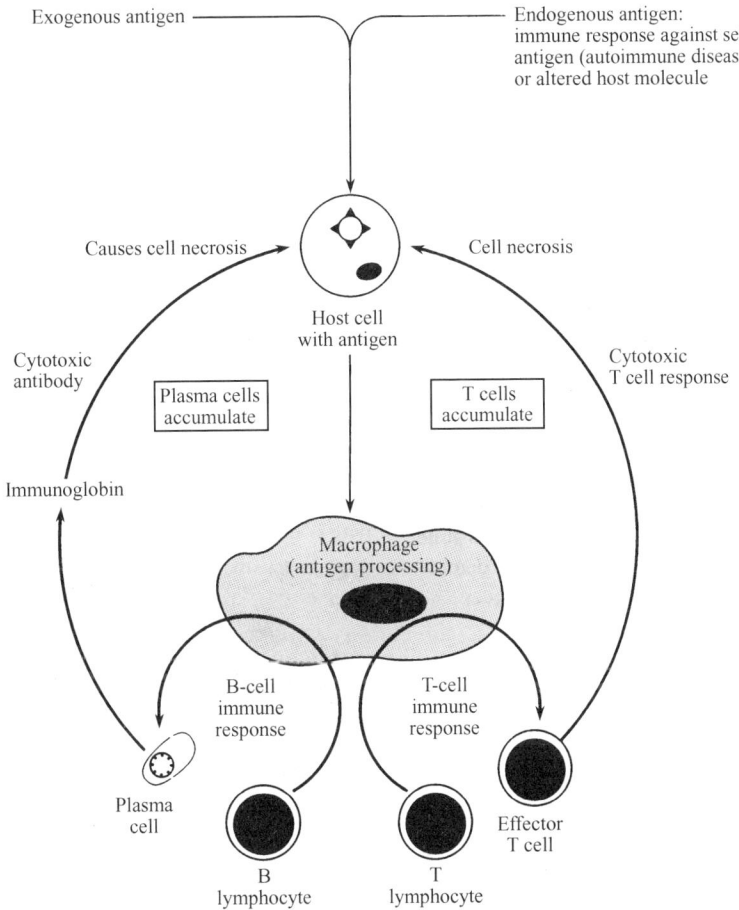

Figure 4-15 Mechanisms of chronic nongranulomatous inflammation due to exogenous antigens or to autoimmune diseases. The process may be exacerbated by abnormalities of the immune response, either (1) an overly vigorous response resulting in further tissue damage – in autoimmune disease and some viral infections, such as chronic viral hepatitis; or (2) an ineffective immune response, allowing unchecked proliferation of microorganisms, as in lepromatous leprosy

b. Chronic autoimmune diseases: A similar type of immune response mediated by cytotoxic antibody and killer T cells occurs in several autoimmune diseases. The antigen involved is a host cell molecule that is perceived as foreign by the immune system. The pathologic result is similar to the nongranulomatous chronic inflammation seen in chronic viral infections, with cell necrosis, fibrosis, and lymphocytic and plasma cell infiltration of the tissue (Figure 4-17).

c. Chronic chemical intoxications: Persistent toxic substances such as alcohol produce chronic inflammation, notable in the pancreas and liver. The toxic substance is not antigenic, but by causing cell necrosis, it may result in alteration of host molecules so that they become antigenic and evoke an immune response. The feature of cell necrosis and repair by fibrosis in such cases dominate the features of the immune response. In many cases of alcoholic chronic pancreatitis, the lymphocytic and plasma cell infiltration is slight.

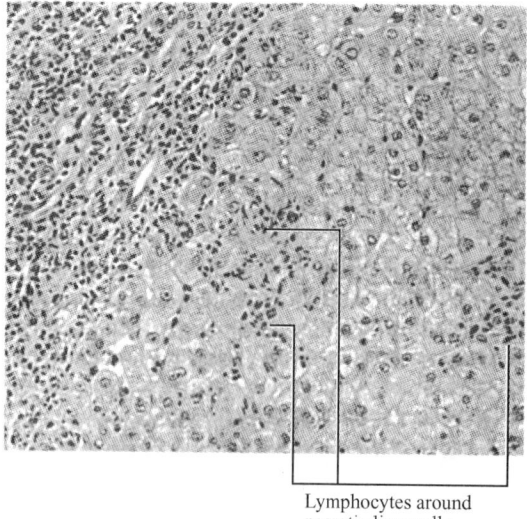

Lymphocytes around necrotic liver cells

Figure 4-16 Chronic viral hepatitis. The periphery of the liver lobule contains numerous lymphocytes and plasma cells. These cells extend into the lobule and are seen there as aggregates around necrotic liver cells. Hepatitis B virus was demonstrated in the cells by immunologic techniques

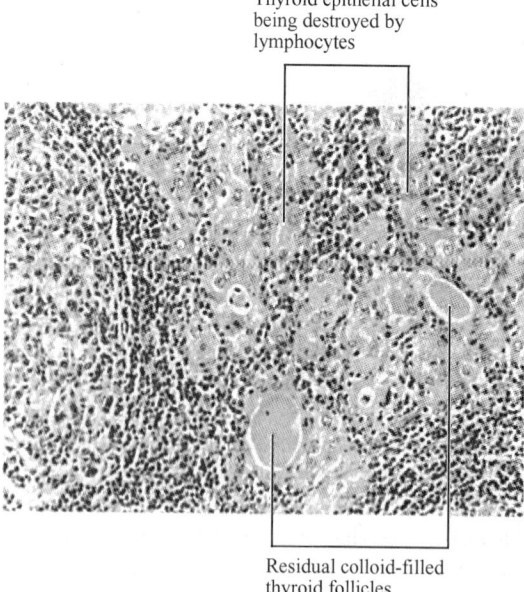

Thyroid epithelial cells being destroyed by lymphocytes

Residual colloid-filled thyroid follicles

Figure 4-17 Autoimmune chronic thyroiditis (Hashimoto's disease). The thyroid is extensively infiltrated by lymphocytes and plasma cells. There is extensive destruction of thyroid follicular epithelial cells

d. Chronic nonviral infections: A specific type of nongranulomatous chronic inflammation is seen with certain microorganisms (Table 4-8) that (1) survive and multiply in the cytoplasm of macrophages after direct phagocytosis and (2) evoke a very ineffective T cell response. This type of infection is characterized by the accumulation of large numbers of foamy macrophages in the tissue (Figure 4-18). The macrophages are present diffusely in the tissue without aggregating into granulomas. The ability of the macrophage to kill the organism is limited because of the poor T cell response, permitting the organisms to multiply in the cell. Typically, large numbers of organisms are present in the cytoplasm of the macrophages. The main defense appears to be direct phagocytosis by the macrophages. Variable numbers of plasma cells and lymphocytes may be present. Accumulation of infected macrophages in the tissue causes nodular thickening of the affected tissue, a clinical feature that is typical of this type of chronic inflammation.

Leprosy is a good example of how the immune response modulates the type of chronic inflammation

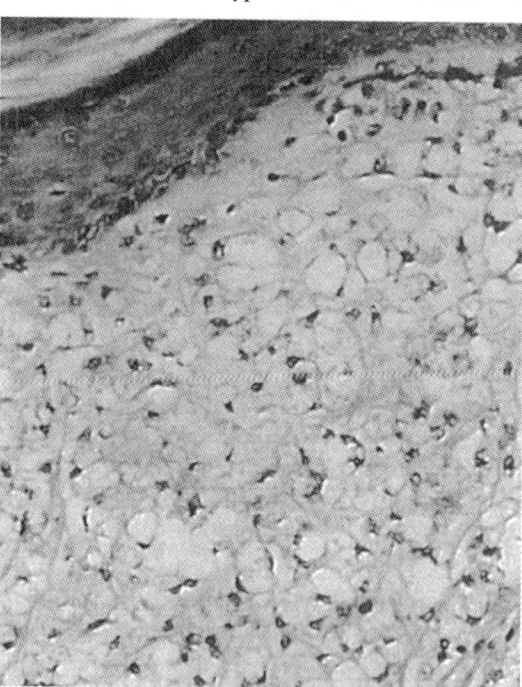

Figure 4-18 Skin in lepromatous leprosy, showing large numbers of foamy macrophages underneath the epidermis. There is no tendency to granuloma formation. Acidfast staining revealed numerous leprosy bacilli in the cytoplasm of the macrophages

that occurs. In patients with a high level of T cell responsiveness against the leprosy bacillus, epithe-lioid granulomas are formed and the multiplication of the organism is effectively controlled (tuberculoid leprosy). In patients with a low level of T cell responsiveness, the organism multiplies unimpeded in macrophages, which accumulate diffusely in the tissue leading to progressive disease (lepromatous leprosy).

e. Allergic inflammation and metazoal infections: Eosinophils typically are present in acute hypersensitivity reactions and accumulate in large numbers in tissues subject to chronic or repeated allergic reactions. It is believed that eosinophils may have evolved as a defense against infection with various metazoal parasites; certainly, eosinophils feature conspicuously in the response against most metazoa. Eosinophils respond chemotactically to complement C5a and factors released by mast cells and in turn release a variety of enzymes and basic proteins. Eosinophils bear high-affinity Fc receptors for IgA and low-affinity receptors for IgE.

Eosinophils are derived from a bone marrow precursor in common with mast cells and basophils. Eosinophils are though to play a role in modulating histamine release or histamine catabolism. Mast cells and basophils have high-affinity Fc receptors for IgE.

CHRONIC INFLAMMATION IN RESPONSE TO NONANTIGENIC INJURIOUS AGENTS

When foreign material that is large (so large as to preclude phagocytosis by a single macrophage), inert (incites no inflammatory response), and nonantigenic (incites no immune response) enters a tissue and persists there, foreign body granulomas form. Nonantigenic material, which includes sutures, talc particles, and inert fibers, is removed by macrophages through nonimmune phagocytosis. Macrophages aggregate around the phagocytosed particles and form granulomas. These frequently contain **foreign body giant cells** characterized by numerous nuclei dispersed throughout the cell (Figure 4-19) rather than arranged around the periphery, as occurs in Langhans-type giant cells. Foreign material is usually identifiable in the center of the granuloma, particularly if viewed under polarized light, when it appears as refractile particles.

Foreign body granuloma is of little clinical significance and indicates only that nondigestible foreign

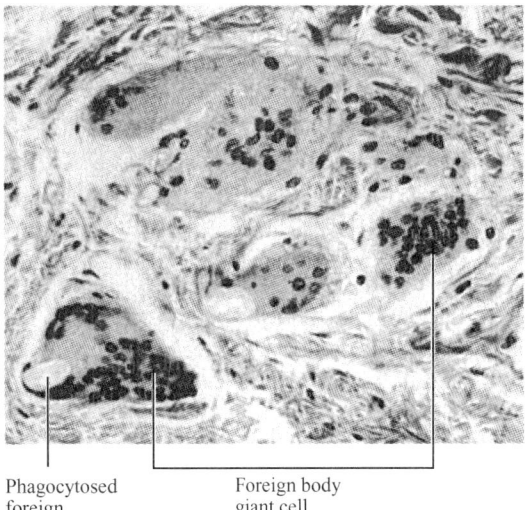

Figure 4-19 Foreign body granuloma, showing macrophages and foreign body giant cells phagocytosing particulate foreign material

material has been introduced into the tissue; e. g. granulomas around talc particles and cotton fibers in alveolar septa and portal areas of the liver are suggestive of intravenous drug abuse (the talc comes from the impure drug preparation and the cotton from the material used for filtering the drug). Tissue necrosis is not an associated feature.

FUNCTION AND RESULT OF CHRONIC INFLAMMATION

Chronic inflammation serves to contain and – over a long period of time – remove an injurious agent that is not easily eradicated by the body. Containment and destruction of the agent are largely dependent on immunologic reactivity, whether these are achieved by (1) direct killing by activated lymphocytes, (2) interaction with antibodies produced by plasma cells, or (3) activation of macrophages by lymphokines produced by T lymphocytes (Figure 4-11).

With the exception of foreign body reactions, chronic inflammation is often associated with tissue necrosis and implies serious illness, e. g. liver failure in chronic active hepatitis. Chronic inflammation is a feature of many chronic diseases that are characterized by total lack of recovery or by a long recovery (months or years).

Associated fibrosis, a repair mechanism is another serous side effect of chronic inflammation if it occurs to an excessive degree. In certain situations, fibrous scarring itself caused disease. For example, fibrosis of the pericardial sac in chronic pericarditis may restrict cardiac filling and cause heart failure, and pulmonary fibrosis may cause respiratory failure.

When removal or neutralization of the injurious agent is ultimately achieved, the tissue heals, usually by fibrosis. The chronic inflammatory cells disappear, and an acellular fibrous scar marks the site of injury.

MIXED ACUTE AND CHRONIC INFLAMMATION

Chronic inflammation may follow acute inflammation, or result from repeated bouts of acute inflammation. In most cases, chronic inflammation begins insidiously and it does not follow an obviously classic acute inflammatory responses. Because acute and chronic inflammation represent different types of host response to injury, features of both types of inflammation may coexist in certain circumstances, as in chronic suppurative inflammation and recurring acute inflammation.

CHRONIC SUPPURATIVE INFLAMMATION

It is difficult to remove the large amounts of pus associated with chronic suppurative inflammation. Infectious agents in pus are basically inaccessible to the actions of antimicrobial drugs and host defense mechanisms because the pus material is avascular. It thus lacks a mechanism for penetration by circulating therapeutic drugs, antibodies, or immune cells. Slow proliferation of the causative agent may therefore continue.

The surrounding viable tissue responds with a longstanding inflammatory process in which areas of suppuration (liquefied necrotic tissue and neutrophils) alternate with areas of chronic inflammation (lymphocytes, plasma cells, macrophages) and fibrosis. Such a pattern occurs in chronic suppurative osteomyelitis and pyelonephritis.

If the area of suppuration localized to an abscess that remains over a long period, a fibrous wall of increasing thickness forms. The difference between an acute and chronic abscess lies in the thickness of the fibrous wall; both forms are filled with pus.

RECURRENT ACUTE INFLAMMATION

Repeated attacks of acute inflammation may occur if there is predisposing cause, e. g. in the gallbladder when there are gallstones. Each attack of acute inflammation is followed by incomplete resolution that leads to a progressively increasing number of chronic inflammatory cells and fibrosis. Depending on the time of examination, the picture may be mainly that of chronic inflammation or of acute superimposed on chronic inflammation. The terms **subacute inflammation** and **acute-on-chronic inflammation** are also used to denote this pattern.

CLINICAL AND PATHOLOGIC DIAGNOSIS

Diagnosis of the nature and cause of chronic inflammatory disease is often difficult because of the insidious nature of the process and the lack of defined separate clinical syndromes for many of the infectious agents involved. Precise diagnosis usually requires recourse to a full range of clinical and pathologic studies (Table 4-9).

Table 4-9 Summary of clinical and laboratory evaluation of chronic inflammation

Systemic features
Fever, usually low-grade and of insidious onset
Peripheral white blood cell count
Usually normal
Sometimes lymphocytosis, monocytosis, eosinophilia
Anemia
Weight loss
Changes in plasma proteins
Elevated levels of plasma immunoglobulins
Association with secondary amyloidosis
Increased erythrocyte sedimentation rate
Local features
Cell necrosis slowly progressive, often extensive
Fibrosis
Presence of effector immune cells (chronic inflammatory cells)
Laboratory evaluation
Biopsy of lesions
Type of chronic inflammation may provide clues to etiology
Microbiologic culture
Immunologic studies
Serologic studies for antibodies against syphilis, fungi
Skin tests for tuberculosis, fungi
Serum autoantibody levels for autoimmune disease

Chapter 5 Neoplasia

Zhou Gengyin, Zhang Qinhui, Meng Bin

CHAPTER CONTENTS
- Definition
- Structure Characteristics of Tumors
- Nomenclature
- Differentiation and Anaplasia of Neoplasms
- Growth, Local Invasion and Metastasis of Neoplasm
    - Excessive Cell Proliferation
    - Invasion
    - Metastasis
- Grading and Staging of Neoplasms
- Difference Between Benign and Malignant Neoplasms
- Effects of Tumors on the Hosts
- Precancerous Lesions, Dysplasia, and Carcinoma in situ
- Mechanisms of Neoplasia
    - Hypotheses of Origin of Neoplasia
    - The Molecular Basis of Neoplasia
    - Multistep Process of Carcinogenesis and Neoplasm Progresses
- Agents Causing Neoplasms
    - Chemical Oncogenesis
    - Radiation Oncogenesis
    - Viral Oncogenesis
- The Role of Inheritance in Oncogenesis
- Tumor Immunity
- Brief Introduction of Common Neoplasms
    - Epithelial Neoplasms
    - Neoplasms of Mesenchymal Cells Origin
    - Neoplasms Arise from Neuro-Ectodermal Tissue

The tumor is a common disease, of which malignant tumor (cancer) is the second leading cause of death in some countries. Only the cardiovascular diseases cause more deaths. With the life span of humankind being much longer, the morbidity and mortality rate of cancer is increasing, despite the progress that has been made in understanding the origins of cancer in the past decades. The only hope to control the dreadful disorder lies in learning more about its molecular origins of cancer.

This chapter deals with the basic morphologic and biologic properties of tumors, the molecular basis of carcinogenesis, also the host response to tumors and clinical manifestation.

DEFINITION

Neoplasia means the process of "the new growth" referred to as a neoplasm, an abnormality of cellular differentiation, maturation, and control of growth. Neoplasms are commonly recognized by the formation of a mass of abnormal tissue (tumor). The term tumor can be applied to any swelling usually caused by inflammation, or hemorrhage into tissue – but today it is used almost solely to denote a neoplastic mass. The study of tumors is called oncology (from oncos, tumor, and logos, study of).

Neoplasms are divided into benign or malignant categories based on several features, chiefly the ability of malignant neoplasm to invade and destroy the adjacent tissue, or metastasize to distant sites to cause death. Cancer is the common term for all malignant neoplasms (the term is thought to derive from the way in which the tumor grips the surrounding tissues with claw-like extensions, much like a crab). Benign neoplasms grow but remain localized, cannot spread to other sites. The patient generally survives after local excision.

Although a neoplasm may not be difficult to recognize, the process of neoplasia is hard to define. In general, neoplasia is an abnormality of cell growth and multiplication characterized by the following features: (1) excessive cellular proliferation that typically but not invariably produces an abnormal mass, or tumor; (2) uncoordinated growth occurring without any apparent purpose and (3) persistence of excessive cell proliferation and growth even after the inciting stimulus that evokes the change has been removed – i.e. neoplasia is an irreversible process.

At molecular level, neoplasia is a disorder of growth regulatory genes (the proto-oncogenes and tumor suppressor genes). It develops in a multistep fashion, such that different neoplasms, even of the same histological type, may show different genetic changes.

STRUCTURE CHARACTERISTICS OF TUMORS

The gross appearance of tumors is varied, reflecting the nature of the tumor to some extent. It may be described as sessile, papillary, nodular, lobulated, cystic, fungating, ulcerated and infiltrating. The variety in tumor shape is usually related to histogenesis, site and biologic behavior. Polypoid and papillary tumors are usually benign. Fungating, ulcerated, annular and infiltrating tumors are more likely to be malignant.

The color and consistency of a benign tumor resembles that of the normal tissue from which it derives. For example, a lipoma is yellow in color and greasy, simulating adipose tissue. The color of the cut surface of a malignant tumor may be gray-white or raddish brown however, often varied due to areas of hemorrhage, degeneration and necrosis, or whether it contains pigment.

The tumors are usually firmer than surrounding tissue, regarding variety of tumor, proportion of parenchyma and stroma, with necrosis and degeneration or not. The lipoma is soft whereas chondroma is hard. The tumor with necrosis is usually softer than that with calcification or osseous metaplasia., and the more numerous the stroma, the harder the tumor.

The benign tumor is usually circumscribed by a clearly defined border, being readily excised. However malignant tumors are invasive and poorly circumscribed, encroaching on the adjacent tissue. All tumors, benign and malignant, have two basic components: the parenchyma and supporting stroma. The parenchyma is made up of transformed or neoplastic cells from which the tumor derives its name, and largely determines its biologic behavior. The classification, nomenclature and histological diagnosis are also made according to the morphology of parenchymal cells.

The supporting stroma, is made up of connective tissue, blood vessels, and possibly lymphatics. It carries the blood supply and provides support for the growth of parenchymal cells and is therefore crucial to the growth of the neoplasm. The growth of a tumor is dependent upon its ability to induce blood vessels to perfuse it. The tumor cells will cease growing if vascular supply to diffuse nutrition into the tumor is limited. Fibroblasts and myofibrobasts offer some mechanical support for the tumor cells and may in addition have nutritive properties. Certain cancers induce a dense, abundant fibrous stroma (desmoplastia) making them hard, so-called scirrhous tumors. The stroma often contain a lymphocytic infiltrate of variable density; this may reflect a host immune reaction to the tumor, patients whose tumors are densely infiltrated by lymphocytes tend to have a better prognosis.

NOMENCLATURE

Benign Tumors

These are generally named after the cell of origin followed by the suffix-oma (Table 5-1). A benign tumor arising in fibrous tissue is a fibroma; a benign neurofibrous tumor is a neurofibroma. The nomenclature of benign epithelial neoplasms is more complex. A benign epithelial neoplasm is called adenoma if it arises within a gland, (e.g. thyroid adenoma, colonic adenoma) or papilloma when arising from an epithelial surface. Papillomas may arise from squamous, glandular, or transitional epithelium (e.g. squamous papilloma, intraductal papilloma of breast, and transitional cell papilloma, respectively). Not uncommonly, descriptive adjectives are incorporated in the nomenclature; e.g. colonic adenomas may be villous or tubular. The hollow cystic masses with papillary pattern are called papillary cystadenoma, they are almost present in the ovary.

Malignant Tumors

A. Carcinoma

Malignant epithelial neoplasms are called carcinomas (adenocarcinomas if derived from glandular epithelium; squamous cell carcinoma and transitional cell carcinoma if originating in those kinds of epithelia). Names may also include the organ of origin and often an adjective as well, e.g. clear cell adenocarcinoma of the kidney, papillary adenocarcinoma of the thyroid, verrucous squamous carcinoma of the larynx.

B. Sarcoma

Malignant neoplasms arising in mesenchymal tissue

Table 5-1 Classification of common neoplasms

Differentiation Potential and Cell Type	Cell or Site	Benign Neoplasm	Malignant Neoplasm
Totipotent cells	Germ cell	Teratoma (mature)	Teratoma (immature), Seminoma (dysgerminoma), embryonal carcinoma, yolk sac carcinoma, choriocarcinoma
Pluripotent cells (embryonic blast cells of organ anlage)	Retinal anlage Retinal anlage Primitive (peripheral) nerve cells Primitive neuroectodermal cells		Retinoblastoma Nephroblastoma (Whilms' tumor) Neuroblastoma Medulloblastoma
Differentiated cells *Epithelial cells*			
Squamous	Skin, esophagus, vagina, mouth, metaplastic epithelium	Squamous papilloma	Squamous carcinoma Basal cell carcinoma
Glandular	Gut, respiratory tract, secretory glands, bile ducts, ovary, endometrium of uterus	Adenoma cystadenoma	Adenocarcinoma Cystadenocarcinoma
Transitional	Urothelium	Papilloma	Transitional cell carcinoma
Hepatic	Liver cell	Adenoma	Hepatocellular carcinoma
Renal	Tubular epithelial cell	Adenoma	Adnocarcinoma
Endocrine	Thyroid, parathyroid, pancreatic islets	Adenoma	Adenocarcinoma
Mesothelium	Mesothelial cells	Benign mesothelioma	Malignant mesothelioma
Placenta	Trophoblast cells	Hydatidiform mole	Choriocarcinoma
Mesenchymal cells Fibrous tissue	Fibroblast	Fibroma	Fibrosarcoma
Cartilage	Chondrocyte	Chondroma	Chondrosarcoma
Nerve	Schwann cell	Schwannoma	Malignant peripheral-nerve-sheath tumor
	Neural fibroblast	Neurofibroma	Malignant peripheral-nerve-sheath tumor
Bone	Osteoblast	Osteoma	Osteosarcoma
Fat	Lipocyte	Lipoma	Liposarcoma
Notochord	Primitive mesenchyme		Chordoma
Vessels	Endothelial cells	Hemangioma lymphangioma	Hemangiosarcoma, Kaposi's sarcoma lymphangisarcoma
Pia and arachnoid	Meningeal cells	meningioma	Malignant meningioma
Muscle	Smooth muscle cells Striated muscle cells	Leiomyoma Rhabdomyoma	Leiomyosarcoma Rhabdomyosarcoma
Melanocytes	Melanocytes	Nevi (various types)	Melanoma (malignant)
Glial cells	Astrocyte		Astrocytomas Glioblastoma mutiforme
	Ependymal cells Oligodendroglial cells		Ependymoma Oliodendroglioma

Differentiation Potential and Cell Type	Cell or Site	Benign Neoplasm	Malignant Neoplasm
Hematopoietic tissue (marrow)	Erythroblasts		Erothroblastic leukemia (Di Guglieimo)
	Myeloblasts		Myeloid leukemia Monocytic leukemias
	Myeloblasts		
Lymphoid tissue	Lymphoblasts, lymphocytes		Malignant lymphoma, lymphocytic leukemias, myeloma
	Histiocytes		Malignant histiocytosis

(Continued)

or its derivatives are named after the cell of origin, to which is added the suffix-sarcoma. A cancer of fibrous tissue origin is fibrosarcoma and malignant neoplasm made up of chondrocytes is a chondrosarcoma.

Exceptions to These Rules

Several neoplasms that do not fit in complicate this simple scheme:

A. Neoplasms That Sound Benign But Are Really Malignant

The names of neoplasms are formed by adding the suffix-oma to the cell of origin, e. g., lymphoma (lymphocyte), plasmacytoma (plasma cell), melanoma (melanocyte), glioma (glial cell), seminoma (germ cell) and astrocytoma (astrocyte). The adjective malignant should be used-malignant lymphoma, malignant melanoma-but if it is not, these neoplasms are assumed to be malignant because there is no benign lymphoma, melanoma, glioma, etc.

B. Neoplasms That Sound Malignant But Are Really Benign

Some tumors derived from primitive tissue are designated blastoma, most of which are malignant, e. g. neuroblastoma, medulloblastoma, nephroblastoma except for two rare bone neoplasms, osteoblastoma and chondroblastoma. The latter may sound malignant because of the suffix-blastoma but are in fact benign neoplasms deriving from osteoblasts and chondroblasts present in adult bone.

C. Leukemia

Neoplasms of blood-forming organs are called leukemia, which are all considered malignant. Leukemias are characterized by the presence of neoplastic cells in bone marrow and peripheral blood; they rarely produce localized tumors.

D. Mixed Tumor

Neoplasms composed of more than one neoplastc cell type, usually derived from one germ cell layer, are called mixed tumors. These may have two epithelial components, as in adenosquamous carcinoma; two mesenchymal components, as in fibrous histocytoma; or an epithelial and a mesenchymal component as in the fibroadenoma of breast and carcinosarcoma of lung.

Mixed tumors containing elements of all three germ layers (e. g. endoderm, ectoderm and mesoderm) is designated teratoma. It is thought to originate from totipotential cells. It is further subdivided into mature teratoma and immature teratoma on the basis of morphologic characteristic.

E. Eponymously Named Tumors

When the cell of origin is poorly understood, the name of the person who first recognized or described the neoplasm is commonly used to name the tumor, e. g. Ewing's sarcoma, Hodgkin's lymphoma and Whilms' tumor. As the histogenesis of these tumors is clarified, the name is often changed: Whilms' tumor is now called nephroblastoma. Some neoplasms of uncertain histogenesis are named descriptively, e. g. granular cell tumor (from Schwann cells?), alveolar soft part sarcoma (from rhabdomyoblasts?).

DIFFERENTIATION AND ANAPLASIA OF NEOPLASMS

Differentiation and anaplasia refer only to the parenchymal cells. When the term differentiation is used to describe the neoplasm, it denotes the degree to which a neoplasm cell resembles the normal mature cells of the tissue both morphologically and functionally; this meaning is distinct from the general use of the word to describe passage of a cell down a particular maturation pathway.

Benign neoplasms are usually fully (well) differentiated, ie, they resemble very closely their normal counterpart. Malignant neoplasms, on the other hand, show variable degrees of differentiation, from well differentiated to completely undifferentiated. The malignant neoplasms that are composed of undifferentiated cells are said to be "anaplastic", which refers to no morphological resemblance whatsoever to normal tissue (Figure 5-1). It is characterized as following:

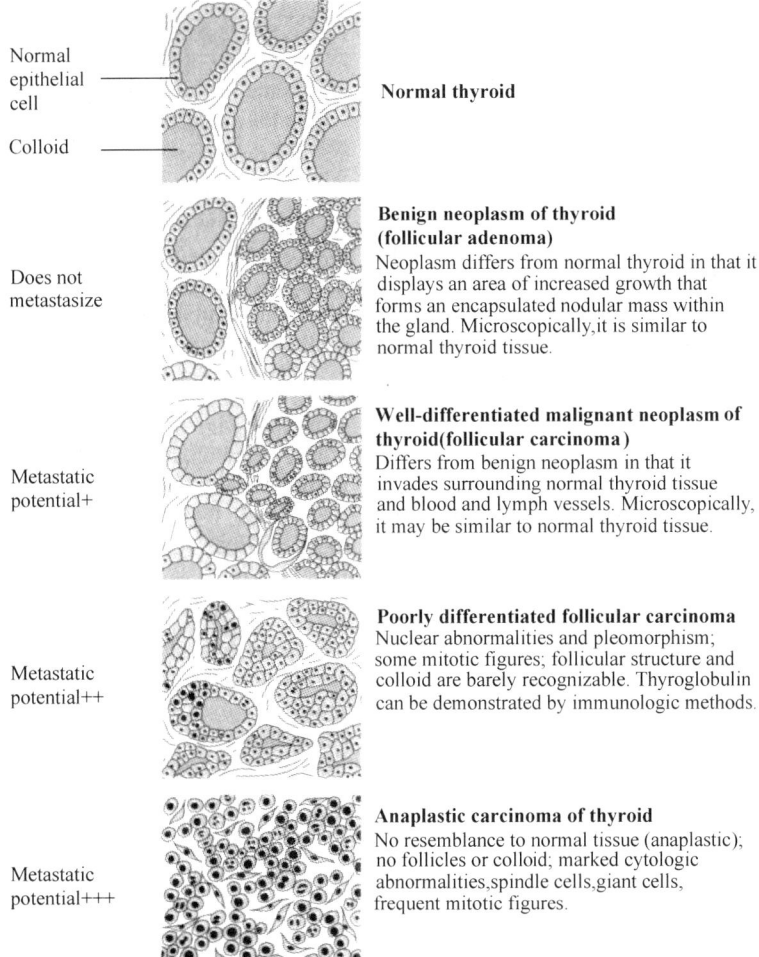

Figure 5-1 Degree of differentiation and anaplasia as exemplified by neoplasms arising in thyroid follicular epithelium. Note that as the neoplasm becomes less well differentiated, its metastatic potential increases

A. Pleomorphism

Both the cells and the nuclei show pleomorphism- variation in cell size and shape. Cells may be many times larger than normal cells, presenting as multinucleated tumor giant cells. Some undifferentiated neoplasms conversely consist of extremely small and primitive appearing cells, e. g. small cell carcinoma of lung.

B. Nuclear Abnormalities

Dysplasia is characterized by increased size of the nucleus, both absolute and relative to the amount of cytoplasm (increased nuclear:cytoplasmic ratio, approaching 1:1 instead of the normal 1:4 or 1:6); increased chromatin content (hyperchromatism ratio); abnormal chromatism distribution (coarse clumping); and nuclear membrane irregularities such as thickening and wrinkling. Large prominent nucleoli are usually present in these nuclei. Undifferentiated tumors usually possess large number of mitoses, especially producing atypical ones, e. g. tripolar, quadripolar or bizarre multipolar mitotic figures. Another feature of dysplasia is to form huge polymorphic nucleus, or having two or more nuclei.

C. Cytoplsmic Abnormalities

Cytoplasmic abnormalities in dysplasia result from failure of normal differentiation, e. g. lack of keratinization in squamous cell and lack of mucin in glandular epithelium.

D. Disordered Maturation

Dysplastic epithelial cells retain a resemblance to basal stem cells as they move upward in the epithelium; normal differentiation (keratin production) fails to occur. The orientation of anaplastic cells are disturbed and lose the normal polarity.

E. Electronic Microscopy of Tumors

No specific determinants of the nature of a neoplasm, whether it is benign or malignant, are detectable by electronic microscopy. On the other hand, organelles and specialized cytoplasmic components may be identified in poorly differentiated cancers, e. g. neuroendocrine granules in neuroendocrine tumors, desmosomes and tonofilament in squamous carcinomas, myofilaments and dense bodies in tumors of smooth muscle origin, melanosomes in melanoma, so as to distinguish them from each other.

(Zhou Gengyin)

GROWTH, LOCAL INVASION AND METASTASIS OF NEOPLASM

The cellular growth abnormality associated with neoplasia is one of its chief attributes and serves to distinguish benign from malignant neoplasms.

EXCESSIVE CELL PROLIFERATION

Neoplastic cells may multiply more rapidly than their normal counterparts. The resulting accumulation of cells in tissue commonly takes the form of a tumor, although in leukemia (cancer of white blood cells), the accumulated cells are spread throughout the bone marrow and peripheral blood and do not form a localized tumor mass. It is important to realize that the overall number of neoplastic cells can increase even if the rate of proliferation is slow; in chronic lymphocytic leukemia, the accumulation of neoplastic cells is due to an arrest in maturation of neoplastic lymphocytes. Such cells fail to complete the cell cycle and therefore do not mature and die as normal cells do.

- **Rate of growth and malignancy:**

The rate of proliferation of neoplastic cells varies greatly. Some neoplasms grow so slowly that growth is measured in years; Others proliferate so rapidly that an increase in size can be observed in days. As a general rule, the degree of malignancy of a neoplasm correlates with its rate of growth: the more rapid the growth, the more malignant the neoplasm. (Table 5-2).

- **Assessment of growth rate:**

Clinically, the rate of growth of a neoplasm can be measured by the time needed for it to double in

Table 5-2 Assessment of growth rate of neoplasms

Clinical approach: serial palpation of the mass
Radiologic approach: serial x-ray or CT scans of the mass
Microscopic approach:
Cellularity (rapidly growing neoplasms are highly cellular)
Number of mitoses (mitotic count per unit area) (see Figure 5-2)[1]
Immunoperoxidase staining of cell cycle-related antigens
Flow cytimetry: percentage of cells in the S and G_2-M phases of the cycle (high with rapid growth)

[1] The number of high-power field used for assessment varies in different neoplasms.

size. This doubling time varies from a few days in Burkitt's lymphoma, to many months in most malignant epithelial neoplasms, to many years in some benign neoplasms.

A crude histologic assessment of the growth rate is the mitotic count, which is usually expressed as the number of mitotic figures (Figure 5-2) counted in 10 consecutive high-power fields in the most active area of the neoplasm. In general, the higher the mitotic count, the more rapid the growth rate of the neoplasm. There are many exceptions to this general statement.

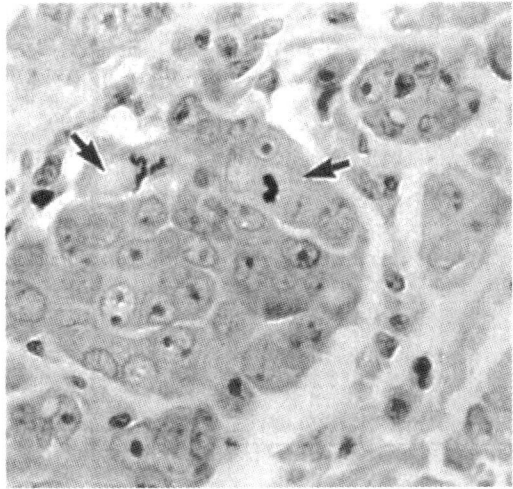

Figure 5-2 Mitotic figures in a malignant neoplasm. Two mitotic figures are present (arrows), one normal (at right) and the other tripolar (at left). Note also the large nuclei, high nuclear: cytoplasmic ratio, and large nucleoli that characterize these malignant cells

More recently, the demonstration of cell cycle-related antigens such as cyclins, ki67 and PCNA (proliferating cell nuclear antigen) promises to be more accurate to assess the growth rate of the neoplasm.

INVASION (INFILTRATION)

Nearly all benign tumors grow as cohesive expansile masses that remain localized to their site of origin and do not have the capacity to infiltrate, invade, or metastasize to distant sites, as do malignant tumors. Because they grow and expand slowly, they usually develop a rim of compressed connective tissue, sometimes called a fibrous capsule, which separates them from the host tissue. This capsule is derived largely from the stroma of the native tissue as the parenchymal cells atrophy under the pressure of expanding tumor. Such encapsulation does not prevent tumor growth, but it keeps the benign neoplasm as a discrete, readily palpable and easily movable mass that can be surgically enucleated. Although a well-defined cleavage plane exists around most benign tumors, in some it is lacking. Thus, hemangiomas (neoplasms composed of tangled blood vessels) are often unencapsulated and may appear to permeate the site in which they arise (commonly the dermis of the skin).

When a benign tumor arises in an epithelial or mucosal surface, the tumor grows away from the surface, because it cannot invade, often forming a polyp which may be either pedunculated (stalked) or sessile; this non-invasive outward direction of growth creates an exophytic lesion.

Malignant neoplasms, in contrast, usually exhibit local invasiveness or infiltration, meaning they extend into adjacent normal structures so as to make the entire mass fixed. In general, malignant tumors are poorly demarcated from the surrounding normal tissue, and a well-defined cleavage plane is lacking. Slowly expanding malignant tumors, however, may develop an apparently enclosing fibrous capsule and may push along a broad front into adjacent normal structures. Histologic examination of such apparently encapsulated masses almost always shows rows of cells penetrating the margin and infiltrating the adjacent structures, a crablike pattern of growth that constitutes the popular image of cancer. They recognize no normal anatomic boundaries. Such invasiveness makes their surgical resection difficult, and even if the tumor appears well circumscribed, it is necessary to remove a considerable margin of apparently normal tissues adjacent to the infiltrative neoplasm. Microscopic examination of rapidly frozen tissue sections must be performed to verify that the margins of resection can be performed while the patient is still in surgery, so that further resection can be undertaken if necessary.

Malignant tumors on epithelial or mucosa surfaces may form a protrusion in the early stages, but eventually invade the underlying tissue, this invasive inward direction of growth gives rise to an endophytic tumor.

Carcinomas and sarcomas demonstrated similar patterns of invasion despite their different tissues of origin. Invasion of the basement membrane (Figure 5-3 and 5-4) by carcinoma distinguishes invasive cancer from intraepithelial (or in situ) cancer. Having penetrated the basement membrane, malignant cells gain access to the lymphatics and blood vessels, the first step toward general dissemination (Figure 5-5). Infiltrating neoplastic cells tend to follow fascial planes along the pathway of the least resistance; eventually, destruction of tissue occurs. The invasiveness of malignant neoplasms is determined by the properties of neoplastic cells within them The mechanisms whereby neoplastic cells invade and destroy tissues are poorly understood, but abnormal or increased cellular motility, loss of contact inhibition of neoplastic cells, protease production, and decreased cell adhesiveness are believed to play a part.

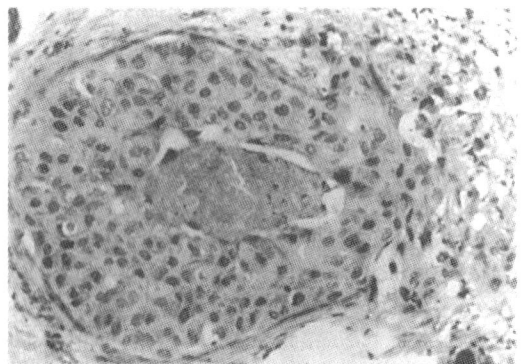

Figure 5-3 Carcinoma of the breast that is predominantly confined within the duct except at the right side, where it has infiltrated through the ductal basement membrane into the surrounding stroma

METASTASIS

Metastasis is the establishment of a second neoplastic mass through transfer of the neoplastic cells from the first neoplasm to a secondary location separate from the original tumor. Metastasis occurs only in malignant neoplasms and explains why they are life-threatening and difficult to eradicate.

A. Route of Metastasis

1. Lymphatogenous metastasis

Metastasis via the lymphatics occurs early in carcinomas and melanomas but is an unusual occurrence in most sarcomas, which tend to spread mainly via the blood stream.

Malignant cells are carried by the lymphatics to the regional lymph nodes (Figure 5-6). The brief that cancerous cells spread first to the regional lymph nodes - where their advanced may be temporarily arrested by the immune response - is the rationale for radical surgery, which removes both the primary neoplasm and the regional lymph nodes to thereby eliminate the most likely sites of early metastases. Removal of lymph nodes is performed only for those neoplasms in which lymphatic metastasis is common, e.g., carcinoma and melanoma. Knowledge of the lymphatic drainage of various tissues enables the clinician to predict the most likely sites of lymph node involvement.

2. Hematogenous metastasis

Entry of cancerous cell into the bloodstream is believed to occur during the early clinical course of many malignant neoplasms. Most of these malignant cells are thought to be destroyed by immune system, but some become coated with fibrin and entrapped in capillaries. (Anticoagulants such as heparin that keep the cell from being coated with fibrin decrease the development of metastases on experimental animals). Metastasis can occur only if enough cancerous cells survive in the tissues to become established and proliferate at a second site (Figures 5-6, 5-7 and 5-8). The production of tumor angiogenesis factor (TAF) by the cancerous cells stimulates growth of new capillaries in the vicinity of tumor cells and encourages vascularization of the growing metastasis.

Certain cancers have a propensity for invasion of veins. Renal cell carcinoma often invades the branches of the renal vein and then the renal vein itself to grow in a snakelike fashion up the inferior vena cava, sometimes reaching the right side of the heart. Hepatocellular carcinomas often penetrate portal and hepatic radicals to grow within them into the main venous channels. Remarkably, such intravenous growth may not be accompanied by widespread dissemination. Histologic evidence of penetration of small vessels at the site of the primary neoplasm is obviously an ominous feature.

The site of metastasis is most commonly the first capillary bed encountered by blood draining the primary site (Figure 5-8). Some types of cancer apparently favor particular metastatic sites, although the mechanisms responsible are unknown. Skeletal metastases are common in cancer of prostate, thyroid, lung, breast, and kidney. Adrenal metastases are common in lung cancer. Experiments using repeated animal passage have enabled researchers to select clones of human cancer cells that selectively metastasize specific sites.

3. Metastasis in body cavities(seeding)

Entry of malignant cells into body cavities (e.g. pleura, peritoneum, or pericardium) or the subar-

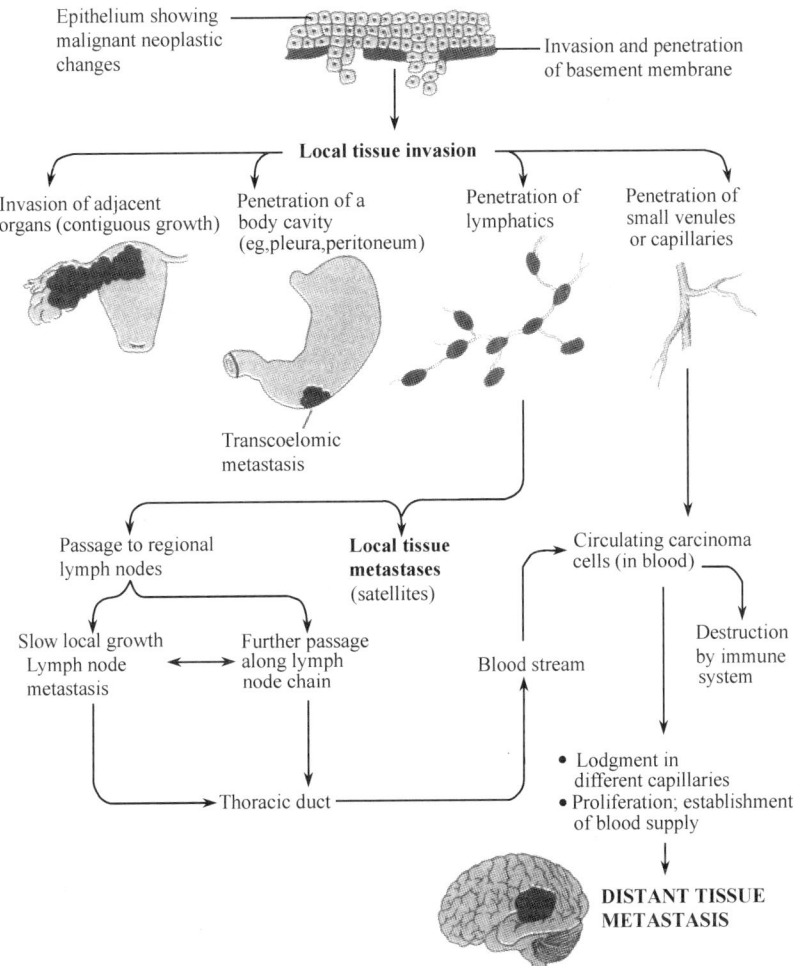

Figure 5-4 Invasion and methods of metastasis as exemplified by a carcinoma. Sarcomas arise in connective tissue and are not limited by a basement membrane. Their properties of invasion and metastasis resemble those of carcinomas, except that sarcomas generally favor hematogenous over lymphatic metastasis

achnoid space may be followed by dissemination of the cells anywhere within these cavities (transcoelomic metastasis); the rectovesical pouch and ovary are common locations for peritoneal metastasis in patients with gastric cancer.

Cytologic examination of the fluid from these body cavities for the presence of malignant cells is an excellent method of confirming the diagnosis of metastasis.

4. Dormancy of metastases

Cancerous cells that spread to distant sites may remain dormant there (or at least remain slowly growing and undetectable), sometimes for many years. The presence of such dormant cancerous cells (or slowing growing subclinical metastases) has led to attempts to eradicate them by means of systemic chemotherapy after treatment of the primary tumor. While results have been encouraging in some types of disseminated cancer, including malignant lymphoma, choriocarcinoma, and testicular germ cell tumors, the overall cure rate is so low – and the morbidity of chemotherapy so high – as to question the validity of this approach for most malignant tumors.

Development of delayed metastases makes it difficult to pronounce a patient cured with any confidence. Survival for 5-years after treatment is considered a sign of cure for most cancers. However, 10-

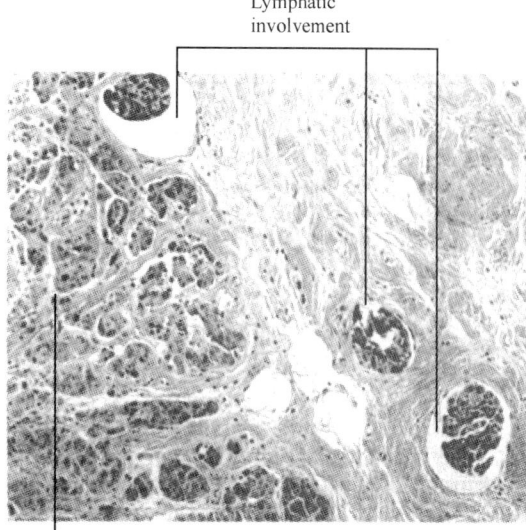

Figure 5-5 Infiltrating carcinoma, showing invasion of lymphatics by the tumor cells

year and 20-year survival rates are almost always lower than the 5-year survival rates, which suggests that many patients experience late metastases.

B. Mechanism of Metastasis

The mechanisms by which malignant tumors leave the primary tumor site, invade lymphatics, bloodstream and metastasize to regional lymph nodes or distant organs are complex. Neoplastic cells must successfully complete a cascade of events before forming a metastatic tumor, only a proportion of the neoplastic cells in a malignant tumor may have the full repertoire of properties necessary for completion of the cascade. Many tumors studied experimentally in animals consist of metastatic and non-metastatic clones, and metastatic tumors in humans often appear histologically less well differentiated than the primary lesion, suggesting that there is clonal evolution of the metastatic phenotype.

There is experimental evidence for the inactivation of anti-metastatic genes, such as nm23, KAI-1, KISS in neoplastic cells capable of metastasis, but their precise role in the metastatic cascade is uncertain.

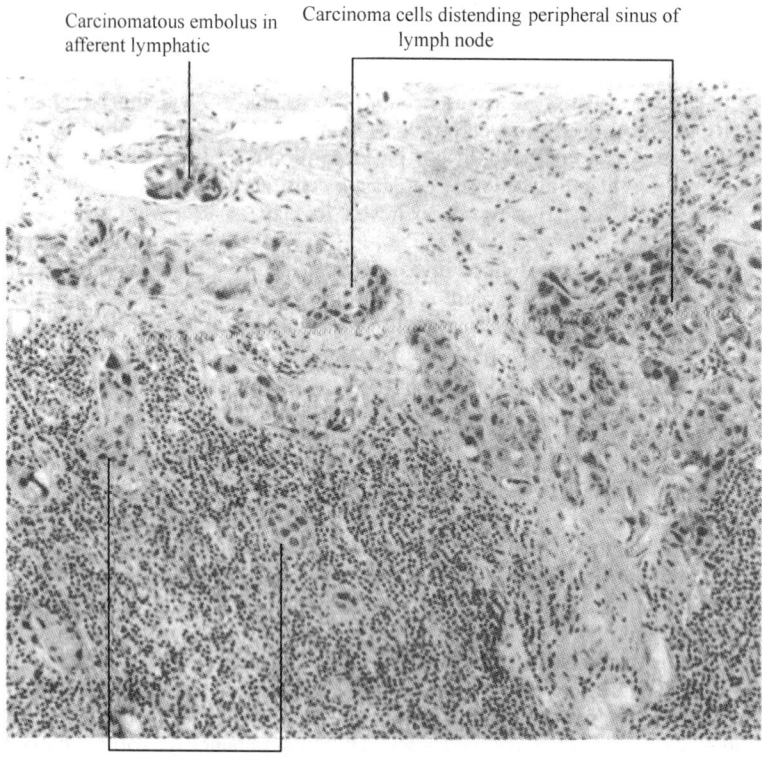

Figure 5-6 Metastatic carcinoma in a lymph node

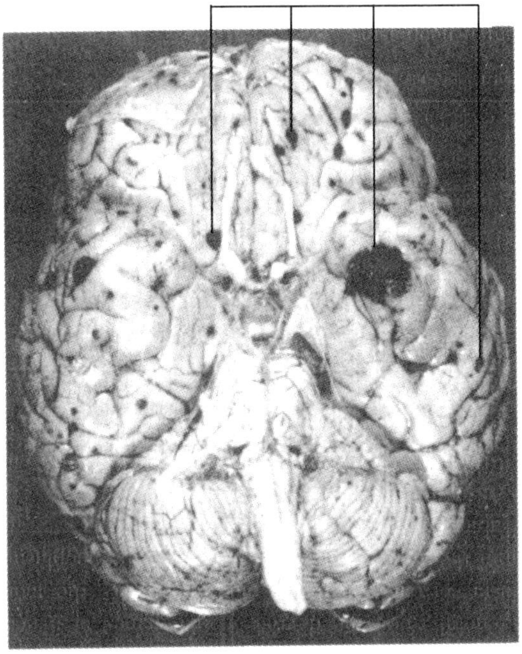

Figure 5-7 Hematogenous metastasis to the brain by a malignant melanoma, showing multiple pigmented tumor deposits

The sequential steps involved in the metastatic cascade are:
- detachment of tumor cells from their neighbours
- invasion of the surrounding connective tissue to reach conduits for metastasis (blood and lymphatic vessels)
- intravasation into the lumen of vessels
- evasion of host defense mechanisms, such as natural killer cells in the blood
- adherence to endothelium at remote location
- extravasation of the cells from the vessel lumen into the surrounding tissue
- neoplastic cell proliferation and form the secondary tumor

On reaching the site of metastasis there is a recapitulation of the events that were required to form the primary tumor. The tumor cells must proliferate and, if they are to grow to form a nodule larger than a few millimeters in diameter, the blood vessels must be elicited by angiogenic factors.

Normal cells are neatly glued to each other and their surroundings by a variety of adhesion molecules. Alterations in cell adhesion molecules are important at several points in the metastatic cascade; these affect cell-cell and cell-substrate adhesion. Studies on experimental and human tumors show that reduced expression of cadherins, which are involved in adhesion between epithelial cells, correlates positively with invasive and metastatic behavior. Increased expression of integrins appears to be important for the invasive migration. Presumably, down-regulation reduces the ability of cells to adhere to each other and facilitates their detachment from the primary tumor and their advance into the surrounding tissues. E-cadherins are linked to the cytoskeleton by the catenins, proteins that lie under the plasma membrane. The normal function of E-cadherin is dependent on its linkage to catenins. In some tumors, E-cadherin is normal, but its expression is reduced because of mutations in the gene for a catenin.

Tumor cells secrete proteolytic enzymes themselves or induce host cells (e.g. stromal fibroblasts and infiltrating macrophages) to elaborate proteases. The activity of these proteases is tightly regulated by antiproteases. At the invading edge of tumors, the balance between proteases and antiproteases is tilted in favor of proteases. Three classes of proteases have been identified: the serine, cysteine, and matrix metalloproteinases (MMPs). MMP9 and MMP2 are collagenases that cleave type IV collagen of epithelial and vascular basement membranes. There is compelling evidence supporting the role of MMPs that degrade type IV collagen in tumor cell invasion:

Once in the circulation, tumor cells are particularly vulnerable to destruction by innate and adaptive immune defenses. Within the circulation, tumor cells tend to aggregate in clumps. This is favored by homotypic adhesions among tumor cells as well as heterotypic adhesion between tumor cells and blood cells, particularly platelets. Formation of platelet-tumor aggregates may enhance tumor cell survival and implantability. Arrest and extravasation of tumor emboli at distant sites involve adhesion to the endothelium, followed by egress through the basement membrane. At the new site, tumor cells need to proliferate, develop a vascular supply, and evade the host defenses.

In some cases, the target tissue may be an unpermissive environment-unfavorable soil, so to speak, for the growth of tumor seedlings. For example, although well vascularized, skeletal muscles are rarely

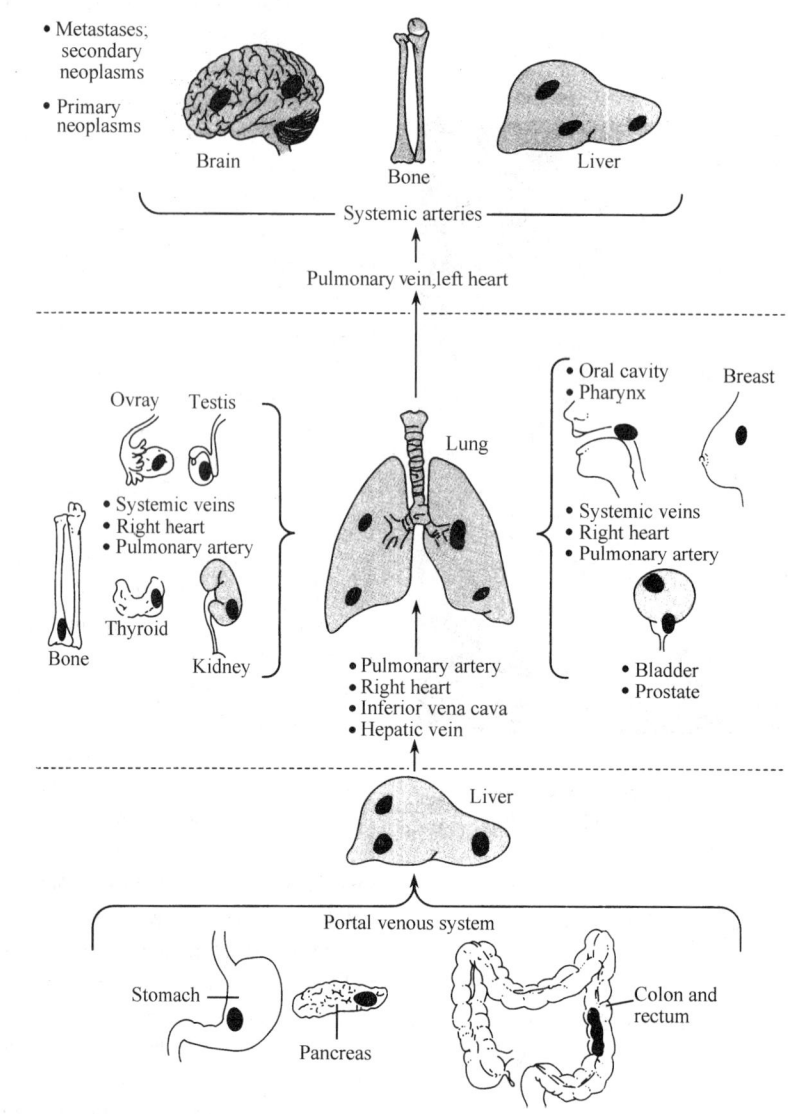

Figure 5-8 Principal anatomic routes of hematogenous metastasis. Primary neoplasms in the gastrointestinal tract and pancreas metastasize via the portal venous system to the liver. Other neoplasms tend to involve the lungs via the systemic circulation. Malignant cells may bypass the liver and lungs and enter the systemic circulation and produce metastases in any organ in the body. Organs such as brain, bone, and liver are the common sites of metastasis of lung cancer

the site of metastases. While primary tumors at various sites have a preferential type of metastatic spread, the precise localization of metastases cannot be predicted with certainty for any form of cancer.

Possible fates of cancer cells in a secondary site, following the arrival of circulating cancer cells in an organ. Cancer cells can exist in a secondary site as solitary cells, small pre-angiogenic metastases or larger vascularized metastases. At each step, only a subset will proceed, and the remainder of cells or micrometastases might either go into a state of dormancy, or die. Only a proportion of vascularized metastases are clinically detectable, solitary cells and micrometastases are generally clinically undetectable. Dormant solitary cells refer to cells that are undergoing neither proliferation nor apoptosis, whereas 'dormant' pre-angiogenic micrometastases refer to those in which active proliferation is balanced by active apoptosis, resulting in no net increase in the size of the metastases.

GRADING AND STAGING OF NEOPLASMS

Once the diagnosis of a malignant is made, it is important to determine the prognosis for the patient. The prognosis depends not only on type of malignancy (some tumor are more aggressive than others), but also on the grade and stage of the tumor. The grade is determined by a pathologist who examines the tumor histologically; the stage is determined by the extent of spread of a cancer within the patient.

Grading

The grade of a malignant tumor is based on the degree of differentiation of the tumor cells, the degree of cytologic atypia and the number of mitoses within the tumor. Cancers are classified as grades I to IV with increasing anaplasia. Criteria for the individual grades vary with each form of neoplasia, but all attempt, in essence, to judge the extent to which the tumor cells resemble or fail to resemble their normal counterparts. In general, low grade tumors are well differentiated, have minimal cytological atypia and low mitotic rates. High grade tumors are poorly differentiated, have marked cytological atypia and high mitotic rates (Table 5-3).

Table 5-3　Guidelines for grading tumors

Grade 1	Well-differentiated (Low grade)
Grade 2	Moderately differentiated (Intermediate grade)
Grade 3	Poorly differentiated (High grade)
Grade 4	Undifferentiated (High grade)

Clinically, lower grade cancers grow more slowly and have a better prognosis, whereas higher grade cancers grow more rapidly and have a poorer prognosis. Nevertheless, some cancers that were once low grade may be transformed over time into high grade, highly malignant tumors.

Staging

The staging of cancers refers to the extent or severity of the cancer and is based on the size of tumor, the extent of invasion into surrounding tissue, the spread to regional lymph nodes and the presence or absence of blood-borne metastases.

The pathologic stage describes the extent of a neoplasm. In a specimen obtained during resection, the pathologic stage is determined by the extent of infiltration and metastasis (eg, depth of invasion of the wall of a viscus; lymph node, bone marrow, or organ involvement). Pathologic staging is important because it determines what further treatment a patient may be given, and it is a valuable guide to prognosis. An attempt to standardize pathologic staging is the so-called TNM classification, which classifies neoplasms on the basis of size of the primary tumor (T), lymph node involvement (N), and distant metastases (M).

Each tumor is assigned a series of identifiers, which include a T, an N and an M component. Together these labels give insight into the severity of the cancer. This set of values is then used to establish a simpler, overall stage for the cancer, which is then described as stage I, II, III, or IV. As would be expected, a mild T, N and M grading corresponds to a lower stage number and a less severe cancer, for example a T1, N0, M0 tumor is most likely labeled as a stage I cancer. This simplified staging method can help physicians and patients make treatment decisions and also gives an indication of the prognosis.

DIFFERENCE BETWEEN BENIGN AND MALIGNANT NEOPLASMS

Treatment of neoplasms is based on their biological behavior. Benign neoplasma are cured by excision of the tumor locally. Aggressive neoplasms must be treated by excising the tumor along with a wide margin of surrounding tissue to ensure that infiltrating cells are removed. Malignant neoplasms require local wide removal, frequently including regional lymph nodes as well as systemic treatment for neoplastic cells that may have metastasis.

The pathologist classifies a neoplasm as benign or malignant on the basis of histological and cytologic features in association with the accumulation clinicopathologic experience gained with various types of neoplasms. There are no absolute criteria for distinguishing benign from malignant neoplasms, and the characteristics listed in table serve as general guideline only (Table 5-4).

Table 5-4 Comparisons between benign and malignant tumor

	Benign	Malignant
Differentiation	Well differentiated	Range from well differentiated to undifferentiated
Rate of Growth	Slow growth over a period of years	Rapid growth, sometimes erratic
Type of Growth	Expansile (pushing margins)	Progressive infiltration, invasion, and destruction of surrounding tissue
Separated from surrounding tissue?	Yes Has fibrous capsule composed of stroma of native tissue	Poorly separated
Stromal invasion	No	Yes
Vascular invasion	No	Yes
Metastases	No	Yes
Effect on host	Often insignificant	Significant
Recurrence	Rare	Often
Cell shape	Monomorphic	Pleomorphic Tumor giant cells
Nuclear chromatin	Normal	Increased, hyperchromatic Peripheral clumping
Nucleoli	Not prominent	Prominent, irregular shape

A. Rate of Growth

Malignant neoplasms generally grow more rapidly than benign ones, but there is no critical rate that distinguishes malignant from benign. Assessment of the growth rate is based upon clinical information (e.g., change in size of the mass in serial examinations). On microscopic examination, the number of mitotic figures and then metabolically active appearance of nuclei (enlarged, dispersed chromatin, large nucleoli) correlate positively with the growth rate of the neoplasm.

B. Size

The size of a neoplasm usually has no bearing on its biological behavior. Many benign neoplasm become very large; conversely, highly malignant neoplasms may be lethal by virtue of extensive dissemination even though the original primary tumor is still small. In a few neoplasms, however, size is the deciding factor in distinguishing benign and malignant growths. A carcinoid tumor of appendix is considered benign unless it is large than 2 cm, in which case it is regarded as malignant; this distinction is based on the observation that the risk of metastasis increases with increasing size of the primary neoplasm and that appendiceal carcinoid tumor unless large than 2 cm in diameter do not metastasize. Benign and malignant carcinoid tumors are histologically identical.

C. Degree of Differentiation

Benign neoplasms are usually fully (well) differentiated. Malignant neoplasms, on the other hand, show variable degrees of differentiation and frequently demonstrate little resemblance to normal tissue (i.e. they are poorly differentiated). The importance of these individual criteria varies with different neoplasms. For example, the mitotic rate is the major factor distinguishing benign and malignant smooth muscle neoplasms in the uterus; in many other neoplasms, the mitotic rate is of little relevance. Similarly, pheochromocytoma, a neoplasm of the adrenal medulla, may show extreme cytologic abnormalities without demonstrating malignant behavior.

D. Changes in DNA

Neoplasms are associated with abnormalities in their DNA content; this abnormality increases with the degree of malignancy. The degree of hyperchromatism (increased staining of the nucleus) provides a crude assessment of DNA content on microscopic examination; malignant cells are hyperchromatic. When measures precisely by flow cytometry, the DNA content of malignant cells correlates well with the degree of malignancy in malignant lymphoma, bladder neoplasms, and astrocytic neoplasms. Cytogenetic studies demonstrating aneuploidy and polyploidy also are indicative of malignancy. Molecular techniques that demonstrate clonal deletions, translocations, or abnormalities of oncogene expression are of increasing value.

E. Infiltration and Invasion

Benign neoplasms are generally noninfiltrative and are surrounded by a capsule of compressed and fibrotic normal tissue. Malignant neoplasms, on the other hand, have infiltrating margins. Many exceptions to this rule exist, and some benign neoplasms-eg, granular cell tumor, dermatofibroma, and carcinoid tumors-lack a capsule and have infiltrative margin.

F. Metastasis

The occurrence of metastasis (noncontiguous or distant growth of tumor) is absolute evidence of malignancy. The major reason for distinguishing benign and malignant neoplasms is to be able to predict their ability to metastasize before they do so.

Gross and microscopic examination of a neoplasm usually enables a trained pathologist to classify most neoplasms as benign or malignant. In some instances, however, this identification is difficult, and the only reliable evidence of a neoplasm's biologic behavior is the occurrence of metastasis; about 90% of pheochromocytomas are benign, but there are no reliable criteria for identifying the 10% that will metastasize.

EFFECTS OF TUMORS ON THE HOSTS

Neoplasia may be the underlying cause of almost any sign or symptom anywhere in the body. Recognizing the ways in which neoplasms produce symptoms and signs is an important part of diagnosis.

Direct Effect of Local Growth of Primary Tumors

The signs and symptoms arising from local growth of a benign neoplasm or a primary malignant neoplasm vary with the site of the lesion, the nature of the surrounding anatomic structures, and the overall rate of growth of the neoplasm. The growing tumor may compress or destroy adjacent structures, cause inflammation, pain, vascular changes, and varying degrees of functional deficits.

If the tumor is growing near a vital structure (e.g. the brain stem), such local effects may be lethal regardless of whether the neoplasm is classified as benign or malignant.

Neoplasms growing in a confined area, the cranial cavity, from space-occupying lesions that are associated not only with local compressive effects but also with a general - and potentially lethal - increase in intracranial pressure.

Systemic Effects

A. Weight loss and Cachexia

Many factors contribute to the loss of weight as cancer progresses, among them: loss of appetite; malabsorption; increased catabolism; chronic infection. In advanced or terminal stages of cancer, a state of extreme wasting, malnutrition, malaise, and weakness occurs and is called cachexia, the precise cause of which is not clear. The role of the cytokine "cachectin" in human cachexia remains unproved.

B. Fever

Fever in neoplastic disease is usually the result of tissue necrosis and infection.

C. Anemia

Anemia associated with neoplastic disease may be caused by blood loss, underproduction, malnutrition, chronic infection, and so on.

D. Infections

Patients with advanced cancer have decreased resistance to bronchopneumonia and various opportunistic infections as the immune responsiveness becomes weakened by cytotoxic drugs, radiation therapy, tumor products, and tumor-cell invasion of bone marrow and lymphoid spaces.

E. Hormone Production and Paraneoplastic Syndromes

Functioning tumors of endocrine glands, such as adrenal cortex and medulla, parathyroid, pancreatic islets, and other endocrine cells, may produce hormones appropriate for the tissue of origin. Furthermore, some tumors not originating in endocrine glands may produce ectopic hormones inappropriate for the tissue of origin. Clinical constellations of signs and symptoms occurring in patients with neoplastic disease and not explained by local or distant tumor spread or by the presence of functioning tumors of endocrine glands are called **paraneoplastic syndromes**. These syndromes are seen in about 15% of patients with advanced cancer and occasionally are the first manifestation of an otherwise occult tumor. Paraneoplastic syndromes may be classified into those associated, or unassociated, with ectopic hormone production by the tumor. Suggested mechanisms include autoimmune phenomena, the formation of soluble immune complexes, and secretion of substances not yet characterized.

Certain paraneoplastic syndromes are so characteristic of a specific cancer that their presence should prompt a thorough investigation for the existence of the underlying cancer. (e.g. myasthenia gravis - thyrmoma; acanthosis nigricans - gastric cancer).

PRECANCEROUS LESIONS, DYSPLASIA, AND CARCINOMA IN SITU

As we noted that the lag period encompasses that span of time between initiation of the carcinogenic process and the clinical detection of the cancer. The sequential multiple hits that are an essential part of carcinogenesis occur during the first part of this period, extending from a few years through 3 or more decades producing the first neoplastic cell. Repeated division of this cell and its progeny (the malignant clone), sufficient to produce a clinically detectable neoplasm (approximately 10^9 cells), occupies additional months or years constituting the remainder of the lag period. In most instances, no clinical or morphologic abnormalities are apparent throughout the time. However, in some cases, an intermediate abnormal, nonneoplatic growth pattern may be detected. Such an abnormality is a precancerous (preneoplastic) lesion.

Precancerous lesions: A premalignant or precancerous lesion is an abnormality in a tissue area which is just a step away form cancer. Not all premalignant lesions change to cancer, but most have greater potential for doing so than normal tissues. There are many varieties of premalignant lesions (Table 5-5).

It is important to recognize precancerous lesions when they occur because surgical excision is curative (the potentially malignant tissue having been removed). While hyperplasias and metaplasia are not per se premalignant, if sustained they may progress to dysplasia, which does carry a high risk of conversion to malignancy. Most benign neoplasiams progress to malignancy only rarely, but in some the risk is high, and these then also are considered premalignant lesions. Again, the detection of dysplasia in a benign tumor is warning sign.

Table 5-5 Precancerous (Premalignant) Changes

Precancerous Lesion	Cancer
Hyperplasia	
Endometrial hyperplasia	Endometrial carcinoma
Breast-lobular and ductal hyperplasia	Breast carcinoma
Liver-cirrhosis of the liver	Hepatocellular carcinoma
Dysplasia	
Ceviex	Squamous carcinoma of cervix
Skin	Squamous carcinoma
Bladder	Transitional cell carcinoma
Bronchial epithelium	Lung carcinoma
Metaplasia	
Glandular metaplasia of esophagus	Adenocarcinoma of esophagus
Inflammatory lesions	
Ulcerative colitis	Carcinoma of colon
Atrophic gastritis	Carcinoma of stomach
Autoimmune (Hashimoto's thyroiditis)	Malignant lymphoma, thyroid carcinoma
Benign neoplasms	
Colonic adenoma	Carcinoma of colon
Neurofibroma	Malignant peripheral-nerve-sheath tumor (malignant schwannoma)

Many neoplasitic growths are preceded by a non-neoplasiatic proliferation of cells within the epithelium from which they arise. These proliferations are non-neoplastic because they are potentially reversible. Something caused the cells to start proliferating in an abnormal fashion, and if this initiating stimulus is removed the cells may revert to normal. If the cells in these non-neoplastic growths have a disorganized pattern, the growth process is called dysplasia.

Dysplasia is an abnormality of both differentiation and maturation. Use of the term dysplasia should be restricted to abnormalities of cell growth with the characteristics described below. Characteristics of dysplastic epithelium include increased size of the nucleus, both absolute and relative to the amount of cytoplasm (increased nuclear : cytoplasm ratio); increased chromatin contain (hyperchromatic); abnormal chromatin distribution (coarse clumping); and nuclear membrane irregularities such as thickening and wrinkling. In squamous epithelium, an increased rate of cellular multiplication is characterized by the presence of mitotic figures in many layers of the epithelium—in contrast to the normal state, in which mitosis is limited to the basal layer. Individual mitosis are morphologically normal in dysplasia. Dysplastic epithelial cells retain a resemblance to basal stem cells as they move upward in the epithelium; normal differentiation (keratin production) fails to occur. Dysplasia is usually graded as mild dysplasia—dysplasia involving basal one-third of epithelium, moderate dysplasia—dysplasia involving basal two-thirds of epithelium; and severe dysplasia—dysplasia estending in to upper one-thired of epithelium.

In the uterine carrix, the relationship of dysplasia to cervical carcinoma is so intimate that the term cervical intraepithelial neoplasia (CIN) is used synonymously with the term dysplasia (Figure 5-9).

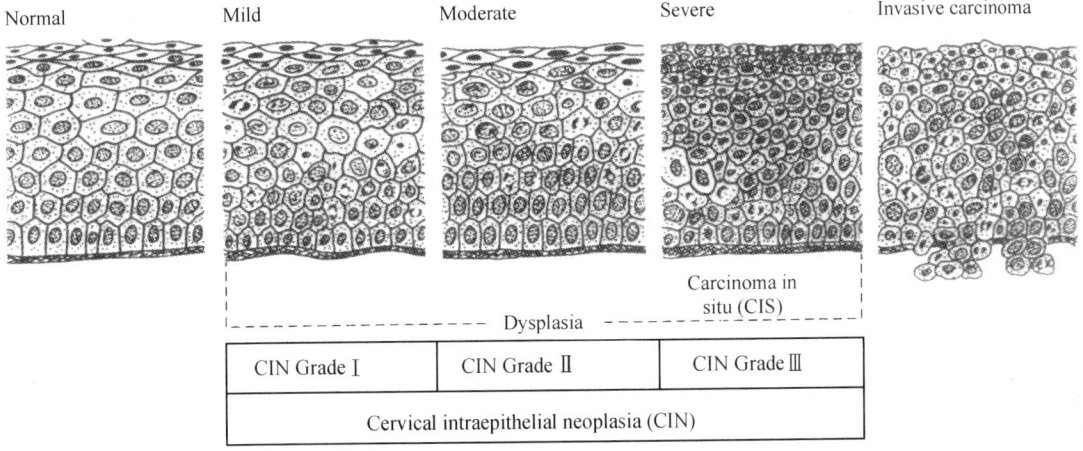

Figure 5-9 Squamous epithelium of the uterine cervix, showing criteria used for grading dysplasia (cervical intraepithelial neoplasia). The maturation defect, the nuclear : cytoplasmic ratio, and the nuclear chromatin abnormalities progressively increase as the grade of dysplasia increases. Note that infiltration of the neoplastic cells through the basement membrane distinguishes invasive carcinoma from dysplasia and carcinoma in situ

Significance of displasia: When it is defined in this manner, epithelial dysplasia is a premalignant lesion, associated with an increased risk of development of cancer. In simple terms, dysplasia is one step short of cancer—with cancer a general term for invasive, aggressive growths that are more properly called malignant neoplasms. A dysplasia may persist, or progress. The risk to developing invasive cancer varies with (1) the grade of dysplasia—the more severe, the greater the risk; (2) the duration of the dysplasia—the longer the duration, the greater the risk; and (3) the site of dysplasia. dysplasia in the urinary bladder is associated with a more imminent risk of cancer than is cervical dysplasia, in which several years may elapse before invasive carcinoma develops. Currently, there are few molecular markers available to identify dysplasias. The abnormality in the microscopic appearance of the cells is the major marker we have. Not all of the lesions we call dysplasia defines a risk of progression.

Carcinoma in situ: The term carcinoma in situ refers to an epithelial neoplasm exhibiting all the cellular features associated with malignancy, but which has not yet invaded with through the epithelial basement membrane separating it from potential route of meatastasis—blood vessels and lymphatics. It is only at this very early stage the excision of a carcinoma will guarantee a cure. Detection of carcinoma at the in situ stage, or of their precursor lesions is the aim of population screening programs for cervical, breast and some other carcinomas. The phase of in situ growth may last for several years before invasion.

Carcinoma in situ may be preceded by a phase of dysplasia, in which the epithelium shows disordered differentiation short of frank neoplasia. Some dysplastic lesions are almost certainly reversible. As there are other applications of word dysplasia as well as some difficulty in reliable distinguishing between carcinoma in situ as dysplasia in biopsies, the term is now less favoured. The term "intraepithelial neoplasia" as in cervical intraepithelial neoplasia (CIN), is used to embrace both carcinoma in situ and the precursor lesion formerly known as dysplasia.

(Zhang Qinghui)

MECHANISMS OF NEOPLASIA

Neoplasia is an abnormality of cell growth and characterized by a uncoordinated, excessive and persistent cellular proliferation. The knowledge about the mechanism of neoplasia strikingly increased in recent decades of years. We know that at the molecular level neoplasia is a disorder of growth-related regulatory genes which include four classes: the proto-oncogenes, the tumor suppressor genes, the genes that regulate programmed cell death or apoptosis, and the genes that regulate repair of damaged DNA. So neoplasm can be called a genetic disease. Neoplasia develops in a multistep process, such that different neoplasms, even of the same histologic type, may show different genetic changes.

HYPOTHESES OF ORIGIN OF NEOPLASIA

Several hypotheses have been advanced to explain neoplasia, many of them reflecting or in response to advances in the basic sciences current at the time. For example, hypotheses of the viral cause of neoplasia coincided with the demonstration of transmission of certain animal neoplasms by ultrafiltrable agents (Rous sarcoma, 1908; Shope papilloma, 1933; Bittner milk factor, 1935). Immunologic hypotheses came to the fore after experiments involving tumor transplantation in animals (Ehrlich, 1908; immune surveillance, Burner, 1950s). DNA mutations as a cause of neoplasia were proposed after the discovery of DNA structure and function (Watson and Crick, 1950s). And now it is believed that the nonlethal genetic damage lies at the heart of carcinogenesis. Such genetic damage (or mutation) may be acquired by the action of environmental agents, such as chemicals, radiation, or viruses, or it may be inherited in the germ line.

For the origin of neoplasia, the genetic evidence implies that a tumor mass results from the clonal expansion of a single progenitor cell that has incurred the genetic damage, i.e., the initial neoplastic change affects a single cell, which then multiplies and gives rise to the neoplasm. The monoclonal origin of neoplasms has been clearly shown in neoplasms of B lymphocytes (B cell lymphomas and plasma-cell myelomas) that produce immunoglobulin, and in some other tumor types by isoenzyme studies in women who are heterozygous for polymorphic X-linked markers, such as the enzyme glucose-6-phosphate dehydrogenase (G6PD) (Figure 5-10).

THE MOLECULAR BASIS OF NEOPLASIA

As mentioned above, the disorder of growth-related regulatory genes caused by nonlethal genetic damage is the molecular basis of neoplasia. Four classes of normal regulatory genes—growth-promoting protooncogenes; growth-inhibiting tumor suppressor genes (antioncogenes); genes that regulate apoptosis; and genes that regulate repair of damaged DNA—are the principal targets of genetic damage.

A. Protooncogene and Oncogene

Protooncogenes are those genes that code for a variety of growth factors, receptors, signal-relay and transcription factors (Table 5-6), which act in concert to control entry into the cell cycle (e.g. the growth promoter effect). In normal condition, the expression of these genes are under-controlled exactly and coordina-

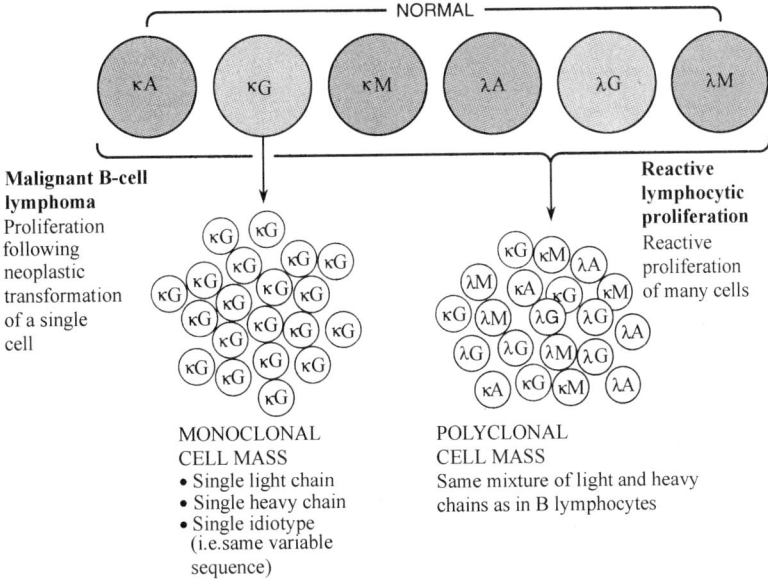

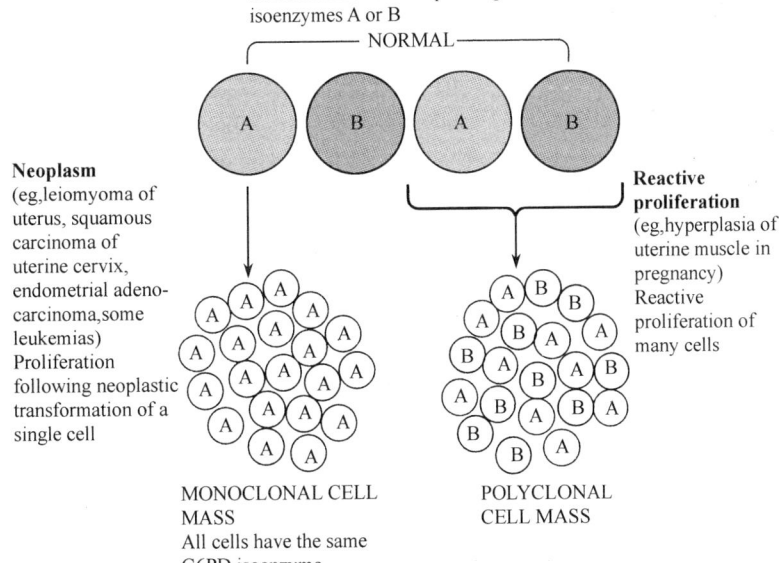

Figure 5-10 Methods of characterization of cell populations as monoclonal or polyclonal. A: Immunoglobulin light and heavy chain distribution in a B lymphocyte population. B: Glucose-6-phosphate dehydrogenase (G6PD) isoenzyme studies may be used in some female patients. G6PD isoenzyme inheritance is X-linked in heterozygous females, one X chromosome codes for the A isoenzyme and the other for the B isoenzyme. Because one X chromosome is randomly inactivated in the adult cell, an adult cell will contain only one of the isoenzymes. A polyclonal population will be composed of cells containing both isoenzymes in approximately equal amounts, whereas a monoclonal population will be composed of cells that express only one isoenzyme

Table 5-6 Oncogenes-growth promoting genes

Functional Category	Oncogene	Action	Tumors
Growth factor	sis	(PDGF truncated) *	Glioma
	int, hst	(FGF like) *	Breast, esophagus
Growth factor receptor	erb-B	(EGFR) *	Breast, ovary
	erb-B2 (Her2/neu)	(EGFR-like)	Breast, ovary
Signal transduction/relay factors	ret, src, abl	Tyrosine Kinase	Thyroid Sarcoma CML; t(9;22)
	N-ras	(GTP binding)	Leukemias
	Ki-ras	(GTP binding)	Lung, pancreas, colon
Transcription factors	c-myc, n-myc, L-myc	(Activate growth promoting genes)	Leukemia, breast, colon Neuroblastoma Lung
Cell cycle control	bcl-1 (PRAD1)	(Codes cyclin-D1)	Breast, squamous cancer
	mdm-2	(p53 antagonist)	Sarcomas
Apoptosis block	bcl-2	(Inhibits programmed cell death)	B cell lymphomas

PDGF, platelet-derived growth factor; FGF, fibroblast growth factor; EGFR, epidermal growth factor-receptor.

ted with the needs of body. They are called oncogenes or cellular oncogenes (c-onc) when their activities are abnormally activated or increased, and have the potential of promoting malignant transformation of cells.

Certain RNA viruses contain nucleic acid sequences that are complementary to a proto-oncogene and can (by reverse transcriptase) produce a viral DNA sequence that is essentially identical, lacking only the introns, of the animal host cell. These sequences are termed viral oncogenes (v-onc). Many, perhaps all, of the oncogenic RNA retroviruses contain such sequences, and they are found in the corresponding neoplasms. Currently, it is thought that the RNA oncogenic virus acquired its v-onc sequence by incorporation of the c-onc from animal cells by a recombination-like mechanism (Figure 5-11).

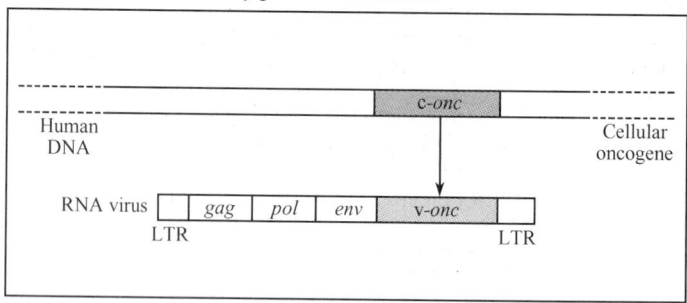

Figure 5-11 Oncogenic RNA viruses, viral oncogenes (v-onc), and cellular oncogenes (c-onc). In the course of evolution, the RNA virus acquires the cellular oncogene (or proto-oncogene) from an animal cell through recombination. The oncogenes are considered growth-regulating genes. Neoplasia thus represents the production of multiple copies or abnormal switching on of these oncogenes

Mechanisms of gene activation and inactivation. It has been suggested that neoplastic transformation occurs as a result of activation (or derepression) of growth promoter genes (proto-oncogenes), or inactivation or loss of suppressor genes. Activation is a functional concept whereby the normal action of growth regulation is diverted into oncogenesis. The resultant activated proto-oncogene is referred to as an activated oncogene (or a mutant oncogene, if structurally changed), or simply as a cellular oncogene (c-onc). Activation and inactivation may occur through several mechanisms (Figure 5-12): (1) mutation, including single nucleotide loss (frameshift) or substitution (nonsense or missense codon), codon loss, gene deletion or more major chromosomal loss; (2) translocation to a different part of the genome where regulatory influences may favor inappropriate expression or repression; (3) insertion of an oncogenic virus at an adjacent site (see Figure 5-16); (4) amplification (production of multiple copies of the proto-oncogenes), which appear as additional chromosome bands or extra DNA fragments (double minutes); (5) introduction of viral oncogenes (see Figure 5-16); or (6) derepression (loss of suppressor control). Oncogenes are considered dominant because they transform cells despite the presence of their normal counterpart—other one of the alleles.

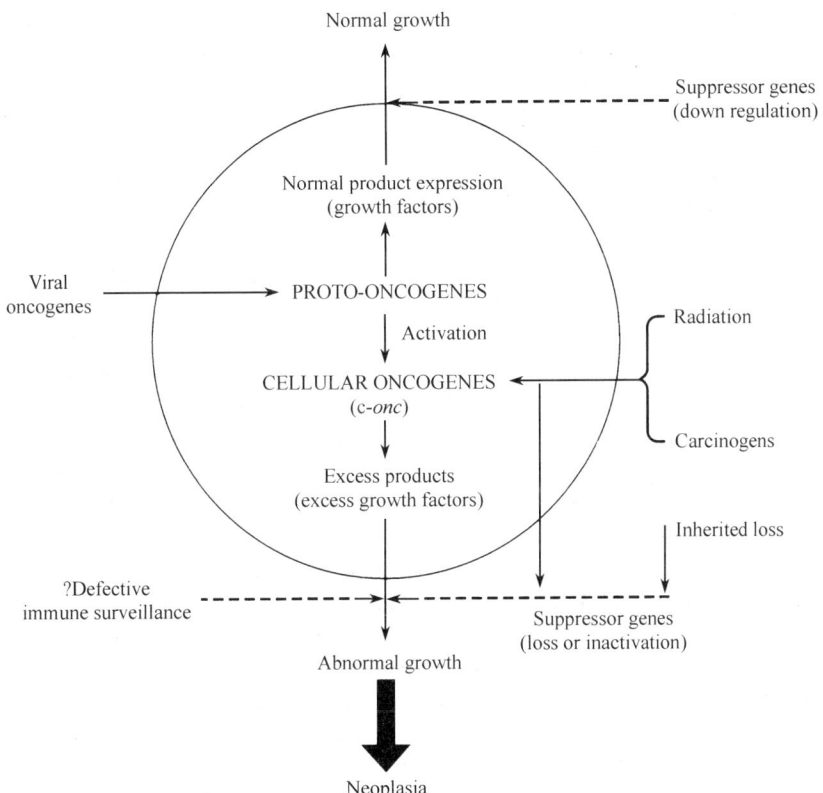

Figure 5-12 Relationship of cellular oncogenes and suppressor genes to normal growth and neoplasia

B. Tumor Suppressor Genes

Although oncogenes encode proteins that promote cell growth, the products of other category of genes, called tumor suppressor genes, exert their opposite reaction (down-regulate the cell cycle) on cell proliferation. The balance and coordination between proto-oncogenes and tumor suppressor genes are the basis of normal cell proliferation. Disruption of tumor suppressor genes renders cells loss of growth inhibition and mimics the growth-promoting effects of oncogenes (Table 5-7). But it is distinctive that both normal alleles of tumor suppressor genes must be lost, ie homozygous loss (inactivated by mutation, loss or methylation), for transformation to occur, so this family of genes sometimes is referred to as recessive oncogenes. The famous *two-hit hypothesis* proposed by Knudson in 1974, which depended on the investigation for a rare cancer of children—retinoblastoma, is an explanation for this phenomina. It has been proved that two mutations (i.e. two hits) are required to produce retinoblastoma (see below).

Retinoblastoma (Rb) gene, located on chromosome 13q14, is the first discovered and prototypic tumor suppressor gene, being discovered initially in retinoblastoma, but it is now evident that homozygous loss of this gene is a fairly common event in several other tumors such as bladder cancer, breast cancer, and small cell cancer of lung. The product of Rb gene is a DNA-binding protein, which exists in an active hypophosphorylated and an inactive hyperphosphorylated state. In its active state, Rb serves as a brake in the advancement of cells from G1 to the S phase of the cell cycle (by binding and possibly sequestering the E2F family of transcription factors). When the quiescent cells are stimulated by growth factors, the Rb protein is inactivated by phosphorylation, and then the E2F transcription factors are released and activate the transcription of several target genes which make the cells transverse the G1→S checkpoint and start the mitosis. If the Rb protein is absent, or its ability to sequester transcription factors is lost by mutations, the molecular brakes on the cell cycle are released, and the cells move into the S phase unblockedly.

There are two types of retinoblastoma, the familial type and sporadic type (see later). In familial cases, children inherit one defective copy of the Rb gene in germ line (first hit) and the other copy is normal. When the normal Rb gene is lost by somatic mutation in the retinoblast (second hit) the retinoblastoma develops, so these cases are much younger and frequently involving both of eyes because just only another mutation (hit) required. In sporadic cases, both normal Rb alleles must be lost by somatic mutation in one of the retinoblasts (two hits) for retinoblastoma developing, so these cases are older than those of familial type and usually just only one eye involved.

p53 tumor suppressor gene is one of the most commonly mutated genes in human cancers. More than 70% of human cancers have a defect in this gene, and the remaining have defects in genes upstream or down-stream of *p53*. With multiple functions, p53 can exert antiproliferative effects and regulate apoptosis. Normal p53 protein is associated with MDM2, a protein that targets it for destruction, and has a short half-life (20 minutes). When the cell is stressed, (including anoxia, inappropriste oncogene expression e.g. *MYC*, and damage to the integrity of DNA), p53 is released from MDM2 and increased its half-life. As a transcription factor, p53 triggers dozens of genes transcription, which involve two broad categories – those that cause cell cycle arrest and those that cause apoptosis.

For example, when DNA damaged by irradiating, p53 triggers the transcription of *p21* (*CDKN1A*), which inhibits cyclic/CDK complexes and prevents phosphorylation of RB that are essential for cells to enter G1 phase. So the cell cycle is arrested in G1 phase and such a pause facilitates the cells to repair DNA damage. P53 also helps the process of DNA repair by inducing certain proteins such as GADD45 (growth arrest and DNA damage). If DNA damage cannot be successfully repaired during the pause, p53 directs the cell to apoptosis by triggering expression of apoptosis-inducing genes such as *BAX*. In view of these activities, p53 can be viewed as a central monitor of stress, directing the cell toward an appropriate response, either cell cycle arrest or apoptosis. So p53 has been called a "guardian of the genome". With homozygous loss of *p53*, DNA damage goes unrepaired, mutations are accumulated and become fixed in dividing cells, and the cell turns onto a one-way road leading to malignant transformation.

Homozygous loss of the *p53* gene is found in virtually every type of cancer. In most cases, the inactivating mutations affecting both *p53* alleles are acquired in somatic cells. Less commonly, some individuals inherit a mutant *p53* allele. As with the *Rb* gene, inheritance of one mutant allele predisposes individuals to develop malignant tumors because only one additional hit is needed to inactivate the second, normal allele. Apart from mutation and amplification of *MDM2*, the inactivation of p53 also can be rendered by certain DNA viruses such as oncogenic HPVs, hepatitis B virus (HBV), and possibly EBV (Epstein-Barr virus), which encode some proteins binding to normal p53 proteins and abolishing their functions.

There are other tumor suppressor genes have been discovered in past decades years, some of them are *NF-1*, *p16*, *APC*, *WT-1*, and so on (Table 5-7). And still others will be discovered in the future.

C. Genes That Regulate Apoptosis and Repair of Damaged DNA

Accumulation of neoplastic cells may result not only from activation of growth-promoting oncogenes

Table 5-7 Tumor suppressor (growth inhibitory) and repair genes

Functional Category	Gene	Tumors
Cell cycle brakes	p53	Bladder, lung, ovary
	Rb	Retinoblastoma, bone, lung
	MTS 1 (p16)	Melanoma, ovary
Other inhibitors	NF-1 (ras antagonist)	Neurofibroma
	BRCA1	Hereditary breast cancer
	BRCA2	Hereditary breast cancer
	WT-1	Wilms' tumor
	APC	Colon
Mismatch repair	MSH2 LH1	Colon, endometrium
	PMS1, PMS2	
Apoptosis inducer	p53	Bladder, lung, ovary

or/and inactivation of growth-inhibiting tumor suppressor genes, but also from mutations in the genes that regulate apoptosis. Just as cell growth being regulated by growth-promoting and growth-inhibiting genes, cell survival being also regulated by genes that promote and inhibit apoptosis. A large family of genes that regulate apoptosis has been identified. It is possible that apoptosis of cancer cells can be frustrated at multiple sites of the apoptosis pathways. For example, CD95 (Fas), a death receptor, when it is bound to its ligand, FasL, it triggers the transduction of apoptotic signals. In hepatocellular carcinoma, the level of CD95 reduced, which renders the tumor cells less susceptible to apoptosis by FasL. Another factor, BCL2, is an anti-apoptosis protein coded by BCL2 gene. In follicular B cell lymphomas, overexpression of BCL2 protects lymphocytes from apoptosis and allows them to survive for long periods, which leads accumulation of B lymphocytes and resulting of tumor.

Genes that regulate repair of damaged DNA are also related with neoplasia (Table 5-7). They affect cell growth or survival indirectly by influencing the ability of the organism to repair nonlethal damage in other genes, including protooncogenes, tumor suppressor genes, and genes that regulate apoptosis. A disability of DNA repair genes can predispose to widespread mutations in the genome and to neoplastic transformation.

MULTISTEP PROCESS OF CARCINOGENESIS AND NEOPLASM PROGRESSES

A. The Lag Period

A constant feature of all known agents that cause neoplasms is the interval (lag period) between exposure and development of the neoplasm. In survivors of the atomic bomb blasts of Hiroshima and Nagasaki, the largest number of cases of leukemia occurred about 10 years after the event, and some cancers developed as late as 20 years afterward. In shipyard workers exposed to asbestos during World War II, neoplasms attributed to asbestos were rare within 15 years of exposure. However, new cases were identified through the 1970s even though exposure stopped in the 1940s. In utero exposure to diethylstilbestrol may give rise to vaginal cancer 15 or more years after birth. These types of long lag periods may account for the difficulty in identifying carcinogenic agents for common neoplasms and also suggest that multiple steps and factors must be needed for neoplastic transformation.

B. Multiple Hits and Multiple Factors

Knudson proposed that carcinogenesis requires two hits. The first event is initiation, and the carcinogen causing it is the initiator. The second event, which induces neoplastic growth, is promotion, and the agent is the promoter. It is now believed that in fact multiple hits occur (five or more), that multiple factors may cause these hits, and that each hit produces a change in the genome of the affected cell that is transmitted to its progeny (i.e. the neoplastic clone). The period between the first hit and the development of clinically apparent cancer is the **lag period.**

The role of the Bittner milk factor (an RNA virus) in mouse mammary carcinoma (Figure 5-13), the genesis of African Burkitt's lymphoma in humans (Figure 5-14), and the sequential changes leading to colon cancer (see Figure 5-15) clearly illustrate that cancer arises through the interaction of many factors.

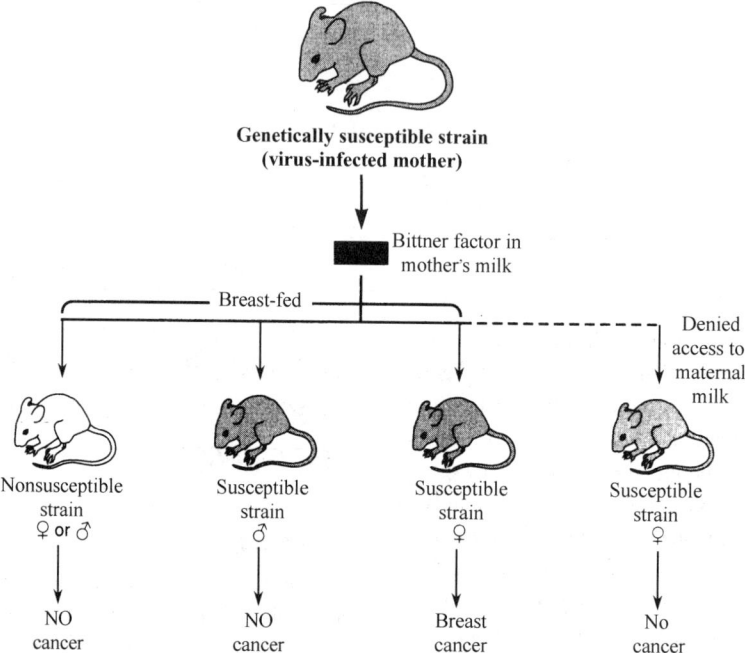

Figure 5-13 Multifactorial causation of breast cancer in experimental mice. Development of breast cancer requires genetic susceptibility, ingestion of the Bittner milk factor (a type B RNA retrovirus) in maternal milk, and an appropriate hormonal environment (female mouse or male mouse injected with estrogens). Absence of any of these factors results in failure to develop cancer

C. Neoplasm Pogression and Heterogeneity

As the description above, carcinogenesis is a multistep process in which several phenotypic attributes of cancer, such as excessive growth, local invasiveness, and the ability of distant metastases, are obtained. This phenomenon that neoplasms become more and more aggressive and acquire greater malignant potential (e.g. accelerated growth, invasiveness, distant metastases, and drug resistance) is called neoplasm/tumor *progression*. Although most malignant tumors are monoclonal in origin, subclones of tumor cells with different characteristics are generated during the process of progression, so by the time that tumors become clinically evident their constituent cells are extremely heterogeneous in morphology, genetics, and biological behavior. This phenomenon is called tumor *heterogeneity*. At the molecular level, tumor progression and associated heterogeneity most likely results from the accumulation of multiple mutations (additional mutations) independently in different cells and immune or nonimmune selection pressures. For example, those cells that require more growth factors are negative selected and highly antigenic subclones are killed by host defenses. With the tumor growing, those subclones that are adept in survival, growth, invasion, and metastasis are enriched, and the progression and heterogeneity of neoplasm are commited.

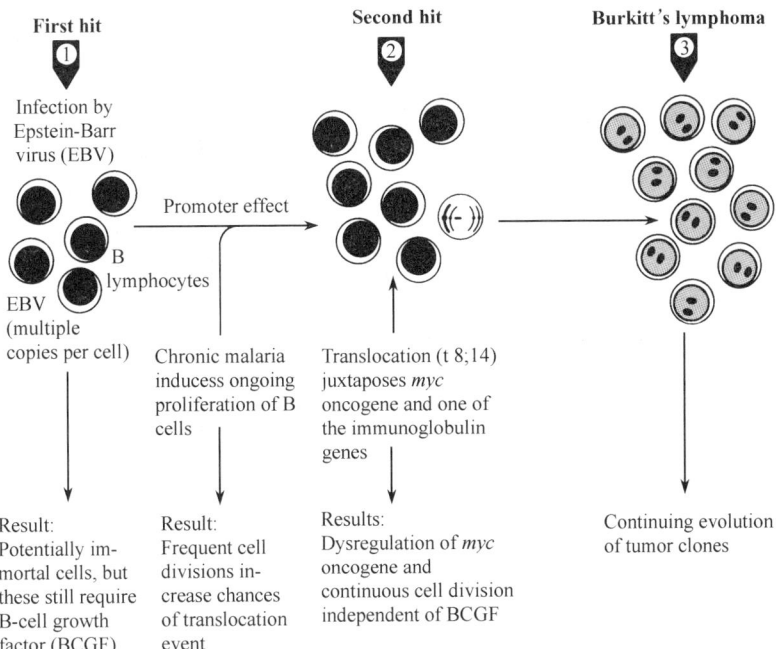

Figure 5-14 Oncogenesis in Burkitt's lymphoma. The first hit is infection of B lymphocytes with Epstein-Barr virus. Chronic malaria induces proliferation of B lymphocytes, increasing the likelihood of the second hit, which is a chromosomal translocation that activates a cellular oncogene and leads to malignant lymphoma

	Normal →	Hyperplasia →	Adenoma →	Adenoma and → Dysplasia	Carcinoma →	Metastasis
Chromosome		5q	12p	18q	17p	
Change		m/del	m	del	m/del	?
Gene		*APC*	*Kras*	*DCC*	p53	?

Figure 5-15 Multi-hit phenomenon with sequential genetic changes leading to carcinoma of the colon. In familial polyposis of the colon, 15 or more years may elapse between the detection of polyps and the diagnosis of cancer (lag period). The full sequence of changes will occur in only one or a few polyps; dysplasia is evident if the right polyps are biopsied. Genes *apc*, *dcc*, and p53 (Table 5-11) are all tumor suppressor genes; typically, both copies must be lost for cancer expression; p53 is exceptional in that loss of one gene copy results in a product that is only partially functional (m, mutation; del, deletion.)

AGENTS CAUSING NEOPLASMS (ONCOGENIC AGENTS; CARCINOGENS)

Carcinogens are substances that are known to cause cancer or at least produce an increased incidence of cancer in an animal or human population. Many carcinogens have been identified in experimental animals, but because of dose-related effects and the metabolic differences among species, the relevance of these studies to humans is not always clear. The following discussion will consider mainly those carcinogens of known importance to humans. It is important to stress that (1) the cause of most common human cancers is unknown; (2) most cases of cancer are probably multifactorial in origin; and (3) except for cigarette smoking, the agents discussed below have been implicated in only a small percentage of cases.

The importance of environmental carcinogens must not be minimized simply because they may not yet have been identified. The marked geographic variation in the incidence of different cancers is thought to result more from the action of different carcinogens than from variations in genetic makeup. If this belief is valid, then still unidentified environmental agents probably play a major role in causing about 95% of human cancers.

Environmental carcinogens identified mainly include three classes: chemicals, radiant energy, and viruses. And other factors such as nutritional and hormonal agents may contribute to carcinogenesis. In few of patients, inheritance may exert significant role on neoplasia. But it is important to note that several agents may act in concert or sequentially to produce the multiple genetic abnormalities of neoplastic cells.

CHEMICAL ONCOGENESIS (TABLE 5-8)

It is difficult to assess the possible carcinogenic effects of the many industrial, agricultural, and household chemicals present in low levels throughout the environment. A significant hazard is also posed by disposal of industrial waste, which may contaminate drinking water and offshore coastal waters (and marine life).

Table 5-8 Major chemical carcinogens in humans[1]

Chemical	Types of Cancer
Polycyclic hydrocarbons	
Soot (benzo[a]pyrene, dibenzanthracene)	Skin; scrotal cancer in chimney sweeps
Inhalation or chewing of tobacco products (mainly cigarettes)[2]	Lung, bladder, oral cavity, larynx, esophagus
Aromatic amines	
Benzidine, 2-naphthylamine	Bladder
Aflatoxins	Liver
Nitrosamines	? Esophagus, ? stomach
Cancer chemotherapeutic agents	
Cyclophosphamide, chlorambucil, thiotepa, busulfan	Leukemias
Asbestos	Lung cancer, mesothelioma
Heavy metals	
Nickel, chromium, cadmium	Lung
Arsenic	Skin
Vinyl chloride	Liver (angiosarcoma)

[1] Most of the chemicals listed here are those for which strong evidence exist for human carcinogenesis; several other compounds exist that are thought to be carcinogenic.

[2] **Note**: Cigarette smoking is responsible for more human cancer than all of the other listed chemicals combined.

One of the major problems associated with the identification of chemical carcinogens is the long lag phase, sometimes 20 or more years between exposure and the development of cancer. Unless the effects produced are dramatic, it is difficult to establish the carcinogenicity of any particular chemical in view of the huge number of substances to which people are exposed during their lives. Table 5-9 summarizes the clinical approach and experimental assays used to detect potential carcinogens.

Most chemical carcinogens act by producing changes in DNA, including abnormal base alkylation, deletions (partial), strand breakages, and cross-linkages. A small number act by epigenetic mechanisms, i.e. they cause changes in growth-regulating proteins without producing genetic changes. Still others may act synergistically with viruses (derepressing oncogenes) or may serve as promoters for other carcinogens.

Chemical carcinogens that act locally at the site of application without having to undergo metabolic change in the body are called **proximate** or **direct-acting carcinogens.** Other chemicals produce cancer only after they are converted into metabolically

Table 5-9 Chemical carcinogenesis: Methods for detecting potential carcinogens[1]

Clinical observation (physicians and patients)
Epidemiologic studies (environment and industry)
Experimental animal bioassays
By chemical and drug industries
By FDA (or equivalent bodies elsewhere)
By university and research groups
Mutagenesis assays
Bacterial mutagenesis (Ames test)
Mammalian cell culture (Syrian hamster embryo; rodent fibroblasts; human cell lines)
In drosophila, mice, and so forth
Cell culture transformation assays
Assays of chromosomal or DNA binding or damage

[1] Modified and reproduced, with permission, from Weinstein IB: The scientific basis for carcinogen detection and primary cancer prevention. CA 1982;32:348.

active compounds within the body; these are termed **procarcinogens** or **indirect-acting carcinogens**, and the active carcinogenic compounds that are produced are called **ultimate carcinogens.**

The potency of carcinogens also varies greatly, at least in experimental systems, expressed as the amount that must be given to induce cancer on a regular basis (i.e. reproducibly). Thus, saccharin requires 10 g/kg/d (a huge dose - low-potency carcinogen); 2-naphthylamine, 10^{-1} g/kg/d; benzidine, 10^{-2} g/kg/d; and aflatoxin B_1, 10^{-6} g/kg/d (making aflatoxin B_1 the most potent known carcinogen).

A. Polycyclic Hydrocarbons

The first recognized carcinogen in humans was soot, the tarry residue of coal combustion. Sir Percivall Putt established in 1775 that soot was the agent responsible for scrotal cancer in London chimney sweeps. Soot from the chimneys tended to collect in the rugose scrotal skin and cause cancer. Much later, it was shown that the active carcinogens in soot and coal tar were a group of polycyclic hydrocarbons, the most active of which were benzo-[a]pyrene and dibenzanthracene. Application of small amounts of these polycyclic hydrocarbons to the skin of experimental animals regularly cause skin cancer.

B. Cigarette Smoking

Cigarette smoking—and to a lesser extent cigar and pipe smoking—is associated with an increased risk of cancer of the lung, bladder, oropharynx, and esophagus. Smoking filtered cigarettes and newer low-nicotine and low-tar cigarettes decreases the risk only slightly. There is also strong evidence that the risk of cancer associated with smoking is not limited to the smoker but may extend to nonsmoking family members, coworkers, and others in close physical proximity to the smoke for long periods (e.g. effect of second-hand smoke). It has been estimated that smoking accounts for more cancer deaths than all other known carcinogens combined.

Cigarette smoke contains numerous carcinogens, the most important of which are probably polycyclic hydrocarbons (tars). Although these are direct-acting carcinogens in the skin, they act as procarcinogens in producing lung and bladder cancer. Inhaled polycyclic hydrocarbons are converted in the liver to an epoxide by a microsomal enzyme, aryl hydrocarbon hydroxylase. This epoxide (the ultimate carcinogen) is an active compound that combines with guanine in DNA, leading to neoplastic transformation. Smokers who develop lung cancer have been shown to have significantly higher levels of aryl hydrocarbon hydroxylase than nonsmokers or smokers who fail to develop cancer. The reported risk of developing cancer has varied in different studies, but it is about ten times higher in someone who smokes a pack of cigarettes a day for 10 years than in a nonsmoker. If a smoker stops smoking, the risk drops almost to that of a nonsmoker after about 10 years of abstinence.

C. Aromatic Amines

Exposure to aromatic amines such as benzidine and naphthylamine is associated with an increased incidence of bladder cancer (first recognized in workers in the leather and dye industries). Similar compounds have been used in many pathology and research laboratories; their use is closely controlled by the FDA (Food and Drug Administration), but as with radiation, there is no safe threshold of exposure.

Aromatic amines are procarcinogens that enter the body through the skin, lungs, or intestine and exert their carcinogenic effects predominantly in the urinary bladder. In the body they are converted to carcinogenic metabolites that are excreted in the urine. Retention of urine in the bladder maximizes the carcinogenic effect on the bladder mucosa.

Different species vary in their susceptibility to the effects of aromatic amines: Humans and dogs are quite susceptible; rats and rabbits, much less so. This variation reinforces the point that procarcinogens (which must be converted in the body to ultimate carcinogens) may have different effects in different species because of different metabolic processes. This is a serious flaw in all animal studies that attempt to establish lack of carcinogenicity of new drugs to be used in humans.

D. Cyclamates and Saccharin

These compounds are artificial sweeteners once widely used by patients with diabetes mellitus. Administration of large amounts of these compounds caused bladder cancer in experimental animals. No carcinogenic effect has been demonstrated in humans, and it is not even known whether humans metabolize these compounds to produce ultimate carcinogens.

E. Azo Dyes

These dyes were extensively used as food coloring agents (scarlet red and butter yellow) until they were shown to cause liver tumors in rats. They have since been withdrawn from commercial use. Less potent relatives, such as trypan blue and Evans blue, remain in use as histologic stains.

F. Aflatoxin

Aflatoxin, a toxic metabolite produced by the fungus *Aspergillus flavus*, is thought to be an important cause of liver cancer in humans. The fungus grows on improperly stored food, particularly grain, groundnuts, and peanuts, producing aflatoxin. In Africa, dietary intake of large amounts of aflatoxin has been shown to correlate with a high incidence of hepatocellular carcinoma. Ingested aflatoxin is oxidized in the liver to an ultimate carcinogen that binds with guanine in the DNA of hepatic cells. In large amounts, the toxin causes acute liver-cell necrosis followed by regenerative hyperplasia and possibly cancer. When lesser amounts (minute amounts, as this is a very potent carcinogen) are ingested over a long period, the carcinogenic effect predominates. There is increasing evidence that aflatoxin induces mutations of *P53*, leading to loss of tumor suppressor function.

G. Nitrosamines

Small amounts of these compounds have been shown to be carcinogenic in experimental animals. Their ability to react with both nucleic acids and cytoplasmic macromolecules provides a theoretic basis for their carcinogenic action, but their role in human carcinogenesis is uncertain.

Nitrosamines are derived mainly from conversion of nitrites in the stomach. Nitrites are ubiquitous in food because of their common use as preservatives, mainly in processed meats, ham, bacon, sausage, and so forth. The direct local action of nitrosamines is thought to be an important cause of esophageal and gastric cancer. The markedly decreased incidence of gastric cancer in the last 2 decades in the United States is believed to be due mainly to better refrigeration of food, which has decreased the need for chemical preservatives. The high incidence of gastric cancer in Japan is thought to be related more to high intake of smoked fish (containing polycyclic hydrocarbons) than to high nitrosamine levels.

H. Betel Leaf

Chewing of betel leaf or betel nut in Sri Lanka and parts of India is responsible for an extremely high incidence of cancers of the oral cavity. The carcinogenic agent has not been identified but is believed to be present either in the Areca (betel) nut or in the crushed limestone or tobacco that is commonly chewed along with the betel leaf.

I. Anticancer Drugs

Certain drugs used in the treatment of cancer (alkylating agents, such as cyclophosphamide, chlorambucil, busulfan, and thio-tepa) interfere with nucleic acid synthesis in normal cells and in cancer cells and may cause oncogenic mutations (direct-acting carcinogens). Leukemia is the most common neoplastic complication of cancer chemotherapy and is a significant problem in patients in whom cure of the primary tumor has been achieved.

J. Asbestos

Asbestos is inhaled into the lung, where it produces fibrosis and chronic lung disease. Crocidolite, the variety of asbestos having the finest diameter fibers (< 0.25 mm), presents the greatest hazard. Asbestosis also leads to fibrous proliferation in the pleura, where it results in fibrous plaques that are a reliable radiologic indicator of previous asbestos exposure. Diffuse pulmonary fibrosis also occurs. Asbestos is associated with two types of cancer.

1. Malignant mesothelioma

This uncommon neoplasm is derived from mesothelial cells, mainly in the pleura but also in the peritoneum and pericardium. Nearly all patients who develop malignant mesothelioma give a history of asbestos exposure.

2. Bronchogenic carcinoma

Patients with asbestos exposure have a risk of lung cancer about twice that of the general population; this risk is greatly magnified by smoking. Although it is not as specifically associated with asbestosis as is mesothelioma, lung cancer is the most common malignant neoplasm in patients with a history of asbestos exposure.

K. Other Industrial Carcinogens

Many other cancer-causing agents have been identified. Miners exposed to heavy metals such as nickel, chromium, and cadmium show an increased incidence of lung cancer. Arsenic exposure, which may occur in agricultural workers exposed to arsenic-containing pesticides, is associated with a high incidence of skin cancer and a lesser risk of lung cancer. Vinyl chloride, a gas used in the manufacture of polyvinyl chloride (PVC), has been shown to be associated with a malignant vascular neoplasm (angiosarcoma) of the liver, mainly in experimental animals.

RADIATION ONCOGENESIS

Several different types of radiation cause cancer, most probably by direct effects on DNA or possibly by activation of cellular oncogenes.

A. Ultraviolet Radiation

Solar ultraviolet radiation is associated with different kinds of skin cancer, including squamous cell carcinoma, basal cell carcinoma, and malignant melanoma. Neoplasms of the skin are especially common in fair-skinned individuals whose occupations expose them to sunlight; farmers in Queensland, Australia, have an extremely high incidence of melanoma. Skin cancer is overall the most common type of cancer in the United States. The incidence of ultraviolet radiation-induced skin cancer, including melanoma, is low in darker-skinned races because of the protective effect of melanin pigment.

Ultraviolet light is believed to induce formation of linkages between pyrimidine bases on the DNA molecule. In normal individuals, this altered DNA molecule is rapidly repaired. Carcinoma occurs when DNA repair mechanisms do not operate efficiently, as occurs in older individuals and in people with xeroderma pigmentosum. Skin cancer due to exposure to sunlight is thus a disorder seen most often in the elderly.

B. X-Ray Radiation

Early radiologists who were exposed to x-rays of low penetration developed radiation dermatitis with a high incidence of skin cancer. As x-rays capable of greater penetration were developed, the second generation of radiologists suffered an increased incidence of leukemia. Present-day radiologists are at minimal risk for cancer because of highly effective protective measures against x-rays.

One complication of radiotherapy for cancer is the occurrence of additional radiation-induced malignant neoplasms, commonly sarcomas, that appear 10 – 30 years after radiation therapy.

Diagnostic x-rays use such small doses of radiation that no increased risk of cancer is believed to be associated with their use. A possible exception is abdominal x-rays during pregnancy, which may slightly increase the incidence of leukemia in the fetus.

C. Radioisotopes

The carcinogenic effect of radioactive materials was first recognized when many cases of osteosarcoma occurred among factory workers who used radium-containing paints to produce luminous watch faces. It was found that these workers shaped their brushes to a point with their tongues and lips, thereby ingesting dangerous amounts of radium. Radioactive radium is metabolized in the body in much the same way as calcium and is therefore deposited in bone, where it induces osteosarcoma.

Occupational exposure to radioactive minerals in the mines of central Europe and the western United States is associated with an increased incidence of lung cancer.

Thorotrast, a radiologic dye containing radioactive thorium, was used in diagnostic radiology between 1930 and 1955. Thorotrast is deposited in the liver and increases the risk for several types of liver cancer, including angiosarcoma, liver cell carcinoma, and cholangiocarcinoma (cancer of the bile ducts).

Radioactive iodine, which is used to treat nonneoplastic thyroid disease, is associated with an increased risk of cancer developing 15-25 years after treatment; the risk is weighed against the nature of the primary disease, the therapeutic benefits, and the patient's age.

VIRAL ONCOGENESIS

Both DNA viruses and RNA viruses can cause neoplasia (Table 5-10). **DNA viruses** insert their nucleic acid directly into the genome of the host cell. Normally, virus replication ensues. In the oncogenic DNA viruses, replication is sporadic or absent. However, viral products may still be formed with 2 observed effects: inactivation of tumor suppressor-gene proteins (p53, Rb), or enhancement of oncogeneaction (see below). **RNA viruses** require RNA-directed DNA polymerase (reverse transcriptase), an enzyme that causes production of a DNA copy of the RNA viral genome; this DNA copy (provirus) can then be inserted in the host genome. Some RNA viruses contain a built-in oncogene that directly activates

Table 5-10 Oncogenic viruses

Group	Virus	Host	Tumor
RNA viruses (retroviruses) type C	Avian leukemia-sarcoma complex	Chicken	Leukosis, Rous sarcoma
	Murine leukemia-sarcoma complex	Mouse, rat, hamster	Leukemia, sarcoma
	Feline leukemia-sarcoma complex	Cat/dog	Leukemia, sarcoma
Type B	Murine mammary tumor virus (Bittner milk factor)[1]	Mouse	Breast cancer
Type C-like	HTLV-1	Human	T cell leukemia
	Human immunodeficiency virus (AIDS virus)	Human	AIDS-related lymphomas
DNA viruses Papovavirus	Papilloma virus	Human, rabbit, cow, dog	Papilloma (laryngeal), condyloma acuminata, verruca vulgaris, ? carcinoma of cervix
	Polyoma virus	Mouse	Many tumors in newborn hamsters
	SV40[3]	Monkey	Tumors in hamsters only
Herpesvirus	Herpes simplex type	Human	? Carcinoma of cervix
	Epstein-Barr virus	Human	Carcinoma of nasopharynx, Burkitt's lymphoma
	Avian	Chicken	Marek's disease
	Rabbit	Rabbit	Lymphoma
Poxvirus	Fibroma-myxoma	Rabbit	Fibromyxoma
	Molluscum contagiosum	Human	Molluscum contagiosum[2]
Parapoxvirus	Hepatitis B	Human, rodent, duck	Hepatocellular carcinoma

[1] See Figure 5-13.
[2] A self-limited proliferative disease of the epidermis: not a true neoplasm.
[3] SV40 = simian virus 40.

the cell; others insert adjacent to an endogenous cellular oncogene, which is thereby activated (Figure 5-16). Insertion of the viral DNA sequence into the host genome is a highly complex process requiring several viral enzymes that cleave the host DNA, insert the viral DNA, and then repair the break.

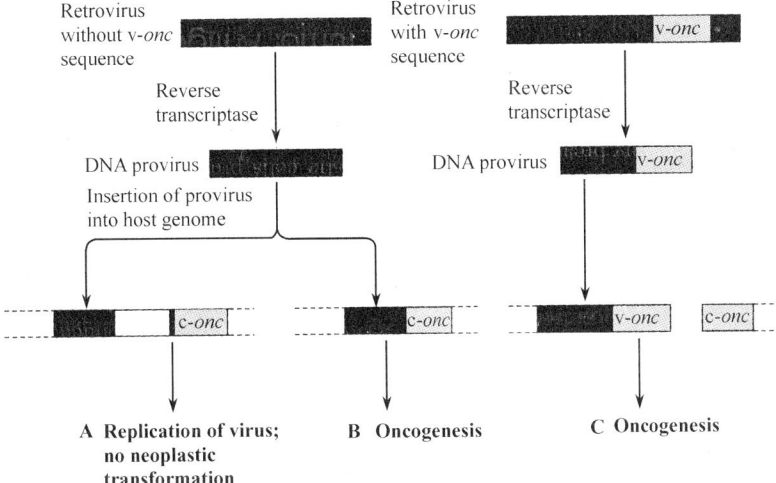

Figure 5-16 RNA virus (retrovirus) oncogenesis. Provirus (from retroviral RNA) can insert at many sites in the host genome. A: When a provirus lacking a v-*onc* gene inserts at some distance from a cellular oncogene, viral replication occurs without neoplastic transformation. B: If the provirus inserts adjacent to a cellular oncogene, it may activate that oncogene and cause neoplasia. C: Retrovirus containing a v-*onc* gene may lead to neoplasia directly on insertion. This is known as a fast transforming retrovirus. The three genes (*gag*, *poi*, *env*) and single-stranded RNA of an oncogenic retrovirus are depicted in Figure 5-11, plus an incorporated v-*onc* sequence; Figure 5-11 is thus equivalent to (C) above

The presence of a viral genome in a cell can be demonstrated in various ways: (1) identification of virus-specific nucleic acid sequences by hybridization with DNA and RNA probes, (2) recognition of virus-specific antigens on infected cells, and (3) detection of virus-specific mRNA.

A. Oncogenic RNA Viruses

Oncogenic RNA viruses (retroviruses) cause many neoplasms in experimental animals, including leukemia and lymphoma in mice, cats, and birds; various sarcomas in birds (Rous sarcoma virus) and primates; and breast carcinoma in mice (Bittner milk factor, or mouse mammary tumor virus). Retroviruses have been implicated in only a few human neoplasms.

1. Adult T cell leukemia

This form of leukemia was first described in Japan. A retrovirus (human T lymphocyte virus type I [HTLV-I]) has been cultured from tumor cells in this disease and may play a direct etiologic role. A related virus (HTLV-II) has been described in cases of hairy cell leukemia.

2. Infection with HIV

Human immunodeficiency virus (HIV) is a retrovirus (lentivirus) that infects human lymphocytes and causes acquired immune deficiency syndrome (AIDS). The malignant B cell lymphomas associated with AIDS may result from HIV oncogenesis.

3. Breast carcinoma

In mice, breast carcinoma is caused by the mouse mammary tumor virus (MMTV), an RNA virus transmitted in breast milk (Figure 5-13). Serum antibodies that are able to neutralize MMTV have been identified in some women with breast cancer, and MMTV or a similar antigen can be demonstrated in some human breast cancer cells. In addition, virus-like particles and RNA resembling that of MMTV have been identified in human breast cancer cells and breast milk. Despite these findings, the hypothesis that an RNA virus is the cause of human breast cancer is still considered unproved.

B. Oncogenic DNA Viruses

Several groups of DNA viruses have been implicated as the cause of human neoplasms.

1. Papilloma viruses

These viruses cause benign squamous epithelial cell neoplasms in skin and mucous membranes, including the common wart (verruca vulgaris), the venereal wart (condyloma acuminatum), and recurrent laryngeal papillomas in children (laryngeal papillomatosis).

DNA hybridization studies have revealed papilloma virus types 6 and 11 in most cases of condyloma acuminata, whereas severe dysplasia and invasive carcinoma of the uterine cervix are associated with types 16, 18, 31, and 33. Furthermore, papilloma viral DNA appears to be present in extrachromosomal episomes in the condylomas but is in an integrated form in severe dysplasia and carcinoma. The E6/E7 transforming proteins of human papilloma virus appear to bind with and inhibit p53 and Rb proteins, thereby removing suppressor function and allowing the cell cycle to proceed unchecked. Polyoma virus acts in a similar manner, but in addition it produces an increase in the tyrosine kinase activity of the c-src oncogene.

2. Epstein Barr virus (EBV)

This herpesvirus causes infectious mononucleosis, an acute infectious disease that occurs worldwide. Epstein-Barr virus is also thought to cause Burkitt's lymphoma in Africa and nasopharyngeal carcinoma in the Far East.

Epstein-Bart virus selectively infects B lymphocytes, binding to membrane receptors on the B lymphocyte that appear to be specific for the virus. Studies using DNA probes show that the Epstein-Barr virus genome is present in over 90% of African Burkitt lymphoma cells. It is thought that infected B lymphocytes undergo neoplastic transformation following chronic immune proliferation induced by malaria (Figure 5-14).

3. Herpes simplex virus (HSV) type 2

Epidemiologic evidence has long pointed toward herpes simplex virus type 2 as a cause of cancer of the uterine cervix. DNA probe studies have identified the herpes simplex virus type 2 genome in some cervical cancer cells. However, a causal relationship has not been established.

4. Cytomegalovirus (CMV)

The nucleic acid of this herpesvirus is present in most cells of the lesions associated with Kaposi's sarcoma, a disorder most commonly found in immunodeficient patients. It is not known whether cytomegalovirus causes Kaposi's sarcoma or whether it is an opportunistic organism.

5. Hepatitis B virus

This virus is believed to be an important cause of hepatocellular carcinoma, which is common in Africa and the Far East—areas with a high incidence of hepatitis B infection and high carrier rates. In some studies, an enormous (200-fold) risk factor has been estimated. The virus can be demonstrated in liver cancer cells in some patients. Sustained liver cell proliferation (regeneration) that occurs in response to virus-induced injury may be the critical factor predisposing to neoplastic change. Important cofactors in a multi-hit sequence include chronic infection with hepatitis C virus and exposure to aflatoxin.

THE ROLE OF INHERITANCE IN ONCOGENESIS

In experimental settings, many animal strains show a genetic susceptibility for development of neoplasms. In many instances, this predisposition appears to result from the inherited loss of one or more tumor suppressor genes (Table 5-11).

A. Neoplasms With Mendelian (Single-Gene) Inheritance

Theoretically, cancer-causing genes may act in a dominant or recessive manner. If dominant, they may produce a molecule that directly causes neoplasia. If recessive, lack of both normal genes may lead to failure of production of a factor necessary for maintaining control of normal growth.

1. Retinoblastoma

This uncommon malignant neoplasm of the retina occurs in children, and 10% of cases are inherited. The morphologic appearance of familial retinoblastoma is the same as that of the non-inherited form. However, the familial form displays other distingui-

Chapter 5 Neoplasia

Table 5-11 Tumor suppressor genes (human)[1]

Name of Gene	Chromosome	Disease
APC (adenomatous polyposis coli)	5q21	Familial polyposis cell
Rb1 (retinoblastoma)	13q14	Retinoblastoma, osteosarcoma, other tumors
WT-1 (Wilms' tumor)	11p13	Wilms' tumor, other tumors (Figure 5-17)
p53	17p12-13	Li-Fraumeni cancer syndrome[2]
NF-1 (neurofibromatosis)[3]	17q11	Von Recklinghausen's neurofibromatosis (type 1)
DCC (deleted in Colon cancer)	18q21	Colon cancer (Figure 5-15)

[1] Tumor suppressor genes give rise to a product that checks growth. As a rule, loss of both genes (alleles) is necessary for initiation of neoplasia, with p53 loss or defect of one gene resulting in an abnormal and malfunctioning product and neoplasia.

[2] High familial incidence of breast cancer, sarcomas, and brain tumors occurring from childhood to old age.

[3] A distinct form of neurofibromatosis (type 2) also exists, producing acoustic neuromas; the NF-2 gene is on chromosome 22.

shing features: (1) it is commonly bilateral; (2) chromosomal analysis consistently shows an abnormality of the long arm of chromosome 13 (13q14, the retinoblastoma [Rb] gene); and (3) spontaneous regression occurs in some cases. Regression enables affected individuals to live into adult life and to reproduce and transmit the gene. Examination of parents of children with familial retinoblastoma frequently reveals signs of the regressed neoplasm in one parent.

The inheritance of retinoblastoma shows an apparent dominant pattern as a result of the high rate of conversion of the inherited single 13q14 (Rb) abnormality to a state in which both Rb genes are lost, allowing expression of the recessive change. The Rb gene is thus an example of a tumor suppressor gene (Table 5-11).

Recent studies reveal the presence of a similar abnormality of chromosome 13 in several other tumors, including osteosarcoma and small-cell undifferentiated carcinoma of the lung. Furthermore, survivors of familial retinoblastoma have been shown to have a high risk of developing small-cell undifferentiated carcinoma of the lung, especially if they smoke cigarettes.

2. Wilms' tumor (nephroblastoma)

Nephroblastoma is a malignant neoplasm of the kidney that occurs mainly in children. Many cases are associated with deletion of part of chromosome 11 (Figure 5-17). Both sporadic and familial cases occur by mechanisms thought to resemble those described for retinoblastoma. Again, 11p13 abnormalities are being identified in other tumor types. WT-1 is also a tumor suppressor gene.

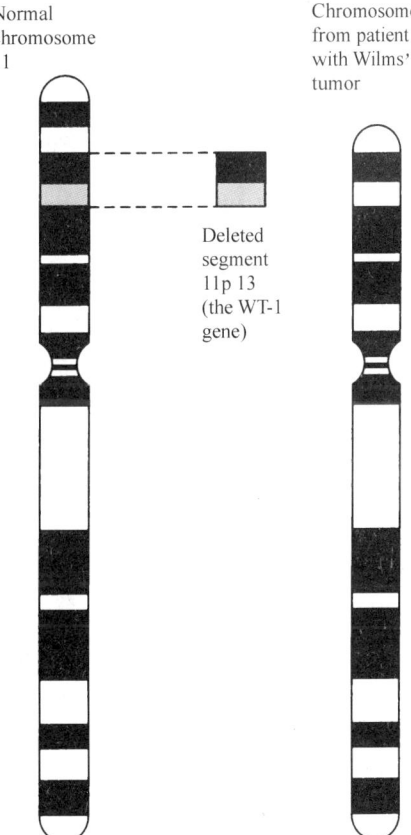

Figure 5-17 Diagrammatic representation of normal chromosome 11 and an abnormal chromosome 11, showing a deleted segment that is commonly found in patients with nephroblastoma (Wilms' tumor). The missing segment is known as the WT-1 gene; its normal function is growth regulation

3. Other inherited neoplasms

Several other neoplasms display a familial pattern.

Most were believed to be dominantly inherited, but this view is being reevaluated since the discovery of recessive tumor suppressor genes.

a. Neurofibromatosis (type I von Recklinghausen's disease): This tumor is characterized by multiple neurofibromas and pigmented skin patches known as café auélait spots. In neurofibromatosis, the NF-1 genes (chromosome 17q11) are absent or defective, leading to loss of NF-1 suppressor protein. NF-1 protein is thought to act by regulating the effect of the products (guanine-binding G proteins) of the *ras* proto-oncogene. Loss of NF-1 allows the growth-promoting effects of G proteins to act unopposed.

b. Multiple endocrine adenomatosis: This disorder is manifested by benign neoplasms in the thyroid, parathyroid, pituitary, and adrenal medulla.

c. Familial polyposis coli: Polyposis coli is characterized by innumerable adenomatous polyps in the colon. (There is loss of heterozygosity on the long arm of chromosome 5, the *APC*—adenomatous polyposis coil – gene). Cancer eventually develops in all patients who do not undergo colectomy. This is a clear example of the multi-hit phenomenon producing sequential changes that lead to malignancy (Figure 5-15). **Gardner's syndrome** is a variant in which colonic polyps are associated with benign neoplasms and cysts in bone, soft tissue, and skin. **Turcot's syndrome**, a very rare disease in which multiple adenomatous polyps of the colon are associated with malignant tumors (gliomas) of the nervous system, is thought to have an autosomal recessive inheritance pattern.

B. Neoplasms With Polygenic Inheritance

Many common human neoplasms are familial to a much lesser degree – i. e. they occur in related individuals more often than would be expected on the basis of chance alone.

1. Breast cancer

First degree female relatives (mother, sisters, daughters) of premenopausal women with breast cancer have a risk of developing breast cancer that is five times higher than that of the general population. The risk is even greater if the patient has bilateral breast cancer.

2. Colon cancer

Cancer of the colon tends to occur in families both as a complication of inherited familial polyposis coli and independently. Some of the cancer families also have other cancers, notably of the endometrium and breast.

As many as one fourth of colon cancer patients display abnormalities of yet another gene (*MSH2*), which present on chromosome 2. *MSH2* normally encodes a DNA housekeeper protein that repairs errors in DNA replication. Defective function of MSH2 therefore allows cancer-causing mutations to accumulate. Still other cancer families show the presence of multiple repeat sequences scattered throughout all of the chromosomes. These dramatically increase replicative errors. It is also possible that the observed familial incidence of tumors may reflect the effects of a common environment.

C. Neoplasms Occurring More Frequently in Inherited Disease

Many inherited diseases are associated with a high risk of neoplasia. They include (1) syndromes characterized by increased chromosomal fragility (e. g. xeroderma pigmentosum, Bloom's syndrome, Fanconi's syndrome, and ataxia-telangiec-tasia), in which neoplasia is due to frequent DNA abnormalities; and (2) syndromes of immunodeficiency, in which failure of immune surveillance may predispose to neoplasia. In these disorders, it is not the neoplasm itself that is inherited but rather some susceptibility to neoplasia.

(Meng Bin)

TUMOR IMMUNITY

The tumor immune encompasses several concepts (1) Neoplastic changes frequently occur in the cells of the body. (2) As a result of alteration in their DNA, neoplastic cells produce new molecules (neoantigen, tumor associated antigen). (3) The immune system of the body recognizes these neoantigens as foreign and mounts a cytotoxic immune response that destroys the neoplastic cells (4) Neoplastic cells produce clinically detectable neoplasms only if they escape recognition and destruction by the immune system.

Tumor Antigen

Tumor antigens are recognized by cellular or humoral effectors of the immune system. Antigens that elicit an immune response have been demonstrated in many experimentally induced tumors and in some human cancers. They were broadly classified into two categories based on their patterns of expression: tumor-specific antigens (TSA), which are present only on tumor cells and not on any normal cells, and tumor-associated antigens (TAA), which are present on tumor cells and also on some normal cells. TSAs can be derived from intracellular or extracellular proteins, and can be presented in a way that they can be recognized by T-cells. TAAs can be used as a marker to categorize the tumor, or to monitor disease progression.

Tumor antigens are particularly well demonstrated by (1) chemical carcinogen-induced tumors, which tend to have specific antigens that vary among tumors, even among tumors induced by the same carcinogen, and by (2) virus-induced tumors, which tend to show cross-reactivity between tumors induced by the same virus. Viral infections may result in "modified self," ie, new antigens recognized in the context of the major histocompatibility complex (MHC).

The mechanisms of origin for these antigens include (1) new genetic information introduced by a virus, such as human papillomavirus E6 and E7 proteins in cervical cancer; (2) alteration of oncogenes by carcinogens, which either generate a novel protein sequence directly or result in the induction of genes that are normally not expressed (except perhaps during embryonic development); (3) uncovering of antigens normally "buried" in the cell membrane because neoplastic cells are unable to synthesize membrane components.

Soluble tumor-associated antigens, which are also released into the blood by human fetal cells, are mentioned elsewhere (refer to: Oncofetel Proteins). These oncofetal antigens include: alpha-fetoprotein associated mainly with hepatocellular carcinomas and carcinoembryonic antigen associated chiefly with colon carcinomas.

Antitumor Mechanisms

Both cell-mediated and humoral immunity have been demonstrated to have anti-tumor activity.

A. Cellular Immunity

The importance of lymphoid cells in tumor immunity has been repeatedly shown in animal experiments. The cytotoxic T-lymphocytes (CTLs) is the primary cell thought to be responsible for direct recognition and killing of tumor cells. CTLs destroy newly transformed tumor cells after recognizing TAAs.

Tumor-specific CTLs have been found with neuroblastomas, malignant melanomas, sarcomas, and carcinomas of the colon, breast, cervix, endometrium, ovary, testis, nasopharynx, and kidney. The significance of immune reactions in controlling tumor growth is not clear, but it seems likely that T-cells can damage tumor cells in vivo under some conditions.

Natural killer (NK) cells are bone-marrow derived lymphocytes ("large granular lymphocytes") which have natural cytolytic activity against tumor cells (and non-tumorous virally infected cells), do not require prior sensitization, and lack MHC restriction. NK cells also mediate antibody dependent cell-mediated cytotoxicity (ADCC). The cytolytic activity of NK cells is increased by various (viral and immune) interferons and by interleukin-2 (IL-2).

Macrophages have natural cytolytic activity against tumor cells, in either the absence or presence of T cells, and also mediate ADCC. Macrophages are activated by lymphokines, such as interferon-gamma, released from sensitized T cells.

B. Humoral Immunity

Humoral mechanisms may also participate in tumor cell destruction. The tumor antigens evoke specific antibodies. These immunoglobins can exert anti-tumor effects by two mechanisms: (1) they can coat tumor cells and render them vulnerable to ADCC by NK cell or macrophages; (2) tumor cells that have been coated with specific antibodies may be lysed by the activation of complement.

Humoral antibodies directed against human tumor cells or their constituents have been shown in vitro in the sera of patients with Burkitt's lymphoma, malignant melanoma, osteosarcoma, neuroblastoma, and lung, breast, and GI carcinomas.

Immune Surveillance

The idea of immune surveillance suggests that there are immune cells that can recognize cancer cells and remove them. In the absence of such surveillance, there would be many more tumors in human.

Evidence supporting the existence of immune surveillance is based on observations of a higher incidence of neoplasia in many immunodeficiency states and in transplant recipients receiving immunosuppressive drugs. About 5% of persons with congenital immunodeficiencies develop cancers, about 200 times the prevalence in immunocompetent individuals. The observation that cancer is a disease of the elderly may then be attributed to progressive failure of immune surveillance in the face of an increased frequency of neoplastic event resulting from the defective DNA repair that accompanies aging.

Most cancers occur in persons who do not suffer from any overt immunodeficiency. It is evident even when a person's immune system is functioning normally, cancer can escape the immune system's protective surveillance.

Tumor cells avoid or escape potential surveillance mechanisms in many conceivable ways, among them: of course, the absence or "subimmunogenic" expression of tumor associated antigens; diminished expression of class I MHC antigens; constant shedding of tumor-cell surface antigens which combine with and neutralize the effector cells; production of "blocking" antibodies which combine with the target antigen and inhibit access by effector cells; formation of soluble tumor antigen-antibody complexes which can block either the target antigen, in an antibody-excess environment, or effector cells, in an antigen-excess environment; generalized immunosuppression of the host; an increased activity of suppressor T cells.

The complexity of interaction between the immune system and tumor is depicted in Figure 5-18.

(Zhang Qinghui)

BRIEF INTRODUCTION OF COMMON NEOPLASMS

EPITHELIAL NEOPLASMS

The epithelia of the body are derived from all three germ-cell layers, which include the cells that cover the surface of the body, line in the tubular or cavitated organs, and consist of various glands. The neoplasms arising from epithelia are the most common tumors in human being, especially the malignancy, called carcinomas, accounting for the largest part of all human malignant tumors.

Benign Epithelial Neoplasms

A. Papillomas

Papillomas can arise from squamous, glandular, or transitional epithelium (e.g. squamous papilloma, intraductal papilloma of the breast, and transitional cell papilloma, respectively). They often grow on the surface of organs such as skin, gastrointestinal or urogenital tract, which produce one or more nipple-like, polypoid, finger-like or villous projections usually with slender stalks. Under microscopy, the finger-like or delicate papillae of tumor project into the surface or lumen, which has a fibrovascular core covered by well-differentiated tumor cells that resemble normal epithelia with or without slight dysplasia. There is a malignant potential when the tumorous cells have severe dysplasia.

B. Adenomas

Adenomas are derived from various glands and usually produce gland patterns. They more often occur in thyroid, ovary, breast, salivary gland and intestines, etc. Adenomas may appear as papillomas (see above) when they arise from mucosal surfaces, or nodular masses often enveloped by fibrous tissue when they arise in glands. The gland patterns of adenomas are similar to their original and secreting function may be remained more or less.

Adenomas can be distinguished to various patterns dependent on their components and structures. *Polypous adenoma* grows on mucosal surface and protrudes into the lumen. It most occurs in colon and rectum. *Cystadenoma* is a hollow cystic mass, which typically occurs in ovary and sometimes in thyroid and pancreas. The hollow cyst is formed by the accumulation of secretion. *Fibroadenoma* of the female breast contains a mixture of proliferated ductal elements embedded in a loose fibrous tissue, which was believed as a mixed tumor in the past. Although studies suggest that only the fibrous component is neoplastic, the term fibroadenoma remains in common usage. *Pleomorphic adenoma*, also called mixed tumor, mainly arises in salivary gland and accounts for over 50% of salivary gland tumors. Pleomorphic adenoma is a firm, solid mass. Histologically, the tumor presents a greatly varied appearance. Uniform epithelial and myoepithelial cells are distributed in cords, nests, and strands within a matrix of mucoid material (Figure 5-19), which frequently resembles cartilage (hence the mistaken notion that this was a mixed mesenchymal and epithelial tumor). Although the lesion is benign and well circumscribed, encapsulation is incomplete, and simple enucleation is followed by a high rate of local recurrence due to regrowth of residual tumor. Wide excision is necessary for cure.

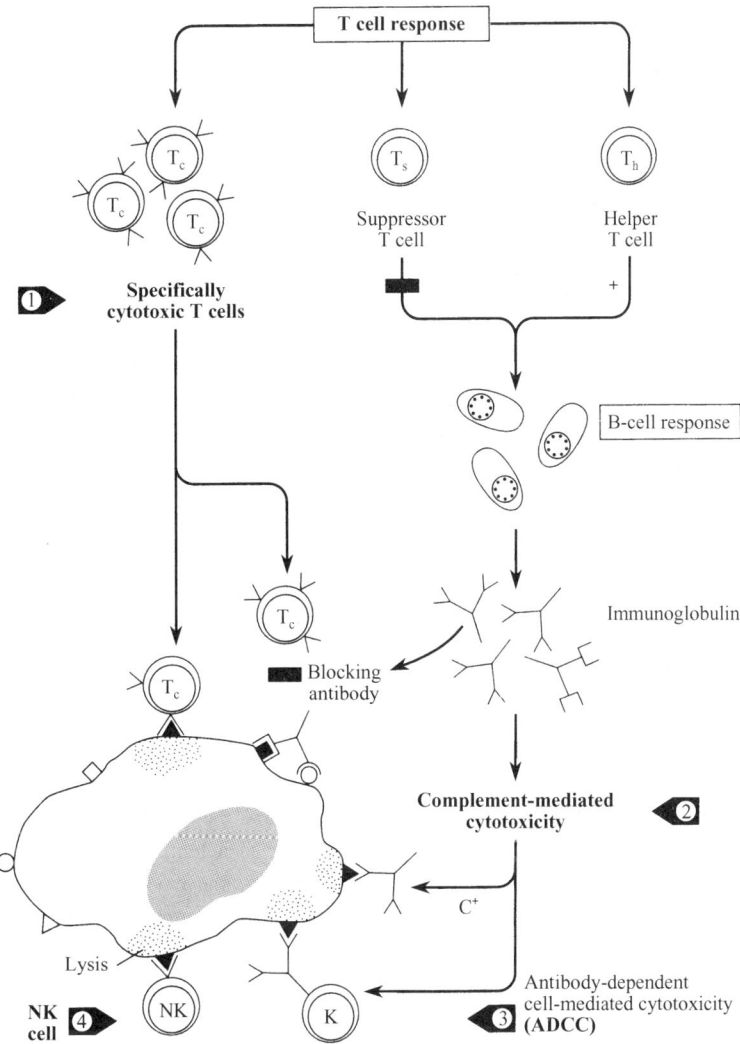

Figure 5-18　The immune response and cancer. The net effect of the immune response on neoplastic cells varies. Neoplastic cells may be killed by (1) cytotoxic T cells (T_c), (2) antibody and complement(C^+), (3) antibody-dependent cell-mediated cytotoxicity (ADCC), or (4) activity of natural killer(NK)cells. On the other hand, blocking antibodies or inappropriate suppressor T cell activity may interfere with these effects and thus enhance growth of the neoplastic cells

Malignant Epithelial Neoplasms

　　Malignant epithelial neoplasms, called carcinomas, are the most common malignant tumors in human being and often occur in people over age 40 years. The growth patterns of progressive infiltration, invasion, destruction and penetration of the surrounding tissue, and metastasis preferred by lymphatic spread are the biological natures of carcinomas. When these tumors grow on the surface of skin or mucosa, their appearances show as polypoid or fungating mass often with superficial necrosis and forming cancerous ulcer; when they are within organs, the appearances often show as fixed, stony-hard, irregular and painless nodules with unclear borderline. On the transection, the tumor appears as a dry, gray-white mass without well-defined capsule or borderline. When the tumor is larger or tumor growth is rapid, central necrosis may be occured. Microscopic examination reveals that nests or sheet-like arrangements of cancerous cells (epithelioid

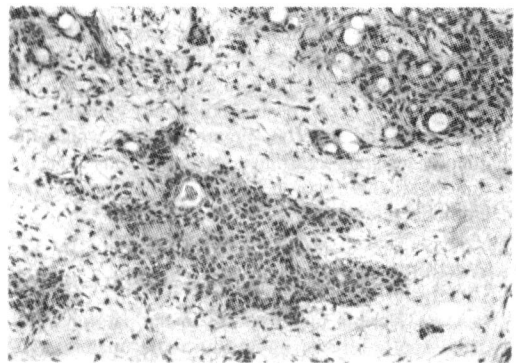

Figure 5-19 Neoplasms of salivary glands. Mixed tumor of salivary gland (pleomorphic adenoma) composed of small, uniform, polygonal cells forming sheets and small glands surrounded by abundant myxomatous intercellular material

arrangement) infiltrate in the fibrous stroma, and in the margin of the tumor, tiny and crablike feet of the parenchyma invade into the surrounding tissue. The stroma is variable in amount and usually there is a clear delimitation between the parenchyma and stroma of carcinomas.

A. Squamous Cell Carcinoma (SCC)

SCC denotes a carcinoma in which the tumor cells resemble stratified squamous epithelium. It is characterized by marked cytologic pleomorphism, intercellular bridges (desmosomes) between tumor cells, and keratinization of the cytoplasm, in addition to the general natures of carcinomas. The tumor cells of well-differentiated SCC are strikingly similar to normal squamous epithelial cells, with intercellular bridges and nests of keratin pearls (round, laminar keratinization), while those of poor-differentiated or undifferentiated SCC are anaplastic, almost without any keratinization and desmosomes. SCCs often occur in the organs covered by stratified squamous epithelium, such as skin, oral cavity, esophagus, and cervix of uterus, etc. They also arise in other organs such as bronchi, bladder and nasopharyn, which epithelia can be transformed to squamous epithelia by metaplasia. (See relative chapters)

B. Adenocarcinoma

Adenocarcinoma denotes a carcinoma in which the neoplastic epithelial cells grow in gland patterns. They originate from glandular epithelia such as glandular acini, ducts or glandular mucosa. Adenocarcinomas often arise in the stomach, colorectum, liver, lung, female breast, ovary, thyroid, prostate, etc. Microscopically, the tumor glands and their cells are atypical with frequent mitotic figures. Adenocarcinomas can be divided different patterns according to their differentiation, structure and components.

For example, *papillary adenocarcinoma* denotes a tumor with a lot of papillary structure, which usually is a well-differentiated adenocarcinoma. When a tumor with one or more cysts, a term of *cystadenocarcinoma* is given; when with papillary structures meantime, *papillary cystadenocarcinoma*. If a poorly differentiated adenocarcinoma, in which the cells do not form glandular structures but are arranged in solid cords or sheet-like separated by interstitial tissue, it is called *solid carcinoma*. A *scirrhous carcinoma* is fibrous and hard, in which the tumor cells are less and presented as a single column of cells or even a single cell scattering in fibrous mesenchyma. On the contrary, a *medullary carcinoma* is soft and brain like in consistency due to a little of mesenchyma.

Some adenocarcinomas, so called *mucinous carcinomas*, can produce large amounts of mucus, in which one type are only a few cancerous cells "floating" in the mucus, in gross they have a semitransparent gelatinous appearance, so a term of *colloid carcinoma* is given; in another type, the most cancerous cells look like signet rings, which are formed because the cytoplasm is extended and the nuclei compressed by the mucus gathered within the cells, therefore the designation "*Signet ring cell*" *carcinoma*. Mucinous carcinomas often arise in colon, stomach, etc.

C. Basal Cell Carcinoma

Basal cell carcinoma is a common skin neoplasm, usually occurring in sun-exposed areas of light-skinned individuals over the age of 40 years. The face is the most common site. Early basal cell carcinoma appears as a waxy papule with small telangiectatic vessels of its surface. Some tumors contain melanin pigment and thus appear similar to nevocellular nevi or melanomas. Advanced lesions may ulcerate with pearly rolled edges (so-called rodent ulcer) (Figure 5-20) because of central necrosis.

Histologically, basal cell carcinoma arises from the basal layer of the epidermis and invades the dermis as nests and cords of cells. The neoplastic cells resemble basal cells, forming a palisade (basal layer) at the periphery of the tumor nests (Figure 5-21).

cells and usually occurs in the urinary bladder, ureter or renal pelvis. According to the newest tumor classification of WHO, this category of carcinoma is called urothelial cell carcinoma. Generally it is papillary in configuration though it may be solid nests of tumor cells without any papillary in poor-differentiated type. The neoplastic cells are similar as transitional epithelia. Transitional cell carcinomas can be divided into three grades according to their differentiation. The higher the grade is, the more malignant the tumor is.

NEOPLASMS OF MESENCHYMAL CELLS ORIGIN

Mesenchymal tissues include bone, cartilage, and so-called soft tissue. The term soft tissue is used to describe any nonepithelial tissues other than bone, cartilage, the brain and its coverings, hematopoietic cells, and lymphoid tissues. The neoplasms arising from these tissues are called soft tissue tumors/neoplasms. Soft tissue tumors are generally classified on the basis of the tissue type that they recapitulate, including fat, fibrous tissue, muscle, and neurovascular tissue. In some soft tissue neoplasms, however, no corresponding normal mesenchymal counterpart is known (Table 5-12).

Neoplasms arising from mesenchymal tissues, including bone, cartilage and soft tissue, may occur at any age. Most of them are benign tumors and common in humans, such as lipomas and hemangiomas. The malignant neoplasms of mesenchymal tissues are less common and some types are apt to arise in children and adolescents. Here only the more common forms will be described.

Benign Mesenchymal Neoplasms

The differentiating extents of benign mesenchymal neoplasms are high and very similar to their original tissues. They are growing slowly and often encapsulated by thin fibrous capsule. Simple surgical excision is usually curative.

A. Fibroma

Fibromas are arising from fibrous tissue and most often occured in the subcutaneous tissue. They usually appear as grey-white nodular masses with complete encapsulation. Histologically, fibromas are composed of slim, well-differentiated fibrous cells

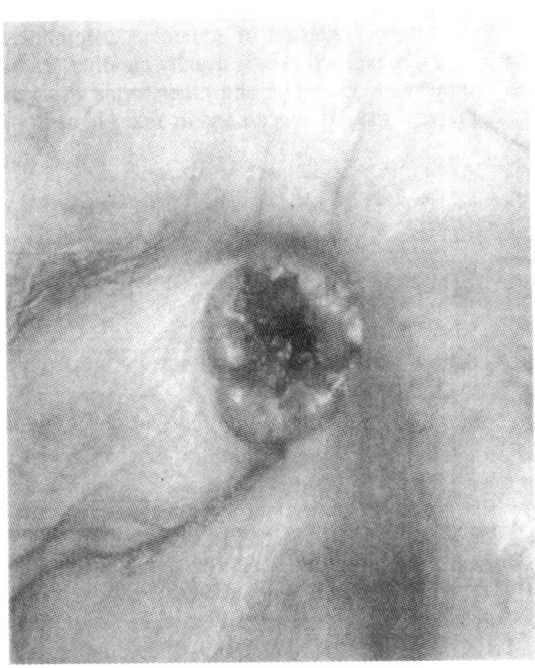

Figure 5-20 Basal cell carcinoma of the eyelid. This is the typical appearance, with a central punched-out ulcer surrounded by a raised edge that has a pearly appearance

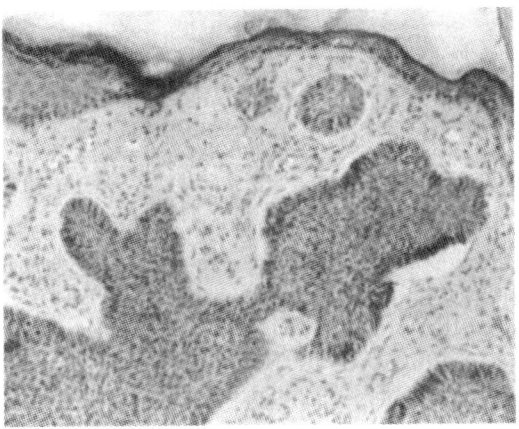

Figure 5-21 Basal cell carcinoma, showing irregular infiltrating nests of carcinoma cells in the dermis. The nests are composed of small cells that show peripheral palisading

Basal cell carcinoma is locally aggressive; it may invade deeply to involve bone and muscle but almost never metastasizes. Wide surgical excision is curative.

D. Transitional Cell Carcinoma

Transitional cell carcinoma arises from urothelial

Table 5-12 Soft tissue neoplasms

Cell of Origin	Benign	Low-Grade Malignant[1] Locally Aggressive	Malignant[1]
Fibroblast	Fibroma	Fibromatosis, fibrosarcoma (low-grade)	Fibrosarcoma (high-grade)
Adipocyte	Lipoma, hibernoma	Liposarcoma (well-differentiated and myxoid)	Liposarcoma (pleomorphic and round cell)
Nerve sheath	Neurofibroma, schwannoma, granular cell tumor		Malignant peripheral-nerve-sheath tumor
Fibrohistiocyte	Fibroxanthoma, dermatofibroma	Atypical fibroxanthoma, dermatofibrosarcoma protuberans	Malignant fibrous histocytoma
Smooth muscle	Leiomyoma	Leiomyosarcoma (low-grade)	Leiomyosarcoma (high-grade)
Skeletal muscle	Rhabdomyoma		Rhabdomyosarcoma
Vascular	Hemangioma	Hemangiopericytoma, hemangioendothelioma (low-grade)	Angiosarcoma, Kaposi's sarcoma
Synovial	Giant cell tumor of tendon sheath		Synovial sarcoma
Melanocyte			Malignant melanoma of soft tissue
Unknown			Ewing's sarcoma (extraskeletal)[2], alveolar soft part sarcoma, epithelioid sarcoma

[1] Benign neoplasms are cured by surgical removal. Low-grade malignant soft tissue neoplasms are locally infiltrative and tend to recur locally after surgical removal. Their metastatic potential is low. Malignant neoplasms have a high metastatic potential as well as local infiltrative properties.

[2] Extraskeletal Ewing's sarcoma probably arises from primitive neuroectodermal cells in connective tissues.

(similar to fibrous cells) with amounts of collagen fibers. They do not recur after surgical excision.

B. Lipoma

Lipomas are the most common soft tissue tumor. It may arise anywhere in the body but is encountered most often in the subcutaneous tissues of adults. The typical lipoma is a soft, yellow mass with thin capsule. Microscopically, the lipoma is composed of mature adipose tissue distinguishable as a neoplasm only because it forms a mass and is encapsulated. Local excision is curative.

C. Hemangioma (angioma)

Hemangiomas are common. About 70% of cases are present at birth, which suggests that they may be hamartomas rather than true neoplasms. The skin, liver, and brain are common sites, but any organ may be involved. Hemangiomas are composed of well-formed vascular spaces lined by endothelial cells that show no cytologic atypia. They are classified as capillary hemangiomas, composed of vessels of capillary size; and cavernous hemangiomas, composed of large thin-walled vascular spaces.

Capillary hemangiomas are usually found in the skin and mucous membranes as small, red to blue plaques or nodules. Most grow slowly with the growth of the child, and many lesions regress spontaneously at or before puberty. Cavernous hemangiomas occur in skin as well as in the viscera, forming a soft spongy mass that may reach 2-3 cm in size. They grow slowly.

Hemangiomas in deep subcutaneous tissues and skeletal muscle (intramuscular hemangiomas) tend to be ill-defined and require wide excision to prevent local recurrence. They do not metastasize.

D. Lymphangioma

Lymphangiomas usually occur in the neck, inguinal region, axilla and tongue. They are the benign lymphatic analogue of the hemangiomas and may also be divided into capillary and cavernous types. Lymphangiomas are composed of neoplastic lymphatic channels filled with lymph fluid. Cavernous lymphangioma (also called cystic hygroma) mainly occurs in the neck in infancy, causing considerable enlargement of the neck. It is common in Turner syndrome. Lymphangiomas also occur in the mediastinum and retroperitoneum in adults. Some of them can grow to large size, making complete surgical removal difficult. They do not metastasize.

E. Leiomyoma

Leiomyomas are common, well-circumscribed neoplasms encountered most frequently in the uterus, although they may arise from smooth muscle cells anywhere in the body. Histologically, they consist of intertwining bands of fairly uniform mature cells with elongated, blunt-ended nuclei.

F. Chondroma

Chondroma is a common benign neoplasm occurring most often in the diaphysial medulla (enchondromas), and less occuring on the surface of the bone. The small bones of the hands and feet are the most common sites, with ribs and long bones affected less frequently. About 30% of patients have more than one lesion. Multiple enchondromas may occur as a familial disease inherited as an autosomal dominant trait (Ollier's disease).

Enchondroma appears as a firm, well-circumscribed, glistening white mass that expands the bone from the center and causes thinning of the cortex. Microscopically, it is composed of lobules of hyaline cartilage of low cellularity.

Malignant transformation does not occur in solitary enchondromas. There is an increased risk of chondrosarcoma in patients with multiple chondroma syndromes.

Malignant Mesenchymal Neoplasms

Malignant neoplasms of mesenchymal cell origin are called sarcomas. They are generally much less common than carcinomas and have some distinctive biologic features. Clinically, some types of sarcomas frequently occur in the young age group, such as osteosarcoma, rhabdomyosarcoma, etc. Sarcomas usually present as a soft tissue mass, often of large size. The cut surface characteristically is homogeneous, whitish, fish-flesh appearance. The extremities and retroperitoneum are the most common sites. Histologically, it is apparently different from carcinoma. In a sarcoma, the tumor cells are usually discrete and mixed with stroma such as blood vessels, no cell nests formed. Necrosis and hemorrhage are fairly common. Table 5-13 show the main differences between carcinoma and sarcoma.

Table 5-13 Differences between carcinoma and sarcoma

	Carcinoma	Sarcoma
Tissue of origin	Epithelium	Mesenchymal tissues
Incidence	More common. Nine time as much as that of sarcoma. More often in adult over forties	Less common. Some types more often occur in children and youngers, some in olders
Gross characteristics	Hard, gray-white color	Softer, moist and fleshy
Histological characteristics	Cancerous cell nests. Distinct demarcation between parenchyma and stroma	Tumor cells distributed diffusely, Parenchyma and stroma mixed, no demarcation
Reticular fiber	Around the cancerous nests	Among the tumor cells
Metastasis	Most often via lymphatics	Often via blood vessels

The biologic behavior of sarcomas is extremely variable. According to their differentiation and biologic behavior, the sarcomas can be divided into two categories: high-grade sarcomas, and low-grade sarcomas.

High-grade sarcomas are highly cellular neoplasms composed of poorly differentiated tumor cells. They show marked nuclear abnormalities and have a high rate of mitotic figures. Because of their anaplasia, high-grade sarcomas are sometimes difficult to classify. High-grade sarcomas grow rapidly, show extensive local invasion, and tend to metastasize early through the bloodstream. Lymphatic spread is uncommon. High-grade sarcomas are usually fatal, and treatment is rarely successful.

Low-grade sarcomas are better differentiated, less cellular, and tend to resemble the tissue of origin to some extent. Cytologic abnormalities are less prominent, and the mitotic rate is usually low. These tumors are characterized by a slower growth rate, a high risk of local recurrence after surgical removal, and a relatively low risk of metastasis. Patients typically survive a long time with repeated local recurrences after surgery.

The follows are some examples of most common sarcomas.

A. Liposarcoma

Liposarcomas usually occur in adults, with a peak incidence in the fifth to sixth decades, and are one of the most common soft tissue malignancies in this age group. In contrast to lipomas, the more common sites of liposarcomas arising are in the deep soft tissues, especially in the lower limbs and retroperitoneum. Liposarcomas can be distinguished several histologic subtypes, including two low-grade variants, the *well-differentiated liposarcoma* and the *myxoid liposarcoma*. The former is composed of well-differentiated tumor cells and easily mistaken for lipoma, the latter characterized by an abundant, mucoid extracellular matrix. High-grade, aggressive variants include the *round cell liposarcoma* which composed of highly undifferentiated vacuolated lipoblasts, and the *pleomorphic liposarcoma* characterized by marked anaplasia with numerous tumor giant cells and only occasional cells bearing fat vacuoles.

B. Rhabdomyosarcoma

Rhabdomyosarcomas denote the malignant mesenchymal tumors that exhibit skeletal muscle differentiation. They predominantly occur in infancy, childhood, and adolescence, with a peak incidence in the first decade of life, and are the most common type of soft tissue sarcoma in the pediatric population. Rhabdomyosarcomas can be divided into three subtypes including: *embryonal rhabdomyosarcoma* which arise most frequently in the head and neck area, genitourinary tract, and retroperitoneum, may present as soft, gelatinous, grapelike mass in gross (so-called sarcoma botryoides), and are composed of small, primitive cells, some of which contain eccentric eosinophilic "straplike" cell processes; *alveolar rhabdomyosarcoma* is less common, and most often occur in the extremities during the adolescency; *pleomorphic rhabdomyosarcoma* is rare, most frequently arises in the deep soft tissues of adults, and may be difficult to distinguish from other pleomorphic sarcomas in histology. All of rhabdomyosarcomas are high-grade sarcomas and have a bad prognosis.

C. Leiomyosarcoma

Leiomyosarcomas may arise in any parts of the body but the most sites are the uterus. Histologically, leiomyosarcomas show a wide range of differentiation, from well-differentiated ones very similar to the leiomyomas to marked atypia lesions approximate to undifferentiated sarcomas. Most leiomyosarcomas arise de novo, rather than transformation from leiomyomas. Well-differentiated leiomyosarcomas can be distinguished from leiomyomas by the infiltrative growth, greater cellularity, pleomorphism, and, most importantly, greater mitotic activity. It is a key point for the treatment of patient to discriminate a leiomyosarcoma from a leiomyoma.

D. Angiosarcoma (Hemangiosarcoma)

Angiosarcomas are rare neoplasms of adults. It may occur anywhere in the body, but the skin, soft tissue, bone, liver, and breast are the common sites. Hepatic angiosarcomas have been etiologically associated with thorium dioxide (Thorotrast), a radiologic dye that was used in 1930-1950, and vinyl chloride, used in the plastics industry.

Angiosarcoma is a malignant neoplasm of endothelial cells, usually presents as a large, hemorrhagic, rapidly growing mass. Histologically, it typically forms interdigitating vascular spaces; less-differentiated angiosarcoma may be solid and composed of anaplastic cells. Angiosarcomas are destructive, infiltrative neoplasms that metastasize early via the bloodstream, and the prognosis is poor.

E. Malignant Fibrous Histiocytoma (MFH)

MFHs include a heterogeneous group of clinically aggressive soft tissue sarcomas that are composed of neoplastic fibroblasts, histiocyte-like, sometimes bizarre and giant cells admixed with variable inflammatory cells. The atypical spindle cells are often arrayed in whorls, a distinctive structure so-called *storiform pattern*. Most MFHs occur in older adults although they may arise in any age. The deep tissues of extremities and retroperitoneal area are the most often occurred but the cell origin of MFH remains obscure. MFHs are highly aggressive tumors that often recur locally and metastasize in about 50% of patients.

F. Fibrosarcoma

Fibrosarcomas are malignant neoplasms arising from fibrous tissue that often occur in adults. The favored sites of origin include the deep tissues of the low limb and retroperitoneal area. Histologically, a typical fibrosarcoma is composed of interlacing fascicles of atypical fibroblasts, often arrayed in a "herringbone" pattern. Low-grade fibrosarcomas are growing slowly, rare metastasis and recurrence after surgical removal; while high-grade variants are easy to metastasis and recur.

G. Osteosarcoma

Osteosarcomas are the most common malignant neoplasm of bone. They mainly affect individuals in the age group from 10 to 25 years. There is a second peak in age incidence in the sixth decade, when osteosarcomas may complicate Paget's disease of bone.

Osteosarcomas arise most commonly in the medullary cavity of the metaphysial region of long bones (Figure 5-22). The lower end of the femur, the upper tibia, and the upper humerus are the most common locations. Rarely, osteosarcomas arise in the periosteum (periosteal osteosarcoma) or on its outer surface (parosteal osteosarcoma).

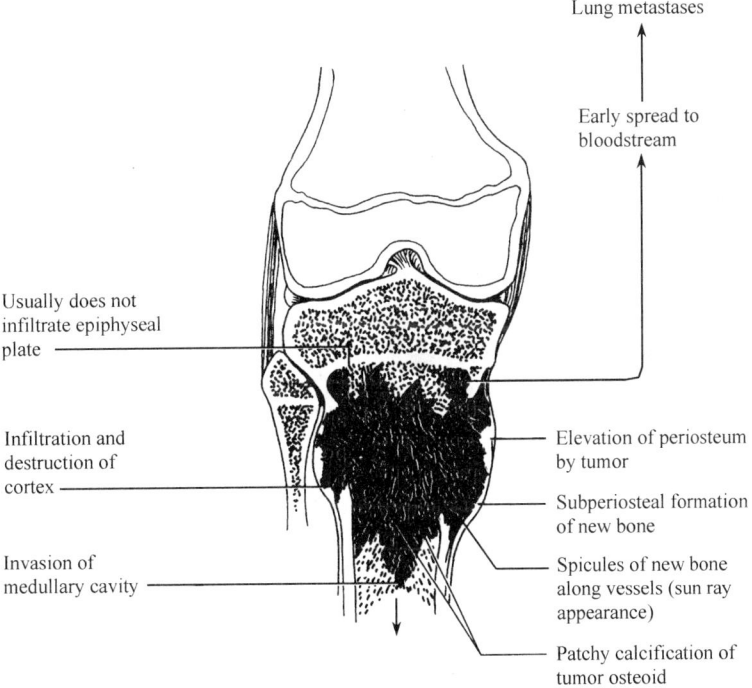

Figure 5-22 Osteosarcoma (diagrammatic), showing the typical metaphysical location of the tumor, which destroys bone and induces reactive subperiosteal bone formation

Grossly, osteosarcoma presents as a fleshy mass with areas of necrosis and hemorrhage (Figure 5-23). The involved bone is expanded by the tumor, which may infiltrate the medullary cavity and the soft tissues outside the bone. The tumor often elevates the periosteum to produce the so-called Codman triangle on radiographs, which is formed by the angle between the elevated periosteum and the surface of the involved bone. Invasion of the epiphyseal plate is uncommon.

Microscopically, osteosarcoma is composed of malignant osteoblasts with anaplasia and a high mitotic rate. Variable amounts of osteoid are produced by the tumor cells and may become calcified (tumor bone). The presence of osteoid in a malignant bone tumor establishes the diagnosis of osteosarcoma.

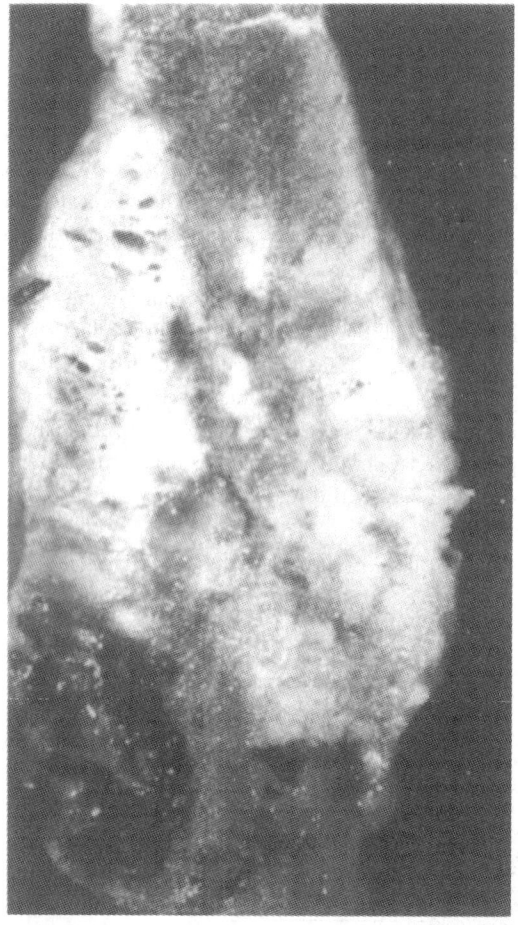

Figure 5-23 Osteosarcoma of the fibula, showing a solid destructive lesion involving the metaphysical region

Cartilage formation also is common and may be extensive (chondroblastic osteosarcoma).

Osteosarcoma usually presents with a bony mass with or without pain. It is a rapidly growing tumor that tends to spread at an early stage via the bloodstream. The availability of effective chemotherapy has altered the treatment and prognosis of osteosarcoma in the past 10 years. The overall 5-year survival in childhood osteosarcoma has increased to 80%. The availability of effective drugs has also permitted less radical limb-sparing surgical procedures in these patients.

H. Chondrosarcoma

Chondrosarcomas most often occur in the group of older age with a peak incidence in the sixth decade. It is second only to osteosarcoma in incidence and males are affected twice as frequently as females. The pelvic girdle, ribs, shoulder girdle, long bones, vertebrae, and sternum are affected – in decreasing order of frequency.

Grossly, chondrosarcoma appears as a large destructive mass with a characteristic translucent whitish appearance because of the chondroid stroma. Microscopically, chondrosarcomas consist of malignant chondrocytes in a chondroid matrix, which vary greatly in appearance. The well-differentiated lesions may be only minimal cytologic atypia, which is difficult to distinguish them from enchondromas; the site of the lesion is helpful to differential diagnosis because cartilaginous neoplasms in the hands and feet are almost always benign whereas those in the axial skeleton are more commonly malignant. The poor-differentiated lesions are composed of highly pleomorphic chondrocytes with frequent mitotic figures and multinucleate cells. Unlike cartilage-forming osteosarcomas, the neoplastic cells in chondrosarcomas do not form osteoid.

NEOPLASMS ARISE FROM NEURO-ECTODERMAL TISSUE

In early embryo, a part of ectoderm develops into the primary nervous system, including neural tube and neural crest, called neuro-ectoderm. The neural tube then develops into brain, spinal cord, retinal epithelia, etc; while the neural crest develops into Ganglia, Schwann cells, melanocytes, chromaffin cells of adrenal medulla, etc. Thus various kinds of neoplasms can arise in neuro-ectodermal tissue. Only a several examples are briefly introduced in following. Some others will be discussed in associated chapters such as the diseases of nervous system, endocrine system, and so on.

Melanocytic Neoplasms

There are two broad categories of melanocytic neoplasms. *Nevi* develop from clusters of melanocyte precursor cells (nevus cells) that are arrested during the terminal phase of their migration from the neural crest to the epidermis, where they form the melanocytes. Nevi develop in childhood but persist into adult life and are benign. *Malignant melanomas*, by contrast, develop by neoplastic transformation of melanocytes in the epidermis and invade the dermis secondarily. They are relatively common in adults and rare in children.

A. Nevocellular Nevus (Melanocytic Nevus)

Melanocytic nevi are usually appear in childhood and stop growing soon after puberty. They are extremely common and are better regarded as hamartomatous growths rather than true neoplasms. They are benign and present clinically as flat, papular, papillomatous or pedunculated pigmented (black or brown) lesions.

Histologically, moles are composed of nests of nevus (melanocytic) cells, which may be found in the dermis (intradermal nevus), at the junction between epidermis and dermis (junctional nevus), or in both locations (compound nevus). Junctional activity (melanocytic proliferation in the junctional zone) usually decreases after puberty; if it is prominent in an older patient or associated with cytologic atypia, malignant melanoma should be considered.

B. Malignant Melanoma

Malignant melanomas, also called melanomas, occur most commonly in fair-skinned people living in sunny climates, in which the most important etiological factor is UV light. Although most of these lesions arise in the skin, other sites of origin include the oral and anogenital mucosal surfaces, the esophagus, the meninges, and the eye.

Malignant melanoma appears clinically as an elevated pigmented nodule (Figure 5-24) that grows rapidly and tends to bleed and ulcerate. Metastasis via the lymphatics and bloodstream tends to occur early. When one of the following signs appears, malignant melanoma should be considered: (1) itching or pain in a preexisting nevus, (2) enlargement of a preexisting nevus, (3) variegation of color within a pigmented lesion, (4) irregularity of the borders of a pigmented lesion, and (5) development of a new pigmented lesion during adult life. Among them, itching and pain may be an early manifestation, while the change in the color or size of a pigmented lesion is more important.

Histologically, malignant melanoma is characterized by melanocytic proliferation originating in the basal epidermis. The cells show marked cytologic atypia, pleomorphism, nuclear hyperchromatism, and increased mitotic activity. Nuclei are large, with prominent nucleoli. The cytoplasm is abundant and usually contains melanin pigment. When no

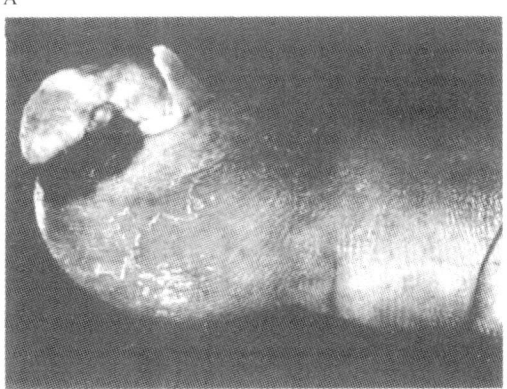

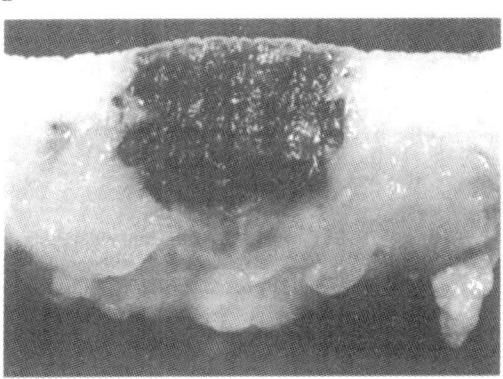

Figure 5-24 Malignant melanoma. A: Occurring in the subungual region. The partially pigmented mass has lifted the nail. B: A cross section of a lesion in the skin of another patient, showing deep dermal invasion

melanin is present, the term amelanotic or achromatic melanoma is used. In these cases, the diagnosis may be established by (1) electron microscopy, which shows premelanosomes and melanosomes; and (2) immunohistochemical demonstration of S100 protein or melanosome-related antigens (e.g. HMB45) in the melanocytes.

Other Neoplasms

A. Retinoblastoma

Retinoblastomas occur in two forms: an inherited form (30%) and a sporadic form (70%) (see the former section of "THE ROLE OF INHERITANCE IN ONCOGENESIS"). They occur almost exclusively in children under 5 years of age, with a frequency of about 1:20,000.

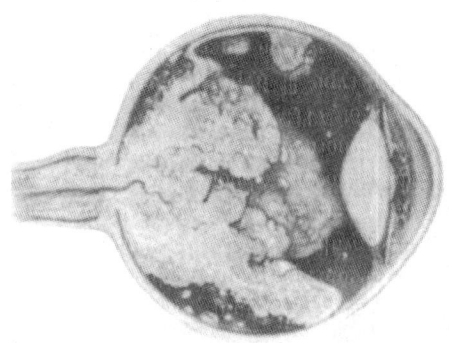

Figure 5-25 Retinoblastoma, showing a large retinal mass extending into the vitreous with multiple satellite nodules and invasion of the optic nerve

Retinoblastoma arises in the retina from primitive neural cells. It is an aggressive neoplasm, infiltrating the retina, extending into the vitreous (Figure 5-25) and along the optic nerve into the cranial cavity. Hematogenous spread also occurs. Microscopically, retinoblastoma is composed of undifferentiated small cells with a high nuclear to cytoplasmic ratio and hyperchromatic nuclei. Mitotic figures are frequent. The presence of Flexner-Wintersteiner rosettes composed of the neoplastic cells arranged in an orderly fashion around a central lumen is a diagnostic feature.

B. Neoplasms of Neural Origin

Include those tumors that arise in the central nervous system such as glioma, medulloblastoma and meningioma, and in the peripheral nervous system such as schwannoma, neurofibroma and ganglioneuroma, etc. All these tumors will be discussed in the chapter 14.

(Meng Bin)

Part B Systemic Pathology

Chapter 6 Diseases of the Cardiovascular System

Song Jingyu, Zhang Jianzhong

CHAPTER CONTENTS
- Structure and Function
- Atherosclerosis
- Medial calcification
- Coronary Atherosclerosis and Coronary Heart Disease
    Coronary Atherosclerosis
    Coronary Heart Disease
    Myocardial Infarction
    Sudden Cardiac Death
    Chromic Ischemic Heart Disease
- Systemic Hypertension
- Aneurysms and Dissections
- Rheumatism
- Infective Endocarditis
- Valvular Heart Diseases
    Mitral Stenosis
    Mitral Regurgitation
    Aortic Stenosis
    Aortic Regurgitation
- Myocarditis and Cardiomyopathy
    Myocarditis
    Cardiomyopathies
- Pericarditis
    Acute Pericarditis
    Chronic Pericarditis

The cardiovascular system is composed of heart, arterials, capillaries and veins. It is the structure foundation for keeping blood circulation, exchanging materials between blood and tissue fluids and transmitting information of tissue fluids. The structure changes of cardiovascular system is responsible for the functional changes that disturb whole and/or local blood circulation. The disorders of cardiovascular system affect the human health and life and are a leading cause of death in the world.

STRUCTURE AND FUNCTION

Structure of the Heart

The heart is composed of (1) the endocardium, which lines the internal surfaces of the cardiac chambers and valves; (2) the myocardium; (3) the pericardium, composed of an inner visceral layer covering the heart and an outer parietal layer completing the pericardial sac; and (4) a specialized conducting system consisting of the sinoatrial (SA) and atrioventricular (AV) nodes, the bundle of His, and the arborizing Pukinje fibers.

The muscular interatrial and interventricular septa divide the heart longitudinally into a right side, which accepts the deoxygenated systemic venous return and pumps it into the low-pressure pulmonary circulation; and a left side, which accepts the oxygenated pulmonary venous blood and pumps it into the aorta.

Each side of the heart is further divided by the atrioventricular valves into an atrium and a ventricle. The muscular atrial walls normally have a thickness not exceeding 2 mm. The right ventricle pumps blood into the relatively low-pressure pulmonary circulation (systolic pressure 15–30 mmHg) and has a wall thickness of less than 0.3 cm. The left ventricle develops a systolic pressure of 100–140 mmHg to maintain the high-pressure systemic circulation. The left ventricle normally has a wall thickness of up to 1.2 cm.

The atrioventricular valves are composed of two (mitral valve) or three (tricuspid valve) cusps. The free edges of the atrioventricular valves are attached to the papillary muscles of the ventricle by fibrous cords (chordae tendineae). Closure of the valves in systole prevents regurgitation of blood into the atrium.

The semilunar (aortic and pulmonary) valves remain closed during diastole, preventing regurgitation of blood from the great vessels into the ventricles.

Myocardial Function

The myocardium is composed of striated muscle fibers that contain myofibrils composed of serially repeating contractile units called sarcomeres. The myofibrils are invested by the sarcolemma. An individual sarcomere is limited by two adjacent Z bands and has a length that varies between 1.6 and 2.2 um. It is composed of regularly overlapping actin and myosin filaments that are connected by cross-bridges in the overlapping zone (Central A band of the Sarcomere). In the relaxed state, these cross-bridges are maintained by troponin C, which acts as a regulatory protein that inhibits contraction. During contraction, troponin C inactivation permits alteration of the cross-bridges, permitting the actin and myosin filaments to slide between one another, leading to contration. In cardiac muscle, all sarcomeres contract during every contraction.

At rest, the interior of the myofibril has (1) a negative charge with respect to the outside with a trans-membrane potential of -80 to -100 mV; (2) a low intracellular Na^+ and a high K^+, maintained by the ATP-driven sodium pump; and (3) a low Ca^{2+}. During activation, there is an influx of Ca^{2+} into the cell through sarcolemmal channels, which causes a rapid Ca^{2+} release from the sarcoplasmic reticulum. The calcium combines with troponin C, producing the conformational changes in the actin-myosin cross-bridges that lead to contraction. After contraction, these events reverse, with reaccumulation of Ca^{2+} in the sarcoplasmic reticulum, reversal of Ca^{2+} troponin binding, and return of the actin and myosin filaments and cross-bridges to the resting state. The energy for most of these reactions is derived from ATP formed from substrate oxidation.

The cardiac (ventricular) output is the product of the heart rate and stroke volume and is normally $2.6-4.2$ (L/min)/m^2. The stroke volume is a function of the extent of shortening of fibers of the ventricular myocardium, which is dependent on the following three independent factors:
• Ventricular preload (ventricular end-diastolic volume), which is the length of the muscle (which in turn is a function of the length of each sarcomere) at the onset of contraction.
• Myocardial contractility (inotropic state) reflects the level of ventricular performance at a given end-diastolic volume.
• Ventricular afterload is the amount of tension the muscle is called upon to develop during contraction. At a given preload and level of myocardial contractility, the extent of shortening of the myocardial fiber is inversely proportionate to the afterload. Afterload in the left ventricle is dependent on the mean pressure in the aorta, the volume of the ventricular cavity, and the thickness of the ventricular muscle wall.

The Systemic Circulation

The systemic circulation supplies arterial blood to the tissues; it begins at the aortic valve and ends with the openings of the venae cavae into the right atrium. The basic constituents of the walls of blood vessels are cells, predominantly endothelial cells (ECs) and smooth muscle cells (SMCs), and extracellular matrix (ECM), including elastin, collagen, and glycosaminoglycans. The three concentric layers - intima, media, and adventitia - are most clearly defined in the large vessels. Based on their size and structural features, arteries are divided into three types of elastic arteries, muscular arteries, and small arteries and arterioles. Its component vessels and their function may be described as follows:
• Elastic arteries - the aorta and its major branches - convert the spasmodic left ventricular output into a more continuous flow distally.
• Muscular arteries - the internal carotid, coronary, brachial, femoral, renal and mesenteric arteries - distribute blood to the tissues.
• Small arteries and Arterioles - by definition, arteries less than 2 mm and $20-100$ μm in diameter, respectively - have muscular walls and a rich sympathetic nerve supply that permits adjustment of luminal size. Arterioles regulate the pressure decrease from aortic to capillary levels (Figure 6-1). Adjustment of resistance within the arterioles is a major factor determining systemic blood pressure and distribution of flow.

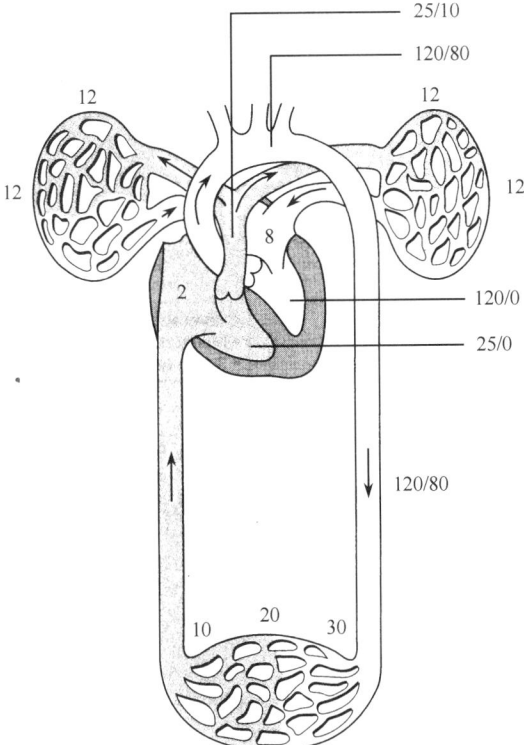

Figure 6-1 Blood pressures (measured in mmHg) in the pulmonary and systemic circulations

- **The microcirculation** consists of capillaries (7 to 8 μm), precapillary sphincters, and postcapillary venules. It is the site of exchange with tissue fluids.
- **Veins** are low pressure capacitance vessels that return blood to the heart. Forward flow in the veins is facilitated by endothelial valves.

The Pulmonary Circulation

The main function of the pulmonary circulation is to effect respiratory gas exchange in the pulmonary capillary bed; it begins at the pulmonary valve and ends in the left atrial openings.

The pulmonary circulation is lower than the plasma osmotic pressure (25/10 mmHg). Because this is lower than the plasma osmotic pressure, there is normally no fluid movement out of the alveolar capillaries, permitting the alveoli to remain dry for effective gas exchange.

Vascular Endothelium

The endothelium is a simple, flat layer of cells that lines the internal surface of the entire vascular system. It covers almost 700 m^2 and weighs 1.5 kg. The vascular endothelium is a versatile multifunctional tissue that has many synthetic and metabolic properties and that is an active participant in blood-tissue interaction, and synthesizes a large number of different substances, the most important of which are prostaglandins (mainly prostacylin, PGI$_2$, and thromboxane A$_2$), thrombomodulin, plasminogen activator, heparin-like molecules, endothelin, nitrous oxide (NO), and coagulation von Willebrand facto (factor VIII-vWF). Pulmonary endothelial cells synthesize angiotensin-converting enzyme.

ATHEROSCLEROSIS

Atherosclerosis (ATH) is a disease of large and medium-size arteries that results in progressive accumulation within the intima of SMCs, lipids and connective tissue. Continued growth of the lesions encroaches on other layers of the arterial wall and narrows the lumen. ATH is the main cause of ischemic heart disease (IHD) and cerebrovascular disease, and it is the major primary cause of death in most developed and developing countries. Global in distribution, ATH overwhelmingly contributes to more mortality – approximately half of all deaths – and serious morbidity in the Western world than any other disorder.

Etiology

The basic abnormality in ATH is the deposition of complex lipids in the intima. The cause is uncertain. Numerous risk factors have been identified (Table 6-1). The major controllable risk factors are discussed here.

A. Hypertension

Hypertension is the most important risk factor in people over 45 years of age. IHD is five times more common in an individual whose blood pressure is > 160/95 mmHg than in one who is normotensive (blood pressure < 140/90 mmHg). The risk is diminished when high blood pressure is controlled with drugs.

B. Cigarette Smoking

People who smoke more than 10 cigarettes per day have a threefold increase in risk. The association of smoking with ATH is thought to be related to the presence of factors such as carbon monoxide (CO) that may cause ECs injury.

Table 6-1 Risk factors for atherosclerotic arterial disease
(Note: The presence of multiple risk factors imposes more than a simple additive risk.)

Increasing age: significant disease is rare under 30 years

Morbid obesity: >30% over ideal body weight

Lack of physical exercise: Incidence greater in persons with sedentary occupations; regular exercise (20 minutes twice weekly) decreases risk

Highly significant factors

    Male sex: Males are affected more than females; sex incidence is equal after age 65 years

    Family history: History of IHD in a parent or sibling under age 55 years

    Hyperlipidemia: The major risk factor in patients under 45 years of age

        Specific lipoproteins involved in increased risk are as follows:

            Total cholesterol > 6 mmol/L (> 240 mg/dL)

            Total TG > 2.8 mmol/L (> 250 mg/dL)

            LDL-cholesterol > 4.2 mmol/L (> 160 mg/dL)

            Low HDL-cholesterol: < 0.9 mmol/L (< 35 mg/dL)

            High lipoprotein(a) in plasma

    Hypertension: The major risk factor in patients over 45 years of age; hypertensives have a fivefold increased risk compared with normotensive persons

    Cigarette smoking: Ten cigarettes per day increases the risk threefold; cessation of smoking decreases risk to normal after 1 year

    Diabetes mellitys: Both type I and type II diabetes mellitus are associated with a twofold increase in risk

C. Diabetes Mellitus

All diabetics who have had the disease for more than 10 years are likely to have significant ATH. Part of the risk in diabetes is due to the coexistence of other risk factors such as obesity, hypertension, and hyperlipidemia. Other suggested reasons for increased risk are (1) increase glycosylation of collagen, which increases low-density lipoprotein (LDL) binding to collagen in ATH lesions; and (2) the fact that glycosylated high-density lipoprotein (HDL) is more easily degraded than is normal HDL. Because the latter two mechanisms are dependent on glycosylation, which is dependent on elevated blood glucose, it may explain how rigid control of diabetes can reduce the risk of ATH.

D. Hyperlipidemia

Hyperlipidemia is a major risk factor for ATH (Table 6-2). Most of the evidence specifically implicates hypercholesterolemia. Both primary and secondary hyperlipidemias increase the risk. Lipoproteins associated with endogenous lipid metabolism such as LDL and intermediate-density lipoprotein (IDL) are much greater risk factors than chylomicrons associated with exogenous lipid metabolism (Figure 6-2). Increased levels of the following components of plasma lipids have been identified as associated with increased risk:

1. Total serum cholesterol

A level of > 240 mg/dL (> 6 mmol/L) imposes a high risk; 200 – 239 mg/dL (5.2 – 6.0 mmol/dL) is borderline; < 200 mg/dL (5.2 mmol/L) is desirable.

2. Low density lipoprotein cholesterol (LDL-C)

A level of > 160 mg/dL (4.2 mmol/L) imposes a high risk; 130 – 159 mg/dL (3.4 – 4.1 mmol/L) is borderline; < 130 mg/dL (< 3.4 mmol/L) is determined by the following formula after direct measurement of plasma levels of total cholesterol, HDL-C, and triglyceride (TG):

$$LDL\text{-}C = C - HDL\text{-}C - TG/5$$

LDL-C levels are greatly elevated in **familial hypercholesterolemia**, which is caused by a mutation in the gene coding for the LDL receptor (LDLr) on the cell surface. Lack (in homozygotes) or decrease (in heterozygotes) of LDL-C receptor leads to failure of clearing of plasma LDL - C receptor leads to

Table 6-2 Hyperlipidemic disorders

Type	Elevated Lipoprotein	Serum Cholesterol	Serum Triglyceride	Basic Defect	Primary Disease (Inherited)	Secondary Diseases
I	Chylomicrons	N	↑	Lipoprotein lipase deficiency	Lipoprotein lipase deficiency (autosomal recessive)	Systemic lupus erythematosus
IIa	LDL	↑	N	Deficiency of LDL receptor	Familial hypercholesterolemia (autosomal dominant)	Hypothyroidism, nephritic syndrome, increased dietary fat, diabetes mellitus
IIb	LDL plus VLDL	↑	↑	Abnormal apoprotein E	Familial type III hyperlipoproteinemia (autosomal dominant; varies)	
III	IDL or chylomicron remnants	↑	↑	Abnormal apoprotein E	Familial type III hyperlipoproteinemia (autosomal redessive)	Obstrucive jaundice
IV	VLDL	N	↑	Unknomn	Familial triglyceridemia (variable)	Diabetes mellitys, alcoholism, increased dietary fat
V	Chylomicrons plus VLDL	N	↑	Defi	Familial combined hyperlipidemia	Alcoholism

Key: VLDL, very-low-density lipoproteins; IDL, intermediate-density lipoproteins; LDL, low-density lipoproteins; N, nomal serum level.

failure of clearing of plasma LDL-C by cells and a subsequent increase in plasma LDL-C. There is also an increased production of LDL in these patients, due to failure of metabolism of IDL by the liver [IDL also uses the LDLr for uptake into the liver cell, and when this fails, IDL is converted to LDL (Figure 6-2)]. As LDL accumulates in the plasma, it is taken up by tissues that do not depend on the presence of LDLr - macrophages (resulting in xanthomas in the skin and connective tissues) and probably the arterial intima. Homozygotes have extremely high LDL-C levels and develop severe atherosclerotic disease in their teens. Heterozygotes are common (1:500 people in the population), have a twofold to threefold elevation of plasma cholesterol, and develop premature ATH. Heterozygous familial hypercholesterolemia is found in 3%-6% of survivors of myocardial infarction (MI).

3. Total plasma triglyceride

A level > 250 mg/dL (> 2.8 mmol/L) imposes a high risk. Accurate risk evaluation for TGs has been difficult because of the associated changes in the more significant cholesterol levels.

4. Low HDL-cholesterol

The risk of ATH bears an inverse relationship to plasma level of HDL-C. An HDL-C level < 35 mg/dL (< 0.9% mmol/L) imposes a high risk. Low HDL-C levels occur more commonly in males, cigarette smokers, diabetics, inactive people who do not exercise regularly, and patients with high TG levels. Regular exercise and a small daily intake of alcohol have been shown to increase plasma HDL-C levels.

HDL are believed to remove cholesterol liberated from cell turnover. It is possible that HDL also removes cholesterol from atheromatous plaques as part of this function, explaining it is protective effect in ATH.

5. Abnormal apoproteins

Apoproteins are proteins that are associated with lipid to form lipoproteins and are genetically determined. Different apoprotein types are associated with different lipoprotein (Table 6-3; Figure 6-2). In addition to being structural components of the lipoprotein molecule, apoproteins function as ligands that interact with cell receptors which bind lipoproteins, and as cofactors of enzymes of lipid metabolism. The following abnormalities of apoproteins, which are inherited, are associated with an increased risk of ATH:

a. **Familial type III hyperlipoproteinemia**, which is associated with an increased plasma level of

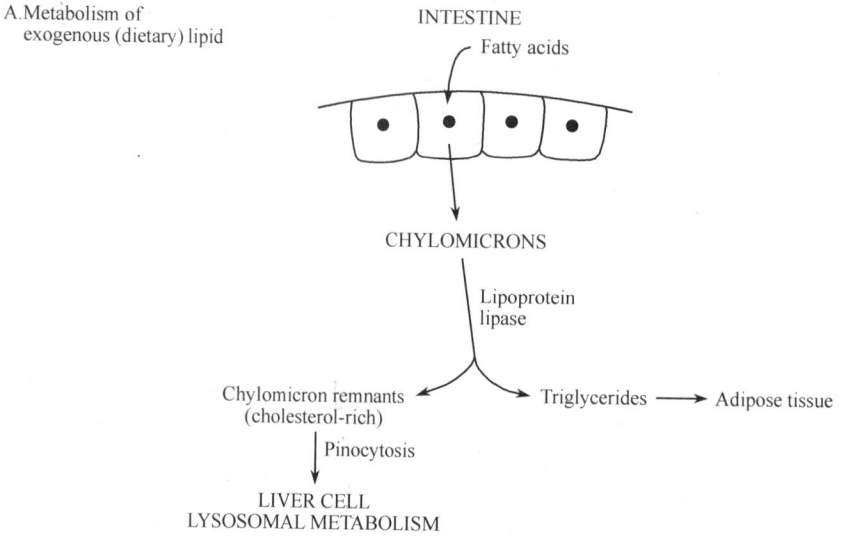

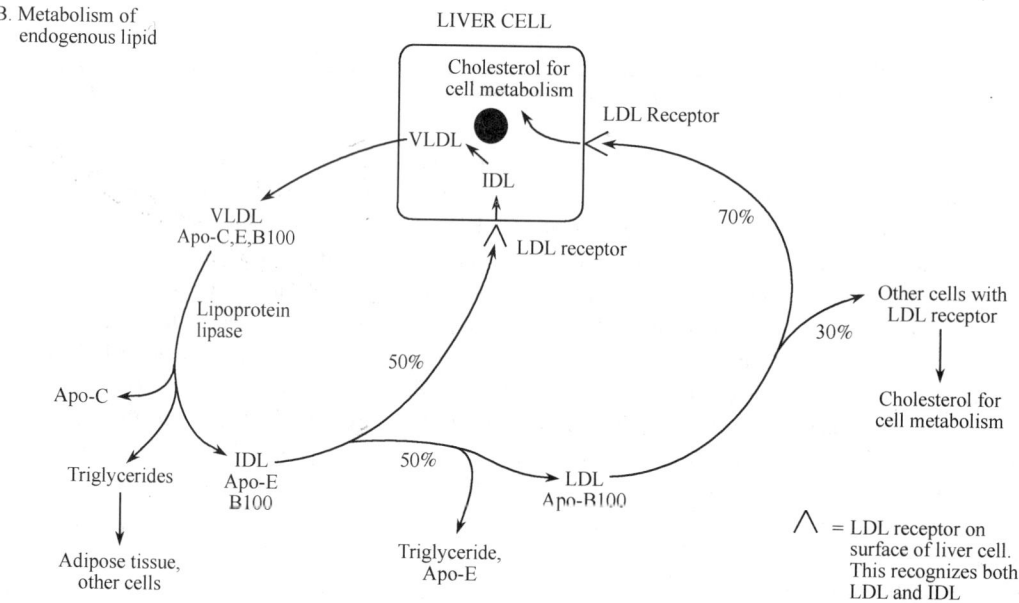

Figure 6-2 Normal metabolic pathways of exogenous (dietary) lipid (A) and endogenous lipid (B)

IDL and accelerated ATH. IDL is normally derived from very low-density lipoprotein (VLDL), which cleaves off TG and leaves the cholesteryl ester-rich IDL (Figure 6-2). IDL is associated with apoproteins B100 and E and is either taken up by the liver cell for recycling into VLDL or metabolized into LDL. Hepatic uptake of IDL is dependent on recognition of IDL by the same receptor that recognizes LDL. The binding of IDL to the receptor is dependent on the presence of apoprotein E. Patients with familial type III hyperlipoproteinemia inherit an abnormal apoprotein E, resulting in failure of IDL uptake by the liver, increased IDL in the plasma, and ATH.

b. Abnormal HDL-associated apoproteins: HDLs are believed to remove excess cholesterol from cells and tissues (probably including atheromatous lesions, explaining their protective effect). HDL is

Table 6-3 Lipoproteins in plasma. Note that chylomicrons represent the main lipoprotein in the metabolism of exogenous (dietary); lipid VLDL, IDL, and LDL represent the lipoproteins associated with metabolism of endogenous TG and cholesterol. HDL is associated with removal of cholesterol resulting from cell turnover

Type of Lipoprotein	Associated Apoproteins	Lipid Content	Source	Metabolism	Atherogenic Potential
Chylomicron	E, C11, B48	90% dietary TG; 10% cholesterol	Intestinal epithelial cell	Conversion to chylomicron remnant (→blood) + TG (→adipose tissue) by endothelial lipoprotein lipase	Minimal
Chylomicron remnant	E, C11, B48	Mainly dietary cholesterol	Degradation of chylomicrons	Taken up by liver cells (pinocytosis) and degraded by lysosomes	High
VLDL	E, C, B100	60% endogenous TG; 25% cholesterol	Liver cell	Conversion by lipoprotein lipase into TG (→ adipose tissue) and IDL	Low
IDL	B100	45% cholesterol; 30%–40% TG	Degradation of VLDL	(1) 50% taken up by liver (via binding to LDL receptor) and recycled into VLDL (2) 50% metabolized (removal of apo-E and TG) into LDL	High
LDL	B100	70% cholesterol	Metabolism of LDL	(1) taken up by cells via LDL-receptro binding (70% liver, 30% other body cells) and metabolized in lysosomes → cholesterol for celluse (2) If present in excess amounts, taken up by macrophages (→xanthomas)	High
HDL	A1, C3, A4	<25% cholesterol	Normal cell turnover of cholesterol	HDL-cholesterol metabolized via lecithin cholesterol acyltransferase (LCAT)	Protective[1]

Key: VLDL, very-low-density lipoprotein; IDL, intermediate-density lipoprotein; LDL, low-density lipoprotein; HDL, high-density lipoprotein. [1] HDL has a protective effect, ie, high levels are associated with a decreased risk of ATH.

associated with several apoproteins, three of which (A1, C3, and A4) are encoded by genes clustered on chromosome 11. Inherited abnormalities of these apoproteins lead to a defect in HDL function and have been associated with ATH. The best-understood component is **defective Apo-AI**. Normally, Apo-AI serves as a cofactor for the enzyme lecithin-cholesterol acyltransferase (LCAT), which is necessary for the metabolism and removal of cholesterol taken up by HDL. With defective Apo-AI, this reaction fails, interfering with the normal protective function of HDL.

c. Increased lipoprotein(a)−(Lp[a]) is associated with an increased risk. Lp(a) is a variant of LDL in which the normal LDL apoprotein (B100) is linked by disulfide bridges to a distinct apoprotein (a) which is encoded by a single gene. Plasma levels of Lp(a) are determined by the amount of apoprotein(a) that is produced. Apo(a) has structural similarity to plasminogen (it contains 37 copies of kringle 4, which is part of the plasminogen molecule that normally binds to fibrin during fibrinolysis). It is known that microthrombi are frequently formed in relation to atherolsclerotic lesions. If these are normally removed by plasminogen, the presence of Apo(a) in the lesions can inhibit this process by competing with plasminogen for kringle 4 receptors on the fibrin molecule.

Pathogenesis

The mechanism responsible for lipid deposition in the intima and formation of the atheromatous lesion is known. At least six hypotheses have been proposed to explain the origins of atherosclerotic plaques.

A. Reaction to Vascular Injury Hypothesis

Ross proposed this more unifying theory. Termed the response-to-injury hypothesis, it postulates that

ATH begins with endothelial injury, making the endothelium susceptible to the accumulation of lipids and the deposition of thrombus. Over the past decade, Fuster and colleagues have proposed that vascular injury starts the atherosclerotic process.

Nondenuding endothelial injury is believed to lead to adherence of blood monocytes, which are activated, imbibe LDL and actively enter the intima, and become macrophages. Active macrophages release free radicals that oxidize LDL. Oxidized LDL (ox-LDL) is toxic to endothelium, causing endothelial loss and exposure of subendothelial connective adhesion and aggregation and to fibrin deposition, forming microthrombi. Platelets release various factors – one of which has been identified as being mitogenic – causing migration of SMCs into the intima and proliferation therein. The activated macrophages and SMCs secrete numerous cytokines that can be found in the early lesion. These include platelet-derived growth factor (PDGF), tumor necrosis factor (TNF), fibroblast growth factor (FGF), and interleukun-1 (IL-1), some of which may also have mitogenic capability.

The SMCs, macrophages, and matrix accumulate LDL from the plasma, a process that is enhanced by the presence of increased LDL in the blood. SMCs and ECs have LDLr on their surfaces, and macrophages are capable of taking up LDL – facts that would explain the high association of LDL with lesions. This sets up a cycle of changes that involves macrophage activation, LDL oxidation, and endothelial damage that cause progression of the atheromatous lesion.

B. Thrombus Encrustation Hypothesis

According to this hypothesis, proposed by Rokitansky in 1851, the primary event is thrombosis. The thrombus becomes incorporated into the intima and then undergoes lipid degeneration to initiate the lesion. Thrombosis is now thought not to be the initial event, but it probably plays a role in the development and enlargement of the lesion. Lp(a) promotes development of ATH by virtue of its inhibition of plasminogen activity, which suggests that removal of fibrin is important in preventing progression of the atheromatous lesion.

C. Monoclonal Hypothesis

The SMC proliferation in the lesion was shown, at least in some cases, to be monoclonal. This suggested that mitogen-induced SMC proliferation was the primary event. This is unlikely, as it has been shown that monoclonality of the SMCs is not a constant feature. However, mitogen-induced SMC proliferation is still thought to be important in the development of the atheromatous lesion.

D. Insudation Hypothesis

In 1856, Virchow proposed that ATH starts with lipid transudation into the arterial wall and its interaction with cellular and extracellular elements, causing "intimal proliferation". This theory states that the lipid in atherosclerotic lesions is derived from plasma lipoproteins.

LDL is the form of lipid in plasma that has been most closely associated with accelerated ATH. ECs have receptors for both LDL and modified forms of LDL. Recent studies of ATH in fat-fed animals have demonstrated that macrophages also play a major role during the early stages of lipid accumulation.

E. Intimal Cell Mass Hypothesis

The location of atherosclerotic lesions has been related to focal accumulation of SMCs in the normal intima at branch points and other sites in certain vessels, particularly the coronary arteries. The distribution of intimal cell masses in children resembles that of atherosclerotic lesions in adults, thereby suggesting that the intimal cell mass is either the early lesion of ATH or its precursor.

F. Hemodynamic Hypothesis

The distribution of atherosclerotic lesions in large vessels and the differences in both the location and frequency of lesions in different vascular beds have encouraged a belief in the role of hemodynamic factors related to turbulence, pressure, and shear forces. That hypertension enhances the severity of atherosclerotic lesions and low blood pressure is generally associated with increased longevity, further encourages the idea that hemodynamic factors somehow play a role in development of sclerotic vascular disease.

Pathology

The lesions associated with ATH are the fatty streak, the fibrous atheromatous plaque, and the complicated lesion. The latter two are definitely pathologic and are responsible for clinically significant disease.

A. The Fatty Streak

Fatty streaks are thin, flat, yellow streaks in the intima. They consist of macrophages and SMCs, the cytoplasm of which has become distended with lipid (to form foam cells). Fatty streaks occur maximally around the aortic valve ring and thoracic aorta. They are present very early in life, often in the first year, and are seen all over the world irrespective of sex, race, or environment. They increase in number until about age 20 years and then remain static or decrease. There is controversy about whether some fatty streaks progress into fibrous atheromatous plaque or whether they are independent of ATH.

B. The Fibrous Atheromatous Plaque

This is the basic lesion of clinical ATH. It consists of three zones: (1) A **fibrous cap** under the endothelium, consisting of dense collagen scattered SMCs and macrophages; (2) the **lipid zone**, which consists of foam cells (lipid-laden macrophages and SMCs) and extracellular lipid and debris; and (3) the **basal zone**, composed of proliferated SMCs and connective tissue. Different plaques contain varying amounts of these three layers; some are mainly fibrous, and others are predominantly fatty.

The fibrous atheromatous plaque appears grossly as a yellow-white elevation on the intimal surface of the artery (Figure 6-3). In cut section, the center of the plaque consists of semisolid yellow material (Gk *ather-* = porridge). Microscopically, the three zones are recognizable and are of varying thickness in different plaques (Figure 6-4). Needle-shaped cholesterol crystals are commonly present in the lipid zone.

Fibrous atheromatous plaques are present in the aorta in most cases, with maximal change most commonly in the abdominal aorta (Figure 6-3). Involvement of muscular arteries such as the coronary, carotid, vertebrobasilar, mesenteric, renal, and iliofemoral arteries is associated with luminal stenosis. This is common and is responsible for many of the clinical manifestations of ATH (Table 6-4). Plaques tend to be most prominent at points of branching of the major arteries. In severe disease, plaques become confluent, involving much of the intimal surface (Figure 6-3).

C. The Complicated Plaque (*Figure 6-5*)

Thrombosis is the most important complication of ATH because it may cause complete occlusion of the artery. Thrombosis is caused by (1) slowing and

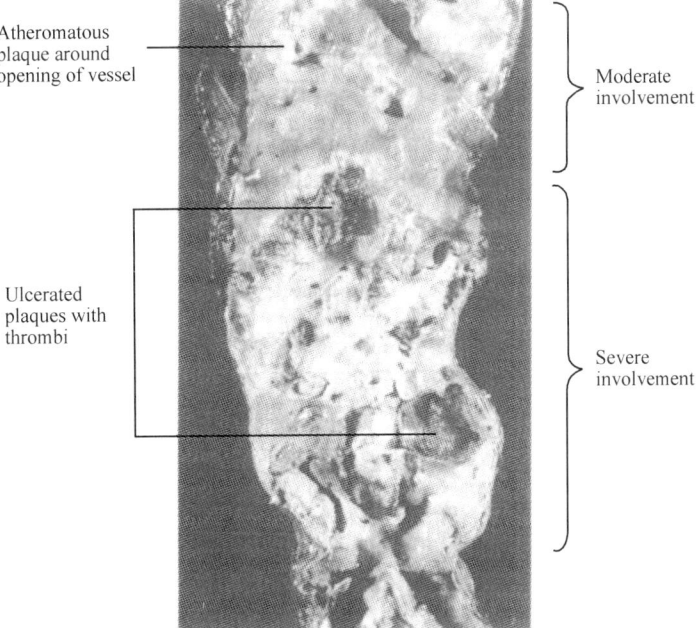

Figure 6-3 Severe atherosclerosis of the lower abdominal aorta. Note multiple areas of ulceration with adherent mural thrombus

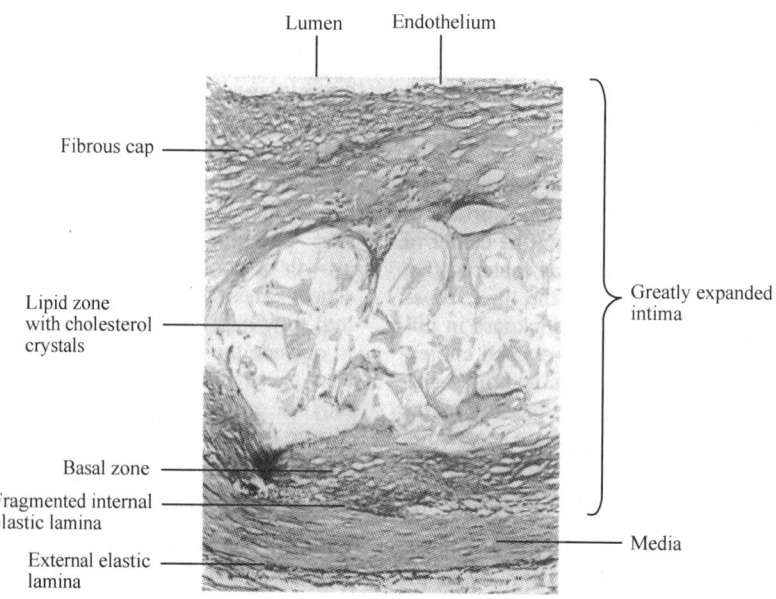

Figure 6-4 Atherosclerotic plaque. Low magnification

Table 6-4 Clinical effects of atherosclerosis related to the major arteries involved

Artery Involved	Clinical Efect
Aorta	Atheroschlerotic aneurysms Acaholesterol embolism
Internal carotid system	Chronic cerebral ischemia Cerebral infarction (stroke) Transient is chemic attacks
Circle of Wilis	Contributes to rupture of berry aneurysms
Vertebrobasilar system	Cerebellar ischemia and infarction Brain stem ischemia and infarction
Coronary arteries	Myocardial infarction Chronic myocardial ischemia Angina pectoris Chronic heart failure Arrhythmias and heart block
Celiac and mesenteric arteries	Intestinal ischemia and infarction Ischemic colitis
Renal arteries	Renal artery stenosis Renovascular hypertension Renal ischemia and infarction
Iliofemaral arteries	Peripheral vascular disease Intermittent claudication Gangrene

turbulence of blood in the artery in the region of the plaque and (2) ulceration of the plaque. **Dystrophic calcification** is very common and occurs in the lipid zone of the plaque. Severely affected vessels (including the aorta) may become converted into calcific tubes. **Ulceration** of the endothelium overlying the plaque may cause the lipid contents of the plaque to be discharged into the circulation as cholesterol emboli. Ulceration of the plaque may also precipitate arterial thrombosis at the site. **Vascularization** of

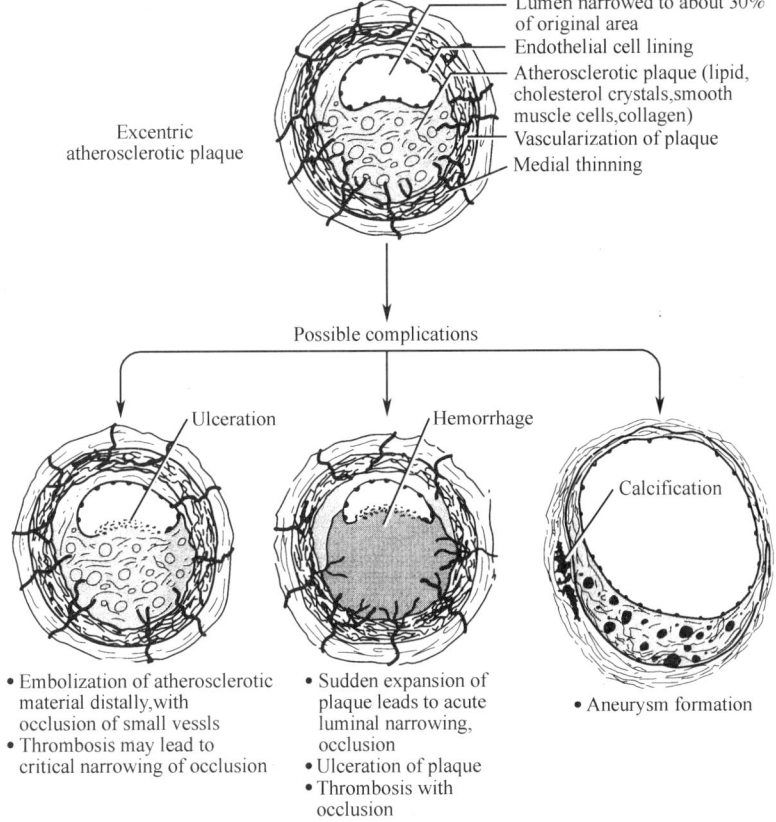

Figure 6-5 Complications of atherosclerosis

the plaque occurs by ingrowth of poorly supported vessels from the medial aspect. These may rupture, leading to **hemorrhage** into the plaque, which may then expand sufficiently to occlude the lumen of the artery. Hemorrhage may also cause ulceration and thrombosis. **Aneurysms** may develop in arteries weakened by extensive plaque formation; the abdominal aorta is the favored site of atherosclerotic aneurysms.

Clinical Features (Table 6-4)

A. Narrowing of Affected Arteries

Ischemia from arterial narrowing is responsible for most of the clinical effects of ATH (Figure 6-6). A decrease in blood flow usually occurs only with severe (>70%) narrowing of the vessel. Aortic narrowing is almost never sufficient to cause symptoms. However, narrowing of coronary, cerebral, renal, mesenteric, and iliofemoral vessels often causes ischemic changes in the organs and tissues supplied. Superimposed thrombotic occlusion of these arteries may cause infarction.

B. Embolism

Ulceration of the atheromatous plaque may result in embolization of the lipid contents of the plaque (Figure 6-5). This is important in the cerebral circulation, where small emboli produce transient ischemic attacks. Emboli can sometimes be visualized in the retinal arteries on funduscopic examination.

C. Aneurysm (Figure 6-7)

In severe atherosclerotic involvement of the aorta, the wall may be weakened to an extent that leads to dilation or aneurysm formation. Atherosclerotic aneurysms occur mainly in the lower abdominal aorta and may appear as a fusiform dilation of the whole vessel circumference or a saccular bulge on one side of it.

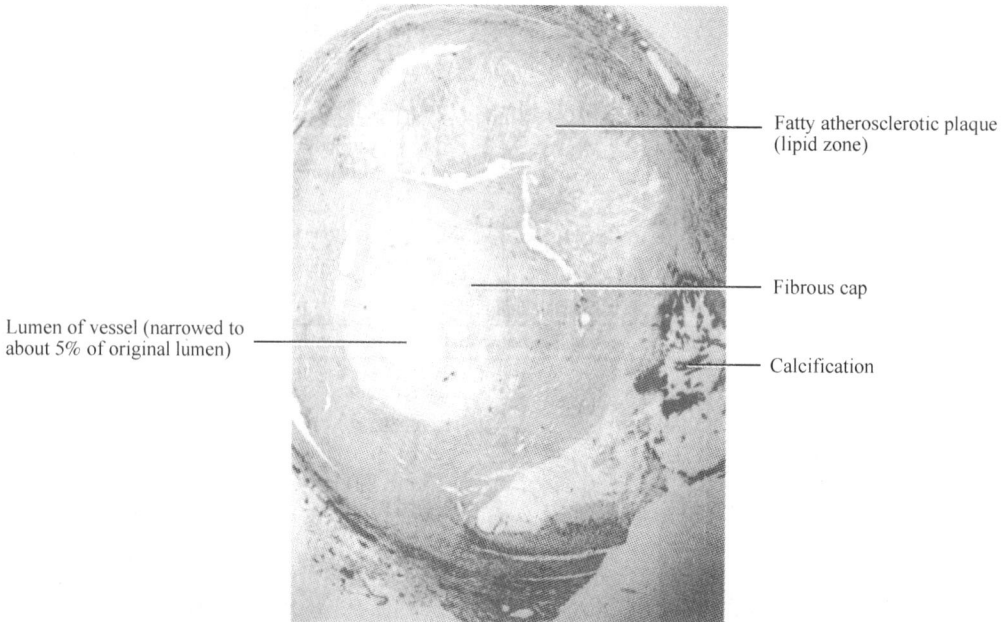

Figure 6-6 Coronary artery narrowing caused by atherosclerosis. Low magnification

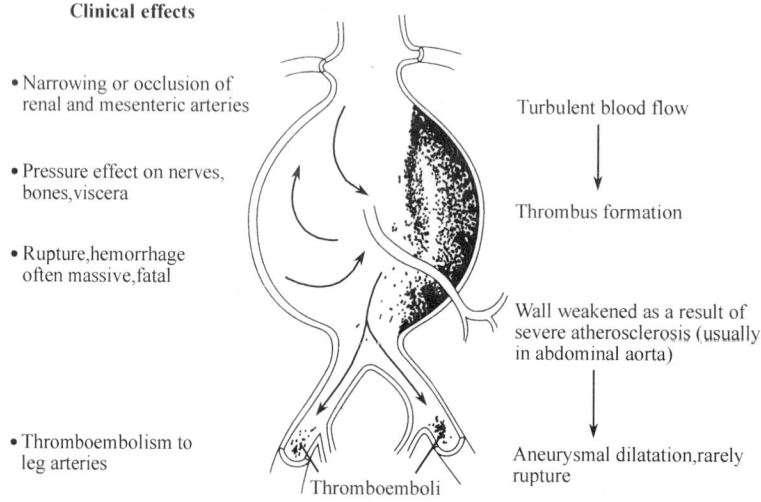

Figure 6-7 Clinical effects of an atherosclerotic aneurysm of the abdominal aorta. This is now the most common type of aortic aneurysm, superseding syphilitic aneurysms that involved the thoracic aorta

MEDIAL CALCIFICATION (MONCKEBERG'S SCLEROSIS)

Medial calcification is a clinically unimportant but very common degenerative change affecting muscular arteries such as the femoral, radial, and uterine arteries. The tunica media shows extensive calcification. There is no luminal narrowing or endothelial damage. Medial calcification does not produce any clinical abnormality – it is seen in elderly persons and is regarded as an aging change.

CORONARY ATHEROSCLEROSIS AND CORONARY HEART DISEASE

CORONARY ATHEROSCLEROSIS

Coronary ATH is the most menaced disease for the human in ATH, and may occur at any age but are most common in older adults, with peak incidence after the age of 60 years in men and 70 years in women. Men are more commonly affected than women until the ninth decade, by which time the frequency of coronary ATH is similar in both sexes.

Coronary ATH is narrowing of the lumina of the coronary artery and accounts for the vast majority of coronary artery disease, and is most marked in the proximal (epicardial) parts of the coronary arteries. The intramural branches may show slight intimal thickening, but are generally free of true ATH.

The location and frequencies of coronary ATH in the right and left main coronary arteries are in turn as follows: (1) left anterior descending coronary artery (40% to 50%); (2) right coronary artery (30% to 40%); and (3) left circumflex coronary artery (15% to 20%). Atherosclerotic plaques, in the coronary arteries are regional crescentic lesion, and progressive enlargement of the lesions which leads to different degree of obstruction of the lumen and results in ischemic heart diseases (angina pectoris, myocardial infarction, sudden cardiac death, and so on). Generally, the obstructive degree of the lumen of the coronary artery is divided into four grades: grade I, ≤25%; grade II, 26%-50%; grade III, 51%-75%; and grade IV, ≥75%.

CORONARY HEART DISEASE

Coronary heart disease (CDH) is one of ischemic heart disease (IHD) that is, in the vase majority of cases, a consequence of ATH of the coronary arteries and develops when the flow of blood is inadequate to provide for the oxygen demands of the heart, and hence IHD is often termed CHD or coronary artery disease (CAD).

IHD is the leading cause of death in most developed countries of the world and is responsible for at least 80% of all deaths from heart disease. Depending on the rate and severity of coronary artery narrowing and the myocardial response, one of four syndromes may develop: (1) various forms of angina pectoris (chest pain), (2) acute myocardial infarction (MI), (3) sudden cardiac death, and (4) chronic IHD with congestive heart failure.

Etiology

IHD is caused by narrowing of one or more of the three major coronary artery branches (Figure 6-8). These are functional end-arteries, and sudden occlusion of any one leads to infarction in the area of supply. However, gradual narrowing may permit development of collaterals that are sufficient to prevent infarction.

ATH accounts for 98% of cases of IHD. The risk factors for IHD are the same as those for ATH.

Other rare causes of coronary artery narrowing include coronary artery spasm (Prinzmetal angina); coronary artery embolism, most commonly in infective endocarditis; coronary ostial narrowing inclusion in aortic dissection of the aorta; and various types of arteritis involving the coronary arteries, including polyarteritis nodosa, thromboangiitis obliterans and giant cell arteriris.

Clinical Features

IHD may be manifested clinically in many ways (Figure 6-9). The more important ones - angina pectoris, MI, sudden death, cardiac arrhythmia, and cardiac failure - are discussed below. An individual patient with IHD may manifest more than one of these conditions.

Angina Pectoris

Angina pectoris is characterized by episodic ischemic cardiac pain not associated with MI. Two types of angina are recognized: angina of effort and variant (Prinzmetal's) angina.

A. Angina of Effort

Angina of effort is a common disorder usually caused by severe atherosclerotic narrowing of the coronary arterial system. The coronary arteries can provide the myocardium with adequate blood supply during rest but not during periods of exercise, stress, or excitement, which precipitate ischemic pain; the pain is relieved by resting or by administration of amyl nitrite or nitroglycerin (glyceryl trinitrate).

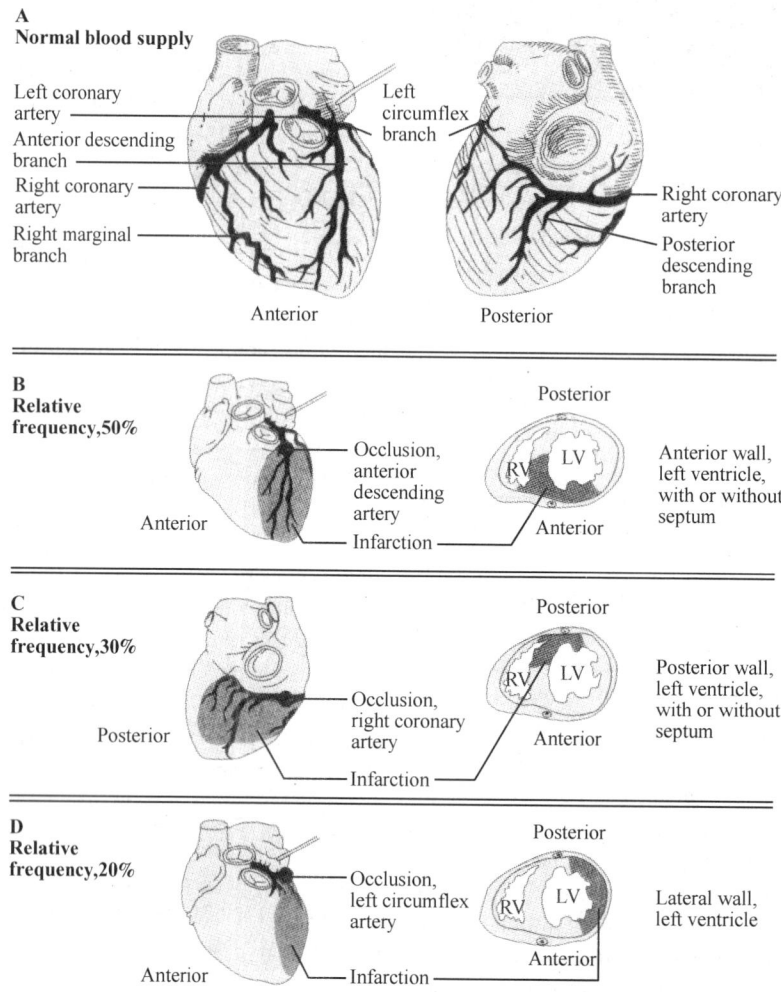

Figure 6-8 Blood supply to the myocardium (A) and areas of infarction resulting from the most frequent sites of coronary artery occlusion (relative frequency expressed as a percentage). (B-D) The exact area of myocardium affected will vary depending on normal anatomic variation in blood supply and the extent of collateral circulation that exists at the time of coronary occlusion

Pathologic changes associated with angina are variable and range from virtually no change in the myocardium to patchy areas of myocardial fibrosis and scars from previous infarcts. Infarction is not present; serum enzyme levels are not elevated; and the electrocardiography (ECG) does not show changes of acute injury. Nonspecific changes in the ST segment such as ST depression and T wave inversion may reflect chronic ischemic damage. ECG during carefully graded exercise (treadmill test) is a sensitive method for detecting IHD.

Patients with angina of effort have an increased risk of MI, which may be preceded by an increase in the severity of anginal stacks (crescendo, or unstable angina).

B. Variant Angina

Variant (Prinzmental's) angina is uncommon and occurs independently of ATH - which is, however, present in 75% of patients. Variant angina occurs at rest and is not relates to myocardial work. It is believed to be caused by coronary artery muscle spasm of insufficient duration or degree to cause MI. Spasm occurs near areas of stenosis in cases associated with ATH.

MYOCARDIAL INFARCTION

Myocardial infarction (MI) is refers to a discrete

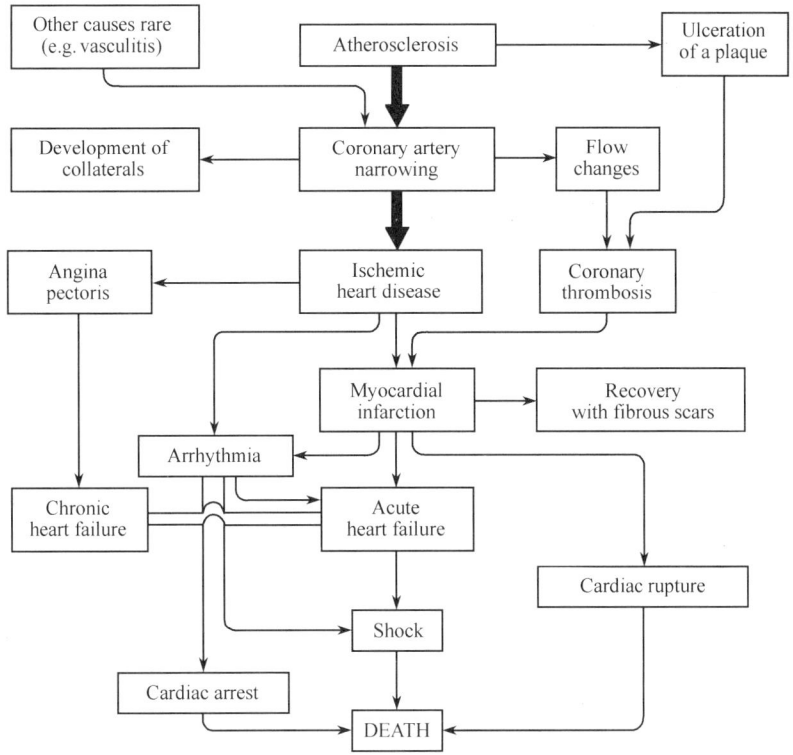

Figure 6-9　Causes and clinical consequences of ischemic heart disease

focus of ischemic necrosis in the heart. Acute MI, also known as "heart attack", is the single most common cause of death in industrialized nations. Among fatal cases, nearly half of the patients die before reaching the hospital. Most patients are over 45 years of age, and men are affected three to five times more frequently than women, paralleling the incidence of ATH.

Etiology

Except in those rare causes of nonatherosclerotic coronary narrowing listed above, most patients who suffer MI have **severe atherosclerotic narrowing** of one or more coronary arteries (Figure 6-10). A fresh thrombus overlying an atherosclerotic plaque is found in 40% – 90% of cases (Figure 6-11), the frequency varying greatly in different studies. Thrombosis may be precipitated by slowing and turbulence of blood flow in the region of a plaque or by ulceration of a plaque.

In cases where no thrombus is found, infarction may be precipitated by increased myocardial demand for oxygen, as occurs during exercise and excitement;

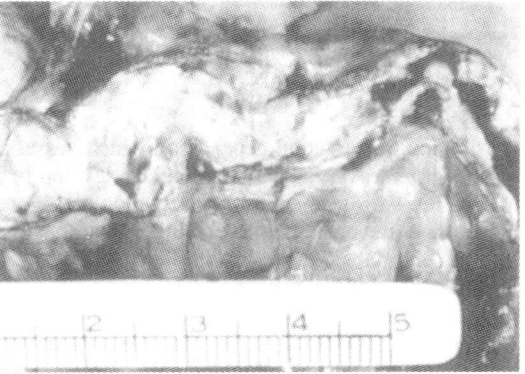

Figure 6-10　Coronary atherosclerosis. The left coronary artery has been opened longitudinally to show extensive plaque formation that has produced marked surface irregularity. Marked narrowing of the vessel was present, but this is better seen in transverse sections

reduction of coronary blood flow through a greatly narrowed artery due to cardiac slowing during sleep; or segmental muscular spasm of coronary arteries. In some cases, the thrombus may undergo lysis by the fi-

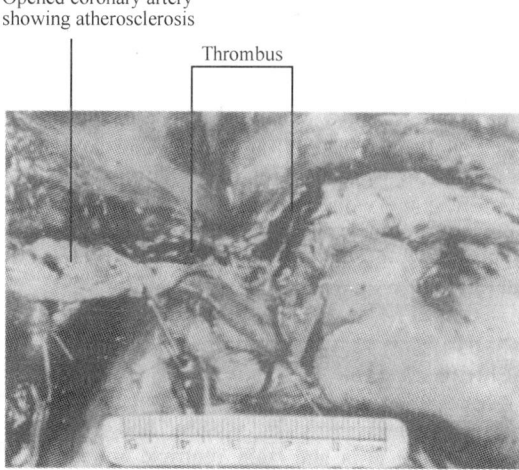

Figure 6-11 Thrombosis in an atherosclerotic coronary artery, resulting in occlusion of the vessel

brinolytic system after infarction has occurred.

Distribution of Infarction (Figure 6-8)

MI involves principally the left ventricle, interventricular septum, and conducting system. The atria and right ventricle are rarely involved, probably because their thin muscle walls derive a considerable part of their nutritional supply directly from the blood in the cardiac lumen. The distribution of infarction depends on which vessel is occluded. However, because collaterals develop in a chronically narrowed coronary circulation, the blood supply may traverse circuitous routes, leading to infarcts in unusual sites (paradoxic infarction).

Infarction may be **transmural**, involving the full thickness of the wall (Figure 6-12), or **subendocardial**. The subendocardial region has the most critical blood supply.

In acute infarction due to coronary occlusion, not all the muscle is necrotic in the early stages (i. e. within the first 3 hours). The critically ischemic but not yet necrotic muscle in the affected region may be salvaged by immediate reperfusion by restoring coronary artery patency. The use of thrombolytic agents (streptokinase and plasminogen activator) reduces the mortality rate by reducing infarct size and left ventricular failure if given within 3 hours after onset of occlusion. Mechanical reperfusion by angioplasty and coronary bypass surgery are usually reserved for cases not suitable for thrombolytic therapy.

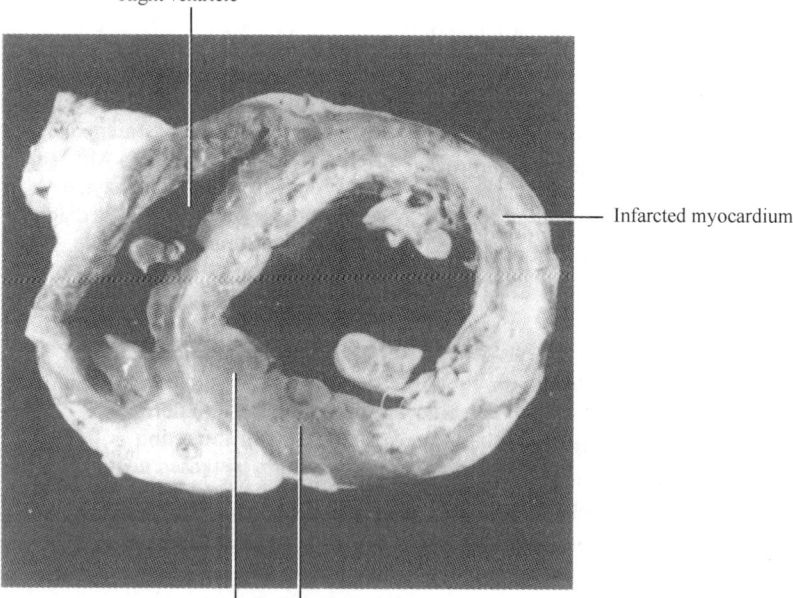

Figure 6-12 Myocardial infarction. The infarcted zone, which is pale, includes the anterior and lateral wall of the left ventricle and the anterior two-thirds of the interventricular septum. This infarct was associated with thrombotic occlusion of the main left coronary artery

Pathology

For 30 min after the onset of MI (as indicated by onset of pain or arrhythmias and shock), reversible changes including mitochondrial swelling, relaxation of myofibrils could be seen by electron microscope (EM). At about 2 hours, EM appears irreversible changes including sarcolemmal disruption, elctron-dense mitochondrial deposits, and fragmentation of myofibrils. Light microscopic changes may appear in 4 - 6 hours but are rarely detectable with certainty before 12 - 24 hours. Coagulative necrosis of the myocardial fibers is recognized by nuclear pyknosis, dark pink staining of the cytoplasm, contraction band and loss of striations in the cytoplasm (Figure 6-13; Table 6-5).

The tetrazolium test. Incubation of a slice of normal myocardium in tetrazolium produces a red-brown color resulting from reaction of tetrazolium with a dehydrogenase enzyme; infracted myocardium remains pale because the enzyme is lost from the cells within hours after infarction. The value of this technique is limited.

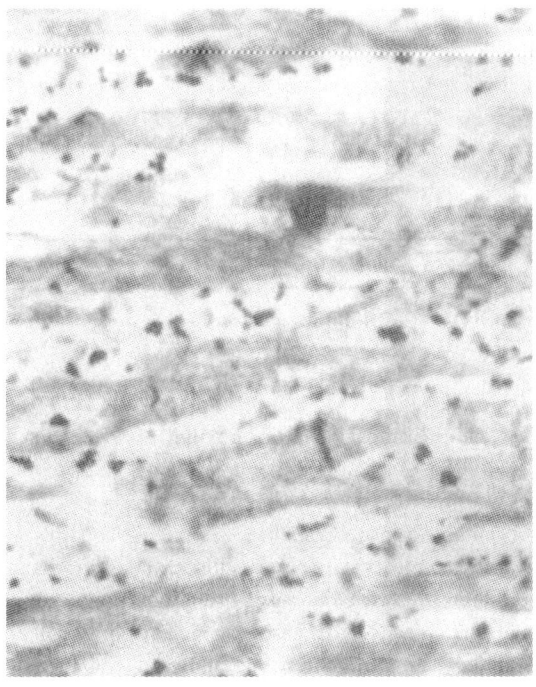

Figure 6-13 Acute myocardial infarction 1 - 3 days after onset. Note loss of striations and lysis of muscle fibers, with acute inflammation. Striations are still visible in a few muscle fibers at the bottom of the figure. High magnification

Clinical Features

Ischemic pain is the dominant symptom of MI - a tightening retrosternal pain that varies in severity from mild to excruciating. It resembles angina but is not relieved by rest or vasodilators. 20% of cases of MI occur without pain (silent infarction). The onset of ischemic pain is sudden and may occur during exercise, excitement, rest, or even sleep. Cardiac pain is often accompanied by signs of autonomic stimulation such as sweating, changes in heart rate, a lowered blood pressure (with or without shock), and additional heart sounds.

The diagnosis of MI, when suspected clinically, is based on ECG and serum enzyme changes. ECG shows elevation of the ST segment above the isoelectric line within a few hours, representing an abnormal electrical potential associated with acute injury. The T wave becomes inverted, and in transmural infarction the dead muscle acts as an electrical window, producing an abnormal Q wave. As healing takes place, the ST segment returns to the isoelectric line, but T wave inversion and the Q wave persist.

Necrotic myocardial fibers release a variety of enzymes into the bloodstream (Figure 6-14). When

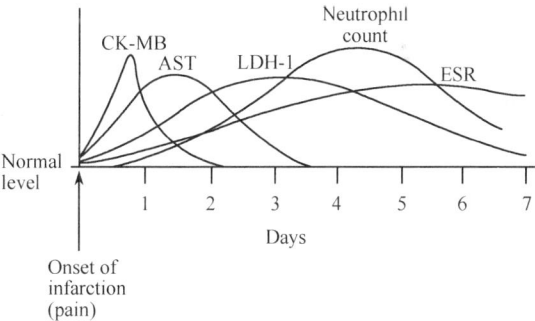

Figure 6-14 Changes in serum enzymes, neutrophil count, and erythrocyte sedimentation rate (ESR) following acute myocardial infarction. The serum level of MB isoenzyme of creatine kinase (CK-MB) rises rapidly, and CK-MB elevation is the test of choice in the first 24 hours. Because CK-MB levels return to baseline rapidly, isoenzyme 1 of lactate dehydrogenase (LDH-1) is the test of choice from 2 to 7 days. A test combination that includes CK-MB and LDH-1 is extremely effective in the diagnosis of acute myocardial infarction. Aspartate aminotransferase (AST) is of limited usefulness because of its lack of specificity; AST is present also in high concentration in liver and skeletal muscle

Table 6-5 Dating of a myocardial infarct[1]

Elapsed Time	Gross or Naked Eye Feature (at Autopsy)	Light Microscopic Features
1 – 2 hr	None	Few "wavy" fibers a margin of infarct
4 – 12 hr	None	Usually none But early coagulation necrosis Minimal edema Occasional neutrophils Minimal hemorrhage
12 – 24 hr	Softening, irregular pallor	Loss of striations Cytoplasmic eosinophilia Nuclear pyknosis disintegration "Contraction band" Mild edema Neutrophils
1 – 3 days	Pale infarct surrounded by a red (hyperemic) zone	As above, plus: Nuclear lysis More neutrophils with early fragmentation of neutrophil nuclei Inflammatory capillary dilatation
4 – 7 days	Pale or yellow (caused by liquefaction by neutrophils), definite red margin	As above, plus: Liquefaction of muscle fibers Neutrophils Macrophages remove debris Ingrowth of granulation tissue from margins
7 – 14 days	Progressive replacement of yellow infarct by red-purple (granulation) tissue	As above, plus: Disappearance of necrotic muscle cells Reduced numbers of neutrophils Macrophages, lymphocytes Beginnings of fibrosis and organization of granulation tissue
2 – 6 weeks	Becomes gray-white	As above, plus: Development of fibrous scar Decreasing vascularity Contraction of scar

[1] The time course is influenced by the size of the infarct.

both creatine kinase (CK)-MB isoenzyme and lactic acid dehydrogenase-isoenzyme 1 (LDH-1) serum levels are elevated, a specific diagnosis of AMI can be made. When a patient with chest pain shows no elevation of either of these enzymes on serial samples, MI can be ruled out. Sequential CK-MB levels are helpful in following the evolution of an infarcteg, a secondary increase indicates new infarction or extension of the area of infarction.

MI is followed by elevation of temperature, increased neutrophil count in the peripheral blood, and changes in plasma proteins. Increases in acute phase reactants such as fibrinogen and haptoglobin cause elevation of the erythrocyte sedimentation rate. These changes are due to the release of chemical mediators in the area of infarction.

Complications

A. Arrhythmias

Abnormalities in cardiac rhythm occur in about 70% of cases of myocardial infarction, mainly during the first few hours. They represent a serious and preventable cause of death.

• **Ectopic electrical foci** develop in the injured myocardium. Ventricular extrasystoles are common; ventricular tachycardia is less common but can lead to impaired ventricular filling and acute left ventricular failure. The most dangerous arrhythmia is ventricular fibrillation, which causes cardiac arrest.

The occurrence of tachyarrhythmias bears no relationship to the size of the infarct. Successful management may therefore be followed by full recovery. Because most arrhythmias occur within the first 2 hours - often before the patient reaches a hospital - traning of the lay community in cardiopulmonary resuscitation (CPR) is an important part of overall management. Community CPR training is recommended by the American Heart Association.

- **Heart block** resulting from involvement of the conduction system occurs more commonly with posterior myocardial infarcts. It is usually due to involvement of the conduction fibers by edema around an infarct, in which case the heart block is temporary. Permanent heart block due to necrosis of the conducting fibers is less common. Complete heart block is characterized by severe bradycardia and reduced cardiac output. Death may occur.
- **Autonomic stimulation** is a common occurrence in acute MI, producing either tachycardia (sympathetic stimulation) or bradycardia (vagal stimulation).

B. Left Ventricular Failure

Acute left ventricular failure results from arrhythmia or massive necrosis of myocardium. The clinical effects are cardiogenic shock, acute pulmonary edema, and sudden death. The first two syndromes have a high mortality rate, even with treatment.

C. Progressive Infarction

Extension of the initial infacted area to adjacent muscle occurs in 5% - 10% of patients in first 10 days after the onset. The muscle around the infracted area has a marginal blood supply that may become inadequate if there is an increased myocardial oxygen demand, e. g. during exercise or under conditions of emotional stress. Vascular supply to the muscle is at risk also if there is a decrease in coronary perfusion, due either to extension of a thrombus or to decreased cardiac output. Progression of an infarct can be diagnosed by following the serum CK-MB levels. Progressive infarction is an indication for mechanical reperfusion by coronary angioplasty or coronary artery bypass surgery.

D. Pericarditis

Fibrinous or hemorrhagic pericarditis complicates MI in about 30% of cases. It usually occurs within the first few days and may cause pericardial pain, pericardia rub, or pericardial effusion. Effusion sufficient to impair cardiac function is uncommon. Dressler's syndrome is a pericarditis that occurs 2 - 6 weeks after the onset of MI. It is believed to be immunologically mediated.

E. Systemic Embolism From Mural Thrombi

Involvement of the endocardium by the infarct leads to the formation of mural thrombi over the area of infarction. Such thrombi may detach to become emboli that enter the systemic arteries.

F. Myocardial Rupture

The infarction muscle represents an area of weakness that is maximal in the first week as the neutrophil enzymes cause liquefaction of the necrotic muscle fibers (Figure 6-15). Rupture may occur into the pericardial sac, producing hemopericardium and rapid death from cardiac tamponade; through the interventricular septum, producing an acute ventricular septal defect, with a left-to-right shunt and acute right ventricular failure; or within the papillary muscles, producing acute mitral regurgitation.

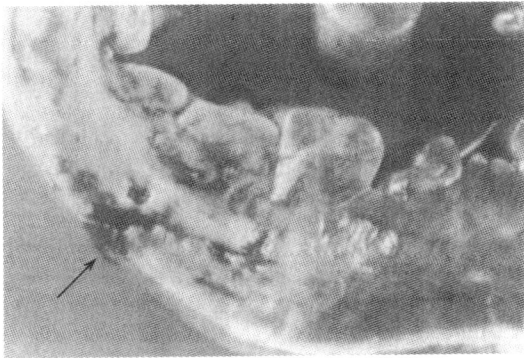

Figure 6-15 Myocardial infarction with rupture of the left ventricular wall. (Courtesy of O Rambo. Reproduced, with permission, from Sokolow M, McIlroy MB: *Clinical Cardiology*, 5th ed. Appleton and Lange, 1990)

G. Ventricular Aneurysm (Figure 6-16)

High intraventricular pressure may cause progressive outward bulging of the area of infarction during systole. This paradoxic motion of part of the ventricular wall during systole is called a ventricular aneurysm. Aneurysms may develop either in the first 2 weeks or after several months in the healed infarct and may cause left ventricular failure. Mural thrombi forming in an aneurysm may become detached as systemic emboli.

SUDDEN CARDIAC DEATH

Sudden death has been defined in many different ways, ranging from instantaneous death to death

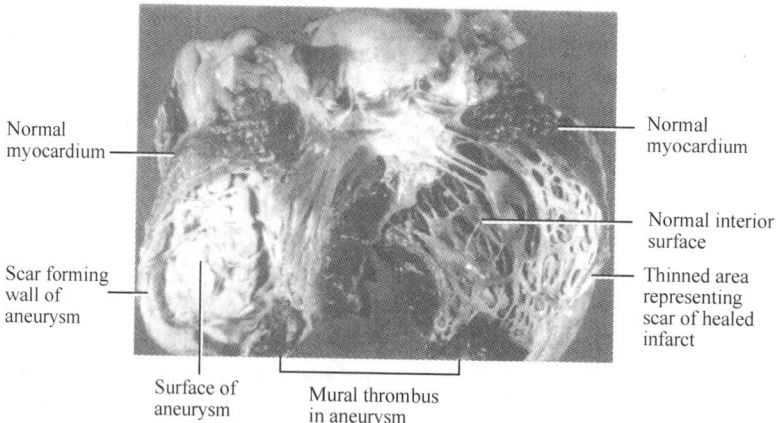

Figure 6-16 Aneurysm of the left ventricle in a patient who died from intractable heart failure 2 months after an acute myocardial infarction. The left ventricle has been cut and the 2 halves splayed out

occuring within 24 hours of the onset of symptoms. Sudden death can be caused by a wide range of diseases, and the most common cause sudden cardiac death is IHD. The most common cardiac lesions in sudden death are those of coronary ATH and its complications. This has been attributed to **ventricular fibrillation**, leading to cardiac arrest. Studies of patients surviving such episodes (ie, in hospitalized patients) have shown that ventricular fibrillation often leads to death before MI can develop. Tragically, however, sudden death is the initial manifestation of IHD in about 50% of patients with the disease.

CHROMIC ISCHEMIC HEART DISEASE

The term chronic IHD is used to describe the development of progressive congestive heart failure as a consequence of long-term ischemic myocardial injury. Patients with severe coronary ATH follow a pattern of increasingly frequent episodes of angina pectoris, reflecting progressive narrowing of one or more coronary arteries. In most patients with chronic IHD, persistently depressed cardiac function reflects the presence of infarcts. In many cases, there are a combination of ischemic myocardial dysfunction, diffuse fibrosis, and multiple small, healed infarcts in chronic IHD. However, there still remains a group of patients who present with left ventricular failure and in whom cardiac dysfunction occurs without tissue necrosis. These patients are said to have ischemic cardiomyopathy.

SYSTEMIC HYPERTENSION

Systemic hypertension has been defined by the World Health Organization (WHO) and International Society of Hypertension (ISH) as being a persistent elevation of blood pressure to greater than 160 mm Hg systolic, greater than 90 mm Hg diastolic or both (Table 6-6). While the concept is clear, the exact pressure that constitutes hypertension is an arbitrary determination based on pressures associated with a statistical risk of developing diseases associated with hypertension.

Hypertension is one of the most common worldwide diseases afflicting humans. Because of the associated morbidity and mortality and the cost to society, hypertension is an important public health challenge. Hypertension is estimated to cause 4.5% of current global disease burden and is as prevalent in many developing and developed countries. Hypertension is the most important modifiable risk factor for coronary heart disease, stroke, congestive heart failure, end-stage renal disease, and peripheral vascular disease. Therefore, health care professionals must not only identify and treat patients with hypertension but also promote a healthy lifestyle and preventive strategies to decrease the prevalence of hypertension in the general population. Control of blood pressure decreases the risk of cardiovascular morbidity.

Chapter 6 Diseases of the Cardiovascular System

Table 6-6 Definitions and Classification of Blood Pressure Levels (WHO-ISH)

Category	Systolic (mmHg)	Diastolic (mmHg)
Optimal	<120	<80
Normal	<130	<85
High-Normal	130-139	85-89
Grade 1 Hypertension ("mild")	140-159	90-99
Subgroup: Borderline	140-149	90-94
Grade 2 Hypertension ("moderate")	160-179	100-109
Grade 3 Hypertension ("severe")	≥180	≥110
Isolated Systolic Hypertension	≥140	<90
Subgroup: Borderline	140-149	<90

When a patients' systolic and diastolic blood pressures fall into different categories, the higher category should apply.

Etiology and Pathogenesis (Figure 6-17)

A. Essential Hypertension

Essential hypertension occurs as a primary phenomenon without known cause. It is the most common type of hypertension, usually occurring after age 40 years, with a familial incidence suggestive of polygenic inheritance upon which environmental factors are superimposed.

The pathogenesis is uncertain. No constant changes have been indentified in plasma levels of angiotensin, renin, aldosterone, or catecholamines – or in the activity of the sympathetic nervous system or baroreceptors – that could account for the elevated blood pressure. Some hypertensive individuals have elevated levels of plasma angiotensin, which has been related to the finding of a variant angiotensin gene. Inhibitors of angiotensin-converting enzyme are effective antihypertensive drugs.

The currently favored hypothesis is that essential hypertension is due to high dietary intake of sodium in a generically predisposed individual. There may be associated failure of excretion by the kidney in the face of a prolonged high sodium load. Sodium retention results in an increase in circulating natriuretic factors. One of these inhibits membrane Na^+-K^+ ATPase, thereby leading to intracellular accumulation of Ca^{2+}. Cytosol Ca^{2+} is increased in essential hypertension; in vascular smooth muscle, increased cytosol Ca^{2+} enhances reactivity and tends to cause vasoconstriction. This effect of Ca^{2+} is inhibited by calcium channel-blocking drugs, which are effective antihypertensive agents.

Endothelium derived factors such as NO are produced in response to shear forces, intraluminal pressure, circulating hormones, and platelet factors. NO acts on the underlying SMCs, causing vasodilation. An abnormality in the NO system has been suggested as causing hypertension. NO donors such as nitroprusside are effective antihypertensive agents.

B. Secondary Hypertension

Secondary hypertension is that due to a preceding defined disease process (Table 6-7). Even though an underlying cause can be identified in less than 10% of cases of hypertension, this group of patients is important because many of their diseases can be treated. Secondary hypertension must be strongly suspected in a patient under 40 years of age who develops hypertension.

Secondary hypertension results from accentuation of one of the many factors (rennin, aldosterone, renalsodium reabsorption, catecholamines, sympathetic stimulation) that may increase cardiac output or peripheral resistance (Figure 6-17 and Table 6-7).

Pathology

A. Benign Hypertension

In the earliest phase of hypertension, vasoconstriction is produced by smooth muscle contraction and there are no microscopic changes in blood vessels. Following sustained vasoconstriction, there is thickening of the media due to muscle hypertrophy, progressing to hyaline degeneration and intimal fib-

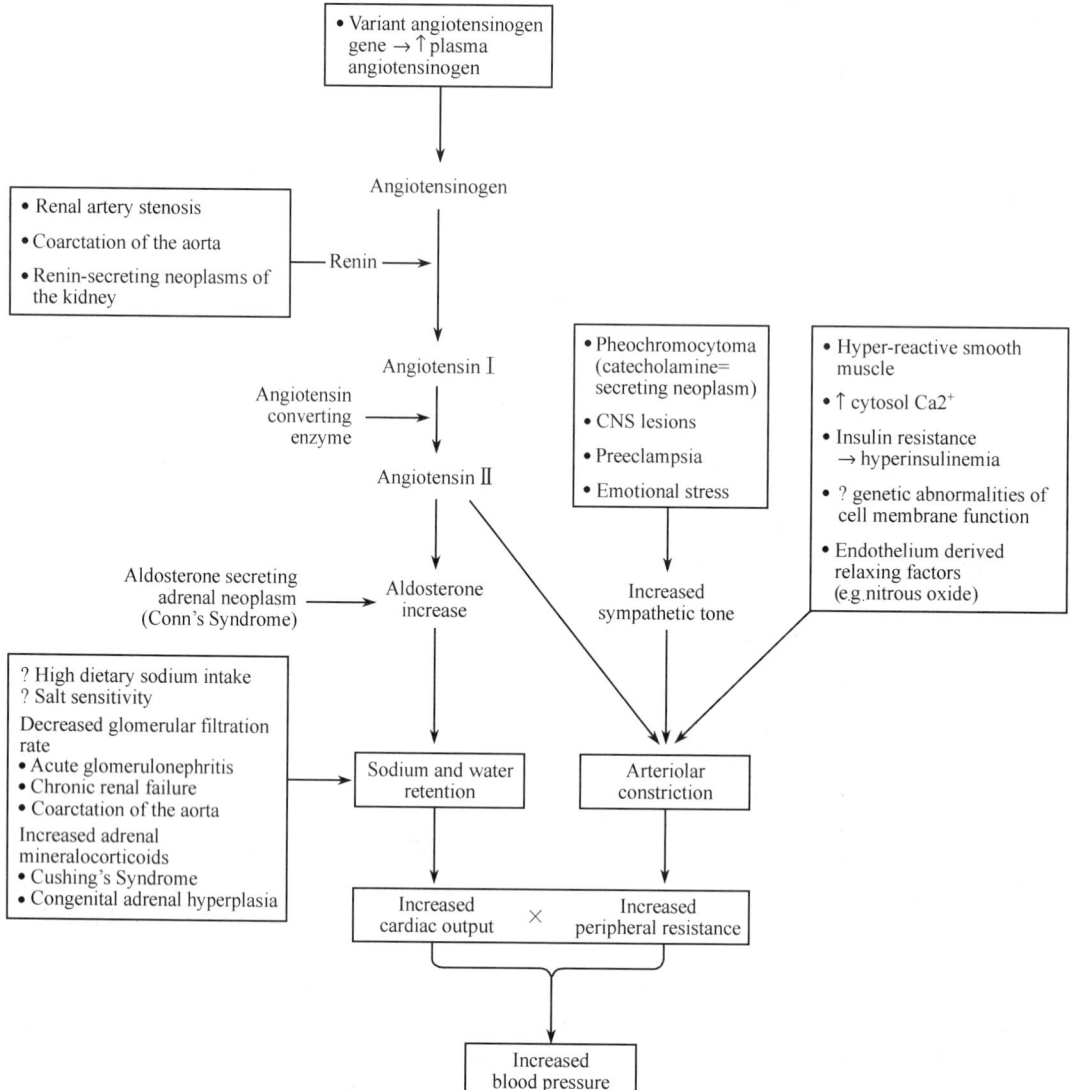

Figure 6-17 Factors involved in the pathogenesis of hypertension. Note that more than one of the factors listed may operate in a given patient

rosis. These changes are known as hyaline arteriolosclerosis and are found with longstanding hypertension of mild to moderate degree (**benign hypertension**). The tissues supplied by affected vessels may show changes of chronic ischemia.

B. Malignant Hypertension

Malignant hypertension is characterized by papilledema (which defines the entity), retinal hemorrhages and exudates, and blood pressures usually > 200/140 mmHg. It is characterized pathologically by the occurrence of **fibrinoid necrosis** of the media with marked intimal fibrosis and extreme narrowing of the arteriole (Figure 6-18). The tissues supplied by affected vessels show acute ischemia with microinfarcts and hemorrhages. Malignant hypertension is frequently associated with elevated serum rennin levels, establishing a vicious cycle that tends toward further elevation of the blood pressure.

Clinical Features (Table 6-8)

A. Early Hypertension

The early phase of hypertension is asymptomatic, and the diagnosis can be made only by detecting the

Table 6-7 Etiology and classification of hypertension and the mechanisms involved in pathogenesis. Percentages shown indicate frequency among hypertensive individuals in the general population. The figures differ in specialty clinics as a consequence of patient selection

Disease	Mechanism
Essential (primary) hypertension (90%–95%)	Unknown; probably mutifactorial
Secondary hypertension (2%–10%)	
Renal diseases (3%–4%)	
Renal vascular diseases (0.2%–4%)	Increased rennin secretion (compensatory)
Renal artery stenosis (ATH, fibromuscular hyperplasia, posttransplantation)	
Arteritis, polyarteritis nodosa	
Renal parenchymal diseases (2.5%–6%)	Sodium retention in kidney
Acute glomerulonephritis	
Chronic glomerulonephritis	
Chronic pyelonephritis	
Polycystic disease of the kidney	
Renal neoplasms	Renin secretion by neoplasm
Juxtaglomerular apparatus neoplasm	
Renal carcinoma	
Wilms' tumor	
Endocrine diseases (1%–2%)	
Pheochromocytoma	Catecholamine excess
Primary aldosteronism (Conn's syndrome)	Aldosterone excess
Cushing's syndrome	Cortisol excess
Congenital adrenal hyperplasia due to 11-hydroxylase deficiency	Mineralocorticoid excess
Coarctation of the aorta	Increased rennin secretion (compensatory)
Drug-induced hypertension	
Corticosteroids	Cortisol excess
Amphetamine use	Increased rennin secretion
Chronic licorice ingestion[1]	Sodium retention
Oral contraceptives	Sodium retention
Neurologic diseases	
Raised intracranial pressure	Increased sympathic tone
? psychogenic	
Hypercalcemia	Arteriolar constriction

[1] Licorice has an aldosterone-like effect (pseudoaldosteronism).

elevation of blood pressure.

B. Hypertensive Heart Disease

The term hypertensive heart disease is used when the heart is enlarged in the absence of a cause other than hypertension. Hypertension causes compensatory left ventricular hypertrophy as a result of the increased workload imposed on the heart. The weight of the heart usually exceeds 375 g in men (normal, 300–350 g) and 350 g in women (normal, 250–300 g). The hypertrophy typically involves the ventricular wall in a symmetric circumferential pattern termed **concentric hypertrophy**, with free wall thicknesses > 1.2 cm and normal size of the chamber. With long-standing and severe hypertension, particularly in the malignant phase, left ventricular dilation and failure occurs.

Hypertension is a major risk factor for coronary ATH and IHD. Ischemia is aggravated by the increased oxygen demand of the hypertrophied myocardium.

C. Hypertensive Renal Disease

Changes in renal arterioles occur in most cases of hypertension, resulting in decreased glomerular filtration rate, progressive fibrosis, and loss of nephrons in the kidneys. Renal ischemia resulting from

TEXTBOOK OF PATHOLOGY

Table 6-8 Clinical features and complications of hypertension

Asymptomatic
Headache: occipital, throbbing, early morning
Heart disease
Left ventricular hypertrophy
Left ventricular failure[1]
Atherosclerotic ischemic heart disease; angina
Myocardial infarction[1]
Renal disease
Chronic renal failure
Ralicly progressive renal failure (malignant nephrosclerosis)[1]
Cerebral disease
Atherosclerotic cerebral cerebral thrombosis and infarction[1]
Cerebral hemorrhage[1]
Hypertensive encephalopathy
Visual disturbances (hypertensive retinopathy)
Aortic dissection

[1] Common causes of death in hypertension.

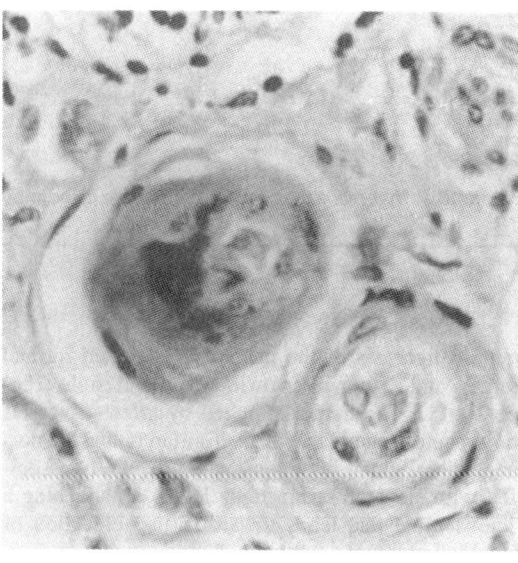

Figure 6-18 Vascular changes in malignant hypertension. The arteriole in the center shows fibrinoid necrosis, which appears as a dark area in the media, with marked luminal narrowing. The adjacent arteriole shows concentric intimal fibrosis. High magnification

these changes sets up a vicious cycle (falling glomerular filtration rate, rennin release, angiotensin production, salt retention) that aggravates the hypertension.

Renal failure with elevation of serum creatinine usually occurs only in patients with malignant hypertension. Fibrinoid necrosis is present in renal arterioles (Figure 6-18). Hematuria occurs, and marked reduction in glomerular filtration rate may progress to acute renal failure.

D. Hypertensive Cerebral Disease

Hypertensive patients have a greatly increased incidence of cerebrovascular disease, both thrombosis and hemorrhage (strokes). Cerebral thrombosis is the result from rupture of microaneurysms in small intracerebral perforating arteries.

Hypertensive encephalopathy is due to spasm of small arteries in the brain induced by very high blood pressures. The temporary spasm, though insufficient to cause infarction, leads to cerebral edema, which produces headache and transient cerebral dysfunction.

E. Hypertensive Retinal Disease

The retinal arterioles show all the changes of hypertension on funduscopic examination (hypertensive retinopathy). Narrow, irregular arteries with thickened walls characterize mild to moderate hypertension. Malignant hypertension leads to papilledema, retinal hemorrhages, and fluffy exudates (cotton wool spots) - ill-defined areas of edema and repair resulting from ischemia (Figure 6-19).

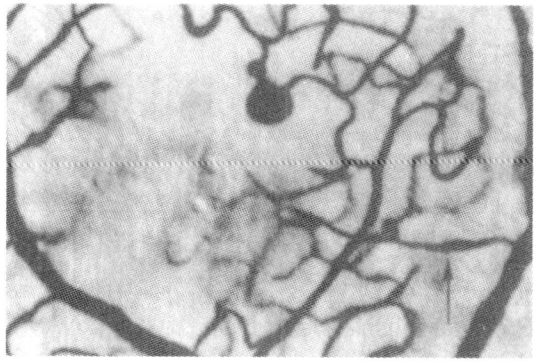

Figure 6-19 Retina of a patient with hypertensive retinopathy showing an exudate and failure of capillary filling in affected area. A microaneurysm is also present. (Injected with India ink; stained with oil red O; magnification ×90.) (Reproduced, with permission, from Ashton N: Pathophysiology of retinal cotton wool spots. *Br Med Bull* 1970; 26: 143)

Diagnosis, Treatment, And Prognosis

The blood pressure should be measured several times over a period of several weeks to make certain that hypertension is sustained. It is important to look for clinical effects due to hypertension and for treatable causes, especially in patients under 40 years, because essential hypertension is uncommon in this age group.

When a treatable cause of hypertension such as renal artery stenosis or an adrenal neoplasm is present, surgery is curative. Patients with essential hypertension must receive lifelong treatment with antihypertensive drugs. The prognosis for patients with essential hypertension depends on how well the blood pressure is controlled. With modern effective drugs, the prognosis is good. Without control of blood pressure, even patients with mild hypertension develop significant complications after 7–10 years. Untreated hypertension shortens life by 10–20 years, usually by increasing the rate of ATH.

ANEURYSMS AND DISSECTIONS

An aneurysm is localized abnormal dilation of a blood vessel or the heart caused by a congenital or acquired weakness in the media. They are not rare, and their incidence tends to increase with age. In fact, aneurysms of the aorta and other arteries are found in as many as 10% of autopsies. The wall of an aneurysm is formed by the stretched remnants of the arterial wall.

Aneurysms are classified by location, configuration, and cause. The classifications themselves are:
- Fusiform aneurysm. An ovoid swelling parallel to the long axis of the vessel.
- Saccular aneurysm. A bubble-like outpouching of the arterial wall at the site of weakened media.
- Dissecting aneurysm. A dissecting hematoma in which hemorrhage into the media separates the layers of the vascular wall by a column of blood.
- Arteriovenous aneurysm. A direct communication between an artery and a vein.

A. Atherosclerotic Aneurysms

Atherosclerotic aneurysm, by definition, is lined by raised, ulcerated, and calcified (complicated) atherosclerotic lesions. Most Atherosclerotic aneurysms of the aorta are distal to the renal arteries and proximal to the bifurcation. They are usually fusiform, although saccular varieties are occasionally encountered. It is the most frequent aneurysms, usually developing after the age of 50 years. They occur much more often in men than in women, and half of these patients are hypertensive. Several studies have implicated genetic factors in pathogenesis of aortic aneurysms.

B. Dissecting Aneurysms

Dissecting aneurysms refers to the entry of blood into the arterial wall and its extension along the length of the vessel. In aortic dissection, there is disruption of the media of the aorta by entry of blood under high pressure through an intimal tear (Figure 6-20). **Hypertension** is present in 70% of patients and is the most important factor, causing tearing of the endothelium and intima and permitting entry of blood at high pressure into the weakened media. Myxomatous degeneration of the media (Erdheim's cystic medial degeneration) is present in 20% of cases.

Aortic dissection is associated with an intimal tear, usually just above the aortic valve or immediately distal to the ligamentum arteriosum. Blood enters the media at this intimal tear and dissects between the layers of smooth muscle in the media. Cystic medial degeneration, when present, facilitates dissection (Figures 6-20 and 6-21).

Cystic medial degeneration appears microscopically as ill-defined mucoid lakes with associated patchy loss of elastin fibers and smooth muscle. Cystic medial degeneration and aortic dissection are more common in patients with Marfan's syndrome.

The clinical effects of aortic dissection depend upon its site and extent. Dissection of the media produces sudden severe pain, which is usually retrosternal and mimics the pain of myocardial infarction. Arteries taking origin from the aorta may become occluded, or rupture may occur leading to massive hemorrhage (Figure 6-18). 30% of patients die within 24 hours. In those who survive, treatment with antihypertensive drugs and surgery has greatly improved survival.

C. Aneurysms of Cerebral Arteries

Aneurysms of cerebral arteries are particularly important, because they lead to fatal subarachnoid hemorrhage. The most common cerebral aneueysm is called a **berry aneurysm**, because as a saccular ancurysm, it resembles a berry attached to a "twig" of the arterial tree. Berry aneurysms are saccular aneurysms that occur at branch points in the carotid system and result from developmental arterial defects.

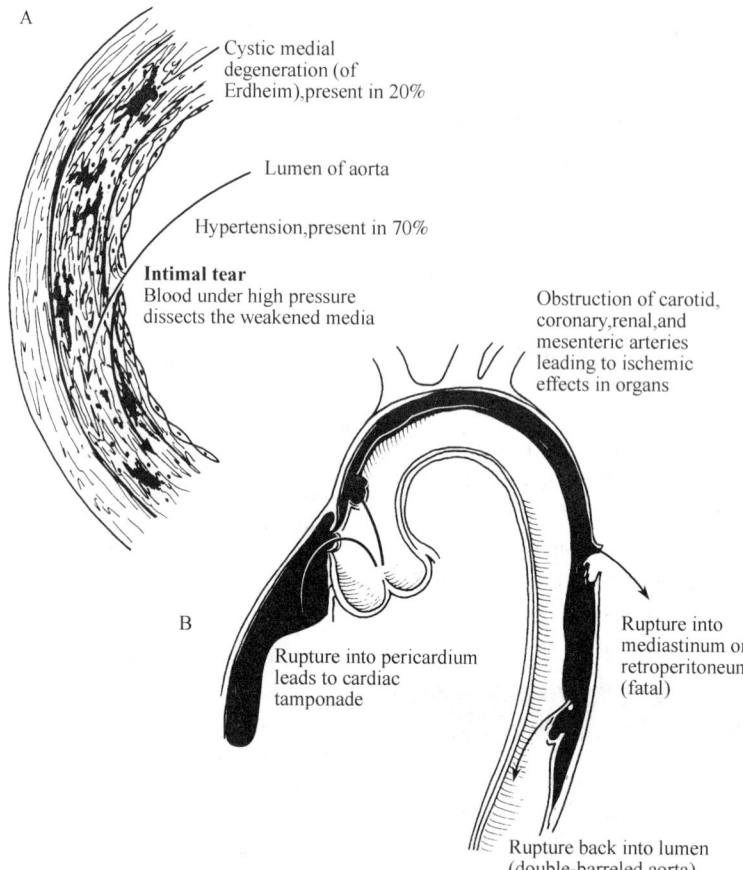

Figure 6-20　Aortic dissection. A: Mechanism of dissection, showing an intimal tear and blood under high pressure dissecting the media, which shows Erdheim's degeneration. B: Possible outcomes of aortic dissection shown here is a type I dissection that involves both ascending and descending aorta. Type II dissection, involves only the ascending aorta, and type III involves only the descending aorta

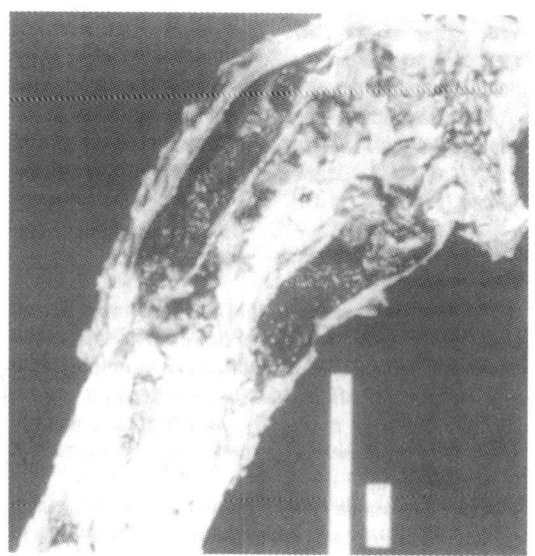

Figure 6-21　Aortic dissection, showing blood clot in the media

They tend to arise at one of the branching angles of the circle of Willis or in one of the arterial branches. The most common sites are (1) between the anterior cerebral artery and anterior communicating artery, (2) between the internal caroid artery and posterior communicating artery, and (3) between the first main divisions of the middle cerebral artery and the bidurcation of the internal carotid artery.

Rupture of a berry aneurysm results in life-threatening subarachnoid hemorrhage, with a 35% mortality rate during the initial hemorrhage. Rupture produces intracerebral or intraventricular hemorrhage in as many as 1/3 of the patients. A sudden, severe headache characteristically heralds the onset of subarachnoid hemorrhage and may be followed by coma.

(Song Jingyu)

RHEUMATISM

Rheumatism is a multisystem inflammatory disease that follows an episode of group A streptococcal infection after an interval of a few weeks. Rheumatism may cause heart disease during its acute phase, called rheumatic fever, characterized by fever, carditis, polyarthritis, high levels of antistreptococcal antibodies (antistreptolysin O), and so on. It occurs in children between 5 and 15 years old. Rheumatic fever may cause chronic valvular deformities that may not manifest themselves until many years after the acute disease.

Etiology and Pathogenesis

Rheumatic fever is an acute, multisystem inflammatory disease that follows an episode of group A streptococcal pharyngitis after an interval of a few weeks. It occurs in children between 5 and 15 years of age, particularly in third world countries and in many crowded, economically depressed urban areas in the Western world, rheumatic fever remains an important public health problem. It is still prevalent in developing countries. It occurs during sporadic epidemics of streptococcal pharyngitis. During such epidemics, approximately 3% of patients develop acute rheumatic fever. Rheumatic fever may cause heart disease during its acute phase, or it may cause chronic valvular deformities that may not manifest themselves until many years after the acute disease.

The pathogenesis of acute rheumatic fever and its chronic sequelae is not fully understood, and that the exact relationship between streptococcal infection and acute rheumatic fever is unknown. It is strongly suspected that acute rheumatic fever is a hypersensitivity reaction induced by group A streptococci. It is proposed that antibodies directed against the M proteins of group A streptococci cross-react with normal proteins present in the heart, joints, and other tissues. While immunologic hypersensitivity is likely, the mechanism remains unknown. The presence of antibodies with activity against both streptococcal antigens and myocardial cells suggests the possibility of a type II hypersensitivity mediated by cross-reacting antibodies. The presence in the serum of some patients of immune complexes formed against streptococcal antigens suggests type III hypersensitivity.

Pathology

A. Early Phase (exudative, degenerative) 1 to 4 Weeks

In acute rheumatic fever, inflammatory infiltrates may occur in a wide range of sites, including synovium, joints, skin, and (most importantly) the heart. The initial tissue reaction is that of focal fibrinoid necrosis. This provokes a mixed inflammatory response, which may take the form of either a diffuse cellular infiltrate or a localized aggregation of cells that resembles a granuloma. Areas of fibrosis eventually develop at sites of inflammation. Fibrosis is particularly common in cardiac tissues, where it is responsible for the valvular deformities.

B. Proliferative Phase (granulomatous phase) 4 to 13 Weeks

Acute rheumatic carditis is characterized by inflammatory changes in all three layers of the heart, and thus it is appropriately designated a pancarditis. The hallmark of acute rheumatic carditis is the presence of multiple foci of inflammation within the connective tissues of the heart, called **Aschoff bodies** (Figure 6-22). They contain a central focus of fibrinoid necrosis surrounded by a chronic mononuclear inflammatory infiltrate and occasional large macrophages with vesicular nuclei and abundant basophilic cytoplasm called Anitschkow cells. Aschoff bodies may be found anywhere in the connective tissues of the heart. In the myocardium, they often lie in close proximity to a small vessel and may encroach on its wall. In addition to Aschoff bodies, the myocardium may also contain diffuse interstitial inflammatory infiltrates. In severe cases, the myocarditis may impair myocardial function sufficiently to cause generalized dilation of the cardiac chambers.

C. Fibrosis Phase (healed phase) 3 to 4 Months

The Aschoff body is fusiform, the cytoplasm of the component cell is diminished in amount, and the cells become spindle shaped. The collagenous fibers fuse to small scars.

Rheumatic Pathological Changes in the Organs

A. Carditis

Carditis is the most serious manifestation and oc-

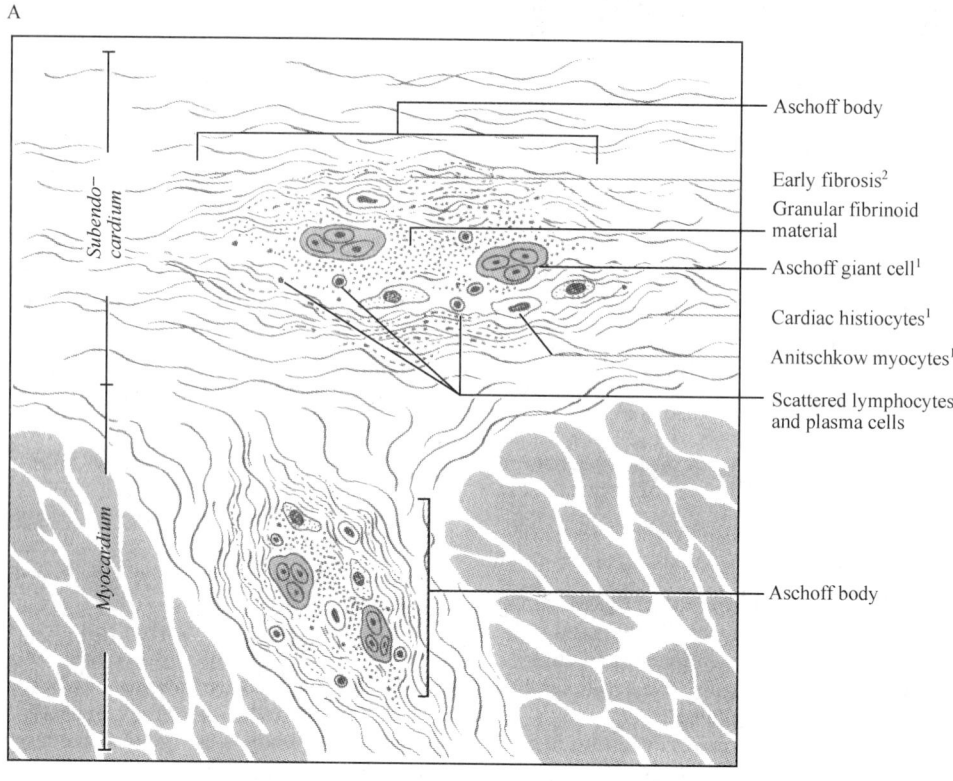

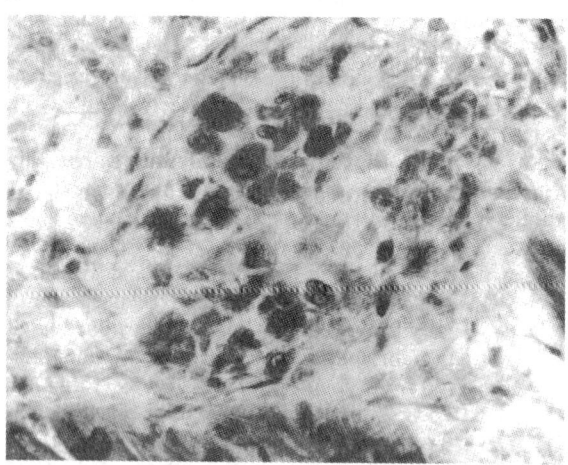

Figure 6-22 A: Diagrammatic representation of Aschoff bodies in the subendocardium and myocardial interstitial tissue in acute rheumatic fever. Note1: Note that many authorities regard Aschoff giant cells, Anitschkow myocytes, and carsult of an Aschoff body is a fibrous scar. B: Aschoff body in myocardial interstitium. Note the typical multinucleated giant cells. High magnification

curs in about 35% of patients with a first attack of rheumatic fever. Cardiac involvement involves all layers of the heart (pancarditis). Endocarditis occurs in all patients with rheumatic carditis, whereas myocarditis and pericarditis are present only in severe cases.

1. Endocarditis (valvulitis)

The valvular endocardium shows maximal involvement. The valves of the left side are affected more often and more severely than those of the right and the mitral valve more than the aortic. Involved valves show edema and denudation of the lining endocardium, particularly in areas of maximal trauma at the line of apposition of the free edge of the valve. Platelet-fibrin thrombi (**rheumatic vegetations**) form in areas of endocardial damage (Figure 6-23). Rheumatic vegetations do not become detached as emboli. Valve edema and vegetations may cause turbulence of blood and produce various transient murmurs (e. g. Carey-Coombs diastolic murmur) ; murmurs occur in most patients with cardiac involvement.

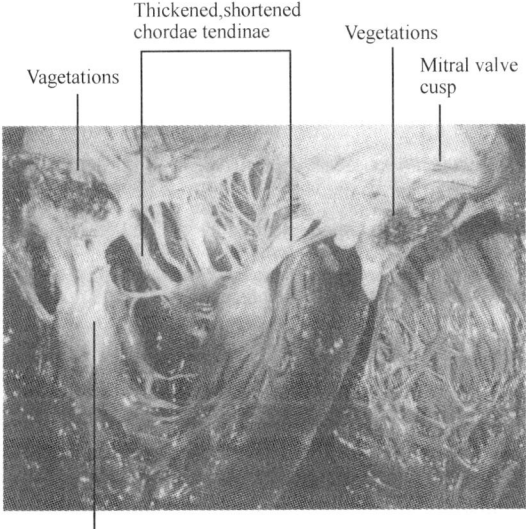

Figure 6-23 Rheumatic heart disease, showing small vegetations typical of acute rheumatic fever at line of apposition of the mitral valve cusps. Note that the chordae tendineae are thickened and shortened, suggesting chronic rheumatic heart disease. This patient gave a history of recurrent attacks of acute rheumatic fever over several years

2. Myocarditis

Acute myocardial involvement, characterized by the presence of numerous Aschoff bodies in the myocardium, causes tachycardia and dilation of the heart. Cardiac failure and arrhythmias occur in a small number of cases.

3. Pericarditis

Acute inflammation of the pericardium (fibrinous pericarditis) occurs only in severe cases, causing chest pain and a pericardial rub. Pericardial effusion is rarely of sufficient magnitude to cause problems.

B. Arthritis

Acute inflammation affecting multiple large joints is the presenting feature in 75% of patients. The joints are involved asymmetrically, and the inflammation tends to move from joint to joint (migratory polyarthritis). Affected joints are swollen, red, warm, and painful.

C. Chorea

Random involuntary movements (chorea) are caused by involvement of the basal ganglia of the brain. Chorea may develop up to 6 months after the streptococcal pharyngitis. It may persist for weeks but has an excellent prognosis.

D. Skin Lesions

Erythema marginatum (a circular ring of erythema surrounding central normal skin) is specific for rheumatic fever but occurs only in about 10% of cases. It is of short duration Erythema nodosum (a nodular, red, tender rash typically seen over the anterior tibia) is less specific but occurs more commonly. Subcutaneous rheumatic nodules occur mainly over bony prominences in the extremities. They are pea-sized, nontender, and last 6 - 10 weeks. Their presence usually indicates concurrent cardiac involvement. Pathologically, rheumatic nodules consist of loci of fibrinoid necrosis with a surrounding granulomatous reaction.

Prognosis

The prognosis of rheumatic fever is determined by (1) the severity of the acute illness; (2) whether or not there is cardiac involvement because all other manifestations, including chorea, resolve completely; (3) the age of the patient - acute rheumatic fever in children under 5 years of age has the highest risk of carditis; and (4) whether or not there are recurrences - the greater the number of recurrences, the higher the incidence of subsequent chronic rheumatic heart disease. This is the rationale for prolonged prophylactic penicillin therapy in patients who have had an attack of acute rheumatic fever.

INFECTIVE ENDOCARDITIS

Infective endocarditis is an infection associated with formation of an adherent, bulky mass of thrombotic debris, and organisms, termed some vegetations on the endocardial surface, usually on a valve. Virtually any type of microorganism is capable of causing endocarditis, although most cases are caused by bacteria. Most cases occur in adults. Patients developing disease in their native valves tend to be over 50 years old. Intravenous drug abusers tend to develop disease in the second and third decades. Endocarditis occurring in prosthetic valves is related to the age of the patient undergoing valve replacement surgery.

Classification

a. Acute infective endocarditis is caused by virulent agents (S aureus group streptococci), which frequently infect previously normal valves. The course is fulminant, characterized by severe destruction of the valve, commonly causing acute valvular regurgitation; severe bacteremia associated with abscesses in the myocardium and throughout the body; and a high mortality rate.

b. Subacute infective endocarditis is commonly caused by less virulent agents such as viridans streptococci and Staphylococcus epidermidis and almost always occurs in a patient with a preexisting cardiac (usually valvular) abnormality. Subacute endocarditis has a more chronic course not characterized by severe valve destruction or abscess formation.

Pathogenesis

Two factors are essential in pathogenesis of infective endocarditis: **bacteremia** and an **abnormality in the endocardial surface** that permits bacterial entry and multiplication. The causative organisms differ somewhat in the three high-risk groups. Endocarditis of native valves is caused most commonly (50% to 60% of cases) by a-hemolytic (viridans) streptococci, which usually attack previously damaged valves. The more virulent S. aureus organisms attack healthy or deformed valves and are responsible for 10% to 20% of cases. The roster of the remaining bacteria includes enterococci and the so-called HACEK group (Haemophilus, Actinobacillus, Cardiobacterium, Eikenella, and Kingella), all commensals in the oral cavity. Prosthetic valve endocarditis is caused most commonly by coagulasenegative staphylococci. In some instances the cause of the hematogenous infection is obvious, as in the case of intravenous drug abusers who inject contaminated material directly into the bloodstream; an infection elsewhere or a previous dental, surgical, or other interventional procedure (e.g. urinary catheterization) may also seed the bloodstream. In other cases, however, the source of bacteremia is occult and presumably related to trivial injuries to the skin or mucosal surfaces. The endocardial abnormality may lead to the formation of sterile fibrin and platelet thrombi on the surface (nonbacterial thrombotic endocarditis). Such sterile thrombi occur in areas of endocardial trauma; over scarred valves; in areas of turbulent flow and high pressure jet effects associated with valvular defects and congenital lesions; and in patients with debilitating chronic diseases, especially cancer. Bacteria that adhere to platelets and fibrin have an advantage, but the adhesion factors are not well understood. Entry of the organism into the thrombus permits multiplication and further deposition of fibrin and platelets, causing an enlarging thrombus (vegetation).

Conditions that increase the risk of infective endocarditis can be segregated into three categories: (1) preexisting cardiac abnormalities; (2) prosthetic heart valves; and (3) intravenous drug abuse.

Pathology

Infected thrombi (vegetations) are the characteristic pathologic finding in infective endocarditis. The hallmark of infective endocarditis is the presence of valvular vegetations containing bacteria or other organisms. The aortic and mitral valves are the most common sites of infection. Vegetations occur principally on the valves of the left side of the heart, following the distribution of chronic rheumatic heart disease (mitral > aortic > tricuspid > pulmonary). The vegetations may be single or multiple and may involve more than one valve. The appearance of the vegetations is influenced by the type of organism responsible for the infection, the degree of host reaction to the infection, and previous antibiotic therapy. The vegetations of infective endocarditis are multiple, large, and friable and commonly become detached from the valve as emboli. Vegetations tend to be larger and more friable in acute than in subacute endocarditis (Figure 6-24).

Clinical Features

The onset of infective endocarditis may be gradual or explosive, depending on the organism responsible

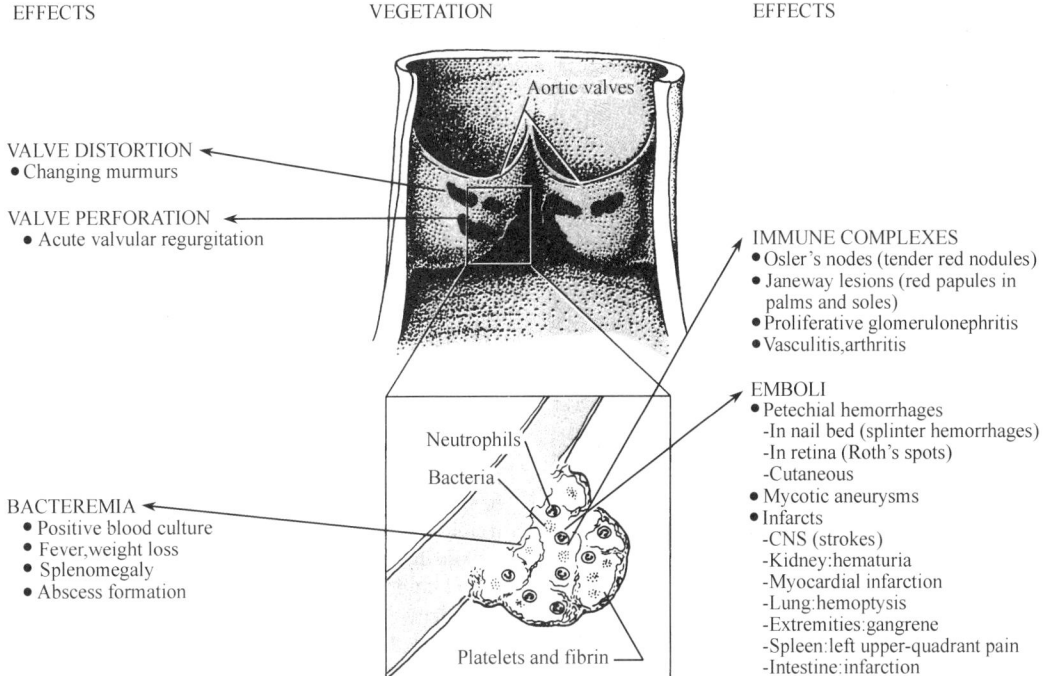

Figure 6-24 Clinical effects of infective endocarditis resulting from infection and formation of vegetations on the valve

for the infection. Low-grade fever, malaise, and weight loss are characteristic of cases caused by organisms of low virulence, while more acute cases, in contrast, typically present as high fevers, shaking chills, and other evidence of overt septicemia. Changing cardiac murmurs are almost always present, although they may be difficult to detect early in the course of acute endocarditis. The spleen is often enlarged, and clubbing of the digits may be seen, particularly in subacute cases. Systemic emboli are very common in all forms of infective endocarditis, manifesting as neurologic deficits, retinal abnormalities, necrosis of the digits, and infarcts of the myocardium and other viscera. Pulmonary emboli may occur in patients with right-sided endocarditis and large vegetations on the tricuspid or pulmonic valves.

A. Bacteremia (or Fungemia)

Blood culture is positive in more than 95% of cases and is the most important diagnostic test. Most patients have constant bacteremia; a few have intermittent bacteremia. Bacteremia also causes **petechial hemorrhages** in the skin, retina (Roth spots), and nails (splinter hemorrhages). When infection is caused by virulent pyogenic organisms, **miliary abscesses** are produced in all organs of the body.

B. Immune Complexes

Antibodies and bacterial antigens combine to form circulating immune complexes. Deposition of immune complexes in the glomerular capillaries causes focal or diffuse proliferative glomerulonephritis. Microscopic hematuria and proteinuria occur in over 50% of patients with infective endocarditis. Cutaneous immune complex-mediated vasculitis is responsible for erythematous papules in the palms and soles (Janeway lesions) and characteristic tender red nodules in the fingers or toes (Osler's nodes). These occur in 25% of patients.

C. Valvular Dysfunction

Large vegetations on the valves impinge on the flow of blood, causing turbulence and **cardiac murmurs.** With changes in size of vegetations, the character of the murmurs changes, a feature that is typical of infective endocarditis. Progressive destruction of the valve may produce valve perforation (Figure 6-25), currently the most common cause of acute mitral and aortic regurgitation.

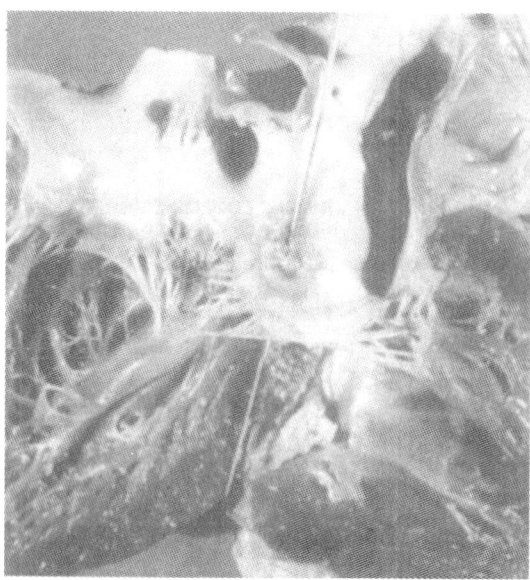

Figure 6-25 Perforation of the mitral valve in infective endocarditis. (Note: A metal probe has been passed through the perforation in the valve.) The perforation has occurred in the area of a vegetation

D. Embolism

Emboli from the friable vegetations are common. With left-sided endocarditis, systemic embolism causes multifocal areas of infarction in the brain, kidney, heart, intestine, spleen, and extremities. With right-sided vegetations, embolism involves the pulmonary vessels.

Prevention And Prognosis

When dental, oral, or urologic procedures are planned in patients with known cardiac valvular disease, antibiotic coverage during and immediately after the procedure is necessary to kill any organisms that enter the bloodstream before they reach the cardiac valves. Such antibiotic prophylaxis is effective in preventing infective endocarditis in these patients.

Antibiotic therapy, based on the antibiotic sensitivity of the organism cultured from the blood, is the mainstay of treatment of infective endocarditis. Even with appropriate antibiotic therapy, 10% - 20% of subacute cases and up to 50% of acute cases end in death. Therapy should be continued for 4 - 6 weeks to eradicate all organisms from the vegetations. Where there is severe valve damage and in prosthetic valve endocarditis, valve replacement is required.

VALVULAR HEART DISEASES

MITRAL STENOSIS

Etiology

Mitral stenosis is almost always the result of chronic rheumatic heart disease. Females are affected more than males in a ratio of 7:1.

Pathophysiology

Mitral stenosis causes resistance to blood flow through the open mitral valve during diastole. The resulting turbulence produces a murmur. With increasing stenosis, the length of the diastolic murmur increases. Normally, the mitral valve opens silently soon after aortic valve closure. However, an abnormal stenotic mitral valve opens with a clicking sound; the shorter the interval between S_2 and OS (Figure 6-26), the higher the left atrial pressure and the more severe the stenosis. Obstruction to flow through the mitral orifice leads to left atrial dilation and hypertrophy.

Blood tends to stagnate in the left atrium, predisposing to thrombus formation, especially if atrial fibrillation develops. Left atrial thrombi may cause systemic embolism, or they may obstruct the narrowed mitral orifice, causing sudden death (ball valve thrombus).

Mitral stenosis leads to increased pulmonary venous pressure and features of left heart failure. If acute, pulmonary edema and pulmonary hemorrhage may occur; if chronic, the results are chronic venous congestion, pulmonary arterial hypertension, and right ventricular hypertrophy.

In mild mitral stenosis, left ventricular filling is normal and cardiac output is normal. With severe stenosis, left ventricular end-diastolic volume and cardiac output are decreased. The left ventricle, which pumps less blood than normal, may undergo mild atrophy.

MITRAL REGURGITATION (MITRAL INSUFFICIENCY)

Etiology

Rheumatic heart disease accounts for about 40%

Chapter 6 Diseases of the Cardiovascular System

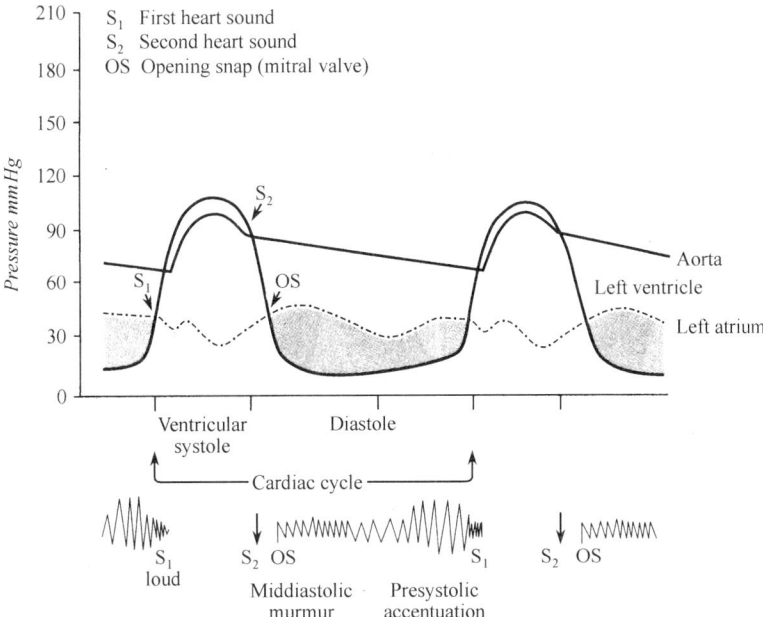

Figure 6-26 Mitral stenosis, showing pressure changes in the left side of the heart and aorta and abnormal heart sounds in a typical case. Compare with normal. Note the pressure gradient between the left atrium and left ventricle during mid-diastole owing to the stenotic mitral opening. This corresponds to the murmur

of cases of mitral regurgitation, usually associated with mitral stenosis. Males and females are equally affected.

Mitral valve prolapse syndrome is a degenerative change that is present in about 1% of the population (especially young women), the result of accumulation of mucopolysaccharides in the valve leaflet. Clinical mitral regurgitation occurs in only a small percentage of cases. A similar abnormality of the mitral valve is present in patients with Marfan's syndrome.

Chronic left ventricular failure with dilation of the mitral valve ring may cause functional mitral regurgitation. Acute mitral regurgitation may occur with rupture of chordae tendineae due to infective **endocarditis** or **trauma** or to rupture of papillary muscles due to **myocardial infarction.** Perforation of the valve leaflet may also occur in infective endocarditis. Rarely, calcification of the valve ring in the elderly may lead to mitral regurgitation.

Pathophysiology

When the mitral valve is incompetent, regurgitation of blood from the left ventricle to the atrium occurs throughout systole, producing a typical **pansystolic murmur.** During diastole, regurgitant blood flows back across the mitral valve, producing a third heart sound and a diastolic flow murmur.

Left ventricular volume is greatly increased, because it is the sum of the cardiac output plus the regurgitant flow; the left ventricle is thus dilated atril hypertrophied.

The left atrium, which accepts both the pulmonary venous return and regurgitant flow, is also dilated in chronic cases. Left atrial pressure and pulmonary venous pressure are increased. In chronic disease, there is pulmonary fibrosis, pulmonary arterial hypertension, and right ventricular hypertrophy followed by failure. Acute mitral valve regurgitation, as occurs with valve perforation or papillary muscle rupture, produces pulmonary edema and acute left heart failure with little left atrial dilation.

AORTIC STENOSIS

Etiology

Rheumatic aortic stenosis is commonly accompanied by mitral valve defects. Isolated aortic stenosis is uncommon in chronic rheumatic heart disease.

Congenital bicuspid aortic valves may undergo progressive fibrosis and calcification; this is now believed to be the cause of more than 50% of cases of aortic stenosis. Calcification of the valve in the elderly may cause mild aortic stenosis.

Congenital narrowing of the left ventricular outflow tract above or below the aortic valve produces the same functional defect as aortic stenosis.

Hypertrophic cardiomyopathy may also produce obstruction of the left ventricular outflow tract.

Pathophysiology

The flow through the stenotic aortic valve is turbulent, producing a rough ejection systolic murmur over the aortic valve (Figure 6-27).

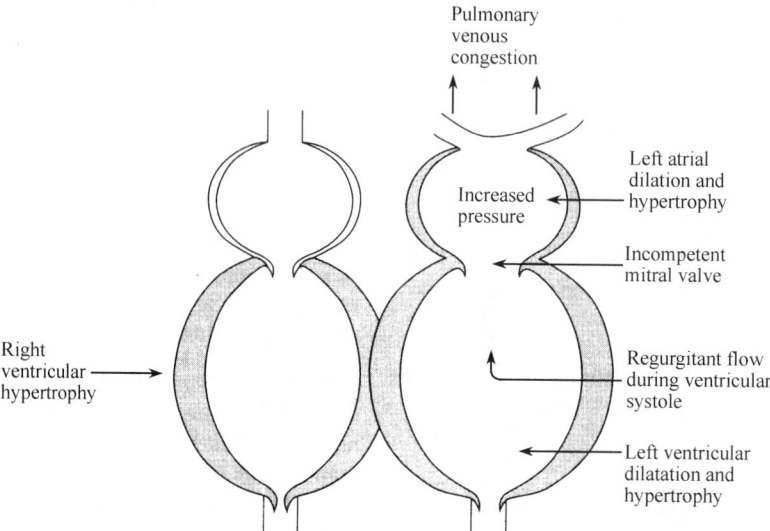

Figure 6-27 Pathophysiology of mitral regurgitation. Regurgitation of blood from left ventricle to left atrium during systole causes dilation and increased pressure in the left atrium. This results in pulmonary venous congestion, pulmonary vascular changes, and pulmonary arterial hypertension, leading to right ventricular hypertrophy. The left ventricle, which must pump out the cardiac output plus the regurgitant flow, undergoes dilation and muscular hypertrophy

Decreased flow of blood through the aortic valve causes decreased cardiac output, hypotension, and syncopal (fainting) attacks, myocardial ischemia, and angina (decreased coronary artery perfusion). Patients with severe stenosis may die suddenly. The systemic blood pressure is decreased, and this results in soft closure of the aortic valve (soft S_2). The peripheral pulse is typically of low amplitude, with the pulse wave rising slowly and being sustained owing to the prolonged left ventricular ejection.

The left ventricle develops increased systolic pressure to overcome the resistance at the aortic orifice and undergoes **hypertrophy**. Increased oxygen demand by the myocardium aggravates the tendency to myocardial ischemia. Features of **left ventricular failure** are common.

AORTIC REGURGITATION (AORTIC INSUFFICIENCY)

Etiology

Rheumatic heart disease accounts for about 50% of cases of aortic regurgitation. In most of these cases, there is associated mitral valve disease as well as aortic stenosis. **Syphilis** was once a common cause of isolated aortic regurgitation but now accounts for less than 10% of cases. Aortic regurgitation in syphilis is caused by dilation of the aortic root and valve ring due to aortitis. The valve itself is not directly affected. **Ankylosing spondylitis**, which also involves the root of the aorta, is an important, although uncommon, cause (5% of cases) of isolated aortic regurgitation.

Rupture of the aortic valve may occur as a complication of blunt chest trauma and infective endocarditis. Infective endocarditis is the most common cause of acute aortic regurgitation.

Myxomatous degeneration of the aortic valve due to accumulation of mucopolysaccharides, similar to that seen in mitral valve prolapse syndrome, is being recognized as a possible cause of aortic regurgitation.

Pathophysiology

Regurgitation of blood across the incompetent aortic valve occurs in diastole (Figure 6-28). The pressure gradient across the valve is greatest in early diastole, and it is in this phase that the murmur is loudest (decrescendo murmur).

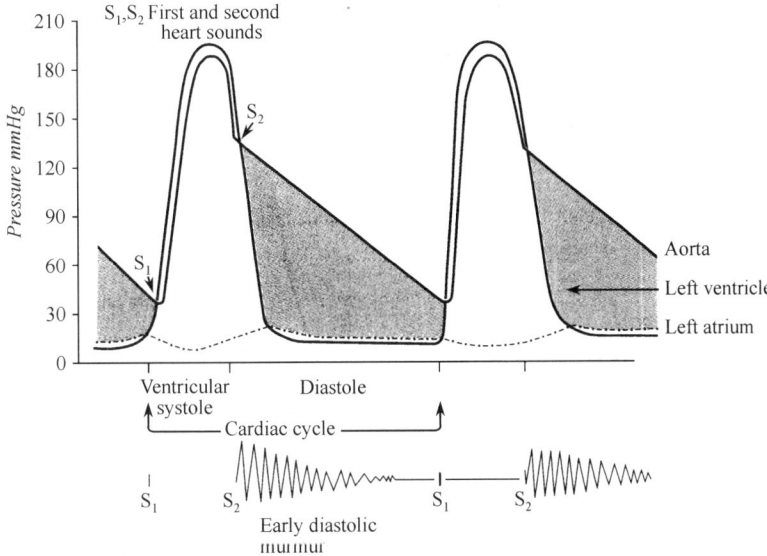

Figure 6-28 Aortic regurgitation, showing pressure changes in the left side of the heart and aorta and abnormal heart sounds in a typical case. Note the rapid fall of aortic pressure in early diastole owing to regurgitation of blood across the incompetent aortic valve. The murmur is produced by the regurgitant blood flow across the pressure gradient

Regurgitation of blood from the aorta in diastole causes decreased diastolic blood pressure, sometimes to zero (which is the ventricular diastolic pressure). At the same time, the systolic pressure is elevated as a result of increased cardiac output. This causes a greatly increased pulse pressure, the typical bounding (water-hammer) pulse and capillary pulsations that are characteristic of aortic regurgitation. Massive dilation and hypertrophy of the left ventricle is typical. Left ventricular failure is common.

MYOCARDITIS AND CARDIOMYOPATHY

Myocarditis and cardiomyopathy are a group of diseases that chiefly involve the myocardium in the absence of hypertensive, congenital, ischemic, or valvular heart disease. The distinction between myocarditis and cardiomyopathy is somewhat arbitrary and not always made. The term myocarditis is generally used to denote an acute myocardial disease characterized by inflammation. The term cardiomyopathy is then reserved for more chronic conditions in which inflammatory features are not conspicuous, including degenerative diseases and various diseases of unknown origin.

MYOCARDITIS

Incidence

The incidence of myocarditis is difficult to establish, in part because of the rarity with which cardiac muscle biopsy is performed as a means of precise diagnosis. Myocarditis is rarely (1% of cases) the cause of death in autopsy studies.

Etiology

A. Infectious Myocarditis

Coxsackie virus B is most frequently implicated; others include mumps, influenza, echo, polio, varicella, and measles viruses. Clinical myocarditis may be seen in certain rickettsial diseases such as Q fever, typhus, and Rocky Mountain spotted fever. Ten percent of patients with Lyme disease develop into myocarditis and conduction abnormalities. Myocardial inflammation in diphtheria is the result of an exotoxin. American trypanosomiasis (Chagas' disease) is endemic in South America. In the acute phase, parasitization of myofibrils leads to focal necrosis and inflammation characterized by the presence of many eosinophils. The chronic phase is characterized by interstitial fibrosis and lymphocytic infiltration.

The myocardium is involved rarely in the acute disseminated form of toxoplasmosis that occurs in immunocompromised patients. Toxoplasma gondii pseudocysts are present in myocardial fibers.

B. Autoimmune (Hypersensitivity) Myocarditis

These disorders include rheumatic fever, rheumatoid arthritis, systemic lupus erythematosus, progressive systemic sclerosis, and polyarteritis nodosa. All are characterized by focal myocardial fiber necrosis, lymphocytic infiltration, and fibrosis; vasculitis may be present. Rheumatic fever may show Aschoff bodies.

C. Toxic Myocarditis

Many drugs may injure the myocardium. The more common ones are ethyl alcohol, doxorubicin, daunorubicin, cyclophosphamide, hydralazine, phenytoin, procainamide, and the tricyclic antidepressants.

D. Sareoid Myoearditis

Sarcoidosis may produce significant cardiac involvement with noncaseaing granulomatous lesions identical to those found elsewhere.

E. Radiation Myocarditis

Radiation myocarditis may develop from large doses of radiation to the mediastinum.

F. Idiopathie Myocarditis

Idiopathie myocarditis may occur without known cause, characterized by diffuse inflammation, sometimes with giant cells (Fiedler's myocarditis) and eosinophils.

Pathology

In acute myocarditis, the heart is dilated, flabby, and pale. There may be small scattering petechial hemorrhages. Microscopically, there is edema, which separates myocardial fibers; hyperemia; and infiltration by lymphocytes, plasma cells, and eosinophils. Neutrophils may also be present if there is necrosis of individual muscle fibers. Recovery from acute myocarditis is associated with resolution. If myofibrillary necrosis has occurred, there may be irregular fibrosis.

Chronic myocarditis is a controversial entity characterized by cardiac failure, ventricular hypertrophy, and the presence of lymphocytes and plasma cells in the interstitium. This pathologic appearance may follow many of the causes listed above.

Clinical Features

The onset is acute, with fever, chest pain, leukocytosis, and elevation of the erythrocyte sedimentation rate. Left ventricular failure may occur, manifested by a third heart sound (gallop rhythm) and mitral regurgitation caused by dilation of the mitral valve ring. Arrhythmias include extrasystoles, atrial and ventricular tachycardia, and atrial and ventricular fibrillation, and they may cause sudden death. Complete heart block is manifested by bradycardia and cardiac failure. Necrosis of myocardial fibers produces injury potentials in the ST segment and elevations of serum concentrations of creatine kinase, lactate dehydrogenase, and aspartate transaminase.

CARDIOMYOPATHIES

As defined above, cardiomyopathies are primary myocardial diseases characterized by a chronic course and minimal features of inflammation. Cardiomyopathy should be suspected in a young normotensive patient who develops cardiac failure in the absence of congenital, valvular, or ischemic heart disease. The term cardiomyopathy is also sometimes used to denote myocardial diseases associated with certain toxic, metabolic, and degenerative diseases, Friedreich's ataxia, and the muscular dystrophies.

Incidence and Etiology

Cardiomyopathy is rare. It may be familial or sporadic. In most cases, no cause can be found (idiopathic), and the disorders listed above account for a relatively small proportion of cases.

Classification

A. Dilated (Congestive) Cardiomyopathy

Dilated cardiomyopathy is characterized by failure of the ventricle to empty in systole. The ventricular end systolic and diastolic volumes are increased, causing bilateral ventricular dilation and failure. Arrhythmias are common and sometimes cause sudden death. Most cases progress slowly to death from heart failure within 2 years from the onset of symptoms.

Histologic features are nonspecific. There is irregular atrophy and hypertrophy of myocardial fibers with progressive fibrosis.

Most cases are sporadic. A few cases are associated with metabolic, toxic, neuromuscular, and late pregnancy (peripartal cardiomyopathy). Chronic alcoholism is the most common cause of secondary dilated cardiomyopathy.

B. Hypertrophic Cardiomyopathy

Hypertrophic cardiomyopathy is characterized by marked hypertrophy of the ventricular muscle with resistance to diastolic filling. Both ventricles are diffusely involved in most cases.

Asymmetric septal hypertrophy (also called hypertrophic obstructive cardiomyopathy, or HOCM; also called idiopathic hypertrophic subaorticstenosis, or IHSS) is a variant characterized by selective hypertrophy of the septum immediately below the aortic valve, obstructing the left ventricular outflow tract. Clinically, this condition mimics aortic stenosis.

About 50% of cases of hypertrophic cardiomyopathy are familial, and in some of these there is a suggestion of an autosomal dominant inheritance pattern. The suspect abnormal gene has been mapped to chromosome 14.

C. Restrictive Cardiomyopathy

Restrictive cardiomyopathy is characterized by decreased compliance of the ventricular muscle, increased resistance to diastolic filling, and cardiac failure. Many cases are now recognized as being due to amyloidosis. Other causes include hemochromatosis and myocardial sarcoidosis.

Cardiac amyloidosis occurs in several different situations, in which the heart is affected infrequently. Amyloid deposition occurs in the myocardial interstitium and around small blood vessels. When involvement is diffuse, the myocardium is thickened and leathery-firm and has a waxy, pale gray color.

D. Obliterative Cardiomyopathy

Obliterative cardiomyopathy is characterized by marked subendocardial fibrosis resulting in encroachment of the lumen, decreased ventricular filling, and cardiac failure. Both left and right ventricles may be involved.

Two different diseases exist within this category. (1) **In endocardial fibroelastosis**, collagen and elastic tissue is laid down beneath the endocardium, with clinical features appearing during infancy. Some cases appear to be familial; others may be secondary to anoxia or fetal viral infection. (2) **Endomyocardial fibrosis** is an acquired disease in which there is fibrosis of the endocardium and inner myocardium.

PERICARDITIS

ACUTE PERICARDITIS

Etiology

Acute pericarditis is relatively common in hospital practice. The common causes are infection, ischemic heart disease, uremia, and the connective tissue diseases. Viruses known to cause pericarditis include coxsackievirus B, echovirus, and the agents of mumps, Epstein-Barr vires, and influenza. Viruses can be cultured from pericardial fluid. Tuberculous pericarditis is due to direct spread of infection from a caseous mediastinal lymph node leading to acute followed by chronic pericarditis. Infection of the pericardium by pyogenic organisms is caused by direct spread from a suppurative focus in the lung or pleura.

Acute pericarditis frequently complicates acute rheumatic fever, myocardial infarction, chronic renal failure (uremia), and connective tissue diseases. Malignant neoplasms may directly involve the pericardium and cause inflammation. Pericarditis may also occur after cardiac trauma and cardiac surgery. Acute pericarditis may follow radiation therapy to the mediastinum in the treatment of cancer.

Pathology

The smooth pericardial surface is transformed into a reddened membrane roughened by adherent clumps of fibrin. Infiltration by neutrophils causes yellow discoloration. The visceral and parietal layers of pericardium are thus thickened and loosely adherent- said to peel apart like two slices of buttered bread (bread and butter appearance). Fluid exudation into the pericardial sac varies from minimal (dry, or fibrinous, pericarditis) to significant (pericarditis with effusion). The fluid is usually serous. Hemorrhagic effusions commonly occur in renal failure, malignant neoplasms, and tuberculosis.

Clinical Features

Pericarditis is an acute-onset illness characterized by fever, pericardial pain, and a pericardial rub. When there is significant effusion, the inflamed pericardial layers separate, and both the rub and the pain diminish. Pericardial effusion causes cardiac enlargement, dullness to percussion, and muffled heart sounds. With large effusions, raised intrapericardial pressure impairs diastolic filling of the right atrium, leading to acute right heart failure (cardiac tamponade). With rapidly developing effusions, cardiac tamponade may cause death very rapidly.

CHRONIC PERICARDITIS

Recovery from acute pericarditis frequently produces fibrous plaques (milk spots) in the visceral pericardium or adhesions between the two pericardial layers (chronic adhesive pericarditis). These are of no clinical significance.

Chronic constrictive pericarditis is uncommon, and in most cases the cause is not known. Tuberculosis and pyogenic infections were common causes in the past. Immunologic mechanisms may account for most noninfectious cases. Chronic constrictive pericarditis is characterized by encasement of the heart in a greatly thickened fibrotic pericardium (Figure 6-29). Chronic inflammatory cells are frequently present, along with dystrophic calcification. The pericardial sac is obliterated.

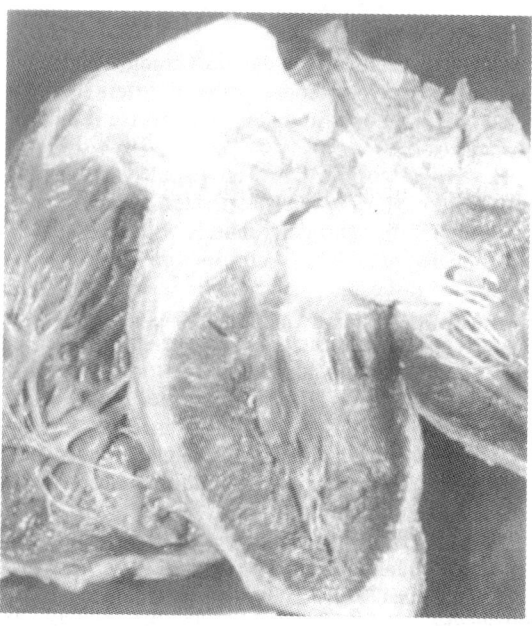

Figure 6-29 Chronic constrictive pericarditis caused by tuberculous pericarditis. The heart is encased by a thickened fibrous pericardium, and the ventricular luminal size is decreased as a result of restriction of filling

The fibrous pericardium constricts the cardiac chambers, particularly reducing right atrial filling. Elevation of jugular venous pressure and decreased cardiac output result Ascites and hepatic enlargement are common clinical features. Chest x-ray frequently shows pericardial calcification. Surgical removal of the thickened pericardial sac (pericardiectomy) is effective treatment.

(Zhang Jianzhong)

Chapter 7 Diseases of the Respiratory System

Qiu Xueshan Han Yuchen

CHAPTER CONTENTS
- Structure of the Respiratory System
- Manifestations of Respiratory Disease
- Infections of the Air Passages
    Acute Tracheobronchitis
    Acute Bronchiolitis
- Acute Infections of the Lung
    Acute Air Space Pneumonia
    Acute Interstitial Pneumonia
- Chronic Obstructive Pulmonary Disease
    Chronic Bronchitis
    Emphysema
    Bronchial Asthma
    Bronchiectasis
- Chronic Diffuse Interstitial Lung Disease
    Pneumoconioses
    Sarcoidosis
- Pulmonary Vascular Disorders
    Acute Respiratory Distress Syndrome
    Pulmonary Hypertension
- Chronic Cor Pulmonale
- Neoplasms
    Carcinoma of the Nasopharynx
    Carcinoma of the Larynx
    Carcinoma of the Lung
- Diseases of the Pleura
    Pleural Effusion
    Malignant Mesothelioma

STRUCTURE OF THE RESPIRATORY SYSTEM

A. The Air Passages

The air passages - nasal cavity, pharynx, larynx, trachea, bronchi, and bronchioles - transmit air from the atmosphere to the alveoli (ventilation).

The bronchi divide dichotomously, becoming gradually smaller and more thin-walled as they progress away from the hilum toward the periphery. When the walls lose their cartilage, they are called bronchioles. Bronchioles are less than 2 mm in diameter, have smooth muscle walls, and terminate in the alveoli. The lining epithelium is ciliated columnar in the larger air passages and ciliated cuboidal in the distal bronchioles. Mucus-producing goblet cells are present, mainly in the larger bronchi. Scattered "small granule cells" are present in the bronchi on the basement membrane between epithelial cells; these are neuroendocrine cells that contain serotonin, bombesin, and other polypeptides. Small domeshaped Clara cells in the terminal bronchioles secrete a protein that lines the small air passages.

B. The Lung Parenchyma

Two units of lung parenchyma are recognized. The **pulmonary lobule** is represented by the structures derived from a small bronchiole, composed of 5-7 terminal bronchioles and the structures distal to them. The lobule is separated from other lobules by connective tissue.

The **pulmonary acinus** is represented by the structures arising from a single terminal bronchiole and consists of respiratory bronchioles and alveoli. Respiratory bronchioles are lined by simple cuboidal epithelium and participate in gas exchange. They lead into alveolar ducts. Alveolar sacs arise as saccular outpouchings from the alveolar ducts and respiratory bronchioles. The alveolar wall is 5 - 10 μm thick and covered by flat type I pneumocytes over 90% of the surface and by type II pneumocytes over the remainder. Type II pneumocytes are cuboidal cells with abundant cytoplasm that contains distinctive granules on electron microscopy. They produce surfactant and proliferate rapidly when there is alveolar injury.

C. The Pleura

The lung is encased by a layer of mesothelial cells, the visceral pleura, which becomes continuous with the internal lining of the chest wall (parietal pleura) at the lung hilum. The pleural cavity is lubricated by a small film of pleural fluid that permits movement of the lung in relation to the chest wall.

D. The Blood Supply

The lung has a dual blood supply. The bronchial arteriolar branches follow the bronchial tree and have a nutritive function. The pulmonary artery divides to produce a network of capillaries, the primary function of which is gas exchange.

MANIFESTATIONS OF RESPIRATORY DISEASE

A. Cough

Cough is a common symptom of respiratory disease. It results from (1) stimulation of the cough reflex by the entry of foreign material into the larynx and (2) the accumulation of secretions in the lower respiratory tract. Cough may be dry (without sputum), as occurs typically in interstitial lung diseases, or productive of sputum in processes involving the air passages and alveoli.

B. Sputum Production

Examination of sputum is very useful in the evaluation of patients with suspected lung disease. A purulent appearance or foul odor suggests bacterial infection; watery, frothy sputum is suggestive of pulmonary edema.

A gram-stained smear of sputum and sputum culture are useful for assessing the presence of bacterial or fungal infections. Cytologic examination may reveal the presence of malignant cells.

C. Hemoptysis

Coughing blood is a symptom of serious respiratory disease. Hemoptysis occurs in a variety of clinical conditions, including (1) left heart failure, due to rupture of pulmonary capillaries under increased hydrostatic pressure; (2) necrotizing parenchymal diseases such as infarcts, tuberculosis, and pneumonia; and (3) lung carcinoma.

D. Dyspnea

Normal ventilation is a process that occurs subconsciously. Dyspnea is any alteration of this normal state and may therefore be a sensation of obstruction or pain associated with breathing or active awareness of the process of breathing. Dyspnea may result from a variety of causes.

E. Cyanosis

Cyanosis is a dusky, bluish discoloration of the skin and mucous membranes caused by the presence in the blood of increased amounts (over 5 g/dL) of reduced hemoglobin.

Two mechanisms may lead to cyanosis:

Central cyanosis is caused by admixture of deoxygenated venous blood with oxygenated arterial blood in the heart and lungs. Central cyanosis occurs in (1) congenital cyanotic heart disease where there is a right to left shunt, e.g. Fallot's tetralogy, transposition of great vessels, and Eisenmenger's syndrome; (2) pulmonary arteriovenous fistula; and (3) extensive right-to-left shunting of blood in the lungs caused by lack of ventilation of adequately perfused alveoli.

Peripheral cyanosis is caused by increased delivery of oxygen to the tissues, resulting in excessive reduction of normally saturated hemoglobin. It usually results from slowing of blood flow, usually in the skin of the extremities, most commonly caused by cold and states of extreme cutaneous vasoconstriction such as shock.

Central cyanosis can be differentiated from peripheral cyanosis by the presence of blue discoloration of mucous membranes such as the tongue in addition to the skin; in peripheral cyanosis, the warm mucous membranes are normal in color.

F. Chest Pain

The lung parenchyma is not sensitive to pain, and most pulmonary diseases do not cause pain. The parietal pleura is sensitive, and diseases that cause inflammation of the parietal pleura, such as bacterial pneumonia and pulmonary infarction, cause chest pain. Pleural pain is characteristically related to ventilatory chest movement and often associated with a pleural friction rub that may be heard on auscultation.

INFECTIONS OF THE AIR PASSAGES

ACUTE TRACHEOBRONCHITIS

Acute tracheobronchitis commonly complicates a severe upper respiratory tract infection, particularly *Haemophilus influenzae* infection of the larynx in young children and influenza in adults and children. Viral tracheobronchitis may also be complicated by secondary bacterial infection, most commonly with *Staphylococcus aureus*.

Pathologic Features

The pathologic spectrum includes an exudative infiltrate of neutrophils and fibrin, vascular congestion, and occasionally severe ulceration. The gross morphologic changes may involve the mucosa uniformly or in patches; commonly, the lower portion of the trachea and the main stem bronchi are involved. Histologically, acute bronchitis is classified into:
- Acute catarrhal tracheobronchitis. The inflammatory exudate on the mucosal surface is chiefly a stringy basophilic mucus only scantily mixed with leukocytes.
- Acute suppurative tracheobronchitis. There is a significant element of leukocytic infiltration.
- Acute ulcerative tracheobronchitis. The inflammatory reaction is more intense, with necrosis of the mucosa in areas; it constitutes an ulcerative form.

With the control of acute inflammation, these inflammatory changes may subside, the epithelium may regenerate and the normal architecture may be restored.

ACUTE BRONCHIOLITIS

Acute bronchiolitis is a common, often epidemic, infection of the small airways that occurs mainly in children under the age of 2 years. Most cases are mild, but 1%-2% require hospitalization, and about 1% of these children die. Most cases are caused by respiratory syncytial virus; more rarely, parainfluenza virus and adenoviruses are responsible.

Patients present with acute-onset tachypnea and wheezing; fever is low-grade and may be absent. Cases caused by adenoviruses tend to have greater degrees of necrosis and a higher mortality rate.

Pathologic Features

The bronchioles show acute epithelial damage and lymphocytic infiltration of the walls. Their lumens are filled with mucus plugs, which cause distal alveolar air trapping. In patients who recover, the bronchiolar epithelium regenerates within 2 weeks. In the more severe bronchiolar involvement, widespread plugging of secondary and terminal airways by cell debris, fibrin, and inflammatory exudates may when prolonged, cause organization and fibrosis, resulting in bronchiolitis obliterans and permanent lung damage.

Bronchiolitis obliterans may occur in viral infections, especially RSV, after inhalation of toxic fumes; it is characterized by polypoid masses of organizing inflammatory exudates and granulation tissue extending from alveoli into bronchioles.

ACUTE INFECTIONS OF THE LUNG (ACUTE PNEUMONIA)

Acute infection of the lung (pneumonia) is common and occurs both as a primary disease or, more commonly, as a complication that affects many seriously ill hospitalized patients. Some degree of pneumonia is present at autopsy in the majority of autopsies of patients who have died of chronic disease, and in many of these cases the pneumonia contributes significantly to death. Many types of pulmonary infections caused by a variety of agents are recognized.

Acute pneumonia is an acute inflammation of the lung parenchyma resulting from infection of alveoli and respiratory bronchioles. Acute pneumonia is characterized clinically by fever, cough, dyspnea, and chest pain. On physical examination and chest x-ray, abnormalities can be demonstrated in the lung parenchyma.

The lung below the main bronchial division is normally sterile despite the frequent entry of microorganisms into the air passages by inhalation during ventilation and by aspiration of nasopharyngeal secretions, the latter occurring to a slight extent even in normal people. Pharyngeal secretions contain the commensal bacteria of the upper respiratory tract, which consist of streptococci (including the pneumococcus), staphylococci, anaerobes (including *Actinomyces*), corynebacteria, neisseriae, and gram-negative bacilli. The commensal flora varies; gram-negative bacilli are rarely present in healthy persons but are common in those who are chronically ill. Sterility of the alveoli is maintained by physical mechanisms and alveolar immune defense mechanisms. Physical mechanisms include (1) the mucociliary mechanism of the bronchi, which physically entraps microorganisms and wafts them up into the pharynx and (2) the laryngeal cough reflex. These prevent entry of organisms into the distal air passages. When organisms enter the alveoli, immune defenses prevent infection. These include the following:

- **Alveolar macrophages**, which phagocytose organisms; phagocytosis is made efficient by the presence of opsonins.
- **Nonimmune opsonins**, such as surfactant produced by type II pneumocytes and fibronectin produced by alveolar macrophages.
- **Immune opsonins**, including complement factor C3b and immunoglobulins. Complement is activated locally by the alternative pathway. IgA is secreted into the bronchial secretions. IgG subclasses in bronchial secretions are present in the same proportions as plasma and are probably derived from the blood. IgG2 in bronchial secretions includes antibodies against capsular bacteria such as *Streptococcus pneumoniae* and *Haemophilus influenzae* and lipopolysaccharide cell-wall components of gram-negative bacilli. Coating of microorganisms by immune opsonins facilitates phagocytosis because macrophages have surface receptors for C3b and the Fc region of the IgG molecule.
- **Immune cells**, mainly T lymphocytes, are normally present in the air spaces. They produce cytokines, the most important of which are γ-interferon and macrophage inhibitory factor. These cytokines are important in the defense against *Mycobacterium tuberculosis*, *Legionella pneumophila*, *Pneumocystis carinii*, and cytomegalovirus.
- **Neutrophils** are normally absent from the air spaces but can be rapidly mobilized by chemotactic factors derived from alveolar macrophages (leukotriene B4) and complement activation (C3a and C5a).

Acute pneumonia occurs when an organism reaches the alveoli, overcomes the alveolar defenses, and starts multiplying. In the majority of cases, the organism is either inhaled during normal ventilation or is present in aspirated pharyngeal secretions. Rarely, the organism reaches the lung via the blood (hematogenous infection) or directly as a result of chest trauma or surgery.

Acute pneumonia may rarely occur in a healthy individual (**primary pneumonia**) and is then the result of infection with a highly virulent agent that is well adapted to causing lung infection, most commonly *S. pneumoniae* and some viruses (Figure 7-1). Most patients who develop acute pneumonia have an underlying abnormality in the lung that predisposes them to infection (**secondary pneumonia**).

Acute pneumonia is manifested in one of two patterns: (1) air space pneumonia, which results from bacterial infection; or (2) interstitial pneumonia, which results from infectious agents that are usually obligate intracellular organisms (Figure 7-2). These two types can be distinguished by clinical and radiologic features. Air space pneumonias show features of consolidation (alveolar pattern) by physical examination and chest x-ray; interstitial pneumonias are characterized by few abnormalities on physical examination and show a reticular (interstitial) pattern on chest x-ray.

ACUTE AIR SPACE PNEUMONIA (ACUTE BACTERIAL PNEUMONIA)

Acute air space pneumonia results from infection by bacteria that multiply extracellularly in the alveoli. This evokes an acute inflammation with dilation of alveolar capillaries, exudation of fluid, and emigration of neutrophils into the alveoli (Figure 7-2). The air spaces become filled with inflammatory exudate, causing the affected lung to become airless (consolidation). The peripheral blood commonly shows a neutrophil leukocytosis.

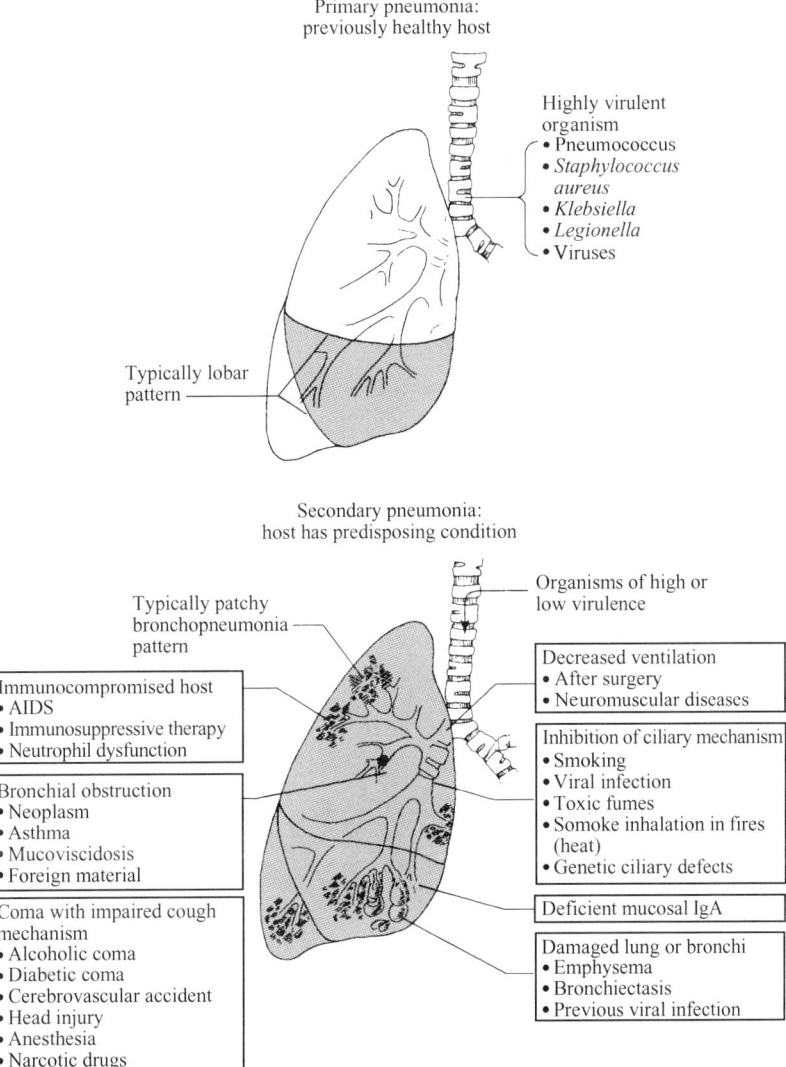

Figure 7-1 Primary versus secondary pneumonia. Note that predisposing diseases (in boxes) are important in the pathogenesis of secondary pneumonia

Acute space pneumonias tend to spread to adjacent alveoli through direct intra-alveolar communications (the pores of Kohn). The facility with which organisms spread directly is a measure of their virulence; highly virulent organisms spread rapidly, causing large areas of lung to become affected, whereas less virulent agents tend to remain localized.

Lobar Pneumonia

In lobar pneumonia, the bronchi are not involved, and large confluent areas (sometimes entire lobes) are consolidated (Figure 7-3). Lobar pneumonia is characterized by a large area of consolidation on chest x-ray associated with air bronchograms that indicate absence of involvement of bronchi. Lobar pneumonia typically occurs with primary pneumonias caused by virulent agents, most commonly pneumococci.

A. Etiology

The most common cause of air space pneumonia is *S. pneumoniae*. This is overwhelmingly the case (60% – 70%) in primary community-acquired pneumonias of lobar pattern, with most of the remainder resulting from *L. pneumophila*.

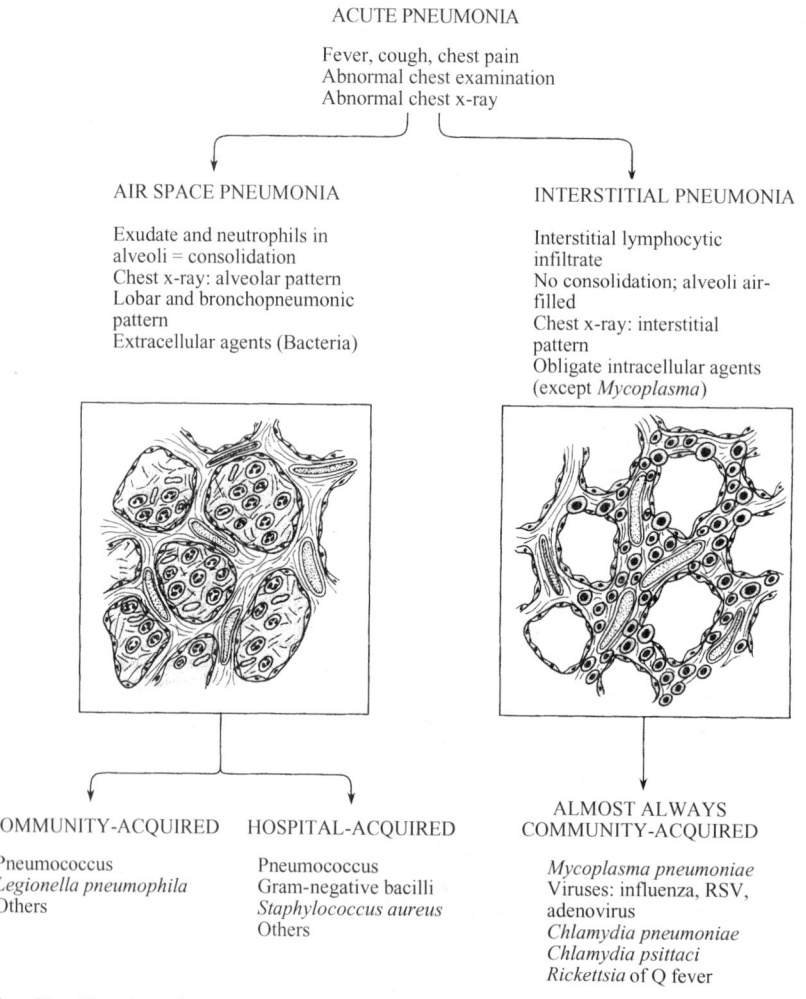

Figure 7-2 Classification of acute pneumonia based on pattern of lung involvement and etiology

B. Pathologic Features

Lobar pneumonia progresses through four stages: acute congestion, red hepatization, gray hepatization, and resolution.

- **Acute congestion** is the early phase of infection, when the bacteria are multiplying in the alveoli and spreading to contiguous alveoli. The normal alveolar defenses have been overcome, and there is early injury to the alveoli. Alveolar macrophages secrete mediators, and there is complement activation resulting in acute inflammation. There is active dilation of alveolar capillaries and early fluid exudation, neutrophil emigration, and erythrocyte diapedesis into the alveoli. Clinically, this stage corresponds to the onset of disease, with high fever and cough. Bacteremia is common. Involvement of the pleura is also common and may result in chest pain, a pleural rub, and pleural effusion.
- **Red hepatization** is characterized by increasing consolidation of the involved lung due to continued exudation and neutrophil emigration (Figure 7-4). Alveolar congestion is still present, and the alveolar air has been replaced by the cellular exudate, red cells, neutrophils, and fibrin, etc. The basic alveolar architecture is maintained, although there is loss of lining cells. The lung lobe has a liver-like consistency. In most patients, the infection is controlled at this stage, either naturally or by antibiotic therapy, which eliminates the bacterium.
- **In gray hepatization**, features of consolidation are present, but the infection has been controlled and there is neither hyperemia nor continued exudation and neutrophil emigration, while the fibrinous exudates persist within the alveoli. The lung is dry, gray and firm. The patient has usually recovered clinically.

Chapter 7 Diseases of the Respiratory System

debris; the exudate is slowly removed and the alveolar injury repaired.

Gray hepatization and resolution correspond to phases of healing, which can go on for several weeks until the lung returns to normal.

C. Clinical Features

Patients with lobar pneumonia present with an acute onset of fever, dyspnea, and cough that is commonly productive of purulent, rust-colored sputum. Chest pain, a pleural friction rub, and effusion are present if there is pleural involvement. When secondary pneumonia occurs in chronically ill patients, these symptoms may not be obvious. Physical examination may show evidence of consolidation. Chest x-ray to confirm an alveolar pattern of pneumonia is essential to differentiate air space pneumonia from interstitial pneumonia. Chest x-ray may also differentiate between lobar and bronchopneumonic patterns, which provides insight to the etiologic agent.

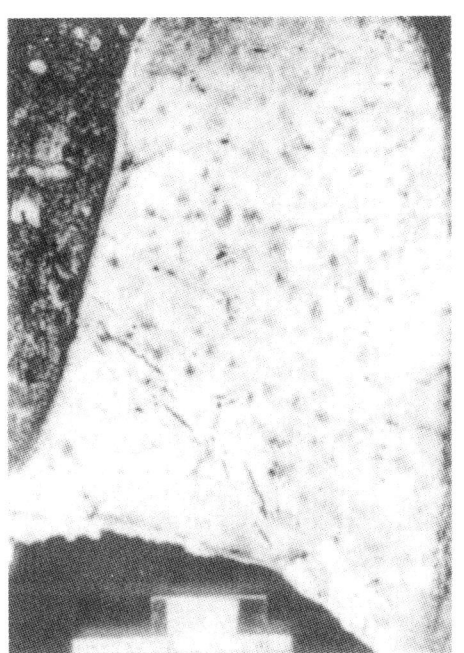

Figure 7-3 Lobar pneumonia. The lobe to the right of the interlobar fissure is pale and consolidated. The lobe to the left of the interlobar fissure is normal

- **Resolution.** This stage represents the resorption of exudate and enzymatic digestion of inflammatory

Lobular Pneumonia (Bronchopneumonia)

In bronchopneumonia, the bronchi are infected, with involvement of adjacent alveoli in a patchy,

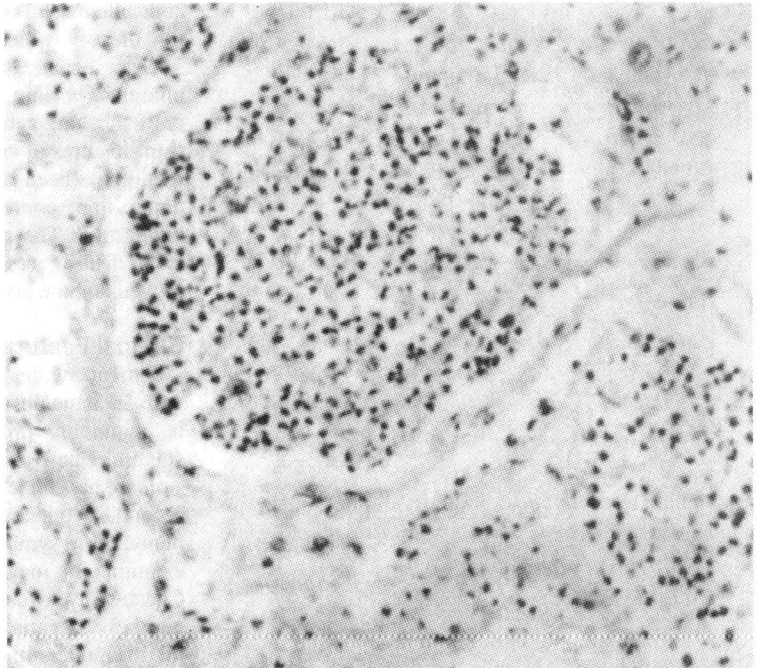

Figure 7-4 Lobar pneumonia – phase of red hepatization. The alveoli are filled with exudate and large numbers of neutrophils

often limited fashion (Figure 7-5). Chest x-ray shows patchy consolidation with absent air bronchograms. Bronchopneumonia occurs typically in secondary pneumonia and is usually caused by less virulent agents. When bronchopneumonia is the result of infection with a virulent agent, infection spreads through the pores of Kohn and becomes confluent, resulting in disease that is very similar to lobar pneumonia.

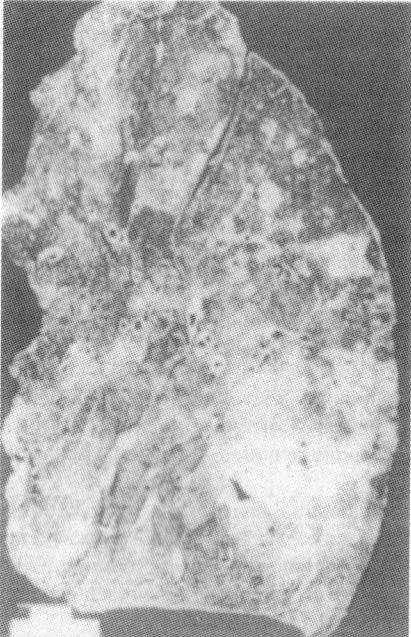

Figure 7-5 Bronchopneumonia. Note the small pale areas of patchy consolidation around bronchioles throughout the lung. There is a larger area of confluent bronchopneumonia at the base

A. Etiology

In patients who develop secondary pneumonias of a bronchopneumonic pattern – many bacteria, such as *Staphylococcus aureus*, gram-negative bacilli, and *H. influenzae* as well as *S. pneumoniae*, can be involved.

B. Pathologic Features

Lobular pneumonia is characterized by foci of acute suppurative inflammation centered on bronchioles. The consolidation may be patchy through one lobe but is more often multilobar and frequently bilateral and basal. Well-developed lesions are slightly elevated, dry, granular, gray-red to yellow, and poorly delimited at their margins. They vary in size up to 0.5 to 1 cm in diameter. Confluence of these foci occurs in the more florid instances, producing the appearance of total lobular consolidation (confluent bronchopneumonia).

The lung substance immediately surrounding areas of consolidation is usually slightly hyperemic and edematous, but the large intervening areas are generally normal.

Histologically, the reaction comprises a suppurative exudate that fills the bronchi, bronchioles, and adjacent alveolar spaces. Neutrophils are dominant in this exudation, and usually, only small amounts of fibrin are present. As expected, the abscesses are marked by necrosis of the underlying architecture.

C. Clinical Features

The clinical picture of lobular pneumonia is seldom as well defined as that of lobar pneumonia, largely because it is frequently overshadowed by the predisposing condition. Moreover the many etiologic agents for this disease have a considerable range of virulence, and patients vary in vulnerability. In general, the onset is insidious; often appearing as a nonspecific worsening of the patient's prior condition, with low-grade fever and cough productive of purulent sputum. Respiratory difficulty is typically not prominent. The course is irregular, but resolution usually occurs if treatment is appropriate and the patient is not severely debilitated. The characteristic radiologic appearance of bronchopneumonia shows focal opacities. The area of affected lung can be identified clinically by hearing crackles (crepitations) on auscultation.

Complications of Acute Air Space Pneumonia

A. Disturbances of Ventilation and Perfusion

Air space pneumonia interferes with gas exchange in the involved area of the lung. There is no ventilation because the alveoli are filled with exudate, and perfusion is abnormal because of the micro-circulatory changes of acute inflammation. In most cases, vital capacity is reduced, but respiratory failure occurs only with extensive disease involving both lungs.

B. Pleural Involvement

Spread of infection to the pleura, with acute inflammation and effusion, commonly accompanies air space pneumonia. In most cases, this resolves with treatment of the pneumonia. Rarely, pleural inflammation becomes progressive and does not resolve, leading to loculation and accumulation of pus (empyema).

C. Bacteremia

Bacteremia is the most serious complication of pneumococcal pneumonia. Its occurrence significantly increases the likelihood of death. Bacteremia may also lead to pneumococcal infections elsewhere in the body, most commonly meningitis and endocarditis.

D. Suppuration (Abscess Formation)

Suppuration is associated with liquefactive necrosis of alveoli leading to areas of destroyed lung replaced by pus. Suppuration is associated with virulent pyogenic bacteria such as *S. aureus*, gram-negative bacilli, and type 3 pneumococci. Suppuration is associated with a high incidence of treatment failure and death. In patients who recover, areas of suppuration heal by fibrous scarring because the destroyed alveoli cannot regenerate.

E. Necrotizing Bacterial Pneumonia

This is a rare complication characterized by extremely severe necrosis of the lung associated with a rapidly progressive disease with a high mortality rate. It is seen with etiologic agents such as *Yersinia pestis* (pneumonic plague) and *Bacillus anthracis* (anthrax), which are rare causes of pneumonia. An acute necrotizing pneumonia may also occur in immunodeficient and malnourished patients secondary to more common pathogens such as *L. pneumophila* and *M. tuberculosis*.

F. Pulmonary Carnification

Organization of the exudate, which may convert a portion of the lung into solid tissue, known as pulmonary carnification.

ACUTE INTERSTITIAL PNEUMONIA

Acute interstitial pneumonia results from infection by agents that are predominantly obligate intracellular pathogens. Infection with these organisms evokes an acute inflammation that is usually restricted to the interstitium without involvement of the alveolar spaces. The peripheral blood commonly shows neutropenia, lymphocytosis, or no change.

Viral Pneumonia

A. Etiology

Most of the agents causing viral pneumonia are obligate intracellular organisms: Influenza and parainfluenza viruses commonly occur in epidemics; respiratory syncytial virus and adenovirus are the most common causes of sporadic viral pneumonia in children and adults, respectively. Cytomegalovirus and herpesviruses are important in immunocompromised patients. Pneumonia may accompany viral exanthems such as measles and chickenpox.

B. Pathologic Features

The alveolar septa are expanded by hyperemia, edema, and a cellular infiltrate composed of lymphocytes and plasma cells (Figure 7-6). The alveolar spaces are airfilled. The infected alveolar epithelial cells may show a variety of cytopathic effects such as necrosis, the presence of inclusion bodies (cytomegalovirus, herpesviruses, chlamydiae), and multinucleated giant cells (respiratory syncytial virus, measles, herpesviruses), which may be useful in identifying the specific agent if tissue biopsies are taken.

C. Clinical Features

Patients with viral pneumonia present with acute onset of fever, cough, and dyspnea. Cough is usually unproductive or produces mucoid sputum. The illness is usually mild and self-limited (walking pneumonia). Physical examination may show scattered rales due to associated bronchiolitis, but there is no evidence of consolidation. Chest x-ray shows the pattern of interstitial involvement that serves to differentiate this disorder from air space pneumonia. Pleural involvement does not occur.

In most cases, patients are not seriously ill, and a specific etiologic diagnosis is not attempted because no specific therapy is indicated.

Severe Acute Respiratory Syndrome (SARS)

SARS is a viral respiratory illness caused by the SARS-associated coronavirus (SARS-CoV), a new member in the family Coronaviridae. Fever, usually greater than 38°C and may be accompanied by chills, malaise, headache, diarrhea, and myalgias giving an overall flu-like picture. Lower respiratory symptoms including cough, shortness of breath, and dyspnea, and can progress to hypoxemia severe enough to require mechanical ventilation. Mortality rates are highest in the elderly and individuals with chronic disease.

Microscopically, the pathologic features are dominated by diffuse alveolar damage in varying phases of organization.

The lungs show bilateral and extensive consolidation, localized hemorrhage and necrosis, desquamative alveolitis and bronchitis, alveolar proliferation and desquamation, accumulation of protein exudates, mononuclear cells, lymphocytes, and plasma cells, as well as hyaline formation in alveoli. In cases that undergo over weeks of the course, the main pattern is organization of intra-alveolar deposit, along with fibroblastic proliferation in the alveolar septa, which leads to obliteration of alveolar space and pulmonary fibrosis.

Extensive consolidation of lungs, formation of hyaline membrane to a large extent, respiratory distress and decrease of immune function are the main causes of death.

Avian influenza ("bird flu")

Avian influenza, commonly called "bird flu," is an infectious disease of birds caused by strains of the influenza virus. The first cases of avian influenza viruses in humans occurred in 1997, when the H5N1 virus triggered an outbreak in Hong Kong. The strain of avian influenza virus that has led to the deaths of 140 million birds and 60 people in Asia appears to be slowly acquiring genetic changes typical of the "Spanish flu" virus that killed 50 million people nearly a century ago.

Avian Influenza is characterized histologically by vascular disturbances leading to edema, hemorrhages and perivascular cuffing, especially in the myocardium, spleen, lungs, brain and wattles. Necrotic foci are present in the lungs, liver and kidneys.

Mycoplasma Pneumonia

Mycoplasma pneumonia is the most common cause of sporadic cases of interstitial pneumonia. Often the patient is an adolescent or a young adult. Respiratory symptoms may be minimal or severe, and the radiographic infiltrate is patchy or segmental in distribution. The diagnosis is often established clinically based on serology with acute and convalesce titers.

Pathologic Features

Microscopic findings are interstitial pneumonia. The alveolar septa and walls of bronchioles are congested, edematous, and infiltrated with mononuclear

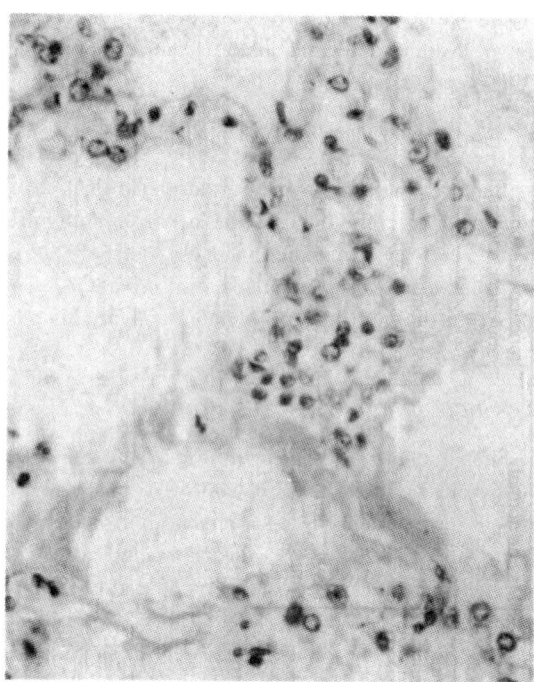

Figure 7-6 Acute interstitial pneumonia in viral infection, showing expanded alveolar septa infiltrated with lymphocytes. Hyaline membranes and exudate are present in the alveoli, indicating severe pneumonia

cells. Epithelial cells degenerate and slough. In fatal cases, edema and hyaline membranes may be seen.

Pneumocystis Pneumonia

Pneumocystis carinii is a common cause of interstitial pneumonia in immunocompromised patients, particularly those with AIDS and to a lesser extent in patients undergoing cancer chemotherapy and in malnourished children. In immunocompromised patients with severe pneumonia specific therapy may be needed.

Pathologic Features

In *P carinii* pneumonia, the interstitial inflammation is associated with the presence of organisms in the alveoli (Figure 7-7A). The organisms are present in large numbers; in routine sections stained with hematoxylin and eosin, they appear as a frothy mass filling the alveoli. The organisms can be demonstrated by methenamine silver stain, where they are seen as 2 μm round and crescent-shaped structures (Figure 7-7B).

Chapter 7 Diseases of the Respiratory System

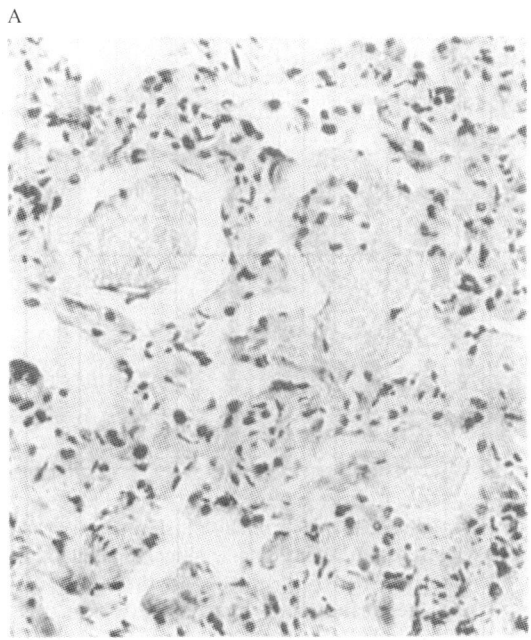

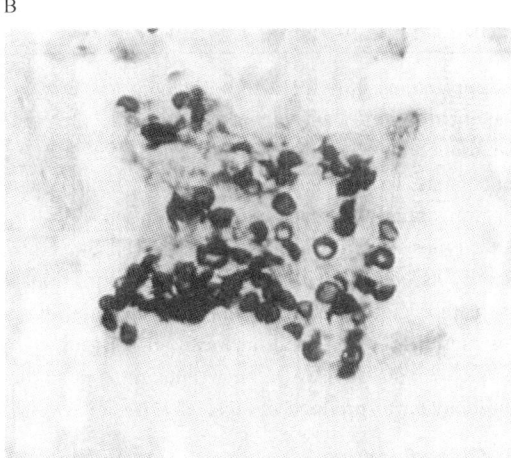

Figure 7-7 *Pneumocystis carinii* pneumonia. A: Routine hematoxylin and eosin stain showing frothy masses of organisms filling the alveoli associated with interstitial inflammation. B: Methenamine silver stain, showing the organisms in the frothy material in the alveolus

Complications of Acute Interstitial Pneumonia

A. Secondary Bacterial Pneumonia

This is the most common complication of interstitial pneumonia, particularly viral pneumonias. It is typically a bronchopneumonia and tends to affect patients at the extremes of age (infants and the elderly). *S. aureus*, pneumococci, other streptococci, *H. influenzae*, and *Moraxella catarrhalis* are most commonly involved. Secondary bacterial pneumonia has a high mortality rate in the elderly and is a common cause of death during influenza epidemics; it is believed to have caused 10 million deaths worldwide during the 1918 influenza pandemic, when antibiotics were not yet available.

B. Spread to Other Systems

Hematogenous spread to other organs such as viral encephalitis and myocarditis is rare. Postviral allergic complications such as Guillain-Barré syndrome are more common.

C. Acute Necrotizing Viral Pneumonia

This complication is rare, occurring most commonly with Influenza and adenovirus infections and most recently in an epidemic of hantavirus infection in the southwestern United States. It is characterized by diffuse alveolar damage associated with hemorrhage and hyaline membrane formation, rapid clinical progression, and a high mortality rate.

D. Reye's Syndrome

Reye's syndrome (acute encephalopathy with acute fatty change of liver and kidney) may rarely complicate influenza and chickenpox, especially when high dosages of salicylates are given to dehydrated children with infection.

CHRONIC OBSTRUCTIVE PULMONARY DISEASE (COPD)

The term chronic obstructive pulmonary disease (COPD) refers to a group of conditions that share a major symptom – dyspnea – and are accompanied by chronic obstruction to air flow within the lungs. These conditions – chronic bronchitis, bronchiectasis, asthma and emphysema – have distinct anatomic and clinical characteristics.

COPD is diagnosed by abnormalities in tests of ventilatory function. The first second of a forced expiration ($FEV1$) : forced vital capacity (FVC) ratio is the most widely used test. Normally, the $FEV1$: FVC ratio is over 75%. In COPD, the ratio is decreased, with the degree of reduction correlating well with disease severity and survival.

Incidence

COPD is a common disease second only to ischemic heart disease as a cause of chronic disability in older individuals. The incidence is increasing.

CHRONIC BRONCHITIS

Chronic bronchitis is defined clinically as a persistent presence of increased bronchial mucus secretion that leads to chronic cough productive of mucoid sputum.

A. Pathogenesis

Chronic bronchitis is 5–10 times more common in heavy **cigarette smokers** than in nonsmokers, even after correction for other factors such as age, sex, place of residence, and occupation. Cigarette smoking acts as a local irritant, causing hypertrophy of bronchial mucous glands, increase in the number of mucous cells, hypersecretion of mucus, and increased numbers of neutrophils. Other inhaled irritants such as sulfur dioxide and oxides of nitrogen associated with heavy air pollution cause exacerbation of chronic bronchitis.

The hypersecretion of mucus increases the susceptibility to bacterial infection. In cigarette smokers, this predisposition is further aggravated by interference with ciliary action that results from smoking. *Haemophilus influenzae*, pneumococci, and *Streptococcus viridans* are common pathogens. These organisms cause both a chronic low-grade inflammation of the bronchiolar wall and acute exacerbations with suppuration manifested clinically as fever and expectoration of purulent sputum. Inflammation leads to progressive destruction of the muscle of the bronchiolar wall, with replacement by collagen.

In heavy smokers, the initial changes of chronic bronchitis are present from an early age, but COPD usually does not become clinically apparent until the fourth or fifth decade of life.

B. Pathologic Features

Pathologic examination shows hypertrophy of bronchial wall mucous glands associated with chronic inflammation and fibrous replacement of the muscular walls of small bronchioles (Figure 7-8). The Reid index – the ratio of mucous gland thickness to bronchial wall thickness – is increased above the normal value of 0.5. Fibrotic bronchioles tend to collapse in expiration under the influence of the positive intrathoracic pressure, resulting in ventilatory obstruction in expiration (chronic obstructive bronchitis).

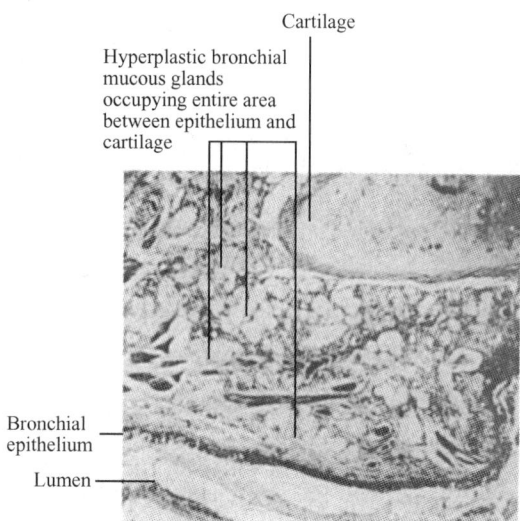

Figure 7-8 Chronic bronchitis, showing marked hyperplasia of the bronchial mucous glands. In this case, the glands occupy almost the entire area between the surface epithelium and cartilage, giving a Reid index of almost 1

EMPHYSEMA

Emphysema is defined in pathologic terms as permanent dilation of the air spaces distal to the terminal bronchiole, usually with destruction of lung parenchyma. To produce clinical COPD, large areas of the lung must be involved by emphysema. Several other types of emphysema are recognized but are not usually associated with COPD. These conditions fit the pathologic definition of emphysema – dilation and destruction of the small airways and alveoli – but usually do not involve a large enough area of lung parenchyma to produce clinical effects.

A. Classification

Emphysema is defined in terms of the anatomic nature of the lesion. There are two major types (Figure 7-9):

• **Alveolar emphysema.** According to the location of the lesions within the pulmonary acinus, three principal types of emphysema are recognized: (1) **centriacinar emphysema**, in which dilation and destruction primarily involve the central part of the acinus formed by the respiratory bronchioles. Centriacinar emphysema occurs predominantly in heavy smokers, often in association with chronic bronchitis; and (2) **panacinar emphysema**, in which dilation and destruction involve the entire acinus, including the alveoli and alveolar ducts as well as the respiratory

Chapter 7 Diseases of the Respiratory System

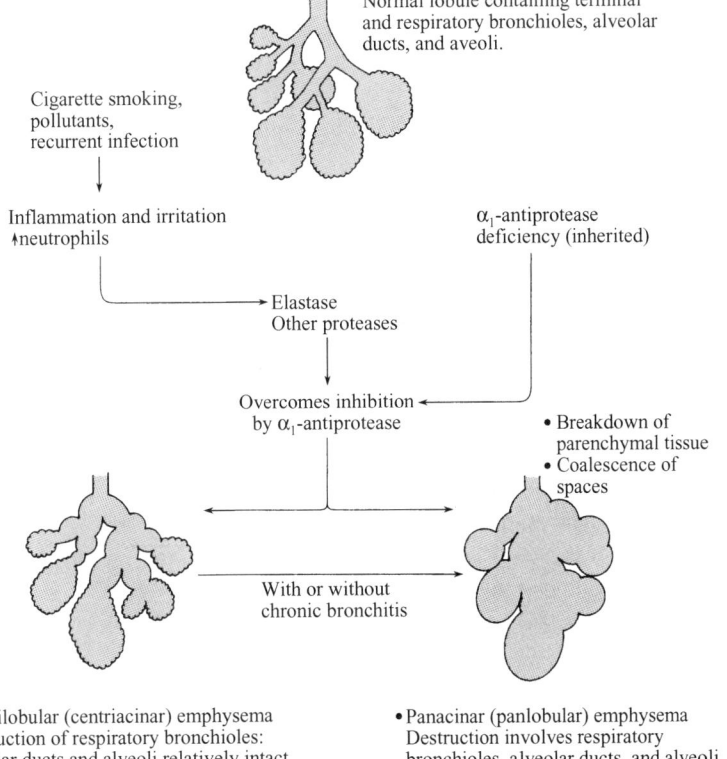

Figure 7-9 Pathogenesis and types of emphysema associated with chronic obstructive pulmonary disease

bronchioles. This type of emphysema is probably associated with α_1-antitrypsin (α_1-AT) deficiency; (3) **periacinar emphysema** can be characterized as distal acinar emphysema. It occurs adjacent to areas of fibrosis, scarring, or atelectasis and is usually more severe in the upper half of the lungs. Since this pattern is accentuated along lobular septa, it is referred to as paraseptal emphysema.

- **Interstitial emphysema.** It refers to the accumulation of air in the interstitial tissues, and is most commonly due to traumatic rupture of an airway or spontaneous rupture of an emphysematous bulla. Typically it begins with the entrance of air into the septa of the lung, which may then dissect its way back to the hilus to reach the mediastinum and thence possibly the subcutaneous tissues of the chest, neck and body, giving the characteristic spongy crepitus on palpation.
- **Other types. Paracicatrical emphysema** is better known as emphysema associated with lung scarring. The precise location of the changes is variable but respiratory bronchioles and sometimes also the alveolar sacs. **Bullous emphysema** is not a specific morphologic pattern of the disease. A **bulla** is an emphysematous space more than 1 cm in diameter. Subpleural bullae may appear in any one of the four well-defined forms of emphysema when severe but are particularly common with the paraseptal form. **Senile emphysema** refers to the extremely common increased volume of the lungs so often found in the aged. It is probably the consequence of skeletal changes that increase the anteroposterior diameter of the chest (barrel chest). With such expansion of the chest cage, the lungs expand to fill the pleural cavities. Because there is no septal wall destruction associated with the process, it is better referred to as senile hyperinflation. **Compensatory emphysema** is a misnomer applied to the alveolar dilatation that follows collapse or loss of lung substance elsewhere, as, for example, the enlargement of remaining lobes following a lobectomy. Because there is no destruction of septal walls, the process is appropriately called compensatory hyperinflation.

Accurate recognition of the gross and microscopic features of emphysema at autopsy requires fixation of the lungs in a state of inflation. This technique permits the gross demonstration of dilated air spaces and microscopic documentation of alveolar destruction (Figure 7-10).

B. Pathogenesis (Table 7-1; Figure 7-9)

The destruction of lung parenchyma in emphysema is believed to be due to the action of **proteolytic enzymes** (proteases, mainly elastase). One important source of these proteases is leukocytes associated with pulmonary inflammation. Normally, antiproteolytic substances such as antitrypsins in the plasma inactivate these proteolytic enzymes as they are released and thereby protect tissues from damage. However, lung destruction - and emphysema - occur in patients who either produce an excess of proteolytic enzymes (chronic neutrophil infiltration) or have too little antiproteolytic activity in the plasma (α_1-antiprotease deficiency; see below). Hypersecretion of mucus in chronic bronchitis and emphysema favors inflammation and local leukocyte enzyme release.

Cigarette smoking is an important etiologic factor in emphysema. Chronic irritation resulting from smoking results in increased numbers of neutrophils, and cigarette smoke directly promotes elastase release from neutrophils. The chronic bacterial infection associated with chronic bronchitis in smokers also contributes to the increased levels of leukocyte-derived proteolytic enzymes. The lungs of heavy smokers show inflammation and destruction of the respiratory bronchioles, with centrilobular emphysema beginning at a relatively young age.

Alpha$_1$-antiprotease (α_1-antitrypsin) deficiency predisposes to emphysema because α_1-antiprotease is responsible for the major part of plasma antiproteolytic activity. The α_1-antiprotease level in serum is determined by inheritance at a single (Pi, or protease inhibitor) locus. A normal individual has two M alleles at this locus (PiMM). The Z allele is the most common of several abnormal alleles that may be inherited. PiZZ homozygotes have severe deficiency of α_1-antiprotease and almost invariably develop panacinar emphysema by age 40 years.

PiZZ occurs with a frequency of 1:4000 and thus is a very rare cause of emphysema; it cannot account for most of the cases of COPD in the population. The heterozygous PiMZ state occurs in about 5% of

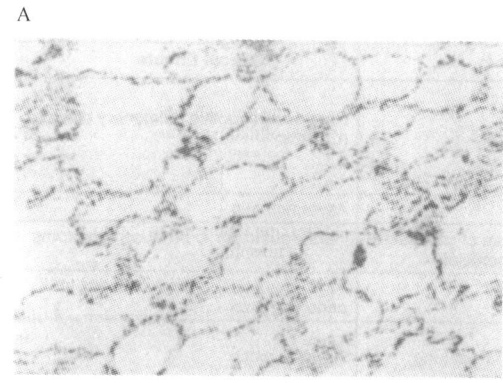
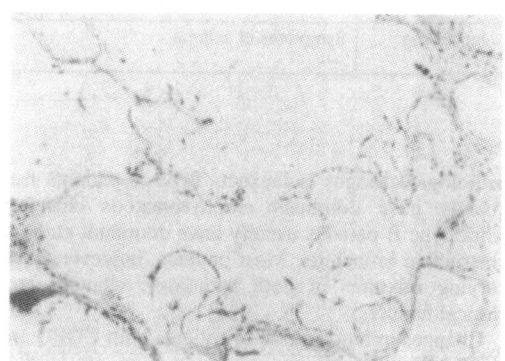
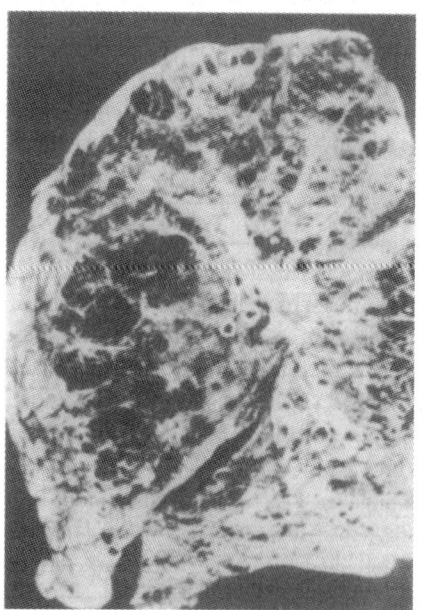

Figure 7-10 Normal lung (A) compared with emphysema (B) at equivalent magnification, showing destruction of lung parenchyma and marked dilation of terminal air spaces in emphysema, both microscopically (B) and grossly (C)

the population in the United States and Europe and is potentially a factor in the genesis of the common type of COPD. The PiMZ state is associated with a moderate reduction in serum α_1-antiprotease. While PiMZ has been associated with emphysema in some families, general population studies have not confirmed a causal association between emphysema and the PiMZ genotype.

Table 7-1 Chronic bronchitis and emphysema

	Causal Factors	Clinical Effects
Destructive lung disease Chronic bronchitis, centrilobular emphysema, panacinar emphysema	Cigarettes Recurrent infection ? Pollutants Alpha$_1$-antiprotease eficiency	Chronic obstructive pulmonary disease (COPD)
Senile emphysema	Aging	Asymptomatic
Paraseptal emphysema (paracicatricial)	Associated with any cause of collapse or fibrosis (scars [paracicatricial])	Rarely sufficient to produce symptoms
Bullous emphysema	Unknown	Asymptomatic, but rupture leads to pneumothorax
Nondestructive lung disease Compensatory emphysema (dilatation without destruction)	Removal or collapse of part of lung; remaining lung expands	Asymptomatic
Focal dust emphysema (dilatation without destruction)	Various dust diseases, pneumoconioses, e.g. coal miner's lung	Usually insufficient to produce symptoms
Dilatation distal to obstruction; no destruction	Acute bronchial asthma; air trapping	Symptoms of asthma

C. Clinical Features

Patients with COPD are asymptomatic in the early stages of the disease because of pulmonary reserve; however, the FEV1:FVC ratio is decreased, as is vital capacity and maximal ventilatory volume. The total lung capacity and residual volume are often increased as a result of air trapping in the distended air spaces.

In the later symptomatic phase, COPD patients present with a spectrum of symptoms, the 2 extremes of which are sometimes designated types A and B. In most cases, features of both type A and type B are present.

Type A patients present with chronic cough – either dry or productive of mucoid sputum – progressive dyspnea, and wheezing. Their lungs are overinflated, with increased anteroposterior diameter of the chest (barrel chest) and flattened diaphragm on chest x-ray. These patients successfully maintain oxygenation of the blood by hyperventilation. Patients with type A COPD are sometimes called "pink puffers."

Type B patients have marked chronic obstructive bronchitis and cannot hyperventilate. There is decreased oxygenation of blood (cyanosis) and increased arterial carbon dioxide content. They also have pulmonary hypertension caused by changes in the microvasculature of the lung parenchyma. This leads to right ventricular hypertrophy and failure (cor pulmonale). Type B patients are sometimes called "blue bloaters."

BRONCHIAL ASTHMA

Bronchial asthma is a disease in which there is increased responsiveness of the tracheobronchial tree to a variety of stimuli. Exposure to these stimuli leads to bronchiolar smooth muscle contraction (**bronchospasm**). The cause of the increased responsiveness of the air passages is unknown but is believed to be related to bronchial inflammation. Bronchospasm causes obstruction to air flow – maximal in expiration – and a high-pitched wheeze. Expiration is prolonged because of airflow obstruction. Attacks of asthma are usually of short duration and reverse completely. Rarely, they may be severe and prolonged (**status asthmaticus**), and may lead to acute ventilatory failure and even death.

A. Etiology and Classification

1. Extrinsic allergic asthma

Extrinsic allergic asthma is a reagin-mediated **type I hypersensitivity** (atopic) reaction. It is common in childhood has a familial tendency. Many different antigens may be involved. Serum IgE is increased, and skin tests against the offending antigens are positive.

2. Intrinsic (nonallergic) asthma

It has been suggested that patients with intrinsic asthma have hyper-reactive airways that constrict in response to a variety of nonspecific stimuli, due in part to abnormal β-adrenergic responses. Aspirin, cold, exercise, and respiratory infections are common precipitants of attacks. Serum IgE levels are normal, and skin tests are negative. Intrinsic asthma occurs in older patients.

B. Pathology

In extrinsic allergic asthma, the inhaled antigen combines with specific IgE on the surface of mast cells in the respiratory mucosa, releasing histamine (Figure 7-11). Other mediators such as bradykinin, leukotrienes, prostaglandins, and platelet-aggregating factor are produced, leading to bronchoconstriction and acute inflammation. Bronchioles show vascular congestion, edema, and infiltration by neutrophils and eosinophils. The bronchioles become filled with thick mucous secretions (Figure 7-12).

Bronchiolar obstruction due to smooth muscle contraction, mucoid plugs, and inflammatory edema is maximal in expiration. This results in distal air trapping and alveolar distention.

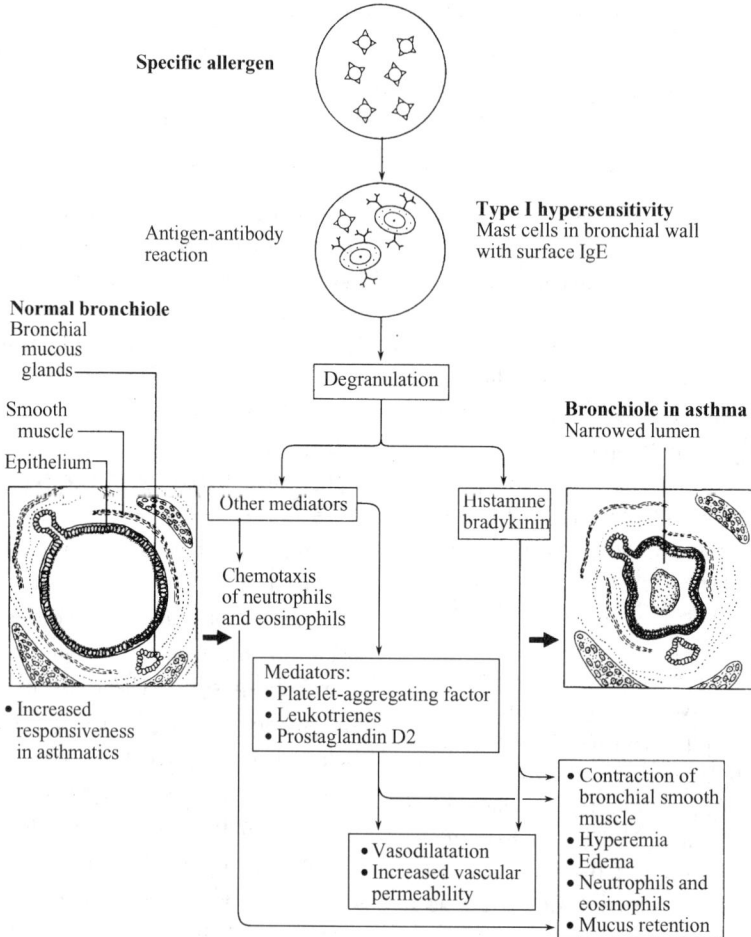

Figure 7-11 Pathogenesis of extrinsic allergic asthma

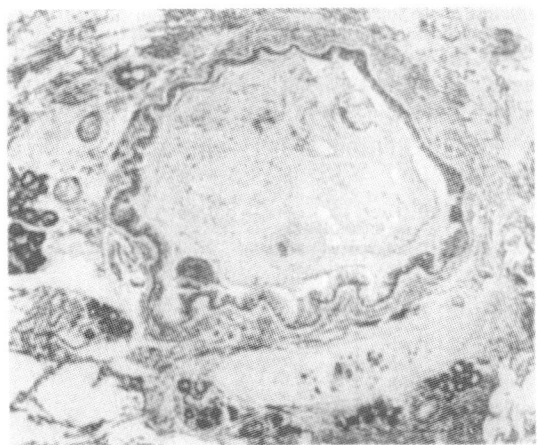

Figure 7-12 Bronchial asthma, showing a small bronchus filled with a plug of viscid mucus and inflammatory cells

C. Clinical Features

Bronchial asthma is characterized by episodic attacks of dyspnea and wheezing. A dry cough is common during the acute attack and may produce thick, tenacious, scanty sputum that is stringy, forming casts of the bronchioles (Curschmann's spirals). In severe attacks, there is frequently secondary bacterial infection. Allergic asthma occurs in childhood and tends to disappear as the child grows. Intrinsic asthma occurs in older individuals and tends to produce a more chronic disease.

BRONCHIECTASIS

Bronchiectasis is abnormal and irreversible dilation of the bronchial tree proximal to the terminal bronchioles – in contrast to emphysema, which involves the bronchial tree distal to the terminal bronchioles.

A. Etiology

Bronchiectasis is the result of chronic infection with resulting parenchymal destruction, fibrosis, and abnormal permanent dilation of damaged bronchi. Several causes act singly or in concert.

1. Long-standing bronchial obstruction

As occurs in bronchial tumors and stenosis. Stagnation of mucus is followed by bronchopneumonia distal to the obstruction, progressing to localized fibrosis and bronchiectasis.

2. Mucoviscidosis (fibrocystic disease of the pancreas)

In this condition, mucus is abnormally thick and viscous; it plugs the smaller bronchi, causing obstruction and predisposing to recurrent infection.

3. Bronchopneumonia

Particularly following childhood infections such as measles and whooping cough, which in the past were common antecedents of bronchiectasis. Bronchiectasis occurs today in immunodeficient children who are susceptible to recurrent pulmonary infections.

4. Kartagener's syndrome

Kartagener's syndrome is due to a congenital defect in ciliary motion caused by absence of the dynein arms in cilia. The lack of ciliary action interferes with clearance of mucus and bacteria in the bronchi, predisposing to bronchopneumonia and therefore bronchiectasis. Chronic infection of the paranasal sinuses also results in absence of the frontal sinuses in this condition. In the male, absence of dynein arms in the microtubules of the sperm tail leads to loss of sperm motility and infertility. Dextrocardia (location of the heart on the right side) completes the syndrome.

5. Intralobar sequestration of the lung (congenital)

In this rare condition a part of the lung receives either no pulmonary arterial supply or no communication with the bronchial tree. The sequestered lobe maintains nutrition via its bronchial arterial supply. The bronchi within the area, however, have no drainage and therefore undergo infection and dilation.

B. Pathology (Figure 7-13)

Bronchiectasis usually has a patchy distribution, depending on the extent of bronchial obstruction. The lower lobes are the most commonly affected. The dilated bronchi and bronchioles may be cylindric, fusiform, or saccular and are made more conspicuous by extensive destruction and fibrosis of the intervening lung parenchyma. An important diagnostic feature is the finding of large bronchi near the pleura.

The walls of the distended bronchi show inflammation and fibrosis. The mucosa may be ulcerated, and the lumen is commonly filled with pus.

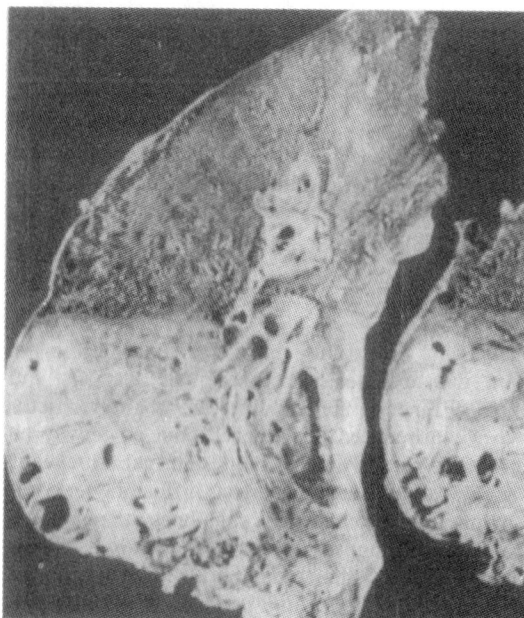

Figure 7-13 Bronchiectasis, showing fibrosis and dilation of bronchi in the lower lobe. Note the dilated bronchi immediately beneath the pleura, a feature of diagnostic value

C. Clinical Features

Bronchiectasis is a chronic illness with cough, usually productive of a large volume of foul-smelling sputum, and episodic fever. The chronic infection commonly causes clubbing of fingers and hyperglobulinemia and may cause secondary amyloidosis.

Common bacteria cultured from bronchiectatic cavities include *Staphylococcus aureus*, *Staphylococcus epidermidis*; streptococci of all types, including pneumococci; *Haemophilus influenzae*; enteric gram-negative bacilli; and anaerobes. Several of these organisms can usually be grown at any one time. Rarely, bacteremia may occur.

CHRONIC DIFFUSE INTERSTITIAL LUNG DISEASE

PNEUMOCONIOSES

The term pneumoconiosis literally means "dust in the lungs" and denotes pulmonary disease secondary to inhalation of various inorganic dusts. Changes that occur in the lung vary with the type and amount of dust inhaled, particle size, and the presence of other lung diseases, most importantly those associated with cigarette smoking. Genetic factors play an uncertain role in susceptibility. Some dusts such as coal dust do not evoke a fibrous response (**noncollagenous pneumoconioses**), whereas others such as silica do (**collagenous pneumoconioses**). In some patients, inhalation of several different kinds of dust results in mixed disease (e.g. anthracosilicosis).

There is a variable latent period between exposure to dust and onset of clinical disease that may be as long as 20 - 30 years. Rarely, acute disease develops within weeks after a massive exposure.

Silicosis

Silicosis is caused by inhalation of crystalline silicon dioxide (silica) dust particles in the range of 1 -5 μm. Silica exists in nature as quartz, chrystobalite, and tridymite. Occupations at increased risk for silicosis are hardrock, gold, tin, and copper mining; sand-blasting; and iron, steel, and granite working. More than 1 million workers in the United States are at risk for developing silicosis. Significant pulmonary disease usually occurs with 10 - 15 years of exposure but may rarely occur after as little as 1 year. Silicotic lesions may be found long after exposure has been terminated.

A. Pathogenesis

Small silica crystals, when inhaled, reach the lung acinus. Larger crystals (>5 μm) are caught in the bronchial mucus layer and wafted upward by the ciliary action to be expelled; particles less than 1 μm remain airborne and are exhaled.

In the alveoli, the silica crystals are phagocytosed by macrophages. Silica is toxic to the internal organelle membranes of the macrophages and causes phagolysosomal disruption, cell death, and liberation of free silica particles. Inflammation and fibrosis follow, leading to formation of a nodule composed of hyalinized collagen around the crystals. Silica crystals are also carried in lymphatics to the hilar lymph nodes, where similar silicotic nodules form. One hypothesis suggests that fibrosis is the result of a fibroblast-stimulating factor liberated by macrophages upon phagocytosis of silica particles. A second hypothesis attributes fibrosis to a lymphokine produced by silica-activated T lymphocytes.

B. Pathology

Grossly, the silicotic nodule is gray-black (due to

associated carbon pigment), hard, and brittle and has concentric rings of hyalinized collagen in cross section. Nodules are found mainly along lymphatic pathways, especially around the hilum and in the upper lobes. Microscopically, the nodules are composed of a solid mass of macrophages, fibroblasts, and collagen (Figure 7-14). Silica particles are recognized as birefringent needle-shaped crystals in the nodules when examined by polarized light.

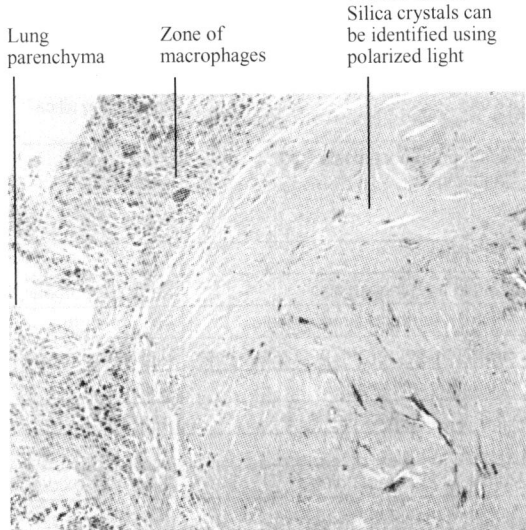

Figure 7-14 Pulmonary silicosis, showing a large fibrotic nodule surrounded by macrophages

C. Clinical Features

Silicosis is often asymptomatic, being found incidentally at chest x-ray or histologic examination of lungs and hilar lymph nodes removed for an unrelated reason. Rarely, when patients are exposed to massive amounts of dust, acute lung disease may occur, with alveolar thickening and accumulation of proteinaceous material in the alveoli (acute silicotic proteinosis). More often, there is chronic pulmonary fibrosis with a mild restrictive ventilatory defect, slowly progressive dyspnea, and pulmonary hypertension (cor pulmonale).

D. Complications

Progressive massive fibrosis may complicate chronic silicosis, particularly when the level of exposure to dust is high. The disorder is characterized by confluence of silicotic nodules into large masses of fibrous tissue that cause obliteration of vessels and bronchioles. Central necrosis and cavitation may occur in these masses as a result of ischemia. Progressive massive fibrosis commonly involves the upper lobes and is associated with a significant ventilatory defect and respiratory failure.

Patients with silicosis have a greatly increased incidence of **tuberculosis**, believed to be due to the adverse effects of silica dust on macrophage function. Tuberculosis causes extensive necrosis in the nodules, and large numbers of tubercle bacilli can be found in such lesions.

Silicosis is also associated with an increased incidence of autoimmune disease, especially progressive systemic sclerosis.

Asbestosis

Asbestos is a fibrous silicate found in nature as the minerals chrysotile, amosite, and crocidolite. It is present in such diverse components of the modern environment as insulation, flame retardants, flooring and roofing materials, water and sewage pipes, and brake linings in vehicles, making low-grade exposure almost universal among urban dwellers.

Asbestos-related disease was first recognized in those with the highest levels of exposure, i.e. workers in shipyards and the construction industry. It is becoming clear, however, that lower levels of exposure are also associated with significant risk. Asbestos-related neoplasms occur in families of shipyard workers - due presumably to the presence in the home of contaminated clothing - and in communities with asbestos-based industries (air pollution by asbestos dust). It is estimated that about 10,000 deaths every year in the United States are due to asbestos-related diseases.

A. Pathology

One of the most common changes associated with asbestos exposure is thickening of the parietal pleura by a plaque-like deposition of hyalinized collagen, maximal in the lateral and diaphragmatic pleura. This change on chest x-ray provides epidemiologic evidence of significant asbestos exposure. Pleural fibrosis does not cause symptoms and does not fall within the definition of asbestos pneumoconiosis because it does not involve lung parenchyma.

Asbestos fibers, when inhaled into the alveoli, are taken up by macrophages and evoke a diffuse interstitial fibrosis. The mechanism of stimulation of pulmonary fibrosis by asbestos is poorly understood. Asbestos, unlike silica, is not cytotoxic to macrophages; there is evidence of activation of macrophages by asbestos. Asbestos, when added to in vitro cultures of fibroblasts, stimulates increased collagen synthesis by these cells. Initially, fibrosis occurs around bronchioles but eventually extends into the alveolar interstitium. Advanced asbestosis causes end-stage fibrosis (honeycomb lung).

Microscopically, asbestos fibers are visible as ferruginous bodies (asbestos bodies) composed of a thin central asbestos fiber 5 – 10 μm long encased in an iron-containing glycoprotein coat which is brown and typically beaded (shish kebab appearance; Figure 7-15). Ferruginous bodies are best seen in sections that have been stained for iron with Prussian blue. While ferruginous bodies are most commonly seen in asbestosis, they are not diagnostic because a similar iron-glycoprotein coat may form on other types of inhaled fibers.

Asbestos fibers that do not have the iron-glycoprotein coat are not visible microscopically, but they outnumber coated fibers 10:1. The amount of asbestos in the lung thus cannot be accurately estimated by microscopy. A quantitative evaluation of asbestos is best made by chemical analysis of lung tissue.

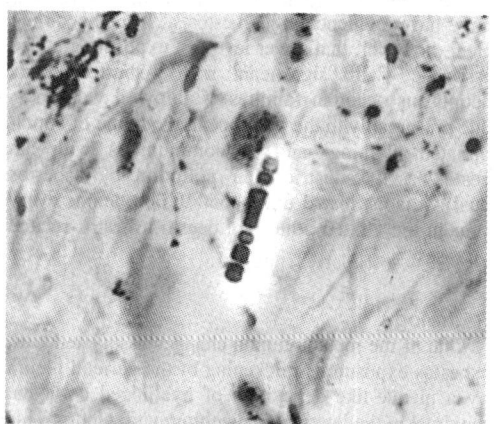

Figure 7-15 Ferruginous body in asbestosis, showing "shish-kebab" appearance of the iron-containing glycoprotein deposit around the linear asbestos fiber. Note that the asbestos fiber at the center of the ferruginous body cannot be seen in routine histologic sections

B. Clinical Features

Asbestos-induced lung disease presents with the features of diffuse interstitial lung disease, i.e. chronic cough, progressive dyspnea, a diffuse infiltrative pattern on chest x-ray, decreased vital capacity with no obstructive element, and blood gas changes of restrictive lung disease (hypoxemia with a normal or reduced arterial Pco_2). Asbestosis rarely causes sufficient lung destruction to result in respiratory failure.

The most significant effect of asbestos exposure is the greatly increased risk of malignant neoplasms. (1) **Bronchogenic carcinoma** is the most common neoplasm associated with asbestosis. Cigarette smoking has a profound additive effect to asbestos exposure in causing bronchogenic carcinoma. (2) **Malignant mesothelioma** of the pleura, peritoneum, and pericardium, although less common than bronchogenic carcinoma, represents the most specific neoplasm associated with asbestos exposure; most patients with malignant mesotheliomas give a history of asbestos exposure. Malignant mesothelioma has a 100% mortality rate, and 90% of patients die within 2 years of diagnosis.

SARCOIDOSIS

Sarcoidosis is a systemic disorder of uncertain cause that is commonly manifested in the lungs. Although the cause is unknown, immunologic mechanisms have been implicated, and abnormalities of the immune system are usually present: (1) **Depressed cell mediated immunity** is manifested by decreased numbers of T cells in the peripheral blood and by anergy (failure of delayed hypersensitivity to antigens injected in intradermal skin tests), (2) **Exaggerated T helper cell activity at sites of disease**, associated with the formation of epithelioid cell granulomas. (3) **Hyperactive humoral immunity** is probably the result of removal of T suppressor activity. There is an increased number of B lymphocytes in the peripheral blood, and most patients have hyperimmunoglobulinemia.

A. Pathology

The hallmark of sarcoidosis is the presence of small, noncaseating epithelioid cell granulomas (Figure 7-16). The granulomas contain Langhans-type giant cells and are associated with fibrosis. Several types of inclusions may be present, but although characteristic of sarcoidosis they are not pathognomonic. Schaumann (conchoidal) bodies are round, calcified, laminated bodies in the cytoplasm of giant cells. Asteroid bodies are smaller and have a central pink zone surrounded by a clear halo that is traversed by fine radial pink lines.

In the lung, granulomas are found in the alveolar

septa (Figure 7-16) and along the pulmonary lymphatics in the bronchial wall. Granulomas are associated with interstitial inflammation and fibrosis. Chronic disease progresses to end-stage honeycomb lung. Granulomas may also be found in lymph nodes, liver, spleen, skin, and many other organs.

The diagnosis of sarcoidosis, is made on clinical grounds. A finding of noncaseating epithelioid granulomas on histologic examination of biopsies provides confirmatory evidence when cultures of these tissues do not grow out mycobacteria and fungi. The cells in the granuloma release angiotensin-converting enzyme into the serum; the detection of elevated levels of this enzyme in serum (seen in 60% of patients) is a useful test for sarcoidosis. High serum levels of angiotensin-converting enzyme indicate activity of sarcoidosis and, when present, provide an important method of monitoring the course of disease.

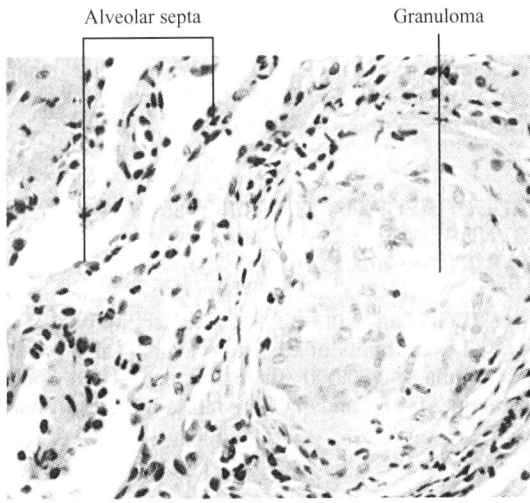

Figure 7-16 Lung in sarcoidosis, showing noncaseating epithelioid cell granuloma in the alveolar septum

B. Clinical Features

Women are more commonly affected, and the most common age at onset is between 20 and 35 years.

An abnormality in the chest x-ray is present in over 90% of patients with sarcoidosis. Bilateral hilar lymphadenopathy is the most common finding. Pulmonary infiltrates due to interstitial pneumonitis may also be present.

Sarcoidosis has a variable course. About 65% of patients with hilar adenopathy alone undergo spontaneous remission. Pulmonary parenchymal involvement usually signifies progressive chronic disease.

Disability and death from pulmonary fibrosis occur in a minority of patients. Steroids are effective in controlling the disease and are indicated when there is symptomatic lung involvement, ocular lesions, cardiac disease, or neurologic disease.

PULMONARY VASCULAR DISORDERS

ACUTE RESPIRATORY DISTRESS SYNDROME (ARDS; "SHOCK LUNG")

ARDS is an acute diffuse alveolar injury that is caused by a variety of etiologic factors. The mortality rate is about 50%.

A. Pathogenesis

The mechanisms by which ARDS occurs are complex and varied. In patients with hypovolemic shock, the acute alveolar injury is secondary to the prolonged vasoconstriction that occurs as a compensatory phenomenon; the vasoconstriction results in ischemic injury to the alveolar epithelium. In gram-negative bacteremia, alveolar damage is caused by endotoxins, which stimulates release of tumor necrosis factor by alveolar macrophages and activates complement. These and other mediators are chemotactic to neutrophils and cause endothelial and alveolar epithelial cell necrosis. In acute pancreatitis, the acute alveolar injury is caused by enzymes liberated into the bloodstream from the injured pancreas. These phospholipases damage alveolar epithelium and antagonize the action of surfactant. With toxic gas inhalation, the alveolar damage is direct; with oxygen at toxic levels, the damage is caused by oxygen-based free radicals.

B. Pathology

ARDS is characterized by acute diffuse alveolar damage leading to necrosis and loss of type I pneumocytes. Endothelial damage also occurs, leading to exudation of protein-rich fluid into the alveoli and resulting in pulmonary edema, hemorrhage, and formation of hyaline membranes. Hyaline membranes are composed of a pink proteinaceous material that lines the alveoli in any condition where there is acute loss of alveolar lining epithelium. They are composed of fibrin together with coagulated cell debris from necrotic cells.

Grossly, the lungs are purple, heavy, and solid. Hemorrhagic fluid exudes from the cut surface.

If the patient recovers, the alveolar epithelium regenerates, initially with hyperplasia of the type II pneumocytes. Residual interstitial fibrosis is present in severe cases.

C. Clinical Features

Patients with ARDS are often seriously ill with some other disease, and the features of ARDS are superimposed. The respiratory symptoms of ARDS are rapidly increasing dyspnea, hypoxemia, and cyanosis. These usually occur 1 - 2 days after the onset of acute injury or disease that has become complicated by ARDS. Chest x-ray shows diffuse interstitial or alveolar edema but may be normal in the early stages. ARDS is commonly the terminal event in many of these patients. Where the underlying cause is reversible, the recognition of ARDS and its aggressive management may reduce the frequency of death.

PULMONARY HYPERTENSION

Pulmonary hypertension is elevation of the mean pulmonary arterial pressure. Most patients with pulmonary hypertension have a recognizable cause for the elevated pressure (**secondary pulmonary hypertension**). In a small number of patients, there is no recognizable cause; this is called **primary (idiopathic) pulmonary hypertension** and occurs mainly in young women in the second and third decades. Primary pulmonary hypertension is frequently associated with immunologically mediated collagen diseases such as rheumatoid arthritis. The pathogenesis of primary pulmonary hypertension is unknown. An intrinsic abnormality of the pulmonary vasculature is the most likely cause.

A. Pathology

The pathologic features of both primary and secondary pulmonary hypertension are similar. There is fibrous thickening of pulmonary arteries of all sizes, with medial hypertrophy and atherosclerosis in the large pulmonary arteries. Atherosclerosis occurs in the pulmonary circulation only in patients with pulmonary hypertension. Abnormal plexiform arteriolar structures may be present in the lungs.

B. Clinical Features

The elevated mean pulmonary arterial pressure causes **right ventricular hypertrophy** and a loud pulmonary valve closure sound with increased separation from the sound of aortic valve closure (split S_2). Pulmonary valve closure is delayed because right ventricular output is prolonged. **Right ventricular failure** with peripheral edema ensues and is the common presenting feature.

Primary pulmonary hypertension is irreversible and slowly progressive. Few patients survive 10 years after diagnosis. In some, disease progression is more rapid. In patients with secondary pulmonary hypertension, treatment of the cause - e.g. surgical replacement of a diseased mitral valve - if it is undertaken early enough, may halt progression of the hypertension.

CHRONIC COR PULMONALE

Chronic cor pulmonary is most frequently secondary to structural cardiopulmonary conditions that increase pulmonary conditions that increase pulmonary blood flow or pressure (or both), pulmonary vascular resistance, or left heart resistance to blood flow. All the above mechanisms lead to cor pulmonary or heart failure caused by respiratory disease, which is manifested by pulmonary hypertension and right ventricular hypertrophy.

A. Etiology and Pathogenesis

Chronic obstructive pulmonary disease, including chronic bronchitis, emphysema, asthma, bronchiectasis, the pneumoconiosis, may lead to cor pulmonale. These entities produce pulmonary hypertension, in part simply through destruction of portions of the pulmonary vascular bed, which results in increased flow through the remaining vessels, and in part through the vasoconstrictive effects of hypoxemia and respiratory acidosis.

Uncommonly, chronic cor pulmonale is caused by disorders affecting chest movement that interfere with normal ventilation, e.g., severe kyphoscoliosis, poliomyelitis, the muscular dystrophies and the Pickwickian syndrome. Presumably these act through pulmonary vasoconstriction induced by the hypoxemia and acidosis that they produce.

Abnormalities of the pulmonary vasculature are a less frequent cause of chronic cor pulmonale. Paramount in this category are multiple or large pulmonary emboli and primary pulmonary hypertension.

Less commonly, disorders inducing pulmonary arteriolar constriction cause cor pulmonale, e.g. metabolic acidosis and hypoxemia.

It is apparent that the common denominator in all

the previously mentioned disorders is pulmonary hypertension. In general, chronic cor pulmonale is asymptomatic until right-sided congestive heart failure ensues.

B. Pathology

The presence of many organizing or recanalized thrombi favors recurrent pulmonary emboli as the cause, and the coexistence of diffuse pulmonary fibrosis, or severe emphysema and chronic bronchitis, points to chronic hypoxia as the initiating event.

The arterioles and small arteries (40 to 300 mm in diameter) are most prominently affected, with striking increases in the muscular thickness of the media (media hypertrophy), muscularization of arterioles and intimal fibrosis, sometimes narrowing the lumina to pinpoint channels. Myocytes of the right ventricle develop hypertrophy with enlarged and deep-staining nucleus.

The right ventricle is thickened with an accompanying increase in the weight of the heart. The right ventricular wall may reach a thickness of more than 1.5cm, and the weight of the heart may be increased to 500 to 700 gm. The thickness of the right ventricular wall exceeding 0.5cm (normal 0.3 - 0.4 cm) under the pulmonary artery valve 2cm is the diagnostic criterion of chronic cor pulmonary in pathology. It may achieve virtually the same dimensions as the left ventricle. When ventricular failure develops, the right ventricle and atrium may also be dilated.

C. Clinical Features

In general, chronic cor pulmonale is asymptomatic until right-sided congestive heart failure ensues. Clinical signs and symptoms include congestion, ascitis, and edema of lower extremities and palpitation or pulmonary encephalopathy. Until then, the picture is usually dominated by the primary disorder.

NEOPLASMS

CARCINOMA OF THE NASOPHARYNX

Nasopharyngeal carcinoma (NPC) represents a morphologic spectrum of neoplasms localized to the nasopharynx and arising from nasopharyngeal epithelium. Nasopharyngeal carcinomas have rather unique clinical, epidemiologic, pathologic, and biologic features. It shows a distinct racial and geographical distribution and a multifactorial etiology. There are certain populations for which the incidence is considerably higher, notably native and foreign-born Chinese, Southeast Asians (e.g. in Thailand, Philippines, and Vietnam), North Africans (e.g. in Algeria and Morocco). The highest incidence of NPC has long been observed in Hong Kong, Guangdong and Guangxi Provinces. NPC incidence rises after the age of 30 years and peaks at 40 - 60 years, and thereafter declines. Rate has a male predilection of about 2 - 3 to 1.

A. Etiology

The specific geographical and demographic distribution of nasopharyngeal carcinoma (NPC), the time trends, and patterns observed in migrants reflect the interplay of infection by Epstein-Barr virus (EBV), genetic susceptibility, and environmental factors in disease causation.

The near constant association of EBV with NPC, irrespective of ethnic background, indicates a probable oncogenic role of the virus in the genesis of this tumor. The incidence includes: (1) raised level of antibodies, especially IgA, against EBV (most commonly viral capsid antigen and early antigen) in most patients with NPC compared with normal controls and patients with other cancer types; (2) higher titers of IgA antibodies against EBV in patients with large tumor bulk; (3) presence of EBV DNA or RNA in practically all tumor cells; (4) presence of EBV in a clonal episomal form, indicating that the virus has entered the tumor cell before clonal expansion; (5) presence of EBV in the precursor lesion of NPC, but not in the normal nasopharyngeal epithelium. Positive serology against Epstein-Barr virus (EBV) is found in close to 100% of patients with non-keratinizing NC. IgA against viral capsid antigen (VCA) and IgG/IgA against early antigens (EA) are the most extensively used diagnostic tool.

B. Pathology

Grossly, the nasopharynx may show fullness or surface granularity, or may reveal an obvious carcinoma, taking the form of nodular, cauliflower, and infiltrative or ulcerative types.

The histological subtypes of nasopharyngeal carcinoma are nonkeratinizing carcinoma, keratinizing squamous cell carcinoma and basaloid squamous cell carcinoma.

Nonkeratinizing comprises solid sheets, irregular

islands, dyscohesive sheets and trabeculae of carcinoma intimately intermingled with variable numbers of lymphocytes and plasma cells. Nonkeratinizing carcinoma is subclassified into the undifferentiated and differentiated subtypes. The undifferentiated subtype, which is more common, is characterized by syncytical-appearing large tumor cells with indistinct cell borders, round to oval vesicular nuclei, and large central nucleoli.

Keratinizing squamous cell carcinoma is an invasive carcinoma showing obvious squamous differentiation. The degree of differentiation can be further graded as: well differentiated (most common), moderately differentiated and poorly differentiated.

Basaloid squamous cell carcinoma has two components, basaloid and squamous cells.

C. Clinical Features

About half of the patients have multiple symptoms, but 10% are asymptomatic. Painless enlargement of upper cervical lymph node is the most common presenting feature. Nearly half of the patients complain of nasal symptoms, particularly blood stained post-nasal drip. Headache and symptoms related to cranial nerve involvement are features of more advanced disease. Obstruction of the opening of the auditory tube may result in otitis media. Only rarely is the primary tumor responsible for early symptoms.

CARCINOMA OF THE LARYNX

A. Incidence and Etiology

Squamous carcinoma is the most common malignant neoplasm of the larynx. Most cases occur after the age of 50 years. Men are affected 7 times more frequently than women. Cigarette smoking and exposure to asbestos have a statistical association with laryngeal carcinoma.

B. Pathology

Laryngeal carcinomas are classified anatomically as (1) glottic, arising in the vocal cord; (2) supraglottic, arising in the aryepiglottic folds and epiglottis; and (3) subglottic, below the vocal cords.

Laryngeal carcinoma often begins as an area of squamous epithelial dysplasia progressing to carcinoma in situ before invasive carcinoma occurs. The noninvasive lesions appear as white areas of thickened plaque-like mucosa. Invasion is associated with nodularity and ulceration.

Microscopically, the majority are well-differentiated squamous carcinomas. A highly differentiated form of squamous carcinoma is characterized by a wart-like exophytic growth pattern with little invasion. This type, called verrucous carcinoma, is successfully treated by surgery.

C. Clinical Features

Laryngeal carcinoma commonly presents with hoarseness, and it is a good rule that carcinoma must be excluded in any patient with persistent hoarseness. Large masses may cause respiratory obstruction and hemoptysis. Metastasis to cervical lymph nodes occurs early. Distant metastases occur late. Diagnosis is diagnosed by laryngoscopy and biopsy. Surgical removal of laryngeal carcinoma is highly successful when the patient has an early neoplasm restricted to the vocal cord. When there is subglottic or supraglottic extension, total laryngectomy and removal of cervical lymph nodes is frequently necessary, and survival rates are considerably reduced. Radiation therapy is effective because squamous carcinoma is a radiosensitive neoplasm.

CARCINOMA OF THE LUNG (BRONCHOGENIC CARCINOMA)

Lung tumor may be primary or secondary. Over 90% of primary lung tumors are carcinoma. Primary tumors other than carcinomas are rare. They can be classified as: benign, e.g. papilloma, alveolar adenoma; malignant, e.g. sarcomas, lymphomas. Secondary tumors are the commonest form of lung neoplasm. With more than 1.1 million deaths annually worldwide, lung cancer is the most frequent and one of the most deadly cancer types.

Incidence

Lung carcinoma is one of the major problems of modern society. The incidence has increased markedly since 1950 (approximately fivefold) and continues to increase. With more than 1.1 million deaths annually worldwide, lung cancer is the most frequent and one of the most deadly cancer types. In men, 85%–90% of cases can be attributed to tobacco smoking. Lung cancer ranks as the commonest lethal cancer in the big cities in China.

Lung carcinoma is more common in males; the

males: female ratio was 7:1 in 1960 but has fallen to about 2:1. Lung cancer has overtaken breast cancer as the leading cause of death by cancer in women. It is a disease of older individuals, being rare under 40 years of age.

Etiology

A. Cigarette Smoking

Cigarette smoking is the main cause of lung carcinoma. Heavy cigarette smokers (over 40 cigarettes a day) have a 20-fold increase in incidence compared to nonsmokers. Cessation of smoking decreases the risk: 10 years after stopping smoking, the risk falls to that of a nonsmoker. The risk is only slightly less with "low-tar" filter cigarettes. Cigar smoking and pipe smoking carry a much lower risk (probably because of less smoke inhalation).

The mechanism by which smoking causes lung carcinoma is not clear. A large number of potent carcinogens are present in cigarette smoke, including polycyclic hydrocarbons, aromatic amines, and heavy metals such as nickel. Any or all of these may be involved in human carcinogenesis.

Cigarette smoking produces changes in the respiratory epithelium of humans. There is loss of cilia and progression from squamous metaplasia through all degrees of dysplasia to carcinoma in situ. Squamous metaplasia alone is not premalignant, but dysplasia is. Dysplasia is very uncommon in nonsmokers. In patients with lung carcinoma, the respiratory epithelium away from the neoplasm frequently shows dysplasia and carcinoma in situ.

Cigarette smoking is most strongly associated with squamous carcinoma and small cell undifferentiated carcinoma and to a lesser degree with adenocarcinoma.

B. Industrial Carcinogens

The best-known occupational lung carcinogen is asbestos, exposure to which increases the risk of lung carcinoma as documented among World War II shipyard workers. The risk of lung cancer following asbestos exposure is compounded by cigarette smoking.

Mining of many different heavy metals (e.g. uranium, nickel, chromate, gold) is also associated with an increased risk of lung cancer.

C. Radiation

Historically, the miners of Schneeberg in Germany were described as developing "mountain sickness" for 4 centuries before it was realized that the sickness was lung carcinoma from exposure to natural radioactive elements in the mines.

D. Urban Pollution

The common urban pollutants are ozone and oxides of nitrogen and sulfur. While there is great concern, most studies to date have failed to demonstrate a significant association between lung carcinoma and urban pollutants.

E. "Scar Cancer"

There is a slightly increased incidence of lung carcinoma - especially peripherally located adenocarcinoma - in areas of scarring due to prior infarcts, granulomas, or diffuse fibrosis.

F. Molecular Genetics

Evidence has accumulated for stepwise accumulation of genetic changes in all major histological types of lung cancers. These changes include allelelic losses (LOH), chromosomal instability and imbalance, mutations in oncogenes and tumor suppressor genes, epigenetic gene silencing through promoter hypermethylation and aberrant of expression of genes involved in the control of cell proliferation. There is a role for dominant oncogenes include c-myc in small cell carcinomas and K-ras in adenocarcinomas. The most frequent one is mutation in the tumor suppressor gene TP53, and the second most common alteration is inactivation of the pathway controlling RB1 (retinoblastoma gene, 13q11), and the third common genetic event that occurs in all lung cancer irrespective of their histological type is LOH on chromosome 3p.

Classification (Figures 7-17 and 7-18)

The International Classification of Lung Carcinoma introduced by the World Health Organization recognizes four major and several minor types.

A. Squamous Cell Carcinoma

Squamous carcinoma arises from the bronchial epithelium. It is characterized by marked cytologic pleomorphism, intercellular bridges (desmosomes) between tumor cells, and keratinization of the cytoplasm (Figure 7-18A). Squamous carcinoma has a strong male predominance, is strongly associated with cigarette smoking, and accounts for 25% - 35% of all lung cancers. There may be a preceding phase of dysplasia and carcinoma in situ. Squamous carcinoma tends to remain localized more than the other types, resulting in large masses in the lung. Central cavitation is common.

B. Small Cell Carcinoma

Small cell carcinoma is composed of small round to oval cells with scant cytoplasm, a high nuclear: cytoplasmic ratio, and hyperchromatic nuclei that do not have prominent nucleoli (Figure 7-18C). Small cell carcinoma is believed to arise from neuroendocrine cells in the bronchial mucosa (Figure 7-17); it stains positively with neuroendocrine immunologic markers such as chromogranin and neuron-specific enolase and has neurosecretory granules in the cytoplasm on electron microscopy. Small cell carcinoma is highly malignant. Bloodstream metastasis occurs early in the course of the neoplasm.

Small cell carcinomas account for 10%-25% of lung carcinomas and are strongly associated with smoking. They are more common in males. They almost always occur in the large bronchi near the hilum of the lung (Figure 7-19).

C. Adenocarcinoma

Adenocarcinoma of the lung, as elsewhere, shows glandular differentiation or secretion of mucin by the tumor cells, showing acinar, papillary, bronchioloalveolar or solid with mucin growth pattern or a mixture of these patterns (Figure 7-18B). Several different forms of adenocarcinoma are recognized: (1) adenocarcinoma arising centrally in large bronchi, (2) adenocarcinoma arising in peripheral scars in the lungs (scar carcinoma), and (3) bronchioloalveolar carcinoma arising in small bronchioles or alveoli, probably from the surfactant-producing Clara cells or from type II pneumocytes. The tumor cells typically line intact alveoli, producing a striking histologic appearance (Figure 7-18B). Bronchioloalveolar carcinoma may be solitary (good prognosis) or multiple (bad prognosis). The histologic appearance of bronchioloalveolar carcinoma may be mimicked by metastatic adenocarcinoma, especially from the pancreas or ovary. Adenocarcinoma constitutes 25%-35% of lung carcinomas, has an equal sex incidence, and is associated with cigarette smoking although not as strongly as squamous carcinoma and small cell carcinoma.

D. Large Cell Carcinoma

This tumor type comprises 5%-20% of lung carcinomas and is composed of large cells that show no squamous or glandular differentiation on light microscopy. In some cases, immunohistochemical or electron microscopic examination is able to detect early glandular, squamous, or neuroendocrine differentiation. Pleomorphic giant cell carcinoma is a highly malignant variant with numerous multinucleated giant cells.

E. Adenosquamous Carcinoma

A carcinoma showing components of both squamous cell carcinoma and adenocarcinoma. The cell of origin is believed to be a pluripotential bronchial reserve cell.

F. Sarcomatoid Carcinoma

A group of poorly differentiated non-small cell lung carcinoma that contain a component of sarcoma or sarcoma-like (spindle and/or giant cell) differentiation. Five subgroups representing a morphologic continuum are currently recognized: pleomorphic carcinoma, spindle cell carcinoma, giant cell carcinoma, carcinosarcoma and pulmonary blastoma.

Pathology

Three distinct gross types of lung carcinoma can be distinguished.

A. Central (Bronchogenic) Carcinoma (75%)

Central carcinomas arise in the first-, second-, or third-order bronchi near the hilum of the lung (Figure 7-19) and tend to be hidden in chest x-rays during their early growth phase. They can, however, be seen and biopsied at an early stage by bronchoscopy. All histologic types occur, but the majority are squamous or small cell carcinomas.

The earliest clearly malignant lesion is carcinoma in situ, which on bronchoscopy may produce no visible change or simply a plaque-like mucosal thickening. However, cytologic examination of sputum shows malignant cells. The term occult carcinoma is used when sputum cytology shows malignant cells and no tumor can be found by radiography and bronchoscopy.

From its mucosal origin, the neoplasm grows into the bronchial lumen (causing ulceration, bleeding, or obstruction) and infiltrates the bronchial wall and adjacent lung parenchyma. Infiltration tends to occur very early. Rarely, tumor growth is mainly endobronchial; in most cases, there is extensive invasion of the bronchial wall and lung parenchyma, forming a large hilar mass with areas of necrosis and hemorrhage.

B. Peripheral Lung Carcinoma (25%)

Peripheral carcinomas arise in relation to small bronchi, bronchioles, or alveoli. These neoplasms are visible on chest x-ray at an early stage as a circumscribed mass but cannot be seen by bronchoscopy.

Peripheral lung carcinomas tend to be adenocarcinomas and, less commonly, squamous carcinomas. Small cell carcinoma rarely occurs in the periphery.

C. Diffuse Type (rare)

On gross examination, this type appears as a diffuse infiltrate of military nodules indistinguishable from lobar pneumonia or tuberculosis.

Early lung cancer can be defined as follows: The diameter of the tumor is below 2 cm; tumor confined to the wall of a bronchus or infiltrate to the bronchial wall and the surrounding tissues; no lymph node metastasis present.

Occult lung cancer refers to both clinical and x-ray examinations are negative, but cytology of sputum smears shows cancer cells, biopsy or surgical materials are certified as in situ carcinoma or early infiltrating carcinoma without lymph node metastasis.

Spread of Lung Carcinoma (Figure 7-20)

A. Local Invasion

With central lung carcinomas, invasion involves vital mediastinal structures such as the superior vena cava and pericardium. Peripheral lung carcinomas tend to extend locally in the lung, with involvement of the pleura occurring early.

B. Lymphatic Metastasis

Lymphatic metastasis to lymph nodes occurs early in all types of lung carcinoma, most commonly in small cell undifferentiated carcinoma and least frequently in well-differentiated squamous carcinoma. Involvement of the hilar and scalene lymph nodes (Figure 7-20) is present in 50% of cases at presentation.

Retrograde permeation of pleural lymphatics (pleural lymphatic carcinomatosis) occurs in advanced lesions, leading to multiple pleural nodules, pleural effusion, and a typical reticular appearance on chest x-ray.

C. Bloodstream Metastasis

Hematogenous metastasis also occurs early, and patients with lung carcinoma frequently present with a distant metastasis. In small cell undifferentiated carcinoma, distant metastases are almost invariably present at the time of diagnosis. Hematogenous metastases occur later in the course of non-small cell carcinomas.

Common sites of metastasis of lung carcinoma are the adrenals (50%), liver (30%), brain (20%), bone (20%), and kidneys (15%).

Clinical Features (Figure 7-20)

The earliest symptoms of bronchogenic carcinoma are cough, hemoptysis, dyspnea, chest pain, and weight loss. Unfortunately, these occur at a relatively advanced stage. A minority of cases of lung carcinoma are detected at an asymptomatic stage by routine chest x-ray.

A. Bronchial Obstruction

A few patients with central lesions present with features of bronchial obstruction, including unresolving pneumonia, lung abscess, and bronchiectasis.

B. Local Invasion

Patients with lung carcinoma may also have symptoms due to local invasion of nearby structures by the neoplasm. Direct invasion of the pleura and pericardium results in pleural and pericardial effusion. The finding of carcinoma cells in aspirated effusion fluid is one method of diagnosis of lung carcinoma. Involvement of the thoracic duct at the lung hilum may result in chylothorax, and superior vena caval obstruction causes edema and congestion of the face and brain (superior vena caval syndrome). Large hilar neoplasms may invade the esophagus, causing dysphagia and tracheoesophageal fistula.

C. Pancoast's Syndrome

This is a specific clinical presentation of lung carcinoma resulting from an apical lung carcinoma (usually squamous) that invades the apical pleura. The tumor causes destruction of the T1 intercostal nerve and leads to a T1 motor and sensory deficit - weakness and wasting of small muscles of the hand and numbness on the medial side of the arm - and the cervical sympathetic trunk, causing Horner's syndromeptosis of the eyelid, pupillary constriction, and absent sweating on the side of the lesion.

D. Distant Metastases

A significant number of patients with lung carcinoma

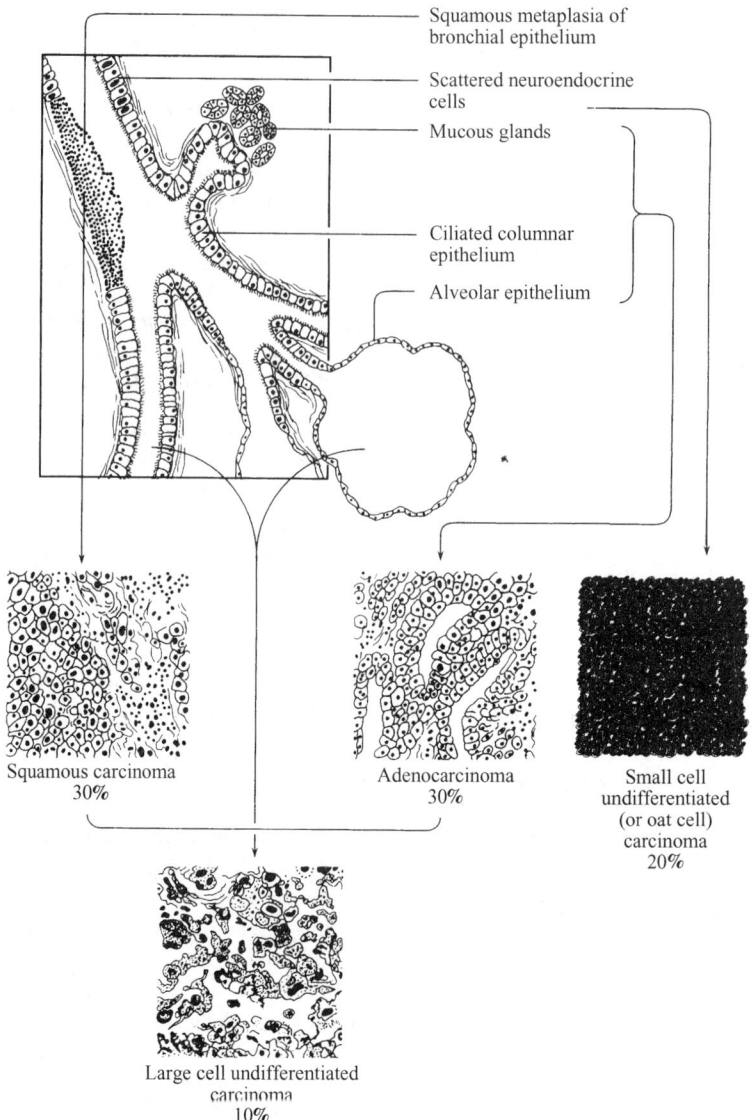

Figure 7-17 Histogenetic classification of bronchogenic lung carcinoma mixed histologic types are present in the remaining 10% of lung carcinomas

present with evidence of lymph node or hematogenous metastases. Cervical lymph node enlargement, pathologic fractures due to bone metastasis, and brain masses are common presenting features.

E. Paraneoplastic Syndromes

A minority of patients presents with a variety of signs or symptoms that cannot be attributed to the direct effects of destruction by primary or metastatic tumors; these conditions are referred to as paraneoplastic syndromes (Table 7-2). These include the effects of secretion of hormones by the neoplasm (ectopic hormone syndromes). The mechanisms that cause many of the other paraneoplastic syndromes are largely unknown, although autoimmune phenomena have been postulated.

Diagnosis

Lung carcinoma must be considered a possibility when a patient presents with any of the protean clinical manifestations described above. This is particularly so if there is a strong smoking history. Chest x-ray and computerized tomography are effective for demonstrating the presence of a mass in the lung, but they do not predict the pathologic diagnosis and

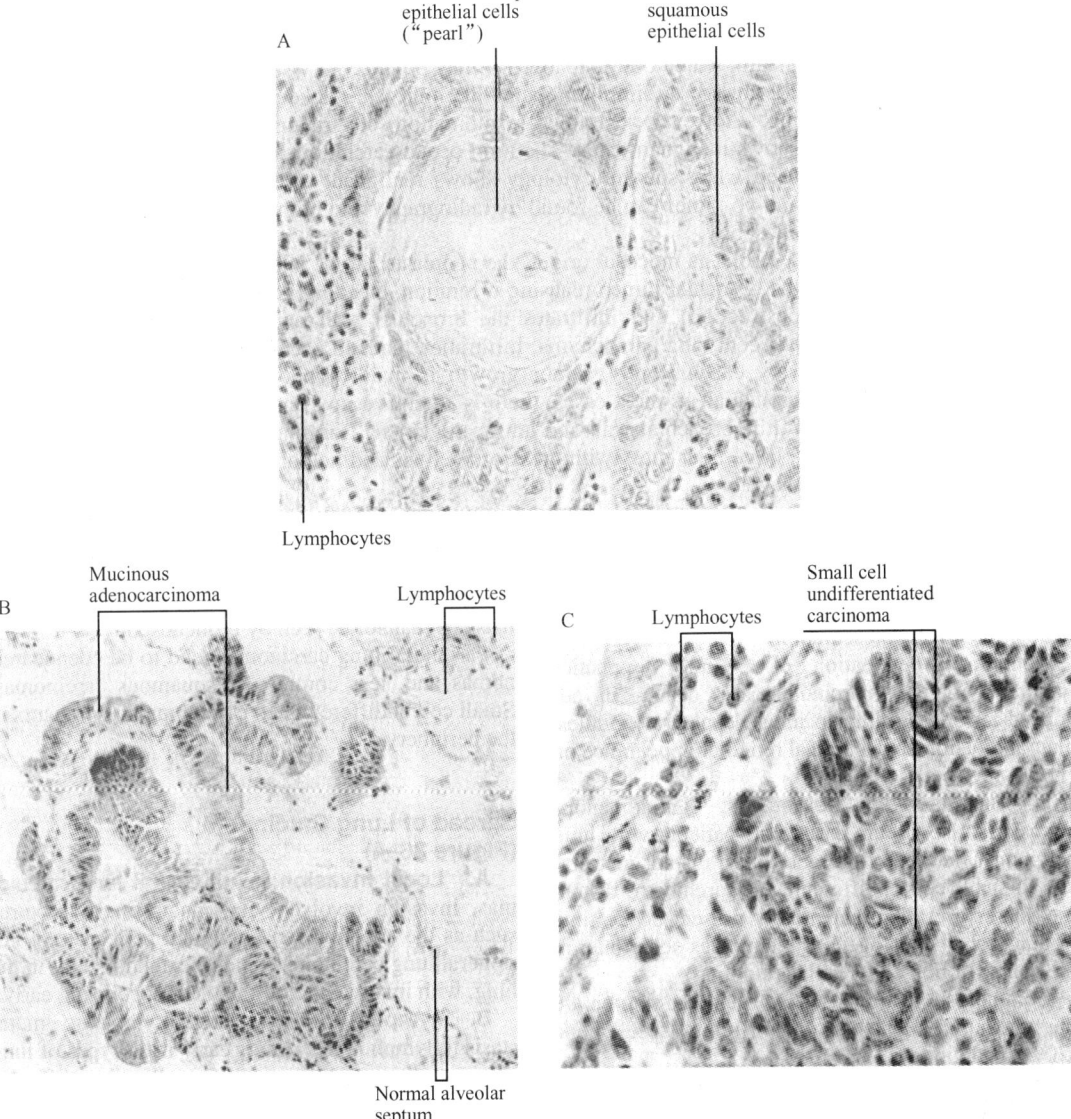

Figure 7-18 Common histologic types of lung carcinoma. A: Squamous carcinoma showing squamous epithelial pearl with keratinization. B: Adenocarcinoma, bronchioloalveolar type, showing malignant glandular epithelium growing along the alveolar basement membrane. C: Small cell undifferentiated (oat cell) carcinoma, showing small oval cells with hyperchromatic nuclei and scant cytoplasm. Note that these pictures are at different magnifications. The best guide to the size of malignant cells is to compare them with lymphocytes present in all three photographs

have a significant failure rate in detection of small hilar lesions.

The diagnosis of lung carcinoma must in every case be substantiated by pathologic examination. In addition to cytologic examination of sputum for malignant cells, bronchoscopy is useful for visualization of central lung cancers, direct biopsy, recovery of brush specimens for cytologic examination, and taking of transbronchial needle biopsies from peripheral lung masses. Percutaneous needle aspiration biopsy may be done under radiologic guidance when a mass lesion is visible on chest x-ray or CT scan. Open lung biopsy may rarely be necessary for diagnosis, especially in peripheral lesions. Biopsy of metastatic lesions in other organs frequently provides the first evidence of a previously undiagnosed lung carcinoma. Aspiration of pleural effusions and biopsy of enlarged cervical lymph nodes and brain masses are examples.

With all of these techniques, both cytologic and histologic examinations provide not only the diagnosis but also the classification of lung carcinoma.

Table 7-2 Paraneoplastic syndromes in lung carcinoma

Ectopic hormone syndromes

    Adenocorticortropic hormone: Small cell carcinoma; causes bilateral adrenal hyperplasia and Cushing's syndrome

    Antidiuretic hormone: Small cell carcinoma; causes hyponatremia

    Parathyroid hormone: Squamous carcinoma; causes hypercacemia

    5-Hydroxytryptamine: Carcinoid syndrome

    Gonadotropins: Gynecomastia

Neuromuscular syndromes

    Peripheral neuropathy

    Myopathy

    Myasthenic syndrome (Eaton-Lambert syndrome)

    Cerebellar degeneration

    Leukoencephalopathy

Others

    Finger clubbing and pulmonary hypertrophic osteoarthropathy

    Dermatomyositis and polymyositis

    Migratory thrombophlebitis

    Skin rashes

DISEASES OF THE PLEURA

PLEURAL EFFUSION

A pleural effusion is a collection of fluid in the pleural cavity. Simple accumulation of small amounts of fluid in the pleural cavity does not cause any symptoms. Large effusions interfere with lung expansion during inspiration, causing a reduction in vital capacity. The presence of a large pleural effusion can be detected clinically by the absence of chest wall movement, shift of mediastinal structures to the opposite side, decreased breath sounds, and dullness to percussion over the effusion. Small pleural effusions cannot be detected clinically and require rad-

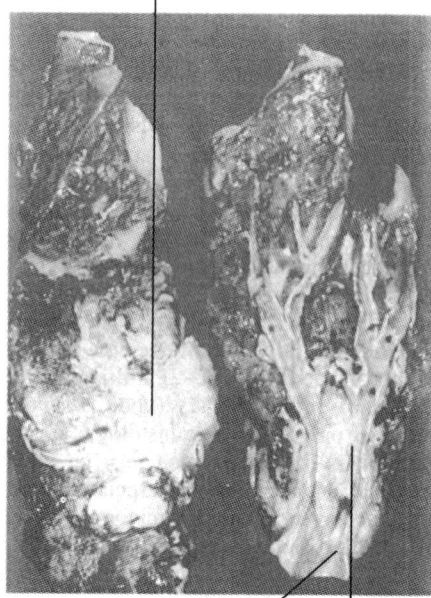

Figure 7-19 Bronchogenic carcinoma, showing the neoplasm in two slices of lung. The lung slice at the right shows the origin of the tumor, seen as an intrabronchial mass; the lung slice at left shows the invasive mass in the adjacent lung

iologic examination. When more than about 300 mL of fluid is present in an adult's pleural cavity, it can be seen on an upright chest x-ray.

Once the presence of an effusion has been established, aspiration of fluid is helpful to identify its cause. Low specific gravity, low protein concentration, and lack of inflammatory cells identify a transudate. Exudates have a specific gravity over 1.015, a protein level of over 1.5 g/dL, and many inflammatory cells. Bacterial infection commonly produces a frankly purulent exudate (empyema). Hemorrhagic exudates occur in malignant effusions, tuberculosis, uremia, and pulmonary infarction. Cytologic examination of effusion sediment for malignant cells is frequently positive when malignant neoplasia is the cause of the effusion.

Pleural biopsy provides a core of pleural tissue for histologic examination and is useful in the diagnosis of tuberculosis or cancer.

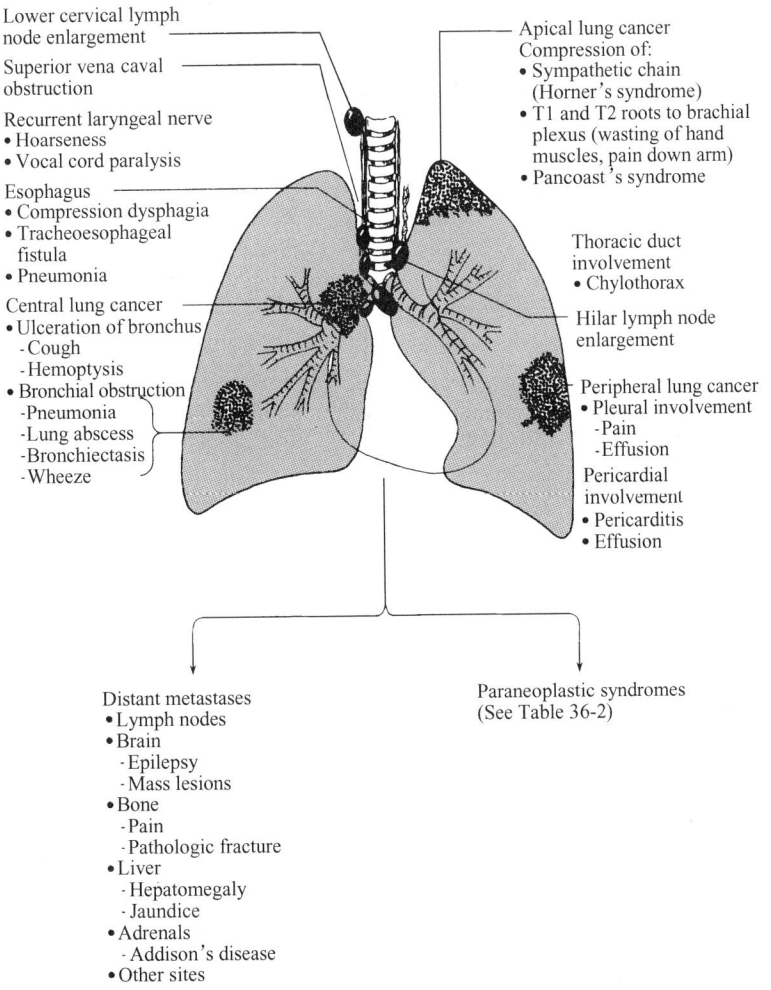

Figure 7-20 Clinical features and spread of lung carcinoma

MALIGNANT MESOTHELIOMA

Malignant mesothelioma is a rare neoplasm strongly related etiologically to asbestos exposure; many cases have occurred in World War II shipyard workers. There is a long lag period (as long as 40 years) between asbestos exposure and tumor development.

Malignant mesothelioma commonly occurs in the over-50 age group. Clinical presentation is with dyspnea and features of pleural effusion. Grossly, the tumor diffusely involves the pleura, encasing large areas of lung as a firm, and grayish, gelatinous mass. Invasion of both lung parenchyma and chest wall occurs frequently. Microscopically, the tumor is biphasic, with a sarcomatoid spindle cell component and epithelial elements that form tubular and papillary structures. When the epithelial component predominates, differentiation from adenocarcinoma may be difficult.

The prognosis is very poor, with 50% of patients dead within 1 year after diagnosis and few survivals of more than 2 years.

Chapter 8 Diseases of the Digestive System

Gan Runliang, Zhang Xianghong

CHAPTER CONTENTS
- Diseases of the Esophagus
    - Structure and Function
    - Inflammatory Lesions of the Esophagus
    - Achalasia of the Cardia
    - Esophageal Diverticula
    - Carcinoma of the Esophagus
- Diseases of the Stomach
    - Structure and Function
    - Inflammatory Lesions of the Stomach
    - Peptic Ulcer Disease
    - Gastric Carcinoma
    - Gastrointestinal Stromal Tumor
- Diseases of the Intestines
    - Structure and Function
    - Congenital Diseases of the Intestine
    - Acute Appendicitis
    - Idiopathic Inflammatory Bowel Disease
    - Colonic Adenoma
    - Carcinoma of the Colon and Rectum
- Diseases of the Liver
    - Structure and Function of the Liver
    - Viral Hepatitis
    - Alcoholic Liver Disease
    - Immunologic Diseases of the Liver
    - Autoimmune Chronic Active Hepatitis
    - Primary Biliary Cirrhosis
    - Cirrhosis of the Liver
    - Neoplasms of the Liver
- Diseases of the Extrahepatic Billary System
    - Structure and Function
    - Cholelithiasis
    - Carcinoma of the Gallbladder
    - Carcinoma of the Bile Ducts
- Diseases of the Exocrine Pancreas
    - Structure and Function of the Pancreas
    - Inflammatory Lesions of the Pancreas
    - Carcinoma of the Pancreas

DISEASES OF THE ESOPHAGUS

STRUCTURE AND FUNCTION

The esophagus is a muscular tube approximately 25 cm long that extends from the neck down the posterior mediastinum and through the diaphragm to the stomach. It is lined by nonkeratinizing stratified squamous epithelium that transforms abruptly to gastric epithelium at the gastroesophageal junction. The junction is usually 37 - 40 cm from the incisor teeth and may be identified endoscopically by a change in appearance from the white squamous mucosa to the tan glandular mucosa.

The esophagus has physiologic high-pressure zones at either end that act as sphincters. There is no anatomic sphincter at either end. The upper cricopharyngeal sphincter prevents entry of air and pharyngeal contents into the esophagus except during swallowing, and the lower esophageal or "cardiac" sphincter prevents reflux into the esophagus of acidic gastric juice.

INFLAMMATORY LESIONS OF THE ESOPHAGUS

Reflux Esophagitis

Reflux of acidic gastric juice into the lower esophagus occurs several times a day even in normal individuals- without producing symptoms or inflammation. Symptomatic esophagitis is believed to occur when there is prolonged exposure of the mucosa to refluxed gastric contents due to (1) excessive reflux, both in number of episodes and volume, resulting from incompetence of the lower esophageal sphincter; and (2) when the normal mechanisms for clearing the lower esophagus are impaired. The composition of the refluxed gastric juice may also be an important determinant of reflux: The levels of acid and pepsin, as well as the presence of bile and pancreatic enzymes refluxed from the duodenum, all may play a part. When bile reflux is present, esophagitis may occur even when the refluxed gastric juice is alkaline (alkaline reflux).

A. Pathology (Figure 8-1)

Reflux esophagitis can be recognized endoscopically as reddening and superficial erosion of the lower esophagus. It may progress to ulceration and fibrous narrowing of the esophagus (stricture).

Histologically, reflux esophagitis is characterized by (1) hyperplasia of the basal cells of the squamous epithelium to more than 15% of mucosal thickness; (2) elongation of lamina propria papillae to more than 70% of mucosal thickness; and (3) the presence of intraepithelial neutrophils and eosinophils. Patients with reflux also show mucosal congestion and inflammation, often severe, in the gastric cardiac mucosa.

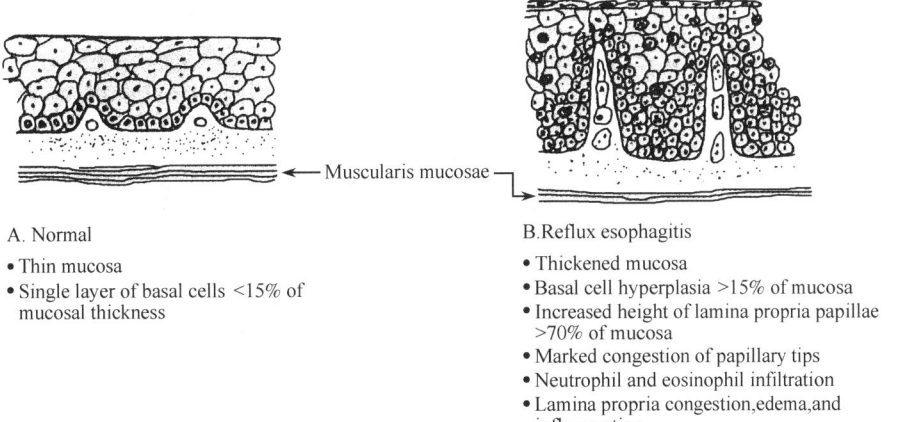

Figure 8-1 Histologic changes in reflux esophagitis (B) compared with normal squamous epithelium lining the esophagus (A)

B. Clinical Features

Reflux of acidic gastric juice into an inflamed esophagus causes a low retrosternal sensation of burning pain (heartburn), typically when the patient lies flat. In chronic cases, pain may be constant and dysphagia may occur as a result of fibrous stricture formation. Reflux into the pharynx occurs in severe cases and may cause spasmodic coughing and hoarseness.

C. Complications

(1) Barrett's esophagus: (Figure 8-2) Prolonged reflux esophagitis commonly leads to metaplasia of the esophageal epithelium from squamous to glandular. Barrett's esophagus is defined as the presence of a glandular mucosa showing intestinal metaplasia. The metaplasia is characterized by the presence of goblet cells and acid mucin on Alcian blue stain, which differentiates intestinal (acid) mucin from gastric (neutral) mucin. Most primary adenocarcinomas of the lower esophagus arise in Barrett's esophagus, which therefore is considered a precancerous lesion. An estimated 5% - 10% of patients with Barrett's esophagus develop adenocarcinoma. (2) Peptic ulceration and fibrous strictures: Severe reflux leads to chronic peptic ulcers in the lower esophagus. Subsequent fibrosis leads to esophageal stricture and dysphagia. (3) Motility abnormality: Prolonged reflux leads to abnormal peristalsis in the lower esophagus. This may decrease esophageal clearing and aggravate reflux disease.

Infectious Esophagitis

Infections are rare in the esophagus except in immunocompromised patients, notably those with AIDS. For example, esophageal candidiasis is one of the common opportunistic infections in patients receiving cancer chemotherapy and those with AIDS. Herpes simplex esophagitis is also common in AIDS patients.

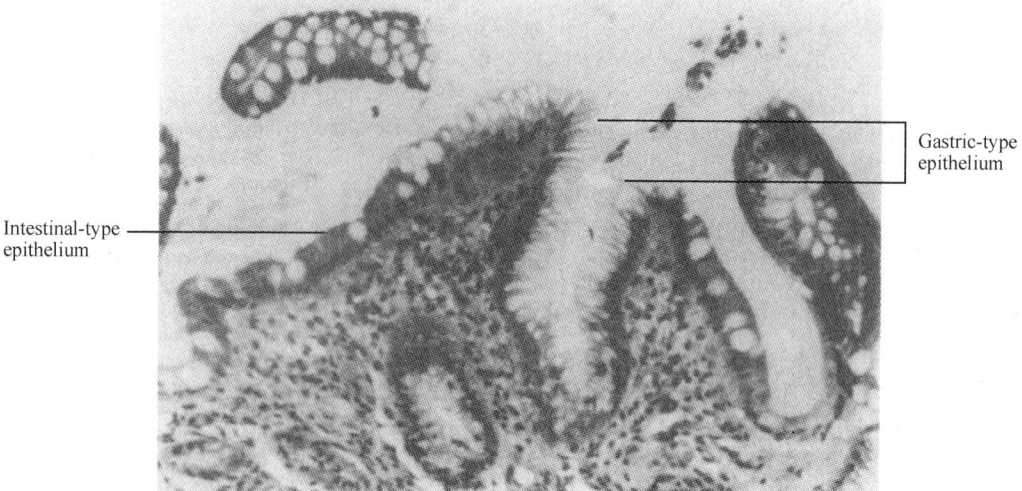

Figure 8-2 Barrett's esophagus, showing the characteristic specialized columnar epithelium composed of a mixture of gastric-and intestinal-type epithelial cells. Note the presence of goblet cells that indicate intestinal metaplasia, the diagnostic criterion for Barrett's esophagus

Traumatic and Chemical Esophagitis

Prolonged feeding through a nasogastric tube frequently causes mucosal inflammation, often with ulceration. Ingestion of corrosives such as phenol, strong acids, and mercuric chloride leads to chemical esophagitis. The strongly alkaline chemical known as lye, which is swallowed in suicide attempts and by unwitting children, causes severe esophagitis with mucosa denudation in the acute phase. Marked fibrous scarring in survivors often requires repeated dilation of the esophagus to overcome resulting obstruction.

ACHALASIA OF THE CARDIA

Achalasia (Greek, unrelaxed) of the cardia (lower esophageal sphincter) is a common disease resulting from loss of ganglion cells in the myenteric plexus of the esophagus. Ganglion cell loss is present throughout the body of the esophagus and is not restricted to the cardia.

The myenteric plexus abnormality leads to failure of propulsive peristaltic waves without which the cardiac sphincter does not relax, creating a zone of high pressure that obstructs the passage of food into the stomach. The esophagus dilates massively above the cardia and becomes elongated and tortuous. The mucosa is usually normal but may show areas of superficial inflammation and ulceration. Patients present with dysphagia. Nutrition is maintained reasonably well. With collection of food in the esophagus, the hydrostatic pressure therein increases and becomes sufficient to physically overcome the sphincter, permitting the intermittent entry of food into the stomach.

An important complication of achalasia is aspiration of the contents of the dilated esophagus into the trachea, leading to recurrent attacks of aspiration pneumonia. Treatment by intraluminal dilation or by surgical myotomy is effective, but many patients need repeated dilations. Achalasia is associated with a slightly increased risk of squamous carcinoma.

ESOPHAGEAL DIVERTICULA

Diverticula (outpouchings of the lumen of a viscus outside the wall of that viscus) are not common, but if large they may cause dysphagia or local inflammation. Pulsion diverticula are believed to occur when internal pressure forces an epithelial sac through a weakened or defective muscle wall. Traction diverticula are due to external inflammatory lesions resulting in fibrosis and traction force that pulls out the full thickness of the esophageal wall as a diverticulum.

CARCINOMA OF THE ESOPHAGUS

A. Incidence

Esophageal carcinoma accounts for over 95% of neoplasms of the esophagus. It is a disease of older people (over 40 years) and is more common in males. Cancer of the esophagus is much more common in China and in certain parts of Asia and Africa. High-risk areas in the world are located in parts of China; the Caspian region of Iran; South Africa; and parts of France. Squamous cell carcinoma remains the most common histologic presentation of esophageal cancer; but in the United States and European countries, the incidence of adenocarcinoma of the lower esophagus associated with Barrett's esophagus (metaplasia) is increasing rapidly.

B. Etiology

The risk factors for esophageal cancer that have been studied extensively include alcohol consumption, tobacco use, and dietary habits. The cause of esophageal cancer in the high-incidence areas of the world is unknown. Hot rice and tea, nitrosamines and aflatoxins in food and water, fungal and mycotoxin contaminants in locally brewed beer and foodstuffs, and smoked fish have all been suggested as causative factors.

A factor of current interest is the possible involvement of HPV. Some esophageal cancers contain HPV in their cells, and viruses of similar subtype can be found in intact and apparently normal esophageal mucosa. It is therefore possible that virus integrated into the host genome can bring about oncogene activation and carcinogenesis.

Many premalignant conditions are associated with an increased risk of esophageal carcinoma. These include lye strictures (squamous carcinoma), Plummer-Vinson syndrome (squamous carcinoma), Barrett's esophagus (adenocarcinoma), and achalasia of the cardia (low risk of squamous carcinoma).

Non-specific chronic esophagitis is common among the general population in high-incidence areas in China, and biopsies will frequently reveal dysplasia. The squamous epithelium shows cellular pleomorphism; there is disordered maturation with immature cells and mitotic activity appearing close to the surface. The degree of atypia can be categorised as low-or high-dysplasia; the latter condition will proceed to invasive carcinoma if surgical resection is not performed.

C. Pathology

Esophageal cancers arise mostly in the middle third of the organ. The early lesion is a plaque-like thickening of the mucosa (Figure 8-3). From its mucosal origin, carcinoma may extend (1) into the lumen as a polypoid, fungating mass that may break down to form a malignant ulcer with raised everted edges (Figure 8-4); (2) transversely in the submucosa, to involve the whole circumference of the esophagus; or (3) into the wall of the esophagus. A marked desmoplastic (fibrotic) response causes fibrosis with esophageal narrowing (malignant stricture). The exact appearance of the carcinoma depends on which of these growth patterns predominates.

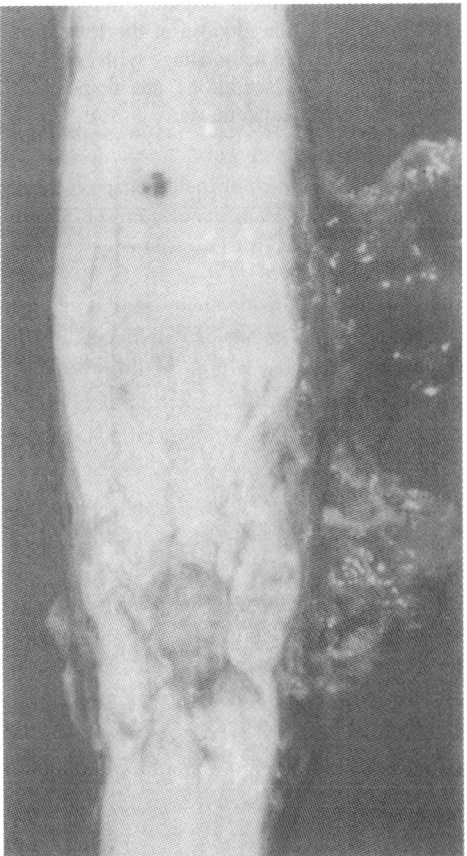

Figure 8-3 Carcinoma of the esophagus, showing ulceration and circumferential involvement of the mucosa

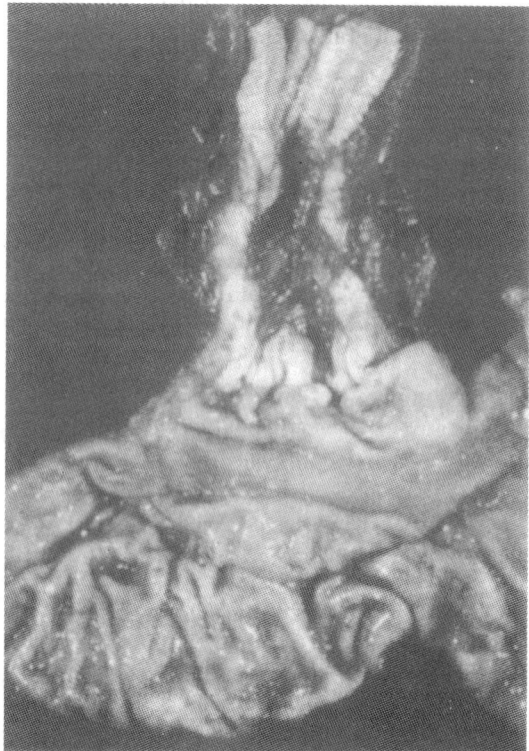

Figure 8-4 Carcinoma of the esophagus, immediately superior to the gastroesophageal junction, showing a large ulcer with everted edges

Microscopically, approximately 90% of esophageal carcinomas are squamous carcinomas in China. Squamous cell carcinomas are usually preceded by a long prodrome of mucosal epithelial dysplasia followed by carcinoma in situ and, ultimately, by the emergence of invasive carcinoma. Adenocarcinoma (arising in Barrett's esophagus) accounts for the rest. Most adenocarcinomas occur in the lower third of the esophagus.

Other rare malignant tumors arising in the esophagus include small-cell carcinoma, primary malignant lymphoma, leiomyosarcoma, and malignant melanoma. However, these tumors are fairly uncommon and account for no more than 1% to 2% of all esophageal cancers.

D. Spread

Local invasion through the esophageal wall to involve adjacent cervical and mediastinal structures occurs early. Invasion of the bronchial wall may rarely result in tracheoesophageal fistula, commonly complicated by necrotizing pneumonia. Invasion of the aorta may lead to massive hemorrhage. Recurrent laryngeal nerve involvement leads to vocal cord paralysis (hoarseness).

Lymphatic spread occurs early, and lymph node metastases are commonly present at the time of diagnosis. Bloodstream spread with metastases to liver and lung also occurs early.

E. Clinical Features and Diagnosis

Most patients present with dysphagia and severe weight loss, and most have large unresectable tumors at this stage. Less often, presentation is with anemia, hematemesis, or melena. The diagnosis is best established by endoscopic visualization of the tumor followed by biopsy.

Regular endoscopic surveillance of patients with Barrett's esophagus is effective in detecting high-grade dysplasia and early cancer.

F. Treatment and Prognosis

Surgery is the primary treatment method. However, many patients with esophageal cancer have unresectable tumors at the time of presentation. The exception is in patients with early cancers detected during surveillance for known Barrett's esophagus. Radiotherapy may cause some regression of tumor. Chemotherapy is not very effective, although new regimens are starting to provide a glimmer of hope.

The overall prognosis is very poor, with 70% of patients dead within 1 year after diagnosis, and about 30% patients surviving after 5 years with surgery treatment. Patients with early cancers restricted to the esophagus that are detected during surveillance for Barrett's esophagus have an excellent prognosis, with over 80% 5-year survival. Often the aim of treatment is palliation to relieve pain and to permit swallowing.

DISEASES OF THE STOMACH

STRUCTURE AND FUNCTION

The stomach lies in the epigastrium and is composed of mucosa, submucosa, a thick muscle layer, and serosa. The mucosa of the stomach is thrown into regular folds, or rugae. The serosa on the lesser and greater curvatures is continuous with the lesser and greater omentum.

The Gastric Mucosa (Figure 8-5)

The epithelial lining of the mucosa is composed of uniform mucous cells without goblet cells. Simple tubular glands open on the surface at epithelial pits. The glands vary in structure in different parts of the stomach: (1) In the cardiac region near the gastroesophageal junction, the glands are composed mainly of mucous cells; (2) in the body and fundus, the glands contain parietal (oxyntic) cells that secrete acid and chief (zymogen, or peptic) cells that secrete pepsin. The parietal cells also probably secrete intrinsic factor; (3) in the pyloric antrum, the glands contain mainly mucous cells.

Neuroendocrine cells are present in the mucosa of the stomach just as they are throughout the remainder of the intestinal tract. These cells are present throughout the mucosa and produce a variety of biogenic amines and peptide hormones. Neuroendocrine cells in the pyloric antral region (G cells) represent the source of gastrin and may be stained by immunohistologic methods using antigastrin antibodies.

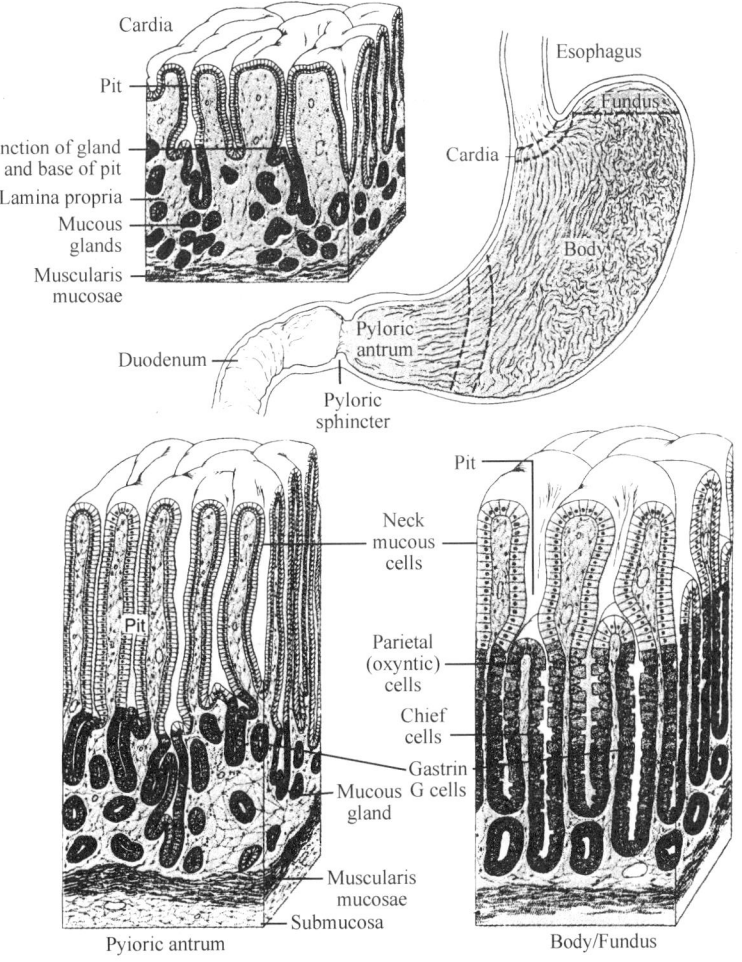

Figure 8-5 Regions of the stomach and their histologic structures

Gastric Mucosal Resistance to Acid

The secretion of acid by the stomach is a continuous process, occurring at a basal rate during fasting periods and increasing markedly in response to a meal.

The gastric mucosa is protected by a variety of mechanisms from the erosive effect of gastric acid:

A. The Anatomic Integrity of the Mucosa

The mucosal cells have a specialized apical surface membrane that resists the diffusion of acid into the cell. Back-diffused hydrogen ions are actively extruded by ionic carrier mechanisms.

B. Gastric Mucus

Mucin and HCO_3^- secreted by surface epithelial cells create a mucous layer that has a pH gradient which is very acid in the lumen to nearly neutral near the cell surface.

C. Prostaglandins (E series)

Prostaglandins are synthesized and secreted by gastric mucosal cells, have a cytoprotective effect on the gastroduodenal mucosa. They act to increase bicarbonate secretion, gastric mucus production, mucosal blood flow, and the rate of mucosal cell regeneration.

D. Mucosal Blood Flow

Ischemia of the mucosa decreases mucosal resistance.

Functions of the Stomach

The main function of the stomach is to serve as a reservoir for meals, presenting food to the duodenum in small regulated amounts. The acid gastric juice contains the proteolytic enzyme pepsin and initiates digestion. The acidity also has an antibacterial action. Simple molecules such as iron, alcohol, and glucose may be absorbed from the stomach.

The stomach has two sphincters. A physiologic sphincter at the cardioesophageal junction prevents reflux of acid gastric contents into the esophagus. The distal or pyloric sphincter is an anatomic thickening of the muscle that controls the rate of gastric emptying and prevents reflux of bile into the stomach.

INFLAMMATORY LESIONS OF THE STOMACH

Acute Erosive Gastropathy

Acute erosive gastropathy is common. It is characterized endoscopically by diffuse hyperemia of the mucosa with multiple small, superficial erosions and ulcers (Figure 8-6). (*Note*: an erosion is a denudation of the surface epithelium with the deep part of the mucosa remaining intact; an ulcer involves the full thickness of the mucosa.) Microscopically, there is surface epithelial injury and denudation and variable necrosis of superficial glands. Hemorrhage may be present in the lamina propria (acute hemorrhagic gastritis). Deep ulceration extending into the wall and resulting in perforation occurs very rarely. Inflammatory cells are not present in large numbers. In the healing phase, the epithelium regenerates rapidly. In some cases, features of regenerative activity dominate (reactive gastropathy).

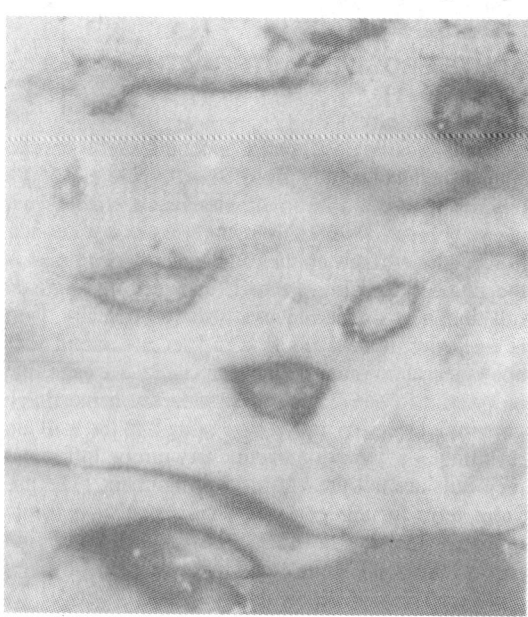

Figure 8-6 Acute erosive gastropathy showing multiple small ulcers in the mucosa

A. Etiology and Pathogenesis

The basic cause of acute erosive gastropathy is damage of the gastric epithelium. Many etiologic agents have been implicated. But in many cases, the mechanism for damage is not known.

1. Drugs

Drugs are the most common cause of acute erosive gastropathy. Nonsteroidal anti-inflammatory drugs (NSAIDs) such as aspirin, ibuprofen, and corticosteroids are the most potent. These probably act by inhibiting prostaglandin synthesis in the mucosa, thus making it more susceptible to acid. Cigarette smoking also inhibits prostaglandin synthesis and tends to aggravate all forms of ulceration, although it is not a primary cause.

2. Luminally acting toxic chemicals

Ethyl alcohol causes acute gastropathy, most commonly after a bout of heavy drinking. The mucosal abnormality in alcoholic "gastritis" is dominated by hemorrhage into the lamina propria. Reflux of bile is believed to be toxic to the gastric mucosa. However, bile reflux commonly occurs in normal people without producing any change in the gastric mucosa. The severe reflux of bile that occurs after partial gastrectomy with removal of the pylorus has been reported to cause gastropathy. Ingestion of corrosives may damage the gastric mucosa, in some cases so extensively as to cause perforation.

3. Stress

Stress of many types causes acute erosive gastropathy. Severe burns (Curling's ulcers), myocardial infarction, intracranial lesions (Cushing's ulcers), and the postoperative period are some of the stressful states associated with gastric erosion. Endogenous corticosteroids may be responsible.

4. Chemotherapy

Chemotherapy, in particular hepatic arterial infusion of cytotoxic drugs, may cause direct mucosal toxicity.

5. Ischemia

Ischemia of the mucosa may be involved in the pathogenesis of erosive gastropathy associated with shock where there is severe vasoconstriction of the splanchnic circulation. Portal hypertension may also cause venous congestion and an element of vascular compromise leading to gastropathy. Gastric antral vascular ectasia caused by antral mucosal prolapse may also result in gastropathy due to vascular compromise.

B. Clinical Features

Mild cases are asymptomatic or associated with mild dyspepsia. Epigastric pain as well as nausea and vomiting occur in moderate to severe cases. Acute gastric hemorrhage causing hematemesis and melena is the most significant symptom; this occurs commonly in cases induced by drugs, stress, shock, and hepatic arterial chemotherapy. In rare cases, hemorrhage can be severe enough to threaten life. Treatment is by withdrawal of the etiologic factor, drug suppression of acid secretion, and supportive fluid care when hemorrhage occurs.

Chronic Gastritis (Table 8-1)

Chronic gastritis is defined histologically as an increase in the number of lymphocytes and plasma cells in the gastric mucosa. The mildest degree of chronic gastritis is chronic superficial gastritis, which involves the subepithelial region around the gastric pits. In the chronic superficial gastritis, there may be some flattening of the mucosa, but it is generally not marked. An inflammatory infiltrate of lymphocytes and plasma cells is typically present within the lamina propria, usually limited to the upper third of the gastric mucosa. More severe cases involve the glands in the deeper mucosa; this is commonly associated with gland atrophy (chronic atrophic gastritis) and intestinal metaplasia. In the chronic atrophic gastritis, the mucosa is more obviously thinned and flattened, with extension of the infiltrate in the lamina propria to the deeper glandular layer. It may appear reddened as the submucosal vessels become more apparent.

Most cases of chronic gastritis are of one of two types – type A, which is an autoimmune gastritis that primarily involves the body and is associated with pernicious anemia; and type B, which primarily involves the antrum and is associated with *Helicobacter pylori* infection (Table 8-1). There are a few cases of chronic gastritis of neither type whose etiology remains unknown.

Table 8-1 Chronic gastritis. Comparison between type A (autoimmune) and type B (antral; *Helicobacter*-associated)

	Type A	Type B
Etiology	Autoimmune	*Helicobacter pylori*
Region most involved	Body and fundus	Pyloric antrum
Endoscopic features	Not distinctive	Not distinctive
Inflammatory cells	Lymphocytes, plasma cells	Lymphocytes, plasma cells, neutrophils
Mucosal atrophy	+	+
Intestinal metaplasia	+	+
Cancer risk	+ +	+
Association with cancer[1]	Low	High
Acid secretion	Decreased or nil	Normal, increased, or decreased
Serum gastrin	Elevated	Usually normal
Endocrine cell hyperplasia	+ +	−
Serum autoantibodies	+ (>90%)	−
Helicobacter pylori infection	−	+ (60%–70%)
Association with peptic ulcers	Ulcers do not occur	High
Serum vitamin B_{12}	Low	Normal
Megaloblastic anemia	+	−

[1] Although the risk of cancer is low in type B gastritis when compared with type A, the high incidence of type B gastritis in the population causes it to be much more frequently associated with gastric cancer than type A chronic gastritis.

A. Type A Chronic Gastritis (*Autoimmune Type Associated with Pernicious Anemia*)

Pernicious anemia results from failure of vitamin B_{12} absorption caused by lack of intrinsic factor due to autoimmune chronic gastritis. The autoimmunity is directed against the parietal cells in the body and fundus of the stomach that secrete both intrinsic factor and acid. Several autoimmune mechanisms exist: (1) a T cell-mediated response against parietal cells, and (2) a humoral response associated with the presence of three different serum autoantibodies that are of diagnostic value: (a) in 90%, antiparietal cell antibody (also called parietal canalicular antibody); (b) in 75%, intrinsic factor blocking antibody (interferes with intrinsic factor complexing to dietary vitamin B_{12}); and (c) in 50%, intrinsic factor binding antibody (binds with the intrinsic factor – vitamin B_{12} complex, preventing absorption of vitamin B_{12}). The antibodies against intrinsic factor are also present in gastric juice.

The autoimmune reaction manifests as a lymphoplasmacytic infiltrate in the mucosa around parietal cells, which progressively decrease in number (Figure 8-7A). Neutrophils are rarely seen, and *H. pylori* is absent. The fundic and body mucosa decreases in thickness, and the glands become lined predominantly by mucous cells. The mucosa frequently shows intestinal metaplasia, characterized by the appearance of goblet cells and Paneth cells. In the end stage of the disease, the mucosa is atrophic, with absent parietal cells (type A chronic atrophic gastritis). Patients with pernicious anemia have an increased incidence of gastric carcinoma – i.e. type A autoimmune chronic gastritis is a premalignant lesion. The epithelial cells show increasing degrees of dysplasia before cancer develops. Regular endoscopic surveillance with biopsy is indicated in all patients with pernicious anemia; recognition of high-grade dysplasia in a biopsy specimen (Figure 8-7B) is an indication for prophylactic gastric resection.

B. Type B Chronic Gastritis (*Chronic Antral Gastritis; Helicobacter pylori Gastritis*)

Type B chronic gastritis has a strong association with *H. pylori*. In 60%–70% of patients, *H. pylori* is demonstrable in biopsies by histologic examination or culture. In many patients in whom the organism is not demonstrable, serologic studies show antibodies against *H. pylori*, indicating previous infection.

Type B chronic gastritis maximally involves the antrum, which is the favored site of infection with *H. pylori*. Early cases show lymphoplasmactyic infiltration of the superficial gastric mucosa. Active infection with *H. pylori* is almost always associated with the presence of neutrophils, both in the lamina propria and the antral mucous glands (Figure 8-8).

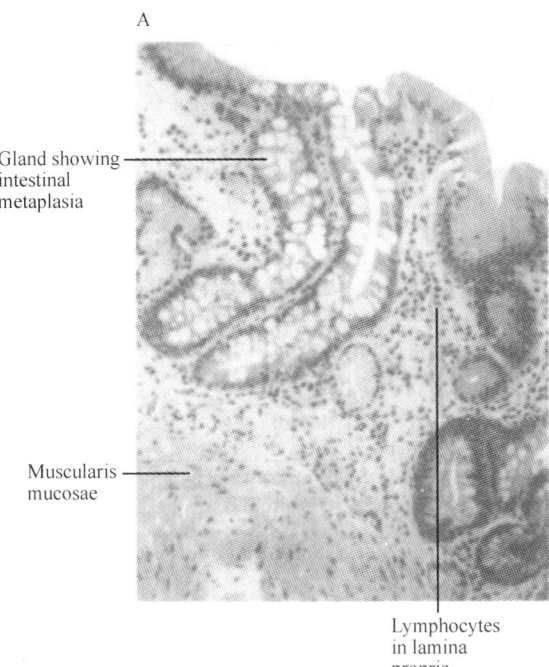
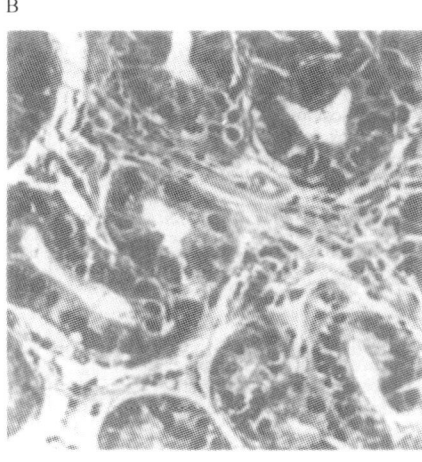

Figure 8-7 Pernicious anemia. A: Chronic atrophic gastritis showing nearly complete loss of parietal cell-containing glands, chronic inflammation, and intestinal metaplasia. B: High-grade dysplasia showing glands lined by cells with enlarged, pleomorphic, hyperchromatic nuclei

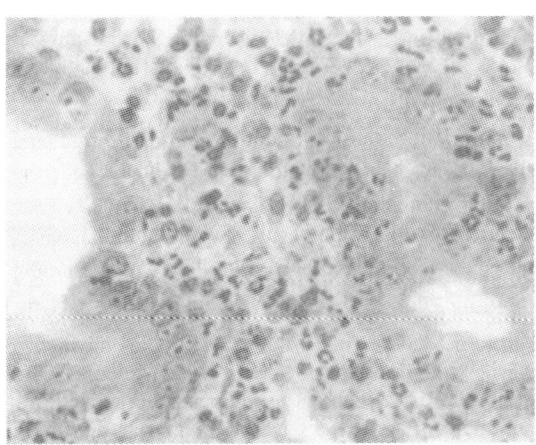

Figure 8-8 Active chronic gastritis. Note neutrophil infiltration of glands and lamina propria

As the lesion progresses, there is extension of the inflammation to involve the deep mucosa as well as the body of the stomach. Deep mucosal involvement is associated with destruction of the antral mucous glands and the appearance of intestinal metaplasia (type B chronic atrophic gastritis). *H. pylori* disappears in glands showing intestinal metaplasia because it cannot survive in the milieu of intestinal epithelium. Reactive lymphoid hyperplasia, characterized by reactive follicles in the mucosa, is common.

Helicobacter pylori is a small, curved vibriolike organism that is present in the surface mucous layer which covers the surface epithelium and the glandular lumina. It can be seen in routine sections but is better demonstrated in sections stained by the genta silver stain. The presence of *H. pylori* correlates best with active inflammation associated with neutrophils. Organisms may be absent in patients with inactive chronic gastritis, particularly when intestinal metaplasia is present.

Helicobacter gastritis is associated with numerous diseases of this region, and the relationships have not been completely clarified. These include (1) chronic duodenal ulcer, which has a nearly 100% association, (2) chronic gastric ulcer (75%), (3) gastric adenocarcinoma (>80%), and (4) malignant lymphoma arising in the mucosa-associated lymphoid tissue.

Most patients with type B chronic gastritis - even severe atrophic gastritis - are asymptomatic. Mild epigastric discomfort and pain, nausea, and anorexia may occur, particularly in the presence of active inflammation. Endoscopic features may be absent or there may be loss of normal rugal folds. Lymphoid hyperplasia may result in rugal thickening and nodularity. The correlation between the presence of symptoms, endoscopic features, and histologic gastritis is poor; 30% of patients with normal gastric mucosa on endoscopy show chronic gastritis.

Patients with type B chronic gastritis have an increased incidence of gastric cancer. The risk is very low and does not justify regular surveillance in all patients with type B chronic gastritis. However, the incidence of type B chronic gastritis in the population is so high that a large number of gastric carcinomas may actually occur in patients with type B chronic atrophic gastritis, as evidenced by the greater than 80% incidence of *H. pylori* infection in patients with gastric adenocarcinoma.

Menetrier's Disease (Hypertrophic Gastritis; Rugal Hypertrophy)

Menetrier's disease is a rare condition of unknown cause that occurs mainly in males over 40 years of age. It is characterized by greatly thickened gastric rugal folds (Figure 8-9) that are visible both radiologically and endoscopically. Hyperplasia and cystic dilation of mucous glands, together with proliferation of the smooth muscle of the muscularis mucosae, suggest that this may be a hamartomatous lesion. Most patients with Menetrier's disease have reduced or normal acid secretion. Overproduction of gastric mucus leads to increased protein loss in the intestine. In the original description of the disease, protein-losing enteropathy was a constant feature.

Enlarged gastric mucosal folds may also occur in gastric neoplasms, notably malignant lymphoma and gastric carcinoma; in Zollinger-Ellison syndrome, in which hypertrophy of parietal cells is associated with hypersecretion of acid; and in eosinophilic gastroenteritis.

PEPTIC ULCER DISEASE

Peptic ulcers are ulcers occurring in any part of the gastrointestinal tract exposed to the action of acidic gastric juice. They occur principally in the duodenum (duodenal ulcer) and stomach (gastric ulcer). Peptic ulcer disease is common all over the world. Duodenal ulcer is two to three times more frequent in males, particularly those under the age of 50 years.

Peptic ulcers occur at all ages; the most common age at onset is 20 – 40 years. A familial tendency exists for duodenal ulcers but not for gastric ulcers. Duodenal ulcers are associated with blood group O, absence of blood group antigens in saliva ("nonsecretors"), and the presence of HLA-B5 histocompatibility antigen.

A. Pathogenesis (*Figure 8-10*)

1. Hypersecretion of acid

Acid is necessary for peptic ulcers to form, and ulcers do not occur in achlorhydric states. The cornerstone of treatment of peptic ulcer is to decrease secretion of acid; histamine H_2 receptor antagonists (e.g. cimetidine, ranitidine, etc) and proton pump inhibitors (e.g. omeprazole) are highly effective.

However, the exact causal role played by the acid is uncertain. Patients with duodenal ulcers have increased acid secretion with heightened responses to normal stimuli, but patients with gastric ulcers frequently have normal or low acid production.

A marked increase in acid secretion occurs in patients with Zollinger-Ellison syndrome, caused by a gastrin-producing neoplasm of the pancreas. The high gastrin levels stimulate continuous maximal acid secretion by parietal cells. These patients have severe intractable peptic ulcers affecting the stomach, duodenum, and jejunum. In Zollinger-Ellison syndrome, high acid output is clearly the primary cause of peptic ulceration.

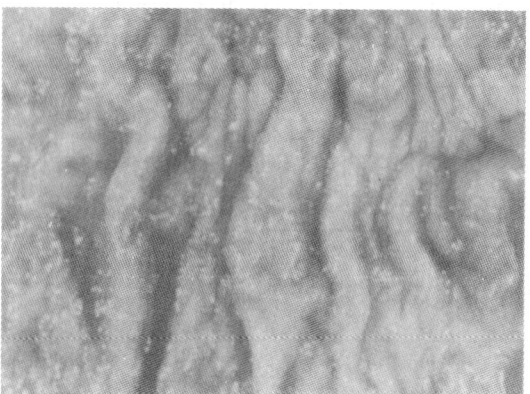

Figure 8-9 Hypertrophic gastritis (Menetrier's disease), showing thickened gastric rugal folds

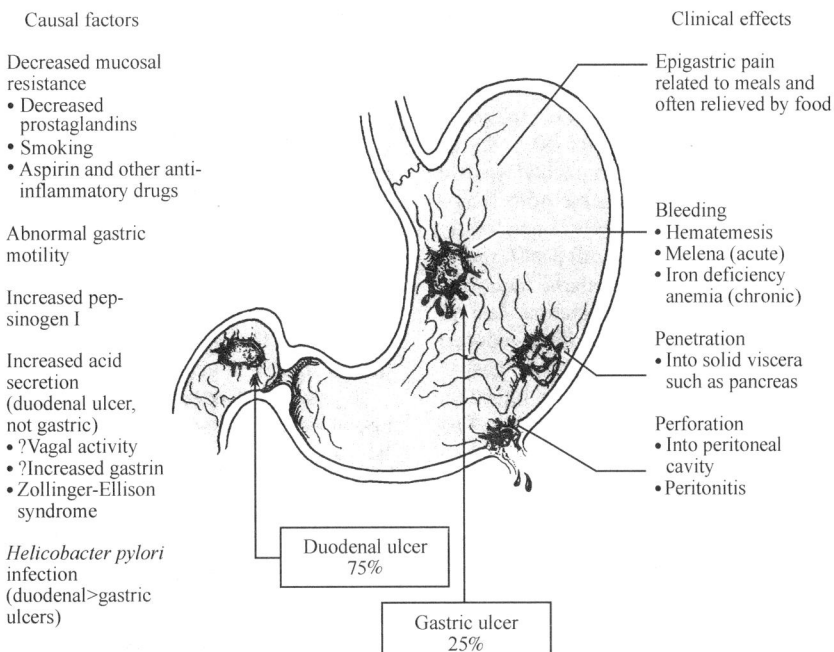

Figure 8-10 Chronic peptic ulcer disease. Causal factors and clinical effects

2. Decreased mucosal resistance to acid

Decreased resistance of the mucosa to acid is believed to be the primary cause of most gastric ulcers. **Prostaglandin E_2** levels in gastric juice have been shown to be consistently decreased in patients with peptic ulcer. PGE_2 levels rise during the healing phase and remain low in patients whose ulcers do not heal. Inhibitors of prostaglandin synthesis such as aspirin and ibuprofen – and cigarette smoking – are known to have an adverse effect on the healing of peptic ulcers. Synthetic PGE_2 analogues like misoprostol have accelerated healing in experimental studies.

3. *Helicobacter pylori* infection

H. pylori infection of the pyloric antrum is present in nearly all patients with chronic duodenal ulcer and approximately 75% of patients with chronic gastric ulcer. In the stomach, the organism grows in the surface mucous layer, which may become altered, decreasing mucosal resistance. The mechanism whereby *H. pylori* infection of the stomach causes duodenal ulcers is unknown. There is no direct infection of the duodenum by *H. pylori*.

B. Pathology

Chronic peptic ulcers are usually solitary, often large (larger than 1 cm, rarely larger than 5 cm), and round-to-oval in shape with a punched-out appearance (Figure 8-11). The margins are either flush with the mucosal surface or slightly raised because of edema. The floor of the ulcer is smooth, and its base is thick and firm because of fibrosis. The mucosa around the ulcer is either normal or – in the stomach – shows changes of chronic gastritis. The mucosal folds around the ulcer appear to radiate outward from it, which is an effect of fibrous contraction of the base of the ulcer.

Chronic peptic ulcer differs from acute erosive gastropathy in its etiologic factors and in the size, number, and distribution of lesions (Table 8-2). Ulcers in acute erosive gastropathy tend to be small (<1 cm), multiple and distributed throughout the stomach, whereas chronic ulcers are large, solitary and usually found on the lesser curvature or pyloric antrum (Figure 8-11)

Microscopically, the base of a chronic peptic ulcer is composed of a surface layer of necrotic, acutely inflamed debris below which is a zone of

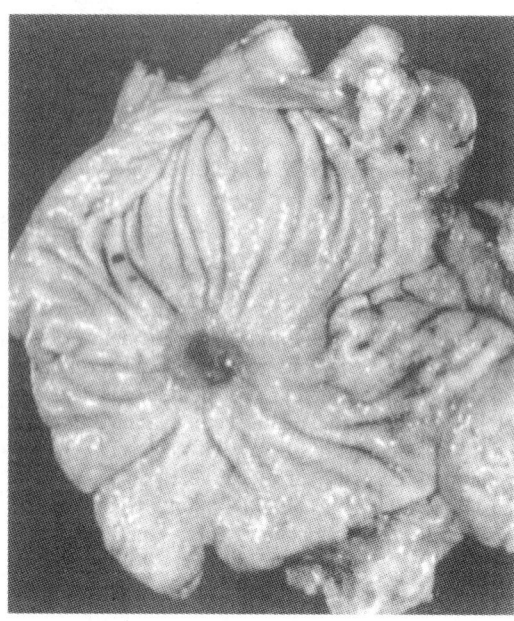

Figure 8-11 Chronic peptic ulcer, showing a large punched-out ulcer below the level of the mucosa. The ulcer edge is flat and flush with the mucosal surface. Note gastric folds radiating from the ulcer

Table 8-2 Differences between acute erosive gastropathy, chronic peptic ulcers, and ulcerative gastric carcinoma

	Acute Erosive Gastropathy	Chronic Peptic Ulcer	Gastric Carcinoma
Etiology	Alcohol, drugs, stress	Hyperacidity, decreased mucosal resistance	Carcinogen (unknown)
Location	Stomach (any part), first part of duodenum	Pyloric antrum, lesser curvature; first part of duodenum	Pyloric antrum, rest of stomach, both lesser and greater curvatures; duodenum spared
Size and form	Small erosions or ulcers	1 – 5 cm; may be larger; deep; flat margins	Commonly > 5 cm; may be smaller; ulcer with raised margins
Number	Multiple	One or two	Solitary
Rest of mucosa	Diffusely erythematous	Chronic gastritis	Chronic gastritis
Complications	Hemorrhagic perforation (rare)	Hemorrhage, perforation, pyloric stenosis (common)	Hemorrhage, pyloric stenosis, metastasis
Result	Healing	Healing, recurrence	Usually fatal
Association with *H. pylori*	–	+ (75% – 100%)	+ (>80%)

granulation tissue. Chronic peptic ulcers typically have extensive fibrosis of the base, with extension of fibrosis into the muscle wall. The muscle wall is commonly drawn up into the ulcer base. The epithelium at the edge of the ulcer shows regenerative hyperplasia, which frequently demonstrates marked cytologic atypia, mimicking neoplastic change. Vessels trapped within the scarred area are characteristically thickened and occasionally thrombosed, but in some instances they are widely patent. With healing, the crater fills with granulation tissue, followed by re-epithelialization from the margins and more or less restoration of the normal architecture. Extensive fibrous scarring remains. Chronic gastritis is extremely common among patients with peptic ulcer disease, and *H. pylori* infection is almost demonstrable in those patients with gastritis.

C. Clinical Features

Peptic ulcer disease is chronic, with remissions and relapses of symptoms, associated with healing and reactivation of the ulcer. Relapses may be precipitated by emotional stress, by drugs such as aspirin, ibuprofen, and steroids, and by cigarette smoking.

Burning or gnawing epigastric pain related to meals is the characteristic symptom of chronic peptic ulcer. Ingestion of food leads to an immediate reduction in pain because the food neutralizes the acid. However, acid secretion is stimulated by the meal, and eating therefore leads to recurrence of pain at a variable time after a meal.

The diagnosis is best established by endoscopy, including biopsy to rule out carcinoma in gastric ulcers.

D. Complications (Figure 8-10)

1. Bleeding

Bleeding is the result of erosion of a blood vessel by the ulcer and occurs in about 30% of patients with peptic ulcer. If slow, it causes occult blood loss in feces, leading to iron deficiency anemia. When bleeding is brisk, as occurs when a large artery like the gastroduodenal artery is eroded, hematemesis or melena occurs. Peptic ulcer disease is the most common cause of hematemesis. Hemorrhage is responsible for 10% of deaths from peptic ulcer disease.

2. Perforation

Perforation occurs in about 5% of peptic ulcer patients and is most common with anterior duodenal ulcers. The entry of gastric juice into the peritoneal cavity results in chemical peritonitis with sudden onset of abdominal pain and board-like rigidity of the abdominal muscles. Perforation is responsible for over 70% of deaths due to peptic ulcer.

3. Pyloric obstruction

The fibrosis associated with an ulcer in the pyloric canal or first part of the duodenum may result in gastric outlet obstruction. Severe vomiting with hypochloremic alkalosis results.

4. Penetration

The ulcerative process may extend through the full thickness of the gut wall into adjacent organs. The fibrotic base of the ulcer is intact in such slow penetration, and there is no perforation. Penetration into the pancreatic substance occurs with posterior ulcers and may lead to constant back pain.

5. Malignant transformation

Although malignant change is claimed to occur in gastric ulcers, this is a very uncommon event (about 1%); as far as duodenal ulcers are concerned it can be assumed that they never become malignant.

E. Treatment

Symptomatic treatment includes dietary change in the form of frequent small meals and avoidance of cigarette smoking, coffee, and alcohol, and the use of antacids. Suppression of acid secretion with drugs such as histamine H_2 receptor blockers and proton pump inhibitors is very effective. Surgical procedures to reduce acid secretion (vagotomy, antrectomy) are needed in rare refractory cases. Treatment of *H. pylori* infection with antibiotics decreases the likelihood of relapse after the ulcer has healed.

If a gastric ulcer does not heal with medical treatment, it must be reexamined by endoscopy and biopsied because ulcerative carcinomas of the stomach can mimic both the symptoms and the gross appearance of peptic ulcers. Biopsy of duodenal ulcers that are slow to heal is not essential because carcinomas are extremely rare in the first part of the duodenum.

GASTRIC CARCINOMA

A. Incidence and Etiology

Gastric carcinoma is the most common cancer in China. Adenocarcinoma accounts for over 90% of malignant neoplasms of the stomach. The favored location of gastric carcinomas within the stomach is the lesser curvature of the antropyloric region.

Gastric carcinoma is a worldwide disease with a widely varying incidence. The incidence of gastric carcinoma is five to ten times higher in China and Japan than in the United States. The incidence is also high in Iceland and Chile. Studies in Japanese immigrants to the United States show a decreased incidence from generation to generation, strongly suggesting that some environmental factor causes gastric cancer in Japan. It has been postulated that polycyclic hydrocarbons in smoked fish may be responsible.

The declining incidence of gastric carcinoma in the United States has been attributed to better refrigeration of meat, thereby decreasing the need for preservatives such as nitrites. Nitrites are converted to nitrosamines, which have been shown to cause gastric carcinoma in experimental animals.

Chronic gastritis associated with *Helicobacter pylori* infection remains a major risk factor for gastric carcinoma. The risk is particularly high in those with chronic gastritis limited to the gastric antrum. These patients develop severe gastric atrophy, intestinal metaplasia, and ultimately dysplasia and cancer. Antibiotic usage, which reduces *H. pylori* infection, may also have contributed to the decline in incidence over time.

Gastric carcinoma is statistically more common in individuals with blood group A. There is no significant familial tendency.

B. Precancerous Lesions

Gastric carcinoma occurs with increased frequency (1) in patients with chronic atrophic gastritis associated with pernicious anemia (high risk); (2) in those with chronic atrophic gastritis associated with *H. pylori* infection, particularly when there is intestinal metaplasia (uncertain risk); (3) in those with adenomatous and hyperplastic polyps (low risk); and (4) in patients who have had subtotal gastrectomy, when the residual gastric stump is believed to be at increased risk. Chronic peptic ulcers of the stomach were at one time believed to carry an increased risk of carcinoma, but that view is no longer held. More important, gastric mucosal dysplasia is the presumed precursor lesion of early gastric cancer.

C. Pathology

1. Gross appearance

Early gastric cancer (defined as gastric carcinoma restricted to the mucosa and submucosa) is increasingly recognized. Cancers can still be 'early' even if spread has occurred to regional lymph nodes. In Japan, where the incidence is high, population screening for gastric cancer is carried out, and early gastric cancer accounts for 30% of cases. In the United States, the incidence is much lower, and screening is not attempted; consequently, less than 10% of cases are detected at this early stage. Early gastric cancer appears as a small, flat mucosal thickening that may have a minimal polypoid and ulcerative component (Figure 8-12). It is thought that there may be a long period (months to years) before invasion of the muscle occurs.

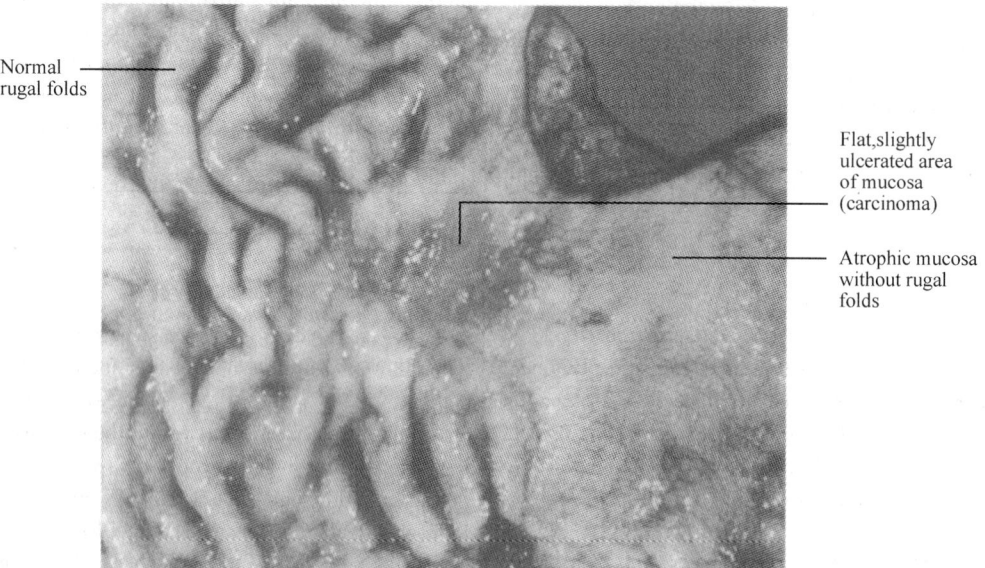

Figure 8-12 Early gastric cancer, showing shallow ulceration of mucosa. Note the difference between the flat mucosa of chronic gastritis (to the right of the carcinomatous ulcer) and normal gastric rugal folds to the left of the ulcer

Late gastric cancer (defined as a gastric carcinoma that has invaded the muscle wall, also called advanced gastric carcinoma) is the stage at which the tumor is commonly diagnosed. Advanced tumors extend into or beyond the main muscle coats. It may present in various ways: (1) as a fungating mass that protrudes into the lumen; (2) as a malignant ulcer with raised, everted edges (Figure 8-13); (3) as an excavated ulcer resembling a chronic peptic ulcer; or (4) as a diffusely infiltrating lesion that causes thickening and contraction of the stomach wall with relatively little mucosal involvement (linitis plastica, or leather-bottle stomach). Differentiation of benign peptic ulcer and ulcerative carcinoma may be difficult without histologic examination (Figure 8-14). Any gastric ulcer that does not heal as expected should be biopsied to rule out carcinoma.

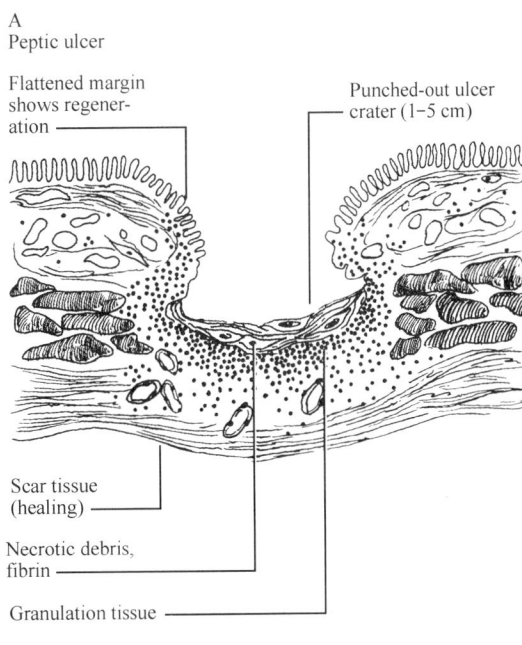

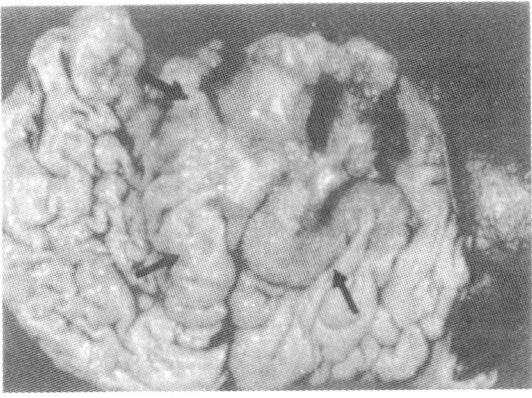

Figure 8-13 Advanced gastric cancer, showing large ulcer in the fundus (arrows). The ulcer has raised, everted edges. The spleen is present in the specimen because the carcinoma infiltrated the splenic hilum

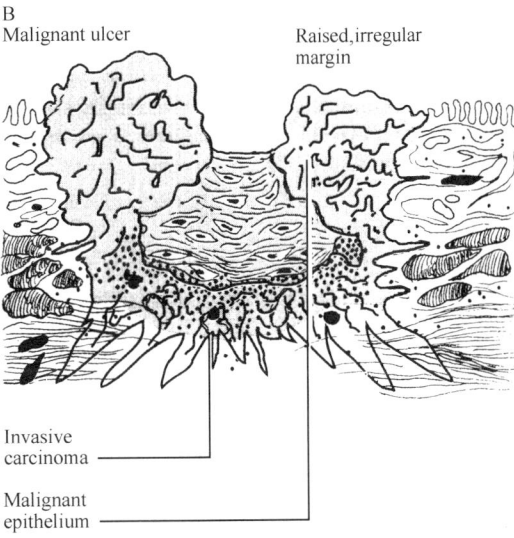

Figure 8-14 Comparative features of benign versus malignant gastric ulcers. A: Chronic peptic ulcer, showing the flat, punched-out ulcer with regenerating epithelium at the edges. B: Carcinomatous ulcer with raised edges composed of malignant epithelial cells

2. Microscopic appearance

Gastric carcinomas are adenocarcinomas of varying differentiation. The most common form is poorly differentiated (diffuse type), with cells distended by intracellular mucin (signet ring cell carcinoma; Figure 8-15). Well-differentiated (intestinal type) adenocarcinoma is less common. A reactive fibrosis is commonly present in relation to the neoplastic cells.

The intestinal variant is composed of malignant cells forming neoplastic intestinal glands resembling those of colonic adenocarcinoma. This pattern of gastric cancer is thought to arise from gastric mucous cells that have undergone intestinal metaplasia in the setting of chronic gastritis. The diffuse variant is composed of malignant gastric-type mucous cells that generally do not form glands but rather permeate the mucosa and wall as scattered individual "signet-ring" cells or small clusters in an "infiltrative" growth pattern. In contrast, the diffuse variant is thought to arise de novo from native gastric mu-

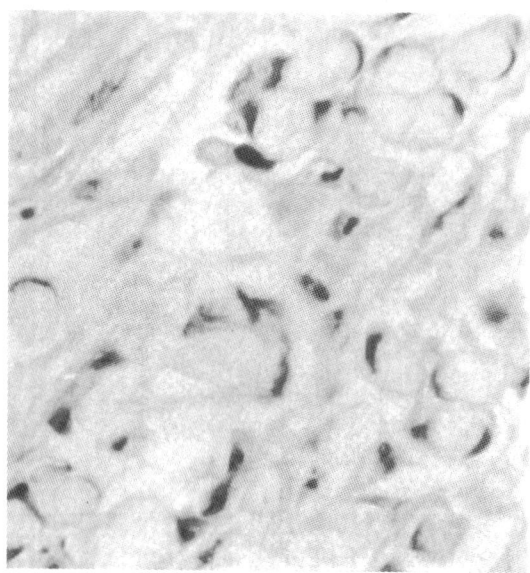

Figure 8-15 Gastric adenocarcinoma, showing signet ring cells

cous cells, is not associated with chronic gastritis, and tends to be poorly differentiated.

The histologic appearances of gastric cancer could be also classified as: papillary adenocarcinoma, tubular adenocarcinoma, poorly-differentiated adenocarcinoma, mucinous adenocarcinoma, and signet-ring cell carcinoma. Whatever the histologic variant, all gastric carcinomas eventually penetrate the wall to involve the serosa, spread to regional and more distant lymph nodes, and metastasize widely.

3. Spread

Gastric carcinoma infiltrates the submucosa and invades through the muscle wall into the omental fat. Involvement of the serosa leads to spread of tumor cells in the peritoneal fluid (transcoelomic spread). Such metastasis occurs to the ovary (Krukenberg tumor) and rectovesical pouch. Involvement of submucosal lymphatics by tumor results in microscopic satellite nodules, often some distance from the main mass. Microscopic examination of frozen sections of the resection margins is therefore very important at the time of surgical removal of tumor. Lymphatic involvement also leads to metastasis to lymph nodes around the stomach. Later, extension of tumor up the thoracic duct may lead to involvement of the left supraclavicular nodes (Virchow's node). Lymph node metastases are present in about 50% of cases at the time of diagnosis. Hematogenous spread to the liver and lungs also occurs early.

D. Clinical Features

Gastric carcinoma is asymptomatic in its early stages and can be detected only by screening of high-risk populations. A few patients with early gastric cancer have symptoms resembling chronic peptic ulcer. Biopsy of a nonhealing gastric ulcer is essential because some of these patients prove to have carcinoma.

Late gastric cancer presents with anorexia, anemia (due to blood loss), and weight loss. Early satiety may occur in a patient with a large mass or a contracted (linitis plastica) stomach. Hematemesis and melena may occur. Tumors near the pylorus may cause gastric outlet obstruction.

Diagnosis may be established by endoscopy and biopsy, which provides a histologic diagnosis; and by radiologic examination - particularly computerized tomography - which provides information about the extent of spread and surgical resectability. Note that radiologic diagnosis of carcinoma must always be confirmed by endoscopic biopsy.

E. Prognosis

The prognosis depends almost entirely on the depth of invasion of the neoplasm. Early gastric cancer restricted to the mucosa and submucosa has a 5-year survival rate of about 85%. Tumors that have invaded the muscle wall (late gastric cancer) but have not involved lymph nodes have only a 30% 5-year survival rate. When there is extension of tumor through the full thickness of the wall and lymph node involvement is present, the 5-year survival rate drops to about 5%.

Histologic features and degree of differentiation are of little prognostic importance.

GASTROINTESTINAL STROMAL TUMOR

Gastrointestinal stromal tumor (GIST), the most common mysenchymal tumor of the gastrointestinal tract, is thought to originate from the interstitial cell of Cajal, or pacemaker cell. Tumors of true smooth muscle, neural (schwannian), fibroblastic, and vascular origin are excluded. Interstitial cells of

Cajal are characterized by expression of KIT. An immunohistochemical marker (CD117) for KIT is now used to distinguish GISTs from non-GIST spindle tumors in the gastrointestinal tract.

GISTs arise most commonly within the wall of the stomach (65%–70%) and small intestine (30%–35%), and are seen far less frequently in the esophagus, colon and rectum. Grossly, tumors vary greatly in size, ranging from 1–2 cm to more than 20 cm in diameter. The tumors are usually well circumscribed and generally unencapsulated, although a pseudocapsule may occasionally be seen. There are two principal histological patterns: a spindle cell or epithelioid character, or a combination of both in variable proportions.

DISEASES OF THE INTESTINES

STRUCTURE AND FUNCTION

The intestine begins at the pylorus and ends at the anorectal junction. It is divided into the small and large intestine, which are separated by the ileocecal valve. The small intestine is composed of the duodenum, jejunun, and ileum and is about 6 meters long in adults; the large intestine is composed of the cecum, ascending, transverse, descending, and sigmoid colon and the rectum, totaling about 1.5 meters in length in adults.

The intestinal wall has four layers:
- **Mucosa**, which is lined by glandular epithelium. The small intestine is characterized by the presence of villi and crypts. The villi increase the surface area for absorption. The colonic mucosa has no villi and is composed only of crypts. The crypts contain proliferating cells that continually divide to replace lost surface epithelial cells.
- **Submucosa**, which contains blood and lymphatic vessels and the submucosal nerve plexus.
- **Muscularis externa**, which is composed of 2 layers in the small intestine. In the large intestine, the longitudinal muscle is attenuated to form the taenia coli. The muscle is responsible for propulsive peristalsis. The myenteric plexus of nerves is situated between the 2 muscle layers and provides the neural impetus to peristalsis.
- **Serosa**, which is the peritoneal lining in those parts of the intestine that lie in the peritoneal cavity.

The intestine digests and absorbs essential components from ingested food, eliminating the waste at defecation. Digestion is effected in the upper small intestine by enzymes contained in the secretions of intestinal juice, pancreatic juice, and bile. The small molecules resulting from digestion – monosaccharides, amino acids, and fatty acids – are absorbed in the small intestine. The colon absorbs water from the liquid ileal effluent to form solid feces.

CONGENITAL DISEASES OF THE INTESTINE

Congenital Megacolon (Hirschsprung's Disease)

Hirschsprung's disease is caused by failure of development of ganglion cells in the myenteric and submucosal plexuses of the colon. The aganglionic segment usually starts at the anorectal junction and extends proximally for a variable distance. In 90% of cases, aganglionosis is restricted to the rectum. Rarely, the aganglionic segment is longer, and in exceptional cases the entire colon lacks ganglion cells.

The absence of ganglion cells in the myenteric plexus results in failure of peristalsis in the affected segment. This segment remains narrow and spastic and represents a zone of functional intestinal obstruction. The colon proximal to the aganglionic segment dilates – often massively – leading to abdominal distention.

Most affected children present soon after birth with failure to pass meconium followed by distention and vomiting. In a few cases, the onset is delayed. The diagnosis may be made by demonstrating absence of ganglion cells in the submucosa of an adequate rectal biopsy. Absence of ganglion cells in the submucosa correlates well with absence of ganglion cells in the myenteric plexus. Treatment consists of surgical removal of the aganglionic segment.

Intestinal Atresia

Atresia is a rare congenital disorder consisting of failure of development of the lumen in one part of the intestine. The jejunum and ileum are most commonly affected, and multiple bowel segments may be affected. Atresia presents with intestinal obstruction in the first week of life. Surgical correction is curative.

Imperforate Anus

Imperforate anus is a common congenital abnormality that results from failure of the endodermal hindgut to open at the anal dimple. Varying degrees of abnormality result, sometimes associated with fistulous communications with the bladder, urethra or vagina.

Meckel's Diverticulum

Meckel's diverticulum is persistence of the intestinal end of the omphalomesenteric duct. It is present in 2% of the population (the most common congenital anomaly of the gastrointestinal tract), is found within 2 feet (1 m) of the ileocecal valve, and is usually 2 inches (5 cm) long.

The diverticulum is usually lined by small intestinal mucosa. About 40% of cases have heterotopic gastric mucosa or pancreatic tissue. Peptic ulceration may occur when there is gastric mucosa. Bleeding from an ulcerated Meckel diverticulum is an important cause of chronic intestinal blood loss, resulting in iron deficiency anemia. Other complications include infection (Meckel's diverticulitis), which presents a clinical picture very similar to that of acute appendicitis and may result in perforation and peritonitis.

ACUTE APPENDICITIS

Acute appendicitis is the most common surgical emergency. It occurs at all ages, with a peak incidence in young adulthood.

In most cases, inflammation of the appendix is preceded by obstruction of the appendiceal lumen (Figure 8-16) by a fecalith (hardened mass of feces), by kinking of the wall, or by submucosal lymphoid hyperplasia. Stagnation distal to the obstruction permits multiplication of colonic bacterial flora, including potential pathogens such as *Escherichia coli*, *Streptococcus faecalis*, and anaerobic bacteria. These bacteria then invade the mucosa and appendiceal wall, causing acute inflammation.

A. Pathology

Acute inflammation of the mucosa is followed by ulceration and inflammation of the muscular wall. Neutrophils are the dominant cells. Suppuration commonly occurs. Grossly, the inflamed appendix app-

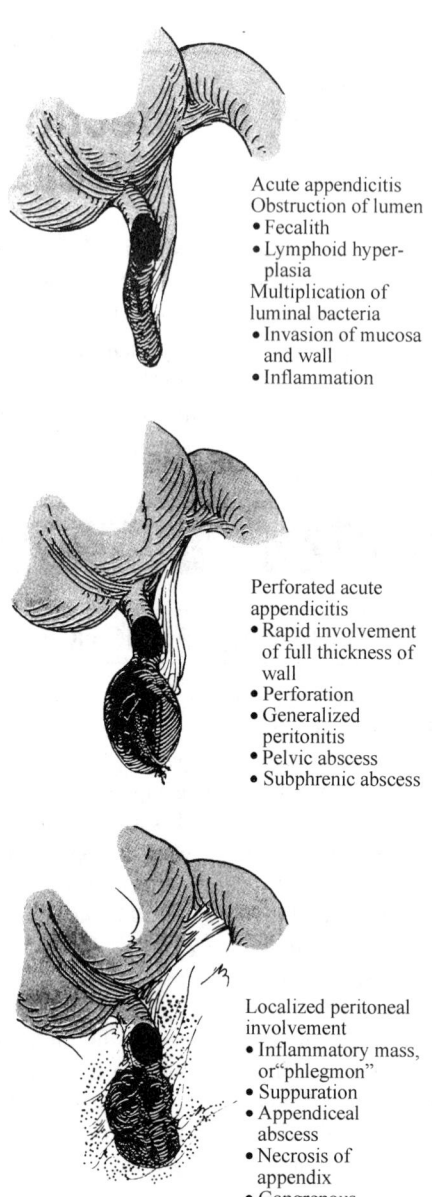

Figure 8-16 Pathogenesis and complications of acute appendicitis

ears swollen and red, with a surface that has lost its normal shiny appearance and frequently is covered by a fibrinopurulent exudate. In a minority of cases, the external appearance is normal, and the diagnosis is confirmed only on histologic examination by finding neutrophil infiltration of the mucosa and wall.

B. Clinical Features

Patients present with acute onset of fever, abdominal pain, and vomiting. Pain is initially periumbilical (referred pain) but becomes localized to the right lower quadrant when the pain-sensitive parietal peritoneum is involved. Tenderness and guarding (reflex muscle spasm during palpation) are commonly present. The peripheral blood shows neutrophilic leukocytosis. Surgical treatment (appendectomy) is curative.

Local extension of the inflammatory process may involve the periappendiceal tissues and result in an inflammatory mass (phlegmon) in the right lower quadrant or in appendiceal abscess. Perforation into the peritoneal cavity may result in acute peritonitis, and distant abscesses may form - commonly in the rectovesical pouch or subphrenic region.

IDIOPATHIC INFLAMMATORY BOWEL DISEASE

The term idiopathic inflammatory bowel disease is used for two diseases - Crohn's disease and ulcerative colitis. Although their causes are still not clear, the two diseases probably have an immunologic hypersensitivity basis. They are recognized as distinct entities with distinct clinical and pathologic features.

Crohn's Disease

Crohn's disease is a chronic inflammatory disorder that most commonly affects the ileum and colon but has the potential to involve any part of the gastrointestinal tract from the mouth to the anus. It is characterized by involvement of discontinuous segments of intestine (skip areas), noncaseating epithelioid cell granulomas, and transmural (full-thickness) inflammation of the affected parts (Figure 8-17).

A. Incidence

Crohn's disease occurs mainly in Western Europe and the United States and is uncommon in Asia and South America. The incidence appears to be increasing.

Both sexes are affected equally. The disease can occur at any age but has its highest incidence in young adults. It is uncommon in young children. Crohn's disease has a familial tendency, with 20%-30% of patients giving a positive family history. There is no inheritance pattern, and the familial tendency is likely to be the result of a shared, common environment.

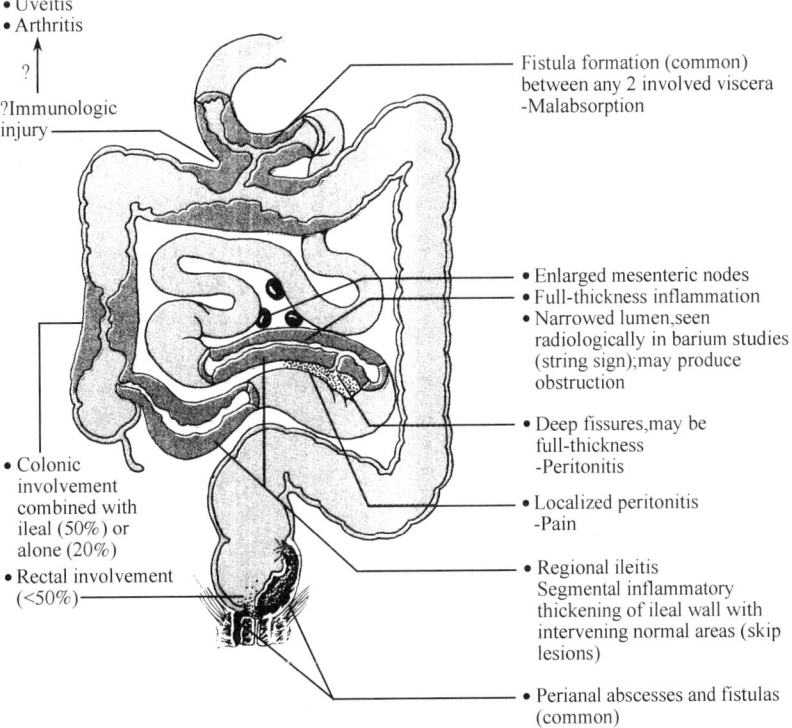

Figure 8-17 Pathologic features of Crohn's disease

B. Etiology

The cause of Crohn's disease is unknown. Despite extensive search, no infectious agent has been found.

There is strong but not conclusive evidence that Crohn's disease is the result of some immunologic injury. Antibodies with activity against intestinal epithelial cells have been identified in the serum and lymphocytes of patients with Crohn's disease. Patients with active Crohn's disease frequently have T cell dysfunction (anergy to tuberculin and mumps antigen, low peripheral blood T cell count).

C. Pathology (Figure 8-17)

1. Sites of involvement

Combined ileal (most commonly terminal ileum) and colonic disease is most common (50%). The ileum alone is involved in 30% of patients and the colon alone in 20%. Involvement of the oral cavity, larynx, esophagus, stomach, and perineum are rare.

Patients with Crohn's disease commonly (in 75% of cases) have perianal lesions such as abscesses, fistulas, and skin tags. Perianal disease occurs in both ileal and colonic disease and is not dependent on the presence of rectal involvement.

2. Gross appearance

Involvement is typically segmental, with skip areas of normal intestine between areas of involved bowel. Normal and affected intestine are sharply demarcated from one another.

In the acute phase, the intestine is swollen and reddened. The mucosa shows diffuse hyperemia, acute inflammation, and shallow, aphthous ulceration. In the chronic phase, the affected segment is greatly thickened and rigid (lead pipe or garden hose appearance; Figure 8-18). Marked fibrosis causing luminal narrowing with intestinal obstruction is common. The serosa is dull and granular. In involved ileal segments, the mesenteric fat creeps from the mesentery to surround the bowel wall (creeping fat). The mucosal surface shows longitudinal serpiginous ulcers separated by irregular islands of edematous mucosa. Fissures (deep and narrow ulcers that look like stabs with a knife that penetrate deeply into the wall of the affected intestine) and fistulas (communications with other viscera) may be present.

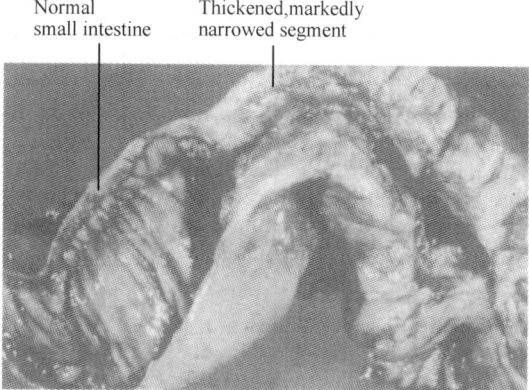

Figure 8-18 Crohn's disease of the terminal ileum, showing marked segmental narrowing and thickening

3. Microscopic features

Crohn's disease is characterized by distortion of mucosal crypt architecture, transmural inflammation, and the presence of epithelioid granulomas on histologic examination; granulomas are present in about 60% of patients. Numerous other histologic changes occur in Crohn's disease, but none are of great diagnostic use. These features include lymphedema of the submucosa, lymphoid follicles at all levels of the bowel wall, and marked fibrosis. Fissure-ulcers and fistulas can be seen microscopically.

The regional mesenteric lymph nodes are frequently enlarged and may contain noncaseating granulomas.

D. Clinical Features

Presentation is extremely variable. In the acute phase, fever, diarrhea, and right lower quadrant pain may mimic acute appendicitis. Chronic disease is characterized by remissions and relapses over a long period of time. Asymptomatic periods may last several months. With the passage of time, weight loss and anemia appear. Thickening of the intestine may produce an ill-defined mass in the abdomen.

Diagnosis is based on a combination of clinical, radiologic, and pathologic findings. In the active phase of the disease, the erythrocyte sedimentation rate and white blood cell count may be elevated, but these are nonspecific findings.

Crohn's disease may be complicated by intestinal obstruction or by fistula formation between involved loops of bowel and adjacent viscera. Crohn's disease carries a slightly increased risk of development of carcinoma of the colon-much less than in ulcerative colitis.

Ulcerative Colitis

Ulcerative colitis is an inflammatory disease of uncertain cause. It has a chronic course characterized by remissions and relapses.

A. Incidence

Ulcerative colitis is common in the 20- to 30-year age group but may occur at any age. The incidence is slightly higher in females than in males. The disease is most prevalent in North America and Western Europe, and less prevalent in Asia, Africa, and South America.

B. Etiology

The cause is unknown; no infectious agent has been identified. Antibodies that cross-react with intestinal epithelial cells and certain serotypes of *Escherichia coli* have been demonstrated in the serum of some patients with ulcerative colitis. Allergy to food proteins has been suggested as a possible cause but without proof.

Psychologic stress frequently precipitates ulcerative colitis, leading to the suggestion that the disease has a psychosomatic basis.

C. Pathology (*Figure 8-19*)

1. Sites of involvement

Ulcerative colitis is a disease of the rectum, which is involved in almost all cases and in some patients remains the only site of disease, and the colon. The disease extends proximally from the rectum in a continuous manner without skip areas. Total colonic involvement is not uncommon. The appendix is involved in about 30% of cases.

2. Gross appearance

Ulcerative colitis involves mainly the mucosa. Even in severe disease, the external appearance of the affected colon shows nothing other than mild hyperemia. There is rarely any thickening of the wall.

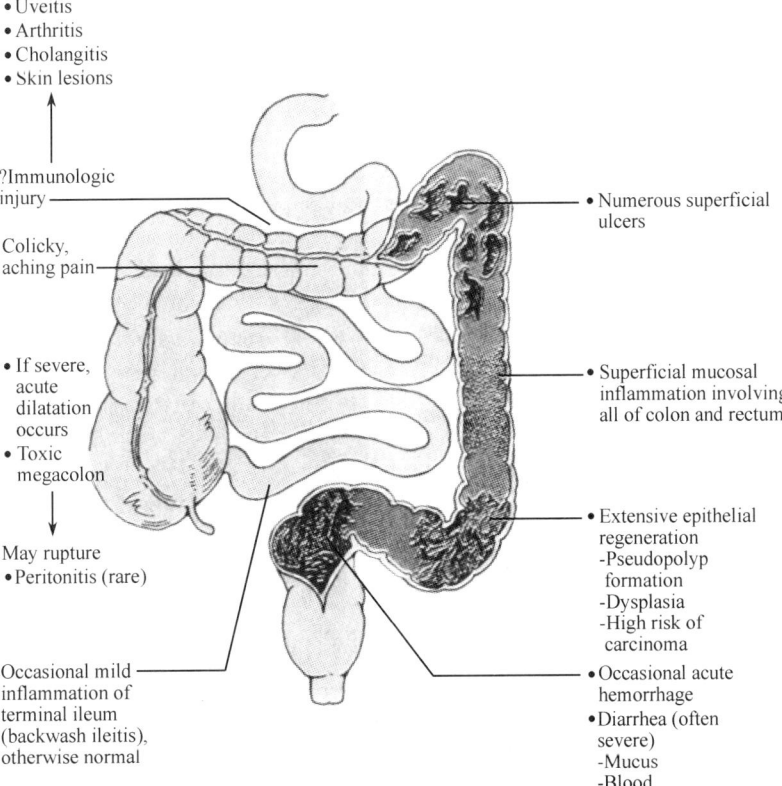

Figure 8-19 Pathologic features of ulcerative colitis

In very rare cases of severe acute ulcerative colitis, toxic dilation (megacolon) occurs.

The mucosal surface shows diffuse hyperemia with numerous superficial ulcerations in the acute phase. The rough, red, velvety appearance on colonoscopy is characteristic but not specific. In the chronic phase of the disease during remission, the mucosa appears flat and atrophic due to re-epithelialization of the ulcers. The regenerated or nonulcerated mucosa may appear polypoid (inflammatory pseudopolyps) in contrast with the atrophic areas or ulcers.

3. Microscopic appearance

In the active phase, the mucosa shows marked inflammation with neutrophils, lymphocytes, and plasma cells. Neutrophils are present in both lamina propria and in glands (crypt abscesses). In the chronic phase, the crypts are decreased in number (crypt atrophy) and show distorted architecture due to abnormal branching (Figure 8-20). There are numerous chronic inflammatory cells in the lamina propria. Active inflammation correlates well with the severity of symptoms. In treated patients, many of the mucosal changes reverse.

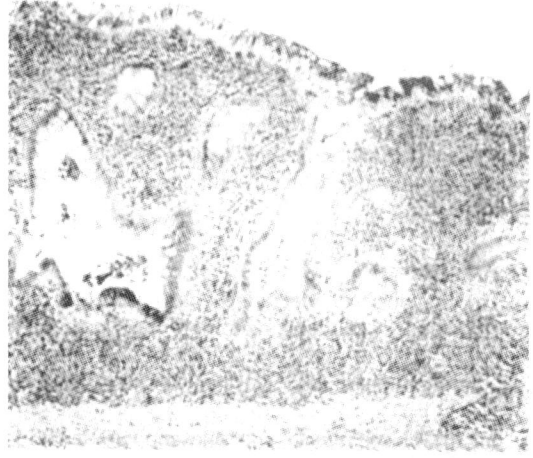

Figure 8-20 Colonic mucosal changes of chronic idiopathic inflammatory bowel disease, showing marked atrophy and distortion of crypts with increased numbers of chronic inflammatory cells in the lamina propria. Note that these changes are present in both ulcerative colitis and Crohn's disease

The inflammation is usually restricted to the mucosa. In severe cases with extensive ulceration, the superficial part of the submucosa may be involved, but the muscle wall is not affected.

D. Clinical Features

In the acute phase and during relapse, the patient has fever, leukocytosis, lower abdominal pain, and diarrhea with blood and mucus in the stool. The disease usually has a chronic course, with remissions and exacerbations; in some cases, the patient has chronic continuous disease with mild diarrhea and bleeding.

The diagnosis of ulcerative colitis is based on a combination of clinical, radiologic, and pathologic findings. The erythrocyte sedimentation rate and white blood count are elevated during the acute phase. Mucosal biopsies taken at endoscopy are useful in diagnosis. The presence of crypt atrophy, distortion of crypt architecture, and an increased number of lymphocytes and plasma cells in the lamina propria are helpful in differentiating ulcerative colitis from other causes of acute colitis. However, these mucosal changes can be seen in both ulcerative colitis and Crohn's disease (Figure 8-20). The only finding on mucosal biopsy that reliably differentiates ulcerative colitis and Crohn's disease is the presence of noncaseating epithelioid granulomas in the latter.

Severe bleeding may occur as a complication in the acute phase. Extraintestinal manifestations occur more commonly in ulcerative colitis than in Crohn's disease. They include arthritis, uveitis, skin lesions (a necrotic skin lesion in the extremities known as pyoderma gangrenosum is typical), and sclerosing pericholangitis (fibrosis around bile ducts), leading to obstructive jaundice.

Patients with chronic ulcerative colitis have an increased risk of developing colon carcinoma. The overall risk is about 10%. The risk increases progressively with disease duration beyond 7 years, with the length of colon involved – greatest with involvement of the entire colon – and the age at onset of disease – the earlier the onset, the greater the risk. Carcinomas occurring in ulcerative colitis tend to be poorly differentiated, infiltrative, and aggressive neoplasms with a poor prognosis.

COLONIC ADENOMA

Adenoma is a common benign epithelial tumor in the intestines. Adenomas of the colon are present in 20%–30% of all individuals over the age of 50 years. They are of two major types: tubular and villous. Because the incidence of adenomas in the small intestine is very low, this discussion focuses on those adenomas that arise in the colon. Colonic adenomas are associated with genetic mutations identical to those seen in colon cancer. The number of mutations in adenomas is less than in carcinoma but increases as the adenoma enlarges and becomes more dysplastic (the adenoma → carcinoma sequence).

Tubular adenomas account for over 90% of colonic adenomas. They are commonly multiple, with 10 - 20 lesions present in some patients, and are pedunculated with a well-defined stalk. Histologically, a tubular adenoma is composed of benign neoplastic glands bunched together above the muscularis. The epithelial cells are hyperchromatic and stratified and show loss of normal mucin content – sometimes termed "adenomatous change." The proliferating epithelium may be composed of tubular glands (tubular adenoma) or a mixture of tubular and villous structures (tubulovillous adenoma). A benign adenoma shows no evidence of invasion and has a clearly defined stalk.

Tubular adenomas are premalignant lesions. Although the risk of cancer is small (1% - 3%), the frequency of these polyps in the population makes them the most important precancerous colonic lesion. The development of carcinoma is preceded by increasing epithelial dysplasia. The risk of developing carcinoma increases with increasing size and number of polyps. Polyps over 2 cm in diameter should be considered highly suspicious. Malignancy of a polyp is most reliably determined by the presence of stalk invasion, which gives the neoplastic cells access to the lymphatics and predisposes to metastasis.

Villous adenomas are uncommon, comprising less than 10% of colonic adenomas. They commonly occur in older individuals as a solitary large, sessile lesion – i.e. have a broad base of attachment to the mucosal surface without a defined stalk. The most common location is the rectum. Villous adenomas appear grossly as soft, velvety, papillary growths that project into the lumen. They are usually 1 - 5 cm in diameter but may be larger. Histologically, villous adenoma is composed of neoplastic proliferation of colonic epithelial cells organized into long finger-like papillary or villous processes (Figure 8-21). Cancer in a villous adenoma (papillary adenocarcinoma) is most reliably determined by the presence of invasion of the muscularis mucosae at the base of the lesion. Villous adenomas have a 30% - 70% incidence of carcinoma.

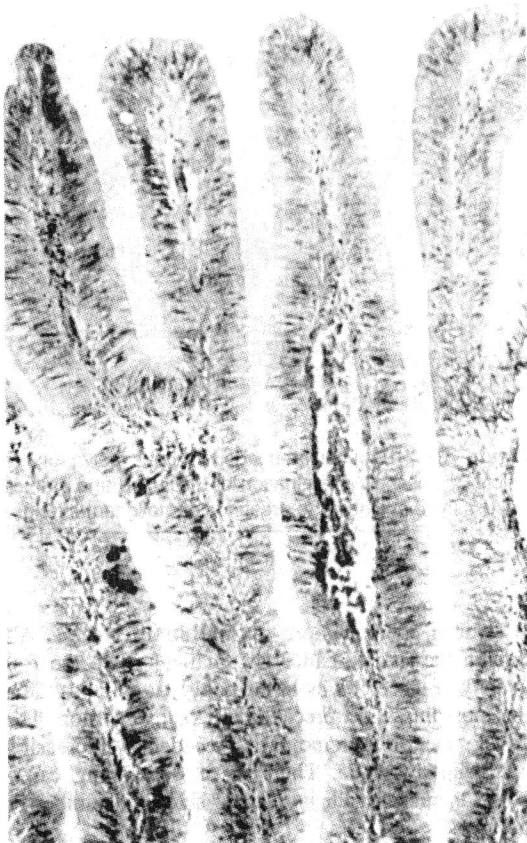

Figure 8-21 Villous adenoma. Note finger-like papillary processes and adenomatous change of the epithelium

CARCINOMA OF THE COLON AND RECTUM

A. Incidence and Carcinogenesis

Colorectal carcinoma accounts for over 90% of malignant neoplasms of the intestine. Colorectal carcinoma is more common in North America and Europe than in Asia, Africa, and South America.

Colorectal carcinoma occurs mainly in older individuals; 90% of cases are in the over-50 age group. A genetic basis for colorectal carcinoma is emerging. In patients with familial polyposis coli, whose disease is related to the deletion of the tumor suppressor gene APC at the locus 5q21, the occurrence of carcinoma has been related to the deletion of another tumor suppressor gene located immediately adjacent to it. The second gene, called the mutated in colon carcinoma (MCC) gene, has also been found in patients with nonfamilial colorectal cancer.

In colorectal cancer that occurs in the general population outside the setting of familial polyposis coli (>98% of all colorectal cancers), many mutations have been reported. These include (1) activation of the oncogene Kras, (2) deletions in chromosome 5q related to the MCC tumor suppressor gene, (3) deletions in chromosome 17 related to the p53 gene, which also behaves in this setting as a tumor suppressor gene, and (4) deletions in chromosome 18q, related to another tumor suppressor gene called deleted in colon carcinoma (DCC). It is likely that many, if not all, of these genetic mutations occur before colorectal carcinoma manifests clinically - a typical multihit phenomenon of carcinogenesis. Premalignant colonic adenomas may show some of these mutations, particularly when they are large and severely dysplastic, forming a genetic basis for the adenoma → carcinoma sequence that has been documented clinically. Clinical tests are becoming available to detect some of these genetic abnormalities and may provide a means of detecting the population at risk for developing colorectal cancer.

Recently, molecular models for carcinogenesis were developed for colon and rectal cancer. It is postulated that loss of one normal copy of the tumor suppressor gene APC occurs early. Indeed, individuals may be born with one mutant allele, rendering them extremely likely to develop colon cancer. This is the "first hit" according to Knudson's hypothesis. The loss of the normal copy of APC follows ("second hit"). Mutations of the oncogene Kras seem to occur next in adenomas. Additional mutations inactivate the tumor suppressor genes DCC and TP53, leading finally to the emergence of carcinoma. Study of colorectal carcinogenesis has provided fundamental insights into the general mechanisms of cancer evolution.

B. Etiology

The cause of colorectal carcinoma is unknown. The high incidence in developed countries is thought to be due to the intake of a diet rich in animal fat and low in fiber content. Such a diet produces a small, hard stool with slow movement through the colon, permitting carcinogenic agents to remain in contact with the mucosa for a longer period of time.

C. Premalignant Lesions

Most colon carcinomas are believed to arise in premalignant lesions, with only a few arising de novo in previously normal mucosa.

The greatest risk for carcinoma is in the heredofamilial adenomatous polyposis syndromes, where the risk is 100%. Villous adenomas also have a high incidence of malignant transformation. In these conditions, colonic resection is justified to prevent carcinoma.

The risk is somewhat less (10% overall) in chronic ulcerative colitis, but prophylactic colectomy is justified when there is total colonic involvement, disease over 10 years in duration, and high-grade epithelial dysplasia on biopsy.

Tubular adenomas have a low risk of carcinoma, but because they are so common they are believed to be the most frequent precursor lesion for colon carcinoma. Clear-cut invasion of the fibrovascular core, particularly when epithelial dysplasia extends through the muscularis mucosae, is the most reliable criterion.

D. Pathology

The rectosigmoid region accounts for about 50% of colon carcinomas, with the remainder distributed throughout the colon (Figure 8-22). Multiple carcinomas are present in 5% of cases.

Carcinomas in the right side of the colon tend to be large polypoid masses that project into the lumen. Left-sided cancers tend to involve the whole circumference and often constrict the lumen (napkin ring or apple core appearance) (Figure 8-23). Rectal carcinomas are most commonly malignant ulcers with raised everted edges (Figure 8-24).

Microscopically, most colon carcinomas are adenocarcinomas of varying differentiation. The majority are well or moderately differentiated (Figure 8-25). Many tumors produce mucin, which is secreted into the gland lumina or into the interstitium of the gut wall. Cancers of anal zone are predominantly squamous cell in origin.

E. Clinical Features

Colon carcinoma is asymptomatic in its early stages. It is recommended that all individuals over the age of 40 years undergo regular examination by sigmoidoscopy or colonoscopy to exclude early colon

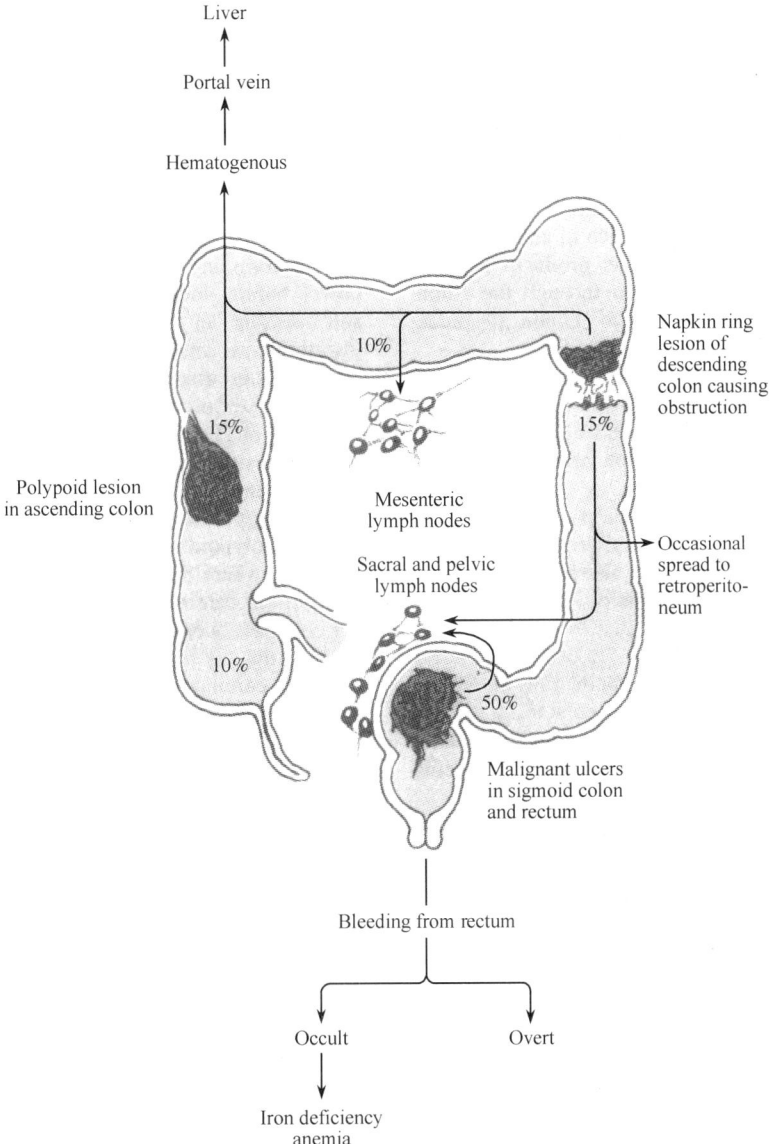

Figure 8-22　Colon carcinoma – sites, gross appearances, and spread

carcinoma. Asymptomatic rectal carcinomas are detected by rectal examination, which should be part of every routine physical examination.

The earliest detectable abnormality is the presence of occult blood in the stools. Examination of stools for occult blood is the only cost-effective means of detecting early colon carcinoma. Chronic intestinal blood loss causes iron deficiency anemia. All patients with iron deficiency anemia must be evaluated for intestinal cancer.

Symptoms in colon carcinoma are any change in bowel habits, including constipation and diarrhea, and bleeding per rectum. Blood is bright red in rectosigmoid cancers and admixed with feces and altered in more proximal lesions.

Left-sided colon cancers commonly present with intestinal obstruction because they tend to be constricting lesions in a narrow part of the colon where the feces are solid. In contrast, right-sided carcinomas rarely present with intestinal obstruction because they are polypoid masses in a more capacious part of the colon where the feces are still semiliquid. Right-sided colon carcinoma commonly presents with abdominal pain, weight loss, anemia,

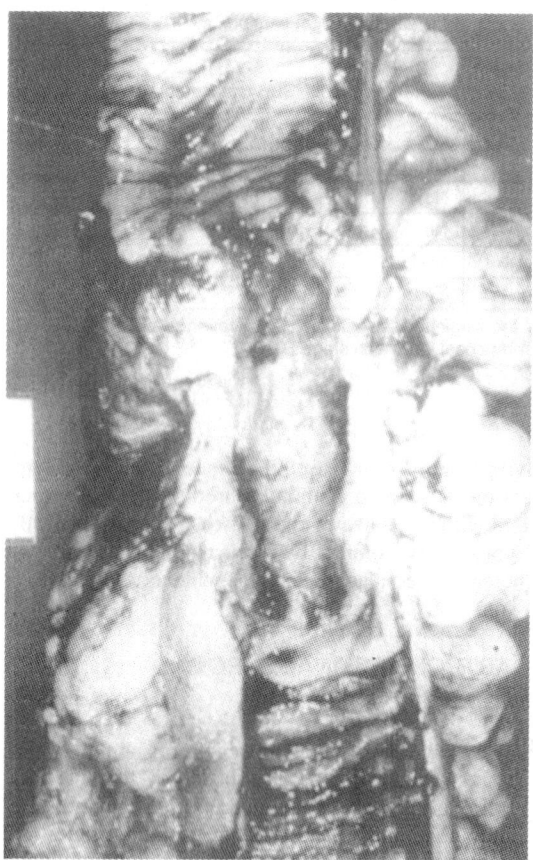

Figure 8-23 Colon carcinoma, showing the circumferential, stenosing type of carcinoma (apple core lesion) that is typically seen in the left side of the colon

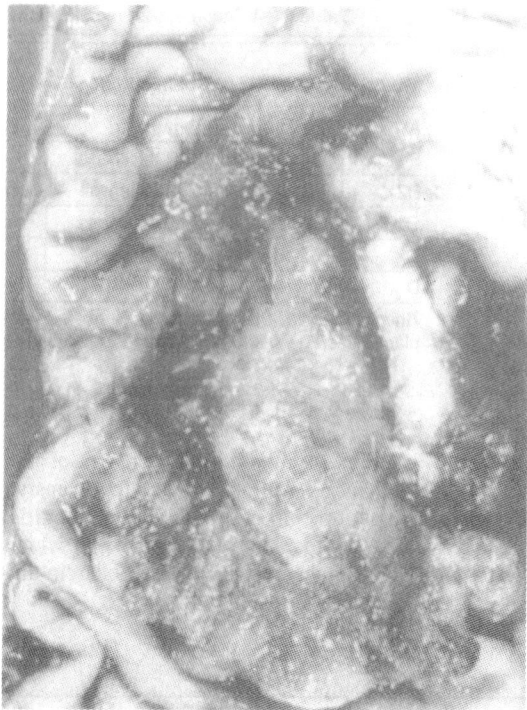

Figure 8-24 Rectal carcinoma, showing the typical malignant ulcer with raised, everted edges

and a palpable abdominal mass is frequently present.

Serum carcinoembryonic antigen (CEA) levels are elevated in about 70% of patients with colon cancer. This is not specific because levels are elevated in many other types of cancer (pancreas, lung). Elevated CEA levels return to normal after surgical resection of colon cancer. Elevation of CEA during follow-up is an indicator of recurrence of tumor.

F. Diagnosis and Treatment

Both colonoscopy and barium enema examination are accurate in detecting colon carcinoma; the former permits biopsy and pathologic diagnosis before surgery. Surgical resection of the involved segment of colon is the mainstay of treatment of colon cancer. Postoperative chemotherapy with levamisole and 5-fluorouracil decreases recurrences by 40% and the risk of death by 33% in patients with stage C (node-positive) colon carcinoma.

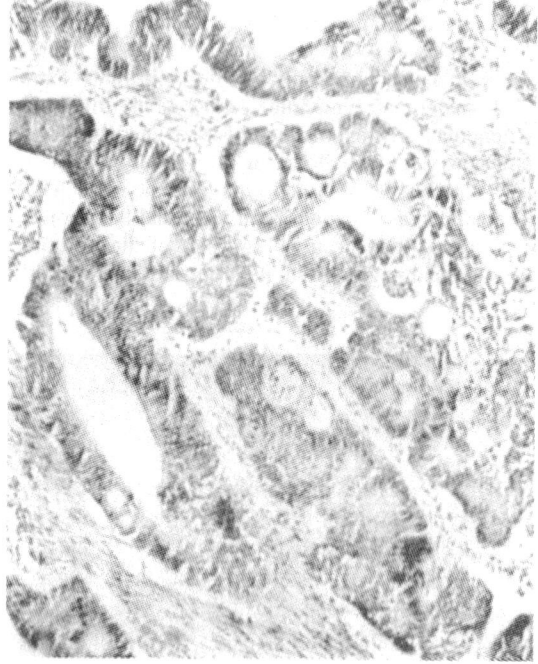

Figure 8-25 Adenocarcinoma of the colon, showing malignant, infiltrating glands. The glandular architecture is complex, with cribriform spaces. The nuclei are arranged irregularly with loss of polarity

G. Prognostic Factors

1. Clinicopathologic stage

The clinicopathologic stage of the disease-assessed by microscopic examination of the resected colon – is the most important prognostic factor. The most commonly used staging system is the modified Dukes system (Table 8-3).

2. Histologic grade

The histologic grade is a numerical expression of the degree of differentiation of the adenocarcinoma. This is a minor prognostic factor. Poorly differentiated (grade III) neoplasms and those with large amounts of extracellular mucin (mucinous carcinoma) have a worse prognosis than well-differentiated (grade I) carcinoma.

(Gan Runliang)

Table 8-3 Astler-Coller modification of Dukes staging system for colon carcinoma

Stage	Invasion of Colonic Wall	Lymph Node Metastases	Distant Metastases	5-Year Survival Rate
A	Mucosa and submucosa[1]	No	No	>90%
B1	Partial muscle wall thickness	No	No	67%
B2	Full thickness of muscle wall	No	No	55%
C1	Partial muscle wall thickness	Yes	No	40%
C2	Full thickness of muscle wall	Yes	No	20%
D	Any	Yes or no	Yes	<10%

[1] Involvement of the submucosa is not addressed in the original Astler-Coller classification and is placed in stage A arbitrarily. Some authorities place submucosal lesions in stage B1.

3. Vascular invasion

Vascular invasion is a minor adverse prognostic factor.

DISEASES OF THE LIVER

STRUCTURE AND FUNCTION OF THE LIVER

Structure of the Liver

The liver is located under the right diaphragm in the lower part of the right rib cage. The left lobe of the liver is in the epigastrium and is therefore not protected by the rib cage. The normal liver is firm and has a smooth surface.

The liver parenchyma is divided into functional units called **lobules** (Figures 8-26 and 8-27). Each lobule is 1 – 2 mm in diameter and is made up of a maze-like arrangement of interconnected plates of hepatocytes separated by endothelium-lined sinusoids (Figure 8-27). The liver cell plates are arranged radially around the central vein; the liver cells that surround a portal tract comprise the **limiting plate**. Liver cell plates are normally one hepatocyte in thickness. Individual hepatocytes are large, with a central round nucleus, a prominent nucleolus, and abundant granular cytoplasm.

The **liver cells** are separated from the sinusoids by a narrow space (space of Disse) that contains connective tissue and represents the scant interstitial compartment of the liver. Specialized cells of the macrophage system (Kupffer cells) are present in the sinusoids scattered among the endothelial cells.

The **biliary system** begins at the biliary canaliculi, which are small channels lined by the complex microvilli of surrounding liver cells. The biliary canaliculi form the intralobular bile ductules (canals of Hering), which drain into the bile ducts in the portal tract.

Functions of the Liver

The normal liver has a huge reserve functional capacity. When the liver is normal, about 80% of it can be removed without compromising function. The liver has synthetic, excretory, and metabolic functions.

A. Synthetic Functions

The liver is the source of plasma albumin; many plasma globulins, including α_1-antitrypsin; and many proteins of the coagulation cascade.

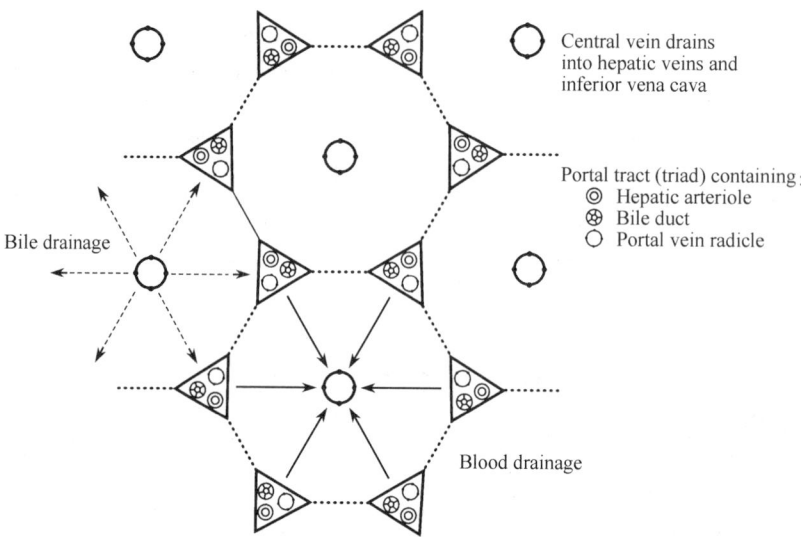

Figure 8-26 Liver lobular architecture, showing blood and bile flow. The sinusoids receive blood from branches of the portal vein and hepatic artery and drain into the central vein (solid arrows). Bile drainage is in the opposite direction, toward the portal tracts (dotted arrows)

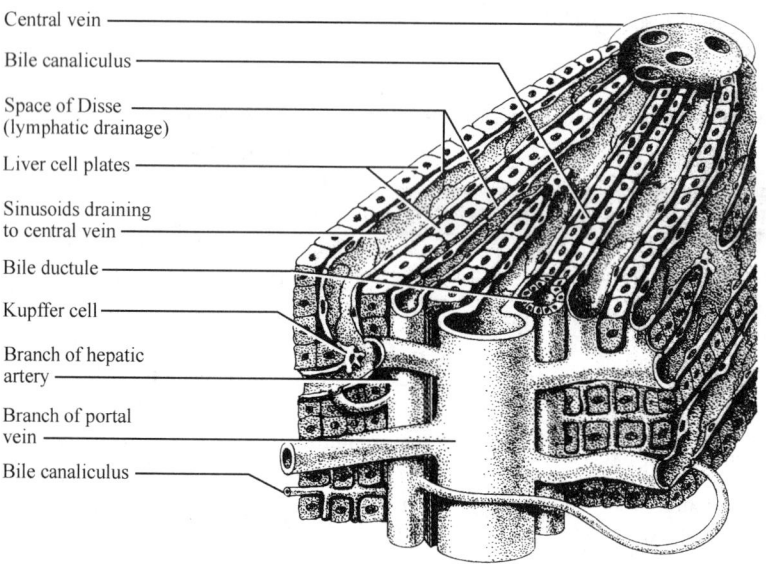

Figure 8-27 Detailed structure of the liver lobule, showing blood and bile flow

B. Excretory Functions

Many substances are excreted by the liver in bile. The main component of bile is bilirubin. Cholesterol, urobilinogen, and bile acids are also present in bile.

C. Metabolic Functions

The liver plays a central role in the metabolism of fat, carbohydrates, and protein and in detoxification.

1. Fat metabolism

Free fatty acids from adipose tissue and medium- or short-chain fatty acids absorbed in the intestine are brought to the liver. Triglycerides, cholesterol, and phospholipids are synthesized in the liver from the fatty acids and complexed with specific lipid acceptor proteins to form very-low-density **lipoproteins** that enter the plasma. The liver also metabolizes intermediate- and low-density lipoproteins.

2. Carbohydrate metabolism

The liver is the main source of plasma **glucose**. Following a meal, glucose is derived from intestinal absorption. In the fasting state, glucose is derived from glycogenolysis and gluconeogenesis in the liver. The liver is the main body storage site for glycogen. When there is a glucose deficiency, the liver metabolizes fatty acids to form ketone bodies, which represent an alternative energy source for many tissues.

3. Protein metabolism

In addition to its synthetic function, the liver is the central organ in protein catabolism and synthesis of urea. Urea is secreted by the liver into the plasma for excretion by the kidney.

4. Detoxification

The liver plays a vital role in detoxifying noxious nitrogenous compounds derived from the intestine, as well as many drugs and chemicals.

VIRAL HEPATITIS

Etiology

Viruses that primarily infect the liver include hepatitis A, hepatitis B, hepatitis C, hepatitis D, hepatitis E and hepatitis G viruses. Hepatitis also occurs as part of systemic viral infection in yellow fever, infectious mononucleosis (Epstein Barr virus), cytomegalovirus infection, herpes simplex, and varicella-zoster infection, but these are not necessarily considered to be 'hepatitis viruses' because the infection is not just confined to the liver.

A. Hepatitis A

Hepatitis A is caused by an RNA enterovirus measuring 27 nm in diameter that has been identified in the stools of patients and infected volunteers. It is usually transmitted via the fecal-oral route and has a short incubation period (2-6 weeks). Explosive epidemics have been recorded after fecal contamination of water, milk, and shellfish. Parenteral transmission is rare, occurring only in the transient acute viremic phase.

Hepatitis A has a global incidence, highest in low socioeconomic populations where fecal-oral transmission is greatest.

Hepatitis A is usually a mild acute illness with recovery occurring in a few weeks. It is rarely fatal in the few cases complicated by massive necrosis, does not progress to chronic hepatitis, and there is no carrier state.

B. Hepatitis B

Hepatitis B is caused by a DNA virus (Figure 8-28) composed of (1) an inner core synthesized in the hepatocyte nucleus and containing the hepatitis B core antigen (HBcAg), hepatitis B e antigen (HBeAg), DNA, and DNA polymerase; and (2) an outer envelope that is synthesized in the hepatocyte cytoplasm and contains the hepatitis B surface antigen (HBsAg). The entire particle measures 42nm in diameter and is called the **Dane particle**. There is excess production of the envelope, free forms of which appear in the blood; these measure 22 nm in size and have a spherical or tubular structure. HBsAg itself is not infective because the nucleic acid core of the virus is required for infection.

The incidence of hepatitis B is quite high in China. Hepatitis B is usually transmitted in blood or blood products from an individual with active disease or a carrier. Transfer may occur with shared needles, during sexual intercourse, by accidental spillage of specimens in the laboratory, and by transfusion of blood products as well as by mother to infant.

Hepatitis B has a long (6 weeks to 6 months) incubation period. Illness is of varying severity and often subclinical. However, the risk of a complicated course, death, chronic disease, or a carrier state is much greater than in hepatitis A.

The appearance of the various hepatitis B antigens and antibodies (Figure 8-29) is important from a diagnostic standpoint. HBsAg appears first, late in the incubation period, and is followed by HBeAg. The presence of HBeAg and hepatitis B-DNA in the serum correlate well with the presence of infective Dane particles in the blood, and they are indications of infectivity. In patients who recover, both HBsAg and HBeAg disappear at the onset of clinical recovery. The first antibody to appear is anti-HBc during the acute illness, followed by anti-HBs. The presence of anti-HBe in the blood indicates absence

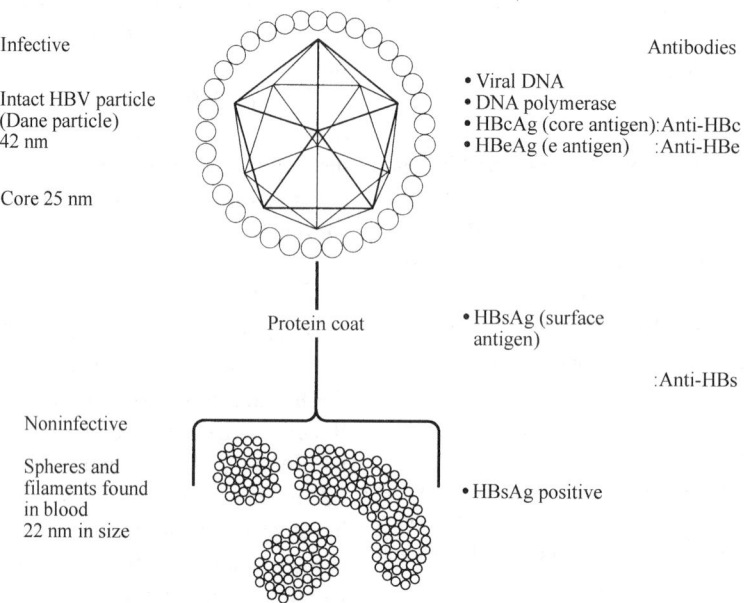

Figure 8-28 Hepatitis B virus. The antibodies that are commonly detected in serum for diagnosis are shown on the right

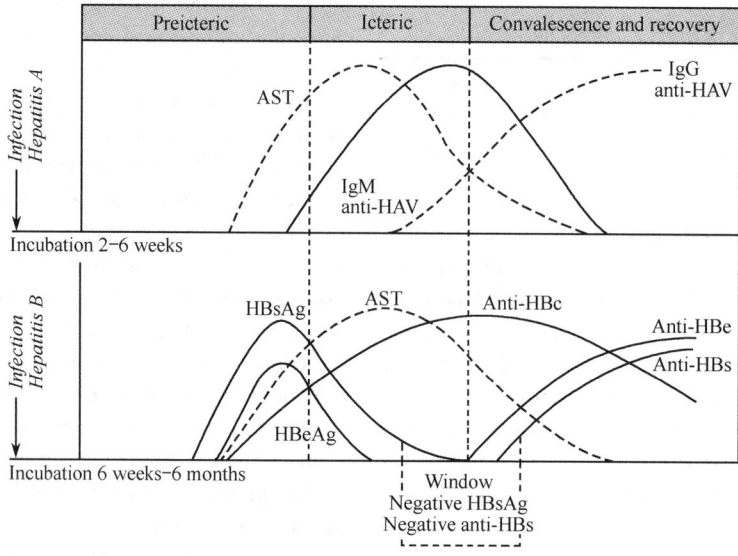

Figure 8-29 Serum antibody and antigen levels in hepatitis A and hepatitis B

of the infective Dane particle; such patients are usually not infective. Testing for all antigens and antibodies permits diagnosis at all stages of the illness. If the testing includes only HBsAg and anti-HBs, there is a window period during the recovery phase when both of these are negative and the diagnosis may be missed.

Hepatitis B-infected hepatocytes may be identified (1) in biopsy material by the presence of hepatocytes with ground-glass cytoplasm (Figure 8-30A); (2) by Shikata orcein stain, which selectively stains hepatitis B-infected cells; and (3) by immunoperoxidase stains using labeled antibodies against HBsAg (Figure 8-30B). The third method is the most specific.

C. Hepatitis C

Hepatitis C virus is a single-stranded RNA virus. Infected patients develop anti-HCV antibodies that can be detected in the serum by immunoassays. Before serologic testing was routinely available, hepatitis C was responsible for over 90% of cases of hepatitis associated with transfusion of blood products. The disease also occurs among drug abusers, in transplant recipients, and in renal dialysis units. The incubation period varies between 2 weeks and 6 months.

Hepatitis C has clinical features almost identical to those of hepatitis B except for a higher incidence of chronic hepatitis, which occurs in 50% of those infected. Cirrhosis complicates 20%. Interferon therapy is useful in controlling chronic hepatitis C.

D. Hepatitis D (Delta Hepatitis)

The hepatitis D virus, also called delta hepatitis agent, is an RNA virus that has the envelope of hepatitis B virus but an antigenically distinct core of delta antigen. It appears to be a "defective" virus that uses hepatitis B virus as a "helper" because it is incapable of causing infection in the absence of hepatitis B virus. HDV is transmitted by the same means as HBV, i.e. sexually, by blood and perinatally.

Hepatitis D occurs (1) as an acute disease along with hepatitis B or (2) as acute or chronic hepatitis in a chronic carrier of HBsAg. The diagnosis is made by demonstration of the antigenically unique delta agent in the blood or in liver cells. HDV increases the severity of an attack of acute hepatitis B and increases the risk of chronic hepatitis and cirrhosis when compared with hepatitis B infection alone.

E. Hepatitis E

Hepatitis E virus is non-enveloped, single-stranded RNA virus tentatively classified as a member of the calicivirus family. Hepatitis E is an uncommon infection occurring mainly in Central America and some Asian countries. Hepatitis E resembles hepatitis A in having a primarily enteric mode of transmission.

F. Hepatitis G

Hepatitis G virus (HGV) was isolated from patients with posttransfusion hepatitis in 1996. HGV is a flavivirus, like HCV to which it is closely related. It is associated with some cases of acute or chronic non-A, non-B, non-C, non-D, non-E hepatitis. Although it seems common in human blood, it may not be a significant cause of hepatitis in human.

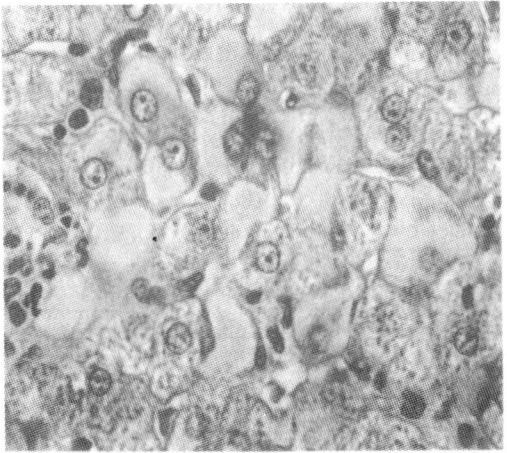

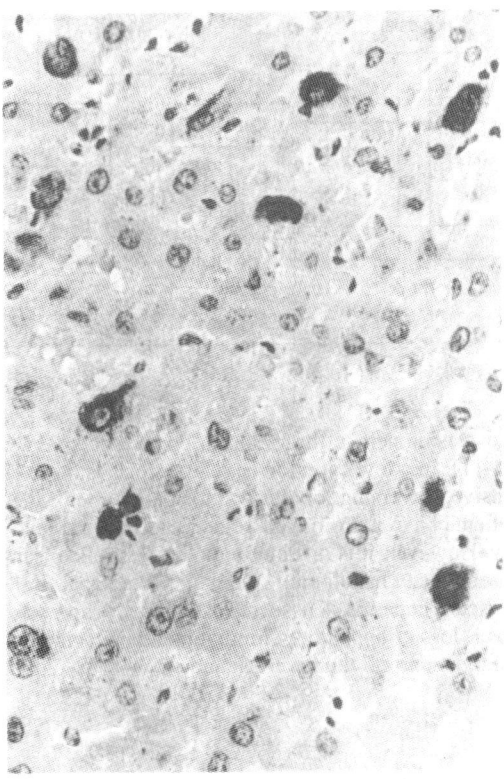

Figure 8-30 A: Hepatocytes infected with hepatitis B virus show a ground-glass appearance that contrasts with the coarsely granular cytoplasm of uninfected hepatocytes; B: Hepatitis B antigens demonstrated in infected hepatocytes by the immunoperoxidase technique (positive cells show black cytoplasmic staining)

Basic Pathological Changes

The basic pathological changes of viral hepatitis include the following:

A. Damages of liver cells

1. Degeneration of liver cells

The most common seen degenerative change is cytoplasmic swelling of liver cells, typically ballooning changes (Figure 8-31).

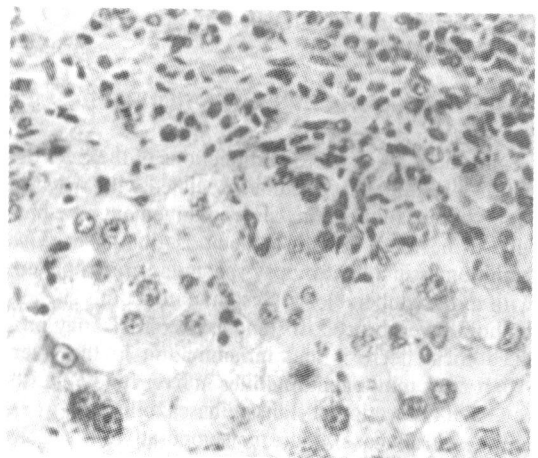

Figure 8-31 Acute viral hepatitis, showing marked edema of hepatocytes and lymphocytic infiltration of the portal areas

2. Apoptosis of individual liver cells

The apoptosis is recognizable by the formation of eosinophilic Councilman bodies (acidophilic bodies).

3. Necrosis of liver cells

Liver cell necrosis is a common manifestation of viral hepatitis, the following types of necrosis could be seen in different viral hepatitis (Figure 8-32).

- **Focal necrosis**: Focal liver cell necrosis is randomly occurring necrosis of single cell or small clusters of cells in all areas of liver lobules. Not all lobules are involved. Its presence is recognized in biopsies by areas of lysed liver cells surrounded by collections of Kupffer cells and inflammatory cells.
- **Zonal necrosis**: Zonal liver cell necrosis is necrosis of liver cells occurring in identical regions in all liver lobules. Centrizonal necrosis, which involves the cells around the central hepatic vein, could be seen in viral hepatitis.
- **Piecemeal necrosis**: Liver cells at the interface between parenchyma and fibrous tissue are destroyed, together with lymphocytic or plasma cell infiltrate (Figure 8-34).

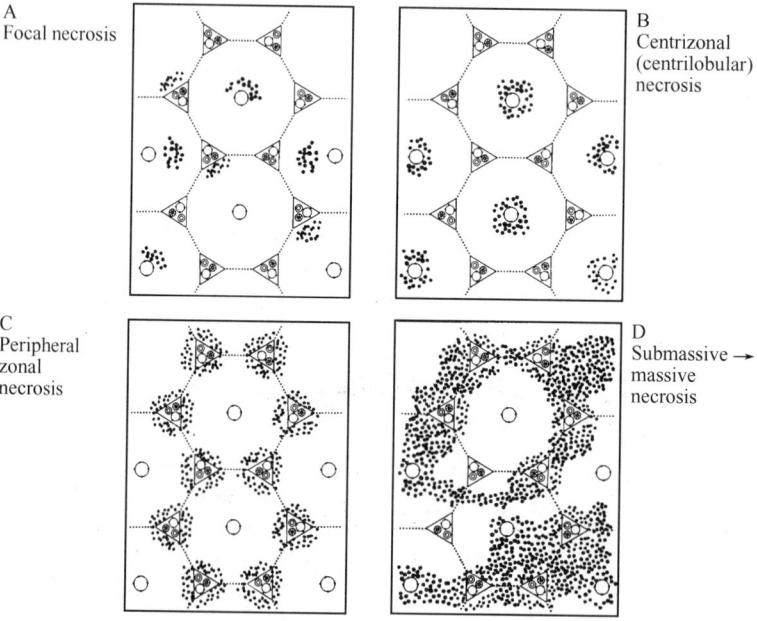

Figure 8-32 Pattern of liver cell necrosis. A: Focal necrosis is a patchy necrosis involving lobules haphazardly. B and C: Zonal necrosis is a necrosis of liver cells in a constant part of every liver lobule. D: Submassive and massive necrosis is extensive necrosis of cells involving multiple adjacent lobules in a contiguous manner

- **Submassive and massive necrosis**: Submassive necrosis is the occurrence of liver cell necrosis that extends across lobular boundaries, often bridging portal areas and central veins (**bridging necrosis**). The most severe form is massive liver necrosis, in which large confluent areas of liver undergo necrosis, leaving only small islands of viable liver cells intact. Massive necrosis is characterized by sudden decrease in size of the liver, which appears soft, yellow, and flabby, with a wrinkled capsule (sometimes called "acute yellow atrophy"). Areas of residual viable liver are seen as mottled dark brown areas contrasting with the necrotic yellow zones.

B. Inflammatory Cell Infiltration

Infiltration of portal tract by mixed inflammatory cells, usually, lymphocyte and plasma cell. In severe cases, chronic inflammation with lymphocytes and plasma cells in the portal tracts may extend into the liver lobule, disrupting the limiting plate of hepatocytes.

C. Parenchymal Regeneration and Interstitial Reaction

Different degrees of liver cell regeneration, hyperplasia of Kupffer cell and stellate cell may be seen in recovery stage and chronic hepatitis. In severe chronic hepatitis, portal fibrosis occurs and progressively increases. Cirrhosis results in the most severe cases.

Clinical Types(Figure 8-33)

The clinicopathologic features of viral hepatitis are considered here as a group (Table 8-4). It is important to note that hepatitis A and probably hepatitis E are mild diseases associated with few deaths and no chronic phase. The other viruses cause much more severe illness with a chronic phase and a carrier state.

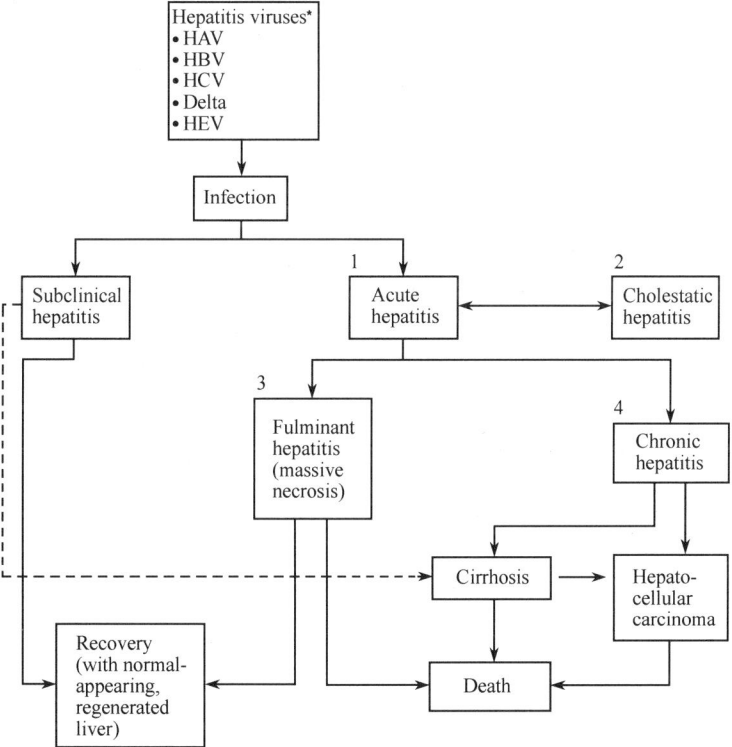

Figure 8-33 Clinical syndromes associated with viral hepatitis. The most common clinical syndrome is acute hepatitis (1), which is sometimes associated with intrahepatic cholestasis (2). Fulminant hepatitis (3) is associated with massive necrosis and with a high mortality rate. Chronic hepatitis (4) may progress to cirrhosis of the liver or hepatocellular carcinoma. * Note that the different viruses have greatly differing tendencies to cause these various clinical syndromes(Table 8-4)

Table 8-4 Hepatitis viruses and the different clinicopathologic forms of liver disease[1]

	Hepatitis A	Hepatitis B	Hepatitis C	Delta Hepatitis	Hepatitis E
Subclinical	+	+	+	+	+
Acute hepatitis	+	+	+	+	+
Fulminant hepatitis (massive necrosis)	+ (rare)	+	+	+	+
Chronic hepatitis	−	+	+	+	?
Cirrhosis	−	+	+ +	+	?
Hepatocellular carcinoma	−	+	+	+	?

[1] The outcome in any given patient is dependent upon age, immunologic status, "dose" of virus, and interactions of viruses such as that between hepatitis B virus and delta virus.

A. Acute Viral Hepatitis

All the hepatitis viruses, replicating within the liver cell, cause damage, either as a direct effect or via an immunologic response against cells bearing viral antigens. Damaged cells show diffuse swelling (ballooning; Figure 8-31). Focal or centrizonal necrosis follows. Single necrotic liver cells have coagulated pink cytoplasm and show pyknosis or karyolysis (Councilman body, **which is now generally considered as apoptosis**). There is a lymphocytic and plasma cell infiltrate in the portal tracts (Figure 8-31). In a few cases, liver cell necrosis is more extensive, traversing lobular boundaries. Some of these patients have a prolonged course and delayed recovery. However, it is difficult to predict chronic disease based on any histologic features in acute hepatitis.

Acute hepatitis is associated with sudden onset of fever, loss of appetite, vomiting, jaundice, and tender enlargement of the liver. Jaundice is caused by a combination of liver cell dysfunction and cholestasis. Bile is present in the urine in most cases, and urinary urobilinogen levels are increased. Liver enzymes (aminotransferases and lactate dehydrogenase) enter the bloodstream from the necrotic cells, appearing early in the course of illness. A few patients develop extrahepatic manifestations such as lymph node enlargement, skin rashes, and joint pains that probably result from circulating immune complexes.

Acute viral hepatitis is frequently subclinical or associated with a flu-like illness (anicteric hepatitis). It can then be diagnosed only by liver function tests (elevated liver enzymes, increased urinary urobilinogen) or hepatitis antibody test. Antibody testing is the only means of identifying the specific virus.

Clinical recovery occurs within 2–3 weeks in most cases. Return of biochemical abnormalities to normal may take months. Recovery is associated with liver cell regeneration.

B. Cholestatic Viral Hepatitis

A clinical variant of acute viral hepatitis is characterized by severe intrahepatic cholestasis, with deep jaundice, bilirubin in the urine, and absence of urobilinogen in urine and feces. The chances of complete recovery are not reduced by this complication.

C. Fulminant Viral Hepatitis

Fulminant viral hepatitis is the most severe form of hepatitis. A fulminant course is characterized by abrupt onset of liver failure associated with massive or submassive liver cell necrosis occurs in about 1% of cases of hepatitis B and hepatitis C and more rarely in hepatitis A. Patients with coinfection with hepatitis B and D have a greater incidence than those with hepatitis B alone.

Patients with fulminant viral hepatitis are divided into two major groups based on morphology, those who have less than a single layer of hepatocyte around the portal areas and no islands of viable parenchyma are classified as having acute massive necrosis; those with larger numbers of hepatocytes, either as islands of regenerating tissue or as evenly distributed periportal cells, are classified as having acute submassive necrosis.

In acute massive necrosis, the liver is shrunken, limp. The capsule is wrinkled. When the liver is sectioned, the portal connective is accentuated, the remaining tissue is deep red and retracted. The liver in acute necrosis simulates the appearance of spleen and thus, is referred as acute red atrophy. In some cases, the liver appears soft, yellow, and flabby, with a wrinkled capsule, and thus referred as acute yellow atrophy. Microscopic study reveals the destruction of hepatocytes. The kupffer cells are large and numerous, and there is a minimum amount of lymphocytic infiltrate and hyperplasia. The stromal collapse is noted. The bile ducts show little hyperplasia unless the fulminant episode occurred late in the course of ordinary hepatitis.

Clinically, acute liver failure may result from sudden severe impairment of hepatic function because of massive parenchymal cell necrosis. The clinical features including (1) rapidly developing jaundice; (2) hypoglycemia; (3) a bleeding tendency due to disseminated intravascular coagulation and failure of synthesis of clotting factors in the liver; (4) electrolyte and acid-base disturbances (hypokalemia is the most dangerous); (5) hepatic encephalopathy; (6) hepatorenal syndrome; and (7) elevation of serum enzymes (LDH, AST, ALT, etc).

The mortality rate of acute massive necrosis is high. Survivors regenerate a normal liver and do not have chronic liver disease.

In acute submassive necrosis, the pathological changes are dependent on the period of survival. Generally, the liver is characterized grossly by islands of yellow liver parenchyma bulging above the surround dark collapsed stroma (subacute yellow atrophy). Microscopically, both large confluent areas of hepatocytic necrosis (submassive necrosis) and nodular regeneration of hepatocytes could be seen.

D. Chronic Viral Hepatitis

Chronic viral hepatitis is defined as the presence, in viral hepatitis, of a clinical, biochemical, or serologic abnormality lasting over 6 months. Chronic hepatitis is caused by viruses B, C, and D, but not by hepatitis A or E. An identical clinicopathologic syndrome occurs as a toxic reaction to certain drugs (oxyphenisatin, methyldopa, isoniazid) and in Wilson's disease, α_1-antitrypsin deficiency, and autoimmune chronic active hepatitis. Diagnosis of viral etiology is by serologic tests for the specific viruses.

Clinically, chronic hepatitis is characterized by a spectrum of disease, which can be characterized in increasing severity as follows: (1) **Asymptomatic carrier state** with normal liver histology. Here, viral serology is positive and virus can be demonstrated in hepatocytes. There are no symptoms, biochemical abnormalities, or histologic evidence of inflammation; (2) **Minimal chronic hepatitis** (previously called chronic persistent hepatitis), which is characterized by minimal symptoms and/or mild biochemical abnormalities (e.g. slightly elevated enzyme levels), and the presence of lymphocytes and plasma cells in the portal triad. Portal chronic inflammation is mild and restricted to the portal triads without extension into the liver lobule across the limiting plate. There is little or no active hepatocyte necrosis and minimal fibrosis; (3) **Chronic active hepatitis**, which is characterized by continuing necrosis of liver cells. The portal areas show severe chronic inflammation with lymphocytes and plasma cells extending into the liver lobule (Figure 8-34), disrupting the limiting plate of hepatocytes. Liver cells in the periphery of the liver lobule are entrapped in the inflammation and undergo necrosis (**piecemeal necrosis**). Portal fibrosis occurs and progressively increases. Cirrhosis results in the most severe cases.

Patients with chronic hepatitis may have disease that progresses at varying rates. Some patients have minimal disease for many years; others pro-

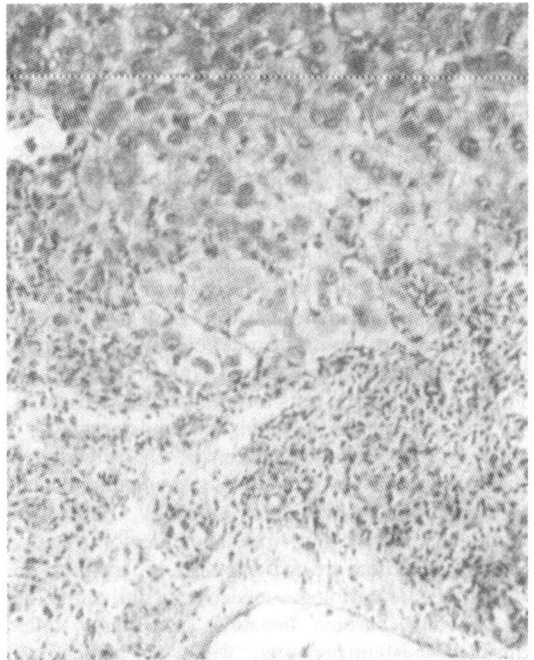

Figure 8-34 Chronic active hepatitis, showing marked lymphocytic infiltration and fibrosis of the portal areas. The lymphocytes extend into the peripheral part of the lobule through the limiting plate. There is ongoing necrosis of hepatocytes in the peripheral part of the lobule (piecemeal necrosis)

gress rapidly through severely progressive active hepatitis to the onset of cirrhosis. The activity of chronic hepatitis may also change, either spontaneously or with treatment. Remission of active disease frequently has histologic features of minimal disease.

The main causes of death in chronic hepatitis are (1) cirrhosis of the liver with chronic liver failure or the effects of portal hypertension and (2) development of hepatocellular carcinoma.

It should be noted that the chronic viral hepatitis in our country is divided into mild, moderate and severe types. The currently used classification for chronic viral hepatitis in China was based on the Protocols for the Treatment and Prevention of Viral Hepatitis determined in the Conference of Viral Hepatitis and Hepatopathy in Xi'an (2000). The classification of chronic hepatitis was based on the grade of inflammation.

1. Mild chronic hepatitis

Mild chronic hepatitis (including the previously called chronic persistent hepatitis and mild active chronic hepatitis) is characterized pathologically by the following: degeneration of hepatocytes, spotty (focal) necrosis or the formation of apoptotic bodies; with (without) inflammatory cell infiltration and expansion of portal areas; with (without) focal piecemeal necrosis; the lobular architectures are intact.

2. Moderate chronic hepatitis

Moderate chronic hepatitis (basically the former moderate chronic active hepatitis) is pathologically characterized by prominent inflammatory changes in portal area with moderate piecemeal necrosis; severe intra-lobular inflammation, confluent necrosis or with a few bridging necrosis; fibrous septa could be seen but the architectures in most lobules remain intact.

3. Severe chronic hepatitis

Severe chronic hepatitis (basically the former severe chronic active hepatitis) is characterized pathologically by severe inflammation in portal area or inflammation with severe piecemeal necrosis; bridging necrosis involving most of the lobules; large amount of fibrous septa formed and lobular architectures destroyed or even early cirrhosis could be seen.

ALCOHOLIC LIVER DISEASE

A. Incidence and Pathogenesis

Chronic alcoholism is a major problem in almost every society. The incidence is quite high in Western countries and is increasing in our country. Alcoholic liver disease is most common in middle-aged men, but there is an increasing incidence among women and in the young.

The greater the amount and the longer the duration of alcohol consumption, the greater the risk of liver disease is. Most patients with chronic alcoholic liver disease have consumed about 150 g or more of ethyl alcohol daily for over 10 years.

Not all heavy drinkers develop liver disease. About 50% of alcoholics have no detectable liver disease, 30% have alcoholic hepatitis, and 20% develop cirrhosis. Prediction of liver disease in individual cases is uncertain.

Alcohol is metabolized in the hepatocyte cytoplasm by the NADH-dependent enzyme alcohol dehydrogenase into acetaldehyde. Acetaldehyde or a related substance is believed to exert a toxic effect on liver cells. Malnutrition, which frequently coexists with alcoholism, may aggravate the liver injury.

B. Clinicopathologic Manifestations

Alcoholic liver disease may be manifested as fatty liver, alcoholic hepatitis, or alcoholic cirrhosis (Figure 8-35). These lesions may coexist.

1. Fatty liver

Fatty liver is a common early manifestation of alcohol injury. It is the result of decreased fatty acid oxidation, increased synthesis of triglycerides, and impaired secretion of lipoproteins by the liver cell. Fat accumulates first as small globules that coalesce, increasing in size and pushing the hepatocyte nucleus to one side.

Clinically, fatty liver causes diffuse liver enlargement. Liver function is normal even when there is severe fatty change. Fatty liver is reversible if the patient stops drinking at this stage.

A
Fatty change

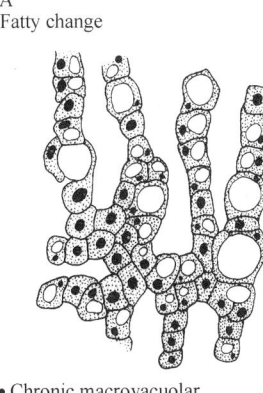

- Chronic, macrovacuolar
- Reversible

B
Acute sclerosing hyaline necrosis

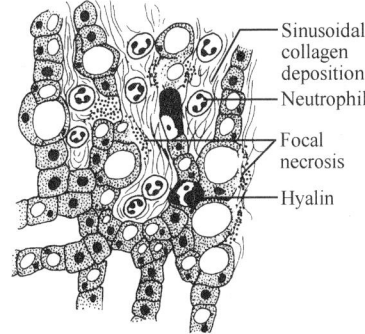

- Sinusoidal collagen deposition
- Neutrophil
- Focal necrosis
- Hyalin

- Focal necrosis with neutrophils
- Cholestasis → jaundice
- Alcoholic hyalin (Mallory bodies)
- Sinusoidal fibrosis
- Reversible unless severe

C
Chronic alcoholic liver disease

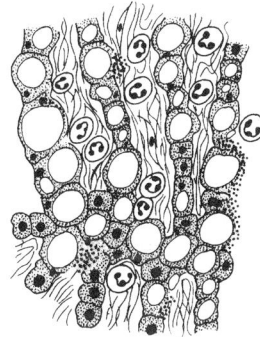

- Ongoing focal necrosis
- Centrilobular and sinusoidal fibrosis
- Some regeneration conserving normal architecture
- ? Irreversible
- ? May not be progressive

D
Alcoholic cirrhosis

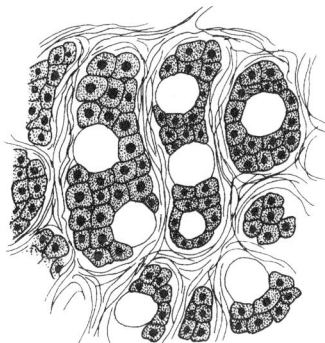

- Ongoing focal necrosis
- Extensive fibrosis
- Regenerative nodules
- Loss of normal architecture
- Progressive and irreversible

Figure 8-35 Alcoholic liver disease. A: Fatty change. B: Acute alcoholic hepatitis (acute sclerosing hyaline necrosis). C: Chronic alcoholic liver disease, precirrhotic. D: Alcoholic cirrhosis

2. Acute alcoholic hepatitis (acute sclerosing hyaline necrosis of the liver)

Acute alcoholic hepatitis is characterized pathologically by (1) focal lytic necrosis of hepatocytes, causing an increase in serum enzyme levels; (2) cholestasis with jaundice; (3) neutrophilic infiltration of the sinusoids and around necrotic liver cells; (4) sclerosis around the central venule, initially as fine fibrils in the space of Disse and later as coarse fibrosis that may obliterate central veins; and (5) the presence of eosinophilic waxy alcoholic hyalin - Mallory bodies - in the cytoplasm of liver cells (Figure 8-36). Hyalin is a fibrillar material derived from the cell's cytoskeleton; it stains positively for cytokeratin and ubiquitin by the immunoperoxidase technique. Hyalin is not specific for alcoholic liver injury as it is also found in biliary cirrhosis, Indian childhood cirrhosis, Wilson's disease, and liver cell carcinoma.

Clinically, patients present with an acute onset of fever, jaundice, tender enlargement of the liver, and ascites, commonly after a recent bout of heavy drinking. With severe alcoholic hepatitis, encephalopathy and death may occur. Symptoms and most of the pathologic features resolve with cessation of

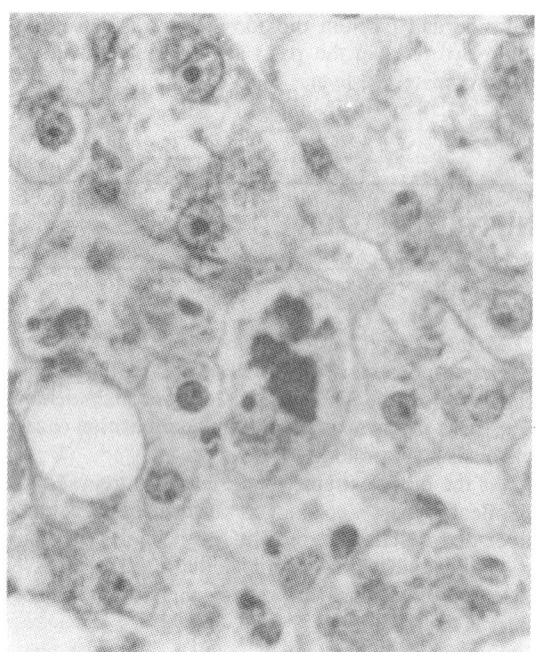

Figure 8-36 Alcoholic hyalin in the cytoplasm of the cell in the center

drinking, but the fibrosis increases progressively with each episode.

3. Chronic alcoholic liver disease

Chronic ingestion of alcohol is associated with progressive fibrosis in the centrizonal region of the liver and distortion of liver architecture by fibrous bands that may connect portal areas and central veins; this differs from cirrhosis in the absence of true regenerative nodules. Progression may slow or come to a halt if alcohol ingestion is discontinued.

4. Alcoholic cirrhosis

Cirrhosis of the liver is discussed below (see Cirrhosis of Liver).

IMMUNOLOGIC DISEASES OF THE LIVER

The role of immunologic hypersensitivity in liver disease is difficult to evaluate. Immune injury probably contributes to the changes seen in viral hepatitis and in several types of drug-induced liver injuries. There is strong evidence that nonviral chronic active hepatitis and primary biliary cirrhosis are the result of injuries mediated by immune mechanisms.

AUTOIMMUNE CHRONIC ACTIVE HEPATITIS

Immune-mediated and viral chronic active hepatitis have identical clinical and pathologic features. Patients with autoimmune chronic active hepatitis have negative viral serologic tests. Anti-smooth muscle antibody and antinuclear antibodies are frequently present in the serum, and the LE cell test is positive (hence "**lupoid**" **hepatitis**). Immune-mediated chronic active hepatitis has no relationship to systemic lupus erythematosus.

In contrast to its viral counterpart, immune-mediated chronic active hepatitis occurs more frequently in women. The disease has a bad prognosis, progressing to cirrhosis in the majority of cases. Corticosteroids are sometimes of value in treatment.

PRIMARY BILIARY CIRRHOSIS

Primary biliary cirrhosis occurs predominantly (over 90% of cases) in middle-aged women. The exact cause is uncertain, but immunologic injury is strongly suspected. Primary biliary cirrhosis is associated with other immunologic diseases such as progressive systemic sclerosis and Sjögren's syndrome and is characterized by the presence in serum of several autoantibodies, the most specific of which is antimitochondrial antibody; when present in the serum in a titer in excess of 1:160, it is diagnostic of primary biliary cirrhosis.

Histologically, the diagnostic changes are in the portal tracts. Lymphocytes and plasma cells surround, infiltrate, and appear to actively destroy the walls of the bile ductules. Epithelioid cell granulomas with Langhans' giant cells occur in 30% of cases. Initial bile duct proliferation is followed by progressive destruction. In the final stage of the disease, bile ducts are absent from the portal tracts, which show marked fibrosis. Even in the terminal phase, primary biliary cirrhosis shows only moderate fibrosis. It does not show nodular regeneration of the liver and is therefore not a true cirrhosis despite its name.

Hepatic parenchymal changes are nonspecific and consist of cholestasis and Kupffer cell hyperplasia. Hyalin may be present in the peripheral zonal liver cells.

Clinically, patients present with slowly progressive biliary obstruction. The onset is insidious; pruritus is the most common first symptom, resulting from accumulation of bile salts in the blood. Portal hypertension and liver failure may occur 5-15 years after onset.

CIRRHOSIS OF THE LIVER

Cirrhosis of the liver is a pathologic entity characterized by (1) necrosis of liver cells, slowly progressive over a long period and ultimately causing chronic liver failure and death; (2) fibrosis, which involves both central veins and portal areas; (3) regenerative nodules, the result of hyperplasia of surviving liver cells; (4) distortion of normal hepatic lobular architecture; and (5) diffuse involvement of the whole liver. A regenerative nodule is an abnormal mass of liver cells without a normal cord pattern or central venule and surrounded completely by fibrosis (Figure 8-37).

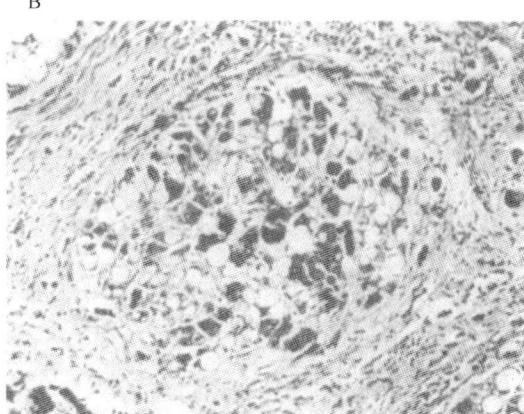

Figure 8-37 Alcoholic cirrhosis of the liver. A: Small regenerative nodules are separated by coarse bands of collagen in which are found blood vessels, bile ducts, and inflammatory cells. B: The regenerative nodule is composed of a disorganized mass of liver cells showing fatty change. There is no central hepatic vein in the nodule

Pathology

Grossly, the liver is enlarged in the early stages, but later it becomes smaller because of cell loss and fibrous contraction. It is much firmer than normal. Nodularity is the most characteristic feature (Figure 8-38). Depending on whether the nodules are more or less than 3 mm in size, cirrhosis is classified as macronodular, micronodular, or mixed.

Figure 8-38 Cirrhosis of the liver (cut surface), showing diffuse nodularity

Histologically, regenerative nodules are characteristic. They are composed of hyperplastic liver cells organized into irregular plates. Liver cells often show enlargement, with atypical nuclei - a picture sometimes called "dysplasia" because of the suspicion that such changes are a precursor of liver cell carcinoma.

The vasculature of the liver is greatly distorted. The fibrous bands obstruct the portal venous radicles and lead to abnormal fistulous communications between portal veins and hepatic arterioles, resulting in portal hypertension.

Clinical Features

Cirrhosis is manifested clinically by features of chronic liver failure and portal hypertension (Figure 8-39). Common presenting symptoms include hematemesis due to rupture of gastroesophageal varices and ascites. Cirrhosis is an irreversible and progressive disease that ultimately causes death. The rate of progression is variable.

Cirrhosis is a premalignant lesion. The risk of hepatocellular carcinoma is greatest in cirrhosis caused by hemochromatosis, virus-induced cirrhosis, cryptogenic cirrhosis, and alcoholic cirrhosis, in order of decreasing hazard.

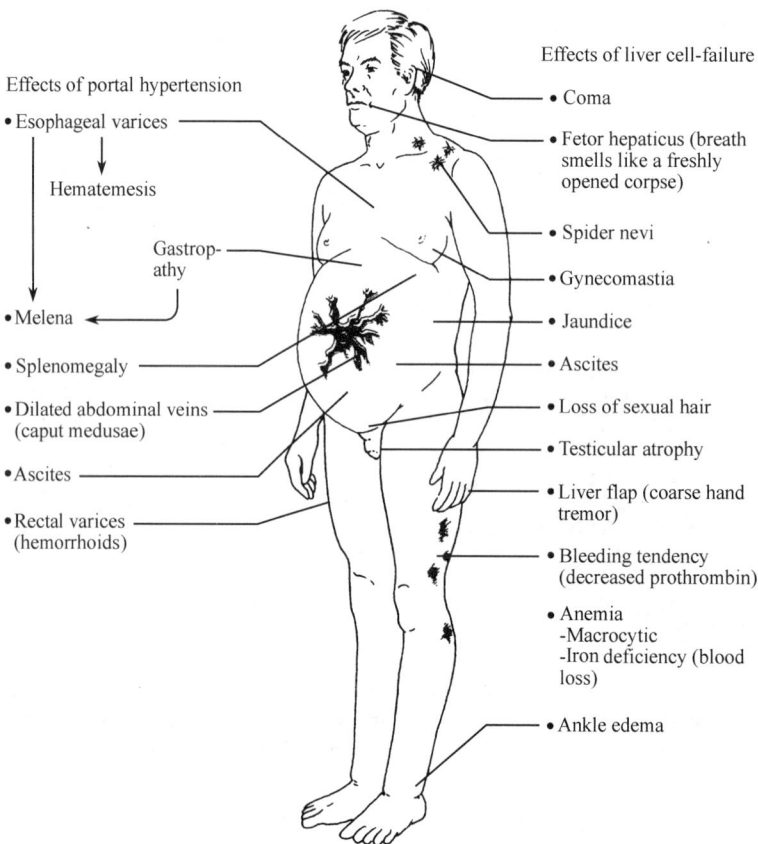

Figure 8-39   Clinical effects of cirrhosis of the liver

A. Chronic Liver Failure

Chronic liver failure usually results from cirrhosis, which is associated with progressive necrosis of liver cells, fibrosis, and nodular regeneration.

The effects of chronic liver failure can be listed as follows:
• Decreased synthesis of albumin, leading to low serum albumin levels, edema, and ascites.
• Decreased levels of prothrombin and of factors VII, IX, and X, resulting in a bleeding tendency.
• Portal hypertension (see below).
• Hepatic encephalopathy.

Hepatic encephalopathy is characterized by cerebral dysfunction (hypersomnia, delirium, flapping tremors of the hands) leading to convulsions, coma, and death. It may occur in both acute and chronic liver disease and is usually accompanied by other evidence of liver failure. In patients with extensive portosystemic venous anastomoses, hepatic encephalopathy may occur in isolation.

Substances suspected of being involved in the pathogenesis of hepatic encephalopathy are (1) ammonia, which is present in high plasma and cerebrospinal fluid concentrations in patients with liver failure; and (2) amides like octopamine, which act as false neurotransmitters.
• Hepatorenal syndrome

Hepatorenal syndrome is the occurrence of acute renal failure in a patient with liver disease. The occurrence of hepatorenal syndrome is an ominous sign in a patient with liver disease.
• Endocrine changes caused by disordered metabolism of certain hormones, testicular atrophy, and small vascular telangiectasias in the skin (spider angiomas). Failure of aldosterone metabolism causes sodium and water retention and contributes to edema. Failure of metabolism of antidiuretic hormone contributes to inappropriately high serum levels of ADH in some cases, causing hyponatremia.
• Fetor hepaticus – a breath like that of "a freshly

opened corpse"-believed to be due to deficient methionine catabolism.

B. Portal Hypertension (Figure 8-40)

Portal hypertension is elevation of portal venous pressure above the upper limit of normal of 12 mmHg. Most cases result from obstruction to the outflow of blood from the portal system. More rarely, portal hypertension results from transmission of arterial pressure to the portal circulation through arteriovenous fistulas, or, in some cases of massive splenomegaly, through dilated splenic sinusoids.

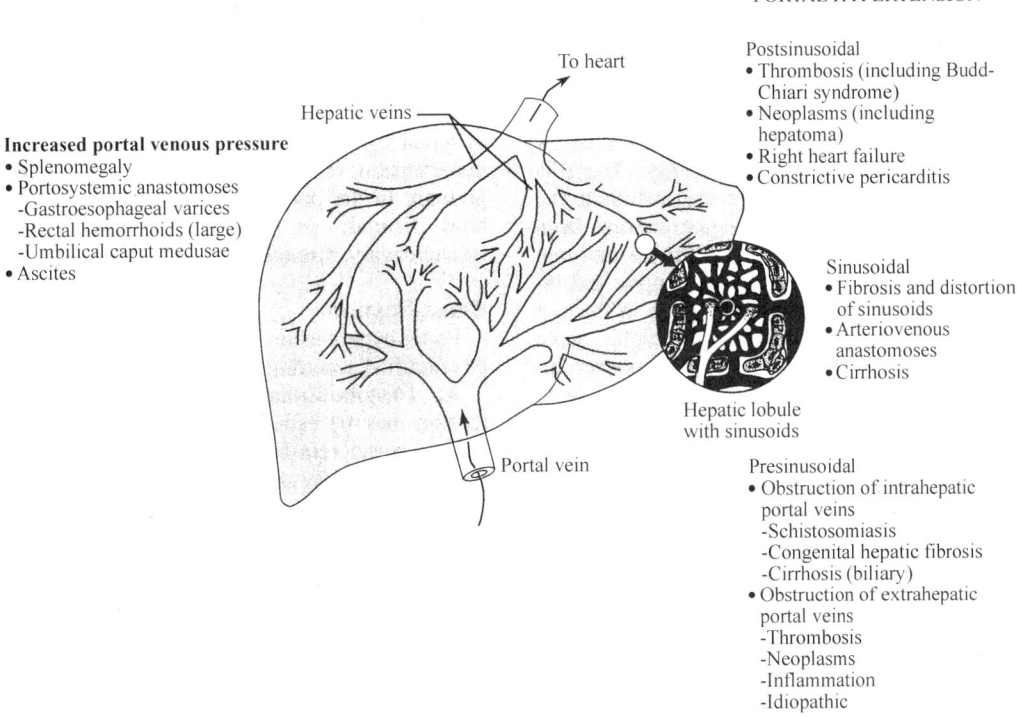

Figure 8-40 Pathogenesis and clinical effects of portal hypertension

1. Splenomegaly

Splenic enlargement is caused by passive venous congestion.

2. Development of Portosystemic Venous Anastomoses, Bypassing the Obstructed Portal Circulation

Venous anastomoses occur wherever the portal and systemic venous drainages commingle, resulting in dilated, tortuous veins at the following sites: (1) in the lower esophagus and stomach (gastroesophageal varices)-these frequently rupture, causing severe upper gastrointestinal bleeding; (2) in the rectum (hemorrhoids); and (3) around the umbilicus, where the collateral veins radiate outward in the abdominal wall (caput medusae).

Entry of portal venous blood into the systemic circulation through these collateral channels may result in **hepatic encephalopathy** because blood bypassing the liver eludes detoxification. Portacaval anastomoses created surgically to relieve portal hypertension may have the same effect.

3. Ascites

Ascites is due to increased transudation of fluid across the peritoneal membrane, particularly over the surface of the liver. The major factor leading to severe ascites in chronic liver disease is a decrease in serum albumin level, with portal hypertension playing only a contributory role.

Classification of Cirrhosis

The terminology of cirrhosis is confusing and unsatisfactory. Characterizing cirrhosis as micronodular and macronodular according to the size of the nodules is of little value because the size of nodules does not correlate with etiology. The terms portal cirrhosis and Laennec's cirrhosis are no longer used; both denoted micronodular cirrhosis of the alcoholic type. The term postnecrotic cirrhosis should no longer be used because all forms of cirrhosis are associated with necrosis of liver cells and are therefore postnecrotic.

Cirrhosis is most usefully classified according to its causes (Table 8-5). All etiologic classifications include a group called cryptogenic cirrhosis (cirrhosis of unknown cause). The incidence of cryptogenic cirrhosis depends on how diligently the cause is sought and how rigorous the criteria are for assigning specific causes to individual cases.

Table 8-5 Etiologic classification of cirrhosis

Type of Cirrhosis	Relative Frequency[1]
Cryptogenic (cause not established)	10%–30%
Alcoholic	30%–60%
Virus-induced (B and C)	10%–30%
Biliary cirrhosis Primary[2] Secondary	10%
Immune-mediated chronic active hepatitis	? 10%
Hemochromatosis	5%
Wilson's disease	Rare
α_1-antitrypsin (-antiprotease) deficiency	Rare
Galactosemia	Rare
Cardiac cirrhosis[2]	Rare

[1] The frequency of these etiologic types of cirrhosis differs greatly in different countries. The commonly quoted figures for the United States are given here. In the United Kingdom, the incidence of cryptogenic cirrhosis is higher. In China, virus-induced cirrhosis is most common etiologic type.

[2] Although traditionally termed cirrhosis, not all of the definitional features are present in these conditions.

A. Cryptogenic Cirrhosis

Hepatic cirrhosis is said to be cryptogenic when complete evaluation of the patient has failed to identify a cause. Cryptogenic cirrhosis may include cirrhosis following immune-mediated chronic active hepatitis or following injury due to drugs or chemicals – because there is no way to identify these causes with certainty. Many patients with cirrhosis give a history of drug ingestion, but it is difficult to establish a causal role for the drugs.

B. Alcoholic Cirrhosis

Alcoholic cirrhosis is frequently associated with evidence of fatty change or acute alcoholic hepatitis. Alcoholic cirrhosis is typically a fatty micronodular cirrhosis (Figure 8-37). In patients who stop drinking, the nodules are not infrequently larger and fat is absent.

Alcoholic cirrhosis tends to have a slow rate of progression, particularly if the patient stops drinking. The disease is irreversible and causes death.

C. Virus-induced Cirrhosis

This is the most commonly seen type of cirrhosis. Cirrhosis may follow chronic active hepatitis resulting from infection with hepatitis B and C viruses. Patients who present with cirrhosis may or may not give a history of hepatitis. Typically, virus-induced cirrhosis is macronodular. Features of chronic active hepatitis may coexist. Virus-induced cirrhosis tends to progress rapidly, with death due to chronic liver failure, portal hypertension, or hepatocellular carcinoma.

Cirrhosis caused by hepatitis B virus may be identified by the presence of HBsAg in the serum and in liver cells; orcein stains and immunoperoxidase stains for HBsAg are positive. A few cases of cirrhosis due to hepatitis B show coinfection with delta hepatitis that can be demonstrated by immunologic techniques. Patients with cirrhosis caused by hepatitis C have anti-HCV antibody in their serum.

D. Biliary Cirrhosis

Primary biliary cirrhosis causes portal fibrosis, but the changes fall short of the definition of true cirrhosis because regenerative nodules are usually absent (Figure 8-41).

Secondary biliary cirrhosis occurs in patients with prolonged large bile duct obstruction (gallstones, stricture, tumor, cholangitis). Marked cholestasis causes liver cell necrosis, and prolonged cholangitis leads to portal fibrosis (Figure 8-41). Biliary cirrhosis causes a fine nodularity (micronodules). Features of chronic liver failure and portal hypertension occur late.

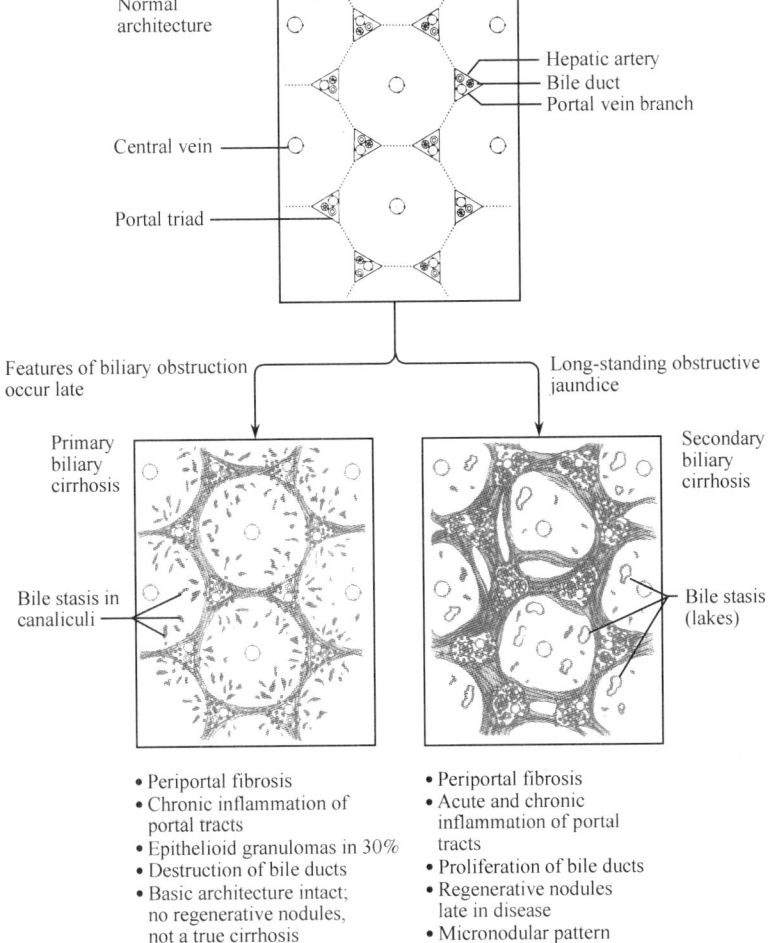

Figure 8-41 Biliary cirrhosis, contrasting the changes of primary versus secondary disease

NEOPLASMS OF THE LIVER

Benign Neoplasms

Benign neoplasms of the liver are not uncommon as incidental findings at autopsy and are becoming increasingly important because modern radiologic imaging procedures are now able to detect small tumors, raising the question of whether such tumors are benign or malignant, primary or secondary. The common seen benign neoplasm of the liver is cavernous hemangioma. Other uncommon benign neoplasms include sclerosing bile duct adenoma, liver cell adenoma, etc.

Malignant Neoplasms

Malignant neoplasms may arise in the liver from (1) hepatocytes (hepatocellular carcinoma), (2) intrahepatic bile ductules (cholangiocarcinoma), and (3) mesenchymal elements such as blood vessels (angiosarcoma and hemangioendothelioma).

A. Hepatocellular Carcinoma

1. Incidence

Hepatocellular carcinoma has a marked geographic variation in incidence, being common in the Far East, especially in China and certain parts of Africa, where in some areas it is the most common type of cancer. It is uncommon in Western Europe and North America.

2. Etiology

The cause is unknown, but several factors have been implicated: (1) **Aflatoxin B_1**, a product of the fungus *Aspergillus flavus*, which grows on improperly stored grain and nuts (including peanuts), is toxic to liver cells. It is present in high levels in grain in Africa and Asia, leading to the suggestion that chronic ingestion of aflatoxin may be at least partially responsible for the high incidence of liver cell carcinoma in these areas; (2) **Hepatitis B virus infection** is strongly suspected of causing hepatocellular carcinoma. African and Far East countries where hepatocellular carcinoma is common have high rates of hepatitis carriers, probably with vertical transmission of the virus from generation to generation; and (3) **Hepatitis C virus infection** is also associated with hepatocellular carcinoma.

Over 80% of patients who develop hepatocellular carcinoma have cirrhosis of the liver. The increased cell turnover in regenerative nodules of cirrhosis is associated with cytologic abnormalities that have been interpreted as premalignant dysplastic changes. While all types of cirrhosis may be complicated by carcinoma, the association is greatest with hemochromatosis, virus-induced cirrhosis, and alcoholic cirrhosis.

3. Pathology

Grossly, hepatocellular carcinoma may present as a large solitary mass (Figure 8-42), as multiple nodules, or as a diffusely infiltrative lesion. Microscopically, the neoplasm is composed of abnormal liver cells of variable differentiation. The better differentiated tumors are composed of cells resembling liver cells arranged in cords separated by sinusoids (Figure 8-43). The cells have enlarged nuclei that show prominent nucleoli and hyperchromatism and may contain bile in the cytoplasm. The less well-differentiated tumors have sheets of anaplastic cells. Invasion of hepatic venous radicles is a typical feature that permits differentiation from adenoma. It may be difficult to distinguish a poorly differentiated hepatocelluar carcinoma from metastatic carcinoma. Rarely, venous involvement is so extensive as to produce Budd-Chiari syndrome. Even more rarely, a tumor thrombus extends along the hepatic vein into the inferior vena cava and up into the right atrium.

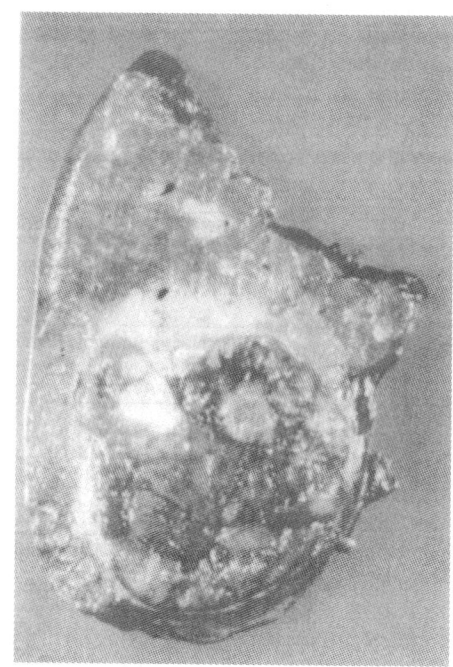

Figure 8-42 Hepatocellular carcinoma, showing a large solitary nodule that is grossly encapsulated except in one area

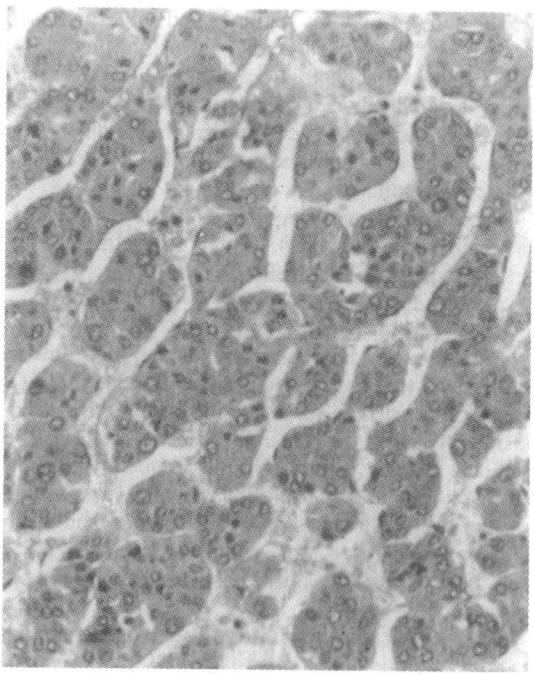

Figure 8-43 Well-differentiated hepatocellular carcinoma, showing trabeculae of malignant hepatocytes separated by sinusoidal spaces. This is characterized by absence of portal areas and greatly expanded trabeculae composed of several layers of malignant hepatocytes

Immunohistochemical stains may show the presence of **alpha-fetoprotein** (**AFP**) in the neoplastic cells. Hepatocellular carcinoma also secretes AFP into the blood; elevated levels are present in 90% of patients, making serum AFP assay an important diagnostic test. (*Note*: AFP levels may be slightly elevated in some cases of hepatitis and cirrhosis, as well as in some germ cell neoplasms of the gonads.)

Hepatocellular carcinoma tends to metastasize early via lymphatics to regional lymph nodes and via the bloodstream to produce lung metastases. Metastases to other sites occur terminally.

A rare variant, fibrolamellar carcinoma, has a better prognosis than the usual hepatocellular carcinoma. This occurs mainly in younger females, has no AFP elevation, and is usually a grossly encapsulated mass. The entity is defined by the presence of large polygonal cells with abundant eosinophilic cytoplasm separated by broad fibrous bands.

4. Clinical features(Figure 8-44)

Hepatocellular carcinoma should be suspected when a patient with known cirrhosis presents with any new symptom such as pain, loss of weight, fever, increasing liver size, or increasing ascites. About 20% of patients present with intraperitoneal hemorrhage. Rarely, hepatocellular carcinoma may secrete an ectopic hormone, causing hypoglycemia (insulin like polypeptide), polycythemia (erythropoictin), or hypercalcemia (parathyroid hormone-like polypeptide).

Surgical resection could be used for the treatment of hepatocellular carcinoma and quite satisfictory results have been achieved in our country. Comprehensive treatments including percutaneous radiofre

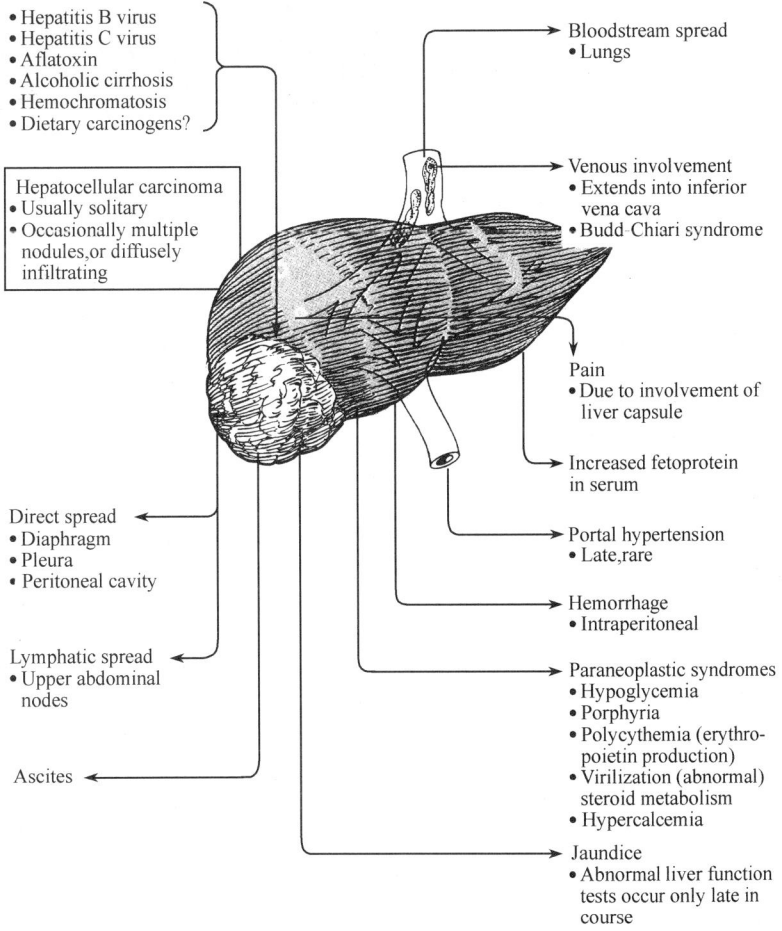

Figure 8-44 Clinical and pathologic effects of hepatocellular carcinoma

quency ablation, transcatheter arterial chemoembolization, biological therapy, etc. are also used in the treatment. Progression is extremely rapid, and most patients are dead within 1 year. The median survival after diagnosis is 2 months; the 5-year survival rate is quite low.

B. Cholangiocarcinoma

Cholangiocarcinoma arises in the intrahepatic bile ductules. It is uncommon in the United States and Europe but has a relatively high incidence in the Far East. Cholangiocarcinoma is not associated with cirrhosis.

Grossly, cholangiocarcinoma presents features indistinguishable from those of hepatocellular carcinoma. Histologically, it is an adenocarcinoma that shows mucin secretion. The presence of cytoplasmic mucin permits differentiation from hepatocellular carcinoma, which does not secrete mucin. Marked sclerosis is common. Differentiation from metastatic adenocarcinoma is almost impossible on histologic grounds alone. Serum AFP levels are normal.

The clinical presentation is with a liver mass. The progress of disease is often slow, but bloodstream spread ultimately occurs, and the prognosis is poor.

C. Metastatic Neoplasms

Metastases account for most neoplasms involving the liver. Virtually any malignant neoplasm in the body can metastasize to the liver; those from the gastrointestinal tract (via the portal vein), breast, and lung and malignant melanoma are most common.

Metastatic carcinoma characteristically produces massive liver enlargement with multiple nodules (Figure 8-45). However, differentiation of hepatocellular carcinoma from metastatic carcinoma is sometimes very difficult. The following features are helpful: (1) Grossly, the nodules of metastatic carcinoma often show central necrosis and umbilication; (2) The presence of cirrhosis favors hepatocellular carcinoma; (3) The demonstration of AFP in tumor cells or in the blood is almost pathognomonic of hepatocellular carcinoma; (4) Invasion of hepatic veins favors hepatocellular carcinoma.

If metastatic spread is from an adenocarcinoma, distinction from primary cholangiocarcinoma of the liver may be impossible unless a primary adenocarcinoma is found elsewhere in the body.

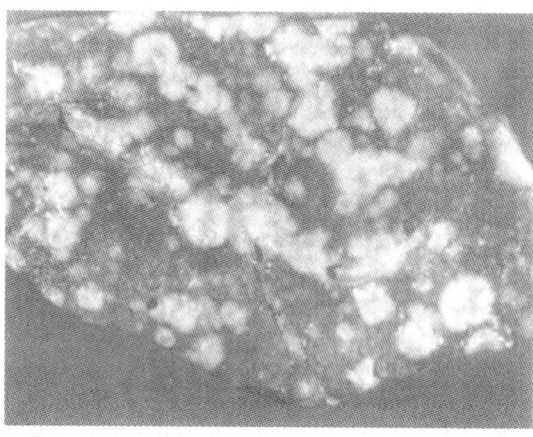

Figure 8-45 Metastatic carcinoma in the liver, showing multiple nodules some of which have central necrosis and umbilication. The patient had a primary carcinoma in the pancreas

DISEASES OF THE EXTRAHEPATIC BILIARY SYSTEM

STRUCTURE AND FUNCTION

The extrahepatic biliary system is composed of the bile ducts and the gallbladder (Figure 8-46). In 70% of patients the common bile duct and pancreatic duct join at the ampulla of Vater and have a common duodenal opening. In the other 30%, the pancreatic and bile ducts open separately. The common bile duct has a luminal diameter of 0.5 - 0.7 cm in the adult.

Histologically, the entire biliary tract is lined by mucus-secreting columnar epithelium. In the gallbladder, the epithelium is thrown up into delicate folds, and mucous glands are buried deeply in the smooth muscle wall (Aschoff-Rokitansky sinuses).

The biliary system stores and delivers the bile secreted by the liver into the duodenum, with the gallbladder acting as a reservoir in which the bile is stored and concentrated (from about 1000 mL/d down to 50 mL/d). The gallbladder is not required for adequate functioning of the system. Bile is an alkaline fluid that contains the excretory bilirubin pigments, bile acids and bile salts, cholesterol, inorganic ions, and mucus. Cholesterol, which is insoluble in water, is maintained in solution by the formation of complexes with the hydrophilic bile salts and lecithin.

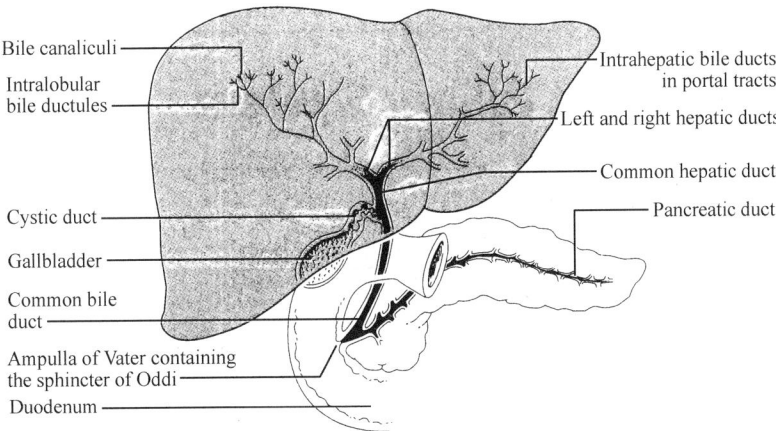

Figure 8-46 Anatomy of the biliary system

CHOLELITHIASIS

Most gallbladder diseases are associated with the formation of gallstones (cholelithiasis). Gallstones are usually formed in the gallbladder and rarely in the common bile duct.

Etiology and Incidence

A. Cholesterol-Based Gallstones

Pure, mixed, and combined cholesterol-based gallstones are common and are formed when the concentration of cholesterol is increased or when bile salts are decreased (Bile salts keep cholesterol in solution). Women are more apt to be affected. Middle age, obesity, and multiparity ("fat, fertile females in their forties and fifties") increase the risk to as high as 20%. Oral contraceptives increase biliary cholesterol excretion and predispose to gallstones.

In patients with terminal ileal disease such as Crohn's disease or those who have undergone ileal resection and ileal bypass surgery, failure of bile salt reabsorption in the terminal ileum is associated with decreased bile salt levels in bile and formation of gallstones.

Patients with diabetes mellitus also have an increased incidence of cholesterol gallstones, probably related to increased cholesterol levels in bile.

B. Pigment (Bilirubin) Stones

These are uncommon and occur (1) in patients suffering from chronic hemolytic anemias such as sickle cell disease and thalassemia, in whom bilirubin excretion is greatly increased; and (2) in patients with parasitic infestations, most commonly Clonorchis sinensis, in whom the parasite ova form a nidus for pigment stones.

In our country, the gallstones are basically classified according to the major constitutes as bile pigment stone, cholesterol stone and mixed stone.

- **Bile pigment stone**: The major constitute is calcium bilirubinate (bile pigment). The stones are usually multiple in numbers, typically black in color and earthy or sandy in shape.
- **Cholesterol stone**: The major constitute of the stone is cholesterol. The stone is yellow or yellow-white in color and round or oval in shape with crystalline surface. It is often solitary and may be as large as several centimeters in diameter. This type of stone is less frequently seen in China than in the North American and European countries.
- **Mixed stone**: The stone is composed of two or more constitutes. Mixed stones with bilirubin as main constitute are common in China. The appearance of the stone is often polygonal or spherical. Mixed stone is usually multiple and seen in gallbladder or larger bile ducts with different size and number. It has a laminated internal structure.

Clinical Manifestations (Figure 8-47)

A. Asymptomatic Gallstones

Thirty percent or more of patients with gallstones have no symptoms, and gallstones are frequently found incidentally at radiologic examination. Only about 25% of gallstones contain sufficient calcium to

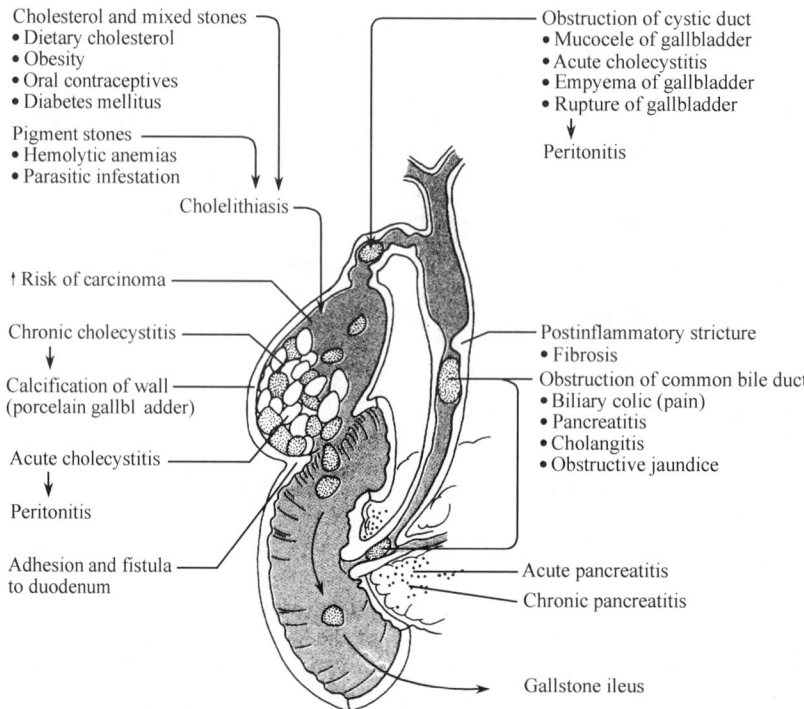

Figure 8-47 Clinical and pathologic effects of cholelithiasis

be visible on plain x-rays, but ultrasonography and computerized tomography are highly effective at detecting gallstones. The presence of asymptomatic gallstones is not an indication for surgical removal.

B. Acute Cholecystitis

Acute cholecystitis rarely occurs in the absence of gallstones. In 80% of cases, a stone is found obstructing the cystic duct, leading to stasis of bile in the gallbladder. The residual bile becomes highly concentrated and causes a chemical acute inflammation. The damaged gallbladder is then susceptible to infection by bacteria; *Escherichia coli* and other gram-negative bacilli are cultured from the bile in 80% of cases.

Pathologically, the gallbladder shows congestion, thickening of the wall by edema, mucosal ulceration, and fibrinous exudation. Large numbers of neutrophils are present. The gallbladder may become filled with pus (empyema of the gallbladder). In severe cases, necrosis of the wall occurs, with greenish black discoloration (gangrenous cholecystitis). Perforation may lead to local abscess formation or to generalized peritonitis.

Clinically, acute cholecystitis produces acute onset of fever and right upper quadrant pain. An enlarged, tender gallbladder is palpable in 40% of cases; mild jaundice may be seen in about 20%. Treatment is with antibiotics and surgical drainage or cholecystectomy.

C. Chronic Cholecystitis

Chronic cholecystitis almost never occurs without gallstones. Pathologically, the gallbladder is contracted and its wall thickened by fibrosis (Figure 8-48), with infiltration by lymphocytes, plasma cells, and macrophages. Calcification may occur in the wall; when extensive, the gallbladder is outlined on abdominal x-ray (porcelain gallbladder). The mucosa of the gallbladder may be near normal or thinned by pressure of a stone, or it may show yellow flecks due to accumulation of cholesterol-filled foamy macrophages in the mucosa (cholesterolosis).

Symptoms are usually vague; abdominal pain, often related to the ingestion of fatty foods, is the most common feature. Biliary colic-severe intermittent right upper quadrant pain-may occur when the cystic duct is obstructed.

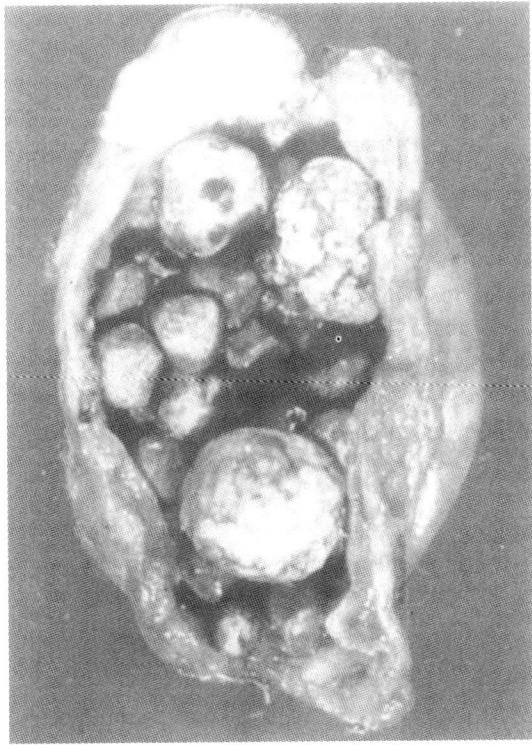

Figure 8-48 Gallbladder filled with multiple mixed gall-stones. The wall shows diffuse thickening due to fibrosis

D. Movement of Gallstones

Migration of gallstones from the gallbladder may cause obstruction or fistula formation.

CARCINOMA OF THE GALL-BLADDER

Carcinomas of the gallbladder and biliary tree are relatively uncommon. Gallbladder carcinoma is much more common in female, following the sex distribution of gallstones (80% of gallbladder carcinomas are associated with gallstones). Chronic cholecystitis with extensive calcification of the wall (porcelain gallbladder) is associated with a 25% incidence of carcinoma.

Grossly, gallbladder carcinoma presents as a polypoid mass that projects into the lumen, with infiltration of the wall (Figure 8-49). In some cases, the infiltrative component dominates, producing thickening of the wall. Histologically, it is an adenocarcinoma of variable differentiation frequently associated

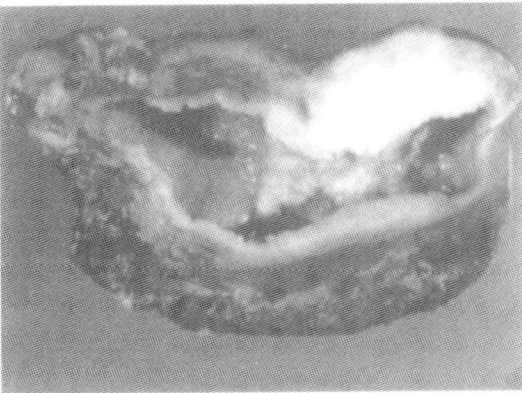

Figure 8-49 Carcinoma of the gallbladder, showing a large mass in the fundus that projects into the lumen and has infiltrated the wall

with marked fibrosis and a tendency to perineural invasion.

Most cases of gallbladder carcinoma are found in patients being evaluated for gallstones. In advanced disease, there is weight loss, a palpable mass, or evidence of metastases. The prognosis depends on the stage. Tumors confined to the gallbladder have a good prognosis. When there is extension through the wall of the gallbladder into the liver or peritoneum with or without evidence of metastatic disease, the 5-year survival rate is close to zero.

CARCINOMA OF THE BILE DUCTS

Although uncommon, bile duct carcinoma represents an important cause of obstructive jaundice in adults. Tumors may involve the hepatic ducts at the hilum of the liver (Klatskin tumor) or the common bile duct, most commonly at its terminal portion (at the ampulla of Vater; Figure 8-50).

Bile duct carcinoma tends to cause obstructive jaundice at an early stage. Histologically, these tumors are usually well differentiated and associated with marked sclerosis.

Bile duct carcinoma grows slowly, with local extension along the biliary system and neighboring structures. Lymph node involvement is early, but bloodstream metastasis usually occurs late. The ultimate prognosis is poor, although many patients have a long survival.

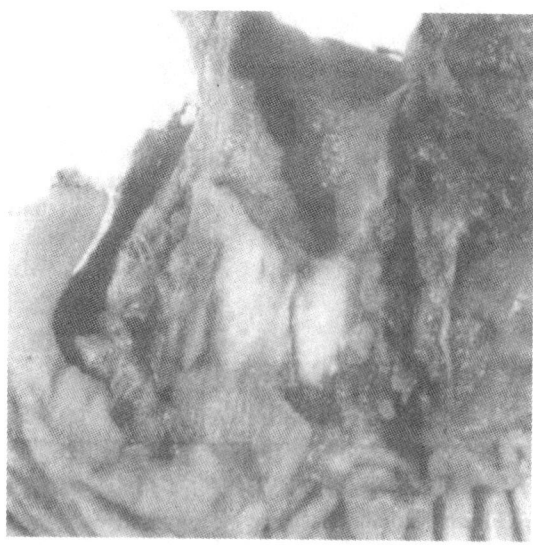

Figure 8-50 Neoplastic stricture of the terminal portion of the common bile duct, causing biliary obstruction. The bile duct proximal to the tumor is markedly dilated. This is the typical appearance of carcinoma of the bile duct

DISEASES OF THE EXOCRINE PANCREAS

STRUCTURE AND FUNCTION OF THE PANCREAS

The pancreas is situated retroperitoneally in the upper abdomen. It is divided into the **head**, which lies in the curve of the duodenum; the **body**, which is situated horizontally in the upper retroperitoneum; and the **tail**, which extends leftward to the hilum of the spleen.

The pancreas has two functional components: exocrine and endocrine.

- **The exocrine pancreas** contains acini that secrete a variety of enzymes into the pancreatic ducts. The main pancreatic duct opens at the duodenal papilla and in 70% of patients joins with the terminal common bile duct at the ampulla of Vater. An accessory (minor) pancreatic duct usually opens independently into the duodenum proximal to the papilla.
- **The endocrine pancreas** is composed of the islets of Langerhans, distributed throughout the pancreas with a maximum density in the tail and containing several different hormone-producing cell types.

INFLAMMATORY LESIONS OF THE PANCREAS

Acute Pancreatitis

Acute pancreatitis is a clinical syndrome resulting from the escape of activated pancreatic digestive enzymes from the duct system into the parenchyma. It is associated with extensive destruction of pancreatic and peripancreatic tissue and acute inflammation. Acute pancreatitis is a common and important medical emergency.

A. Etiology

In about 25% of cases of acute pancreatitis, no etiologic factor can be identified. Infectious agents are usually not involved, although mild non-necrotizing acute pancreatitis occurs in association with some viral diseases – commonly mumps and cytomegalovirus infection.

Factors associated with acute pancreatitis are shown in Figure 8-51 and discussed briefly below.

1. Biliary tract calculi

Biliary tract calculi are present in about 50% of cases and may obstruct the terminal bile duct. Reflux of bile or infected duodenal contents into the pancreatic duct has been suggested as a mechanism leading to pancreatitis in bile duct disease. Obstruction of the pancreatic duct may occur when a calculus becomes lodged in the ampulla of Vater. Acute pancreatitis complicating gallstones is chiefly a disorder of women because of the female preponderance of gallstone disease.

2. Alcoholism

Alcoholism as a cause of acute pancreatitis occurs with varying frequency in different parts of the world. Acute pancreatitis commonly occurs after a bout of heavy drinking. A direct toxic effect of alcohol on pancreatic acinar cells has been postulated.

3. Hypercalcemia

Hypercalcemia, as occurs in primary hyperparathyroidism, is complicated by acute pancreatitis in about 10% of cases. A high plasma calcium concentration is thought to stimulate activation of trypsinogen in the pancreatic duct.

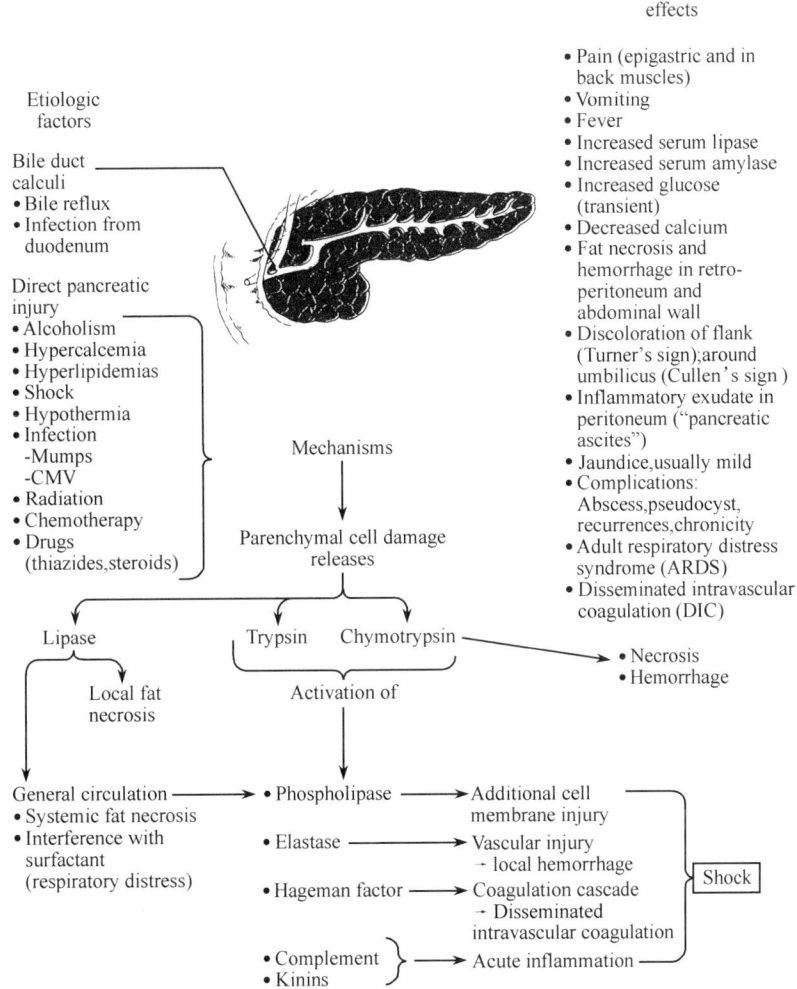

Figure 8-51 Acute pancreatitis - etiologic factors, mechanisms, pathologic changes, and clinical effects

4. Hyperlipidemias

The hyperlipidemias - particularly those types associated with increased plasma levels of chylomicrons - are complicated by acute pancreatitis. It is postulated that free fatty acids liberated by the action of pancreatic lipase produce acinar injury.

5. Shock and hypothermia

In shock and hypothermia, decreased perfusion of the pancreas may lead to cellular degeneration, release of pancreatic enzymes, and acute pancreatitis.

6. Drugs and radiation

Thiazide diuretics, corticosteroids, anticancer agents, and other drugs may also cause acute pancreatitis. Radiation to the retroperitoneum for treatment of malignant neoplasms is an uncommon cause of acute pancreatitis.

B. Pathogenesis

The pathologic changes in acute pancreatitis are the result of the action of pancreatic enzymes on the pancreas and surrounding tissues (Figure 8-51). Trypsin and chymotrypsin activate phospholipase and elastase as well as kinins, complement, the coagulation cascade, and plasmin, leading to acute inflammation, thrombosis, and hemorrhage. Elastase contributes to vascular injury. Phospholipases act on cell membranes, causing cell injury. Pancreatic lipase acts on surrounding adipose tissue, causing enzymatic fat necrosis.

In addition to a local action, pancreatic enzymes enter the bloodstream. Circulating amylase does not contribute to cell injury; however, phospholipases are thought to contribute to the production of adult respiratory distress syndrome by interfering with the normal function of pulmonary surfactant. Rarely, high serum lipase levels are associated with fat necrosis at sites distant from the pancreas.

C. Pathology

Acute pancreatitis is characterized by widespread necrosis in tissues subjected to the effect of extravasated pancreatic enzymes. Necrosis of pancreatic parenchyma is initially coagulative but the necrotic cells rapidly undergo liquefaction. Vascular necrosis and disruption result in hemorrhage. Fat necrosis appears as chalky white foci than may be calcified, usually in and around the pancreas, omentum, and mesentery (Figure 8-52). Rarely, fat necrosis extends down the retroperitoneum and into the mediastinum. In severe cases, massive liquefactive necrosis of the pancreas occurs, resulting in a pancreatic abscess.

In very severe cases, death may occur before an adequate inflammatory response can be mobilized. Neutrophils predominate when the inflammation becomes established.

The peritoneal cavity sometimes contains a brownish serous fluid (pancreatic ascites). This fluid contains altered blood, fat globules ("chicken broth"), and very high levels of amylase.

D. Clinical Features

Acute pancreatitis usually presents as a medical emergency. Patients develop severe constant epigastric pain, frequently referred to the back, accompanied by vomiting and shock. Shock is caused by peripheral circulatory failure resulting from hemorrhage and the entry of kinins into the bloodstream (Figure 8-51). Mild jaundice may be present. In severe pancreatitis, there is discoloration due to hemorrhage in the subcutaneous tissue around the umbilicus (Cullen's sign) and in the flanks (Turner's sign). Activation of the plasma coagulation cascade may lead to disseminated intravascular coagulation.

E. Complications

Most patients recover from the acute attack with proper supportive care, and the pancreas regene-

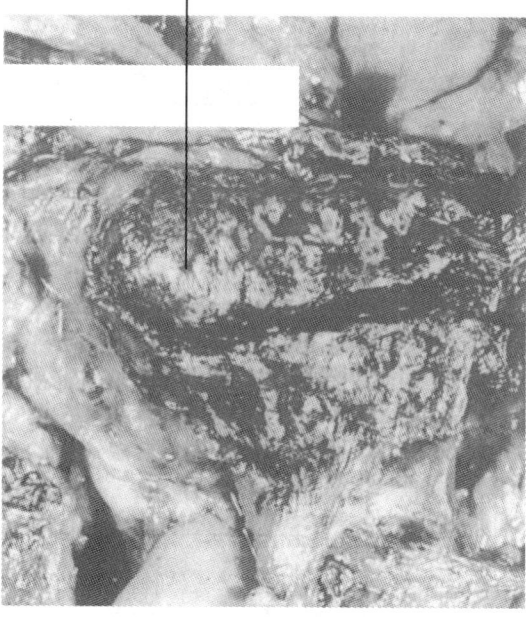

Figure 8-52 Acute pancreatitis, showing marked hemorrhagic necrosis in the upper retroperitoneum around the pancreas

rates and returns almost to normal, with mild residual scarring. In severe cases, death may occur in the acute phase as a consequence of pancreatic abscess, severe hemorrhage, shock, disseminated intravascular coagulation, or respiratory distress syndrome.

Pancreatic pseudocyst may follow weeks to months after recovery from an acute attack.

Chronic Pancreatitis

Chronic pancreatitis is a chronic disease characterized by progressive destruction of the parenchyma with chronic inflammation, fibrosis, stenosis and dilation of the duct system, and eventually impairment of pancreatic function.

A. Etiology

Chronic alcoholism and biliary tract calculi are the two main conditions that are associated with chronic pancreatitis. In 30%-40% of cases, no etiologic factors are identified. Some cases follow recurrent acute episodes; cystic fibrosis is a specific type of chronic pancreatitis described earlier.

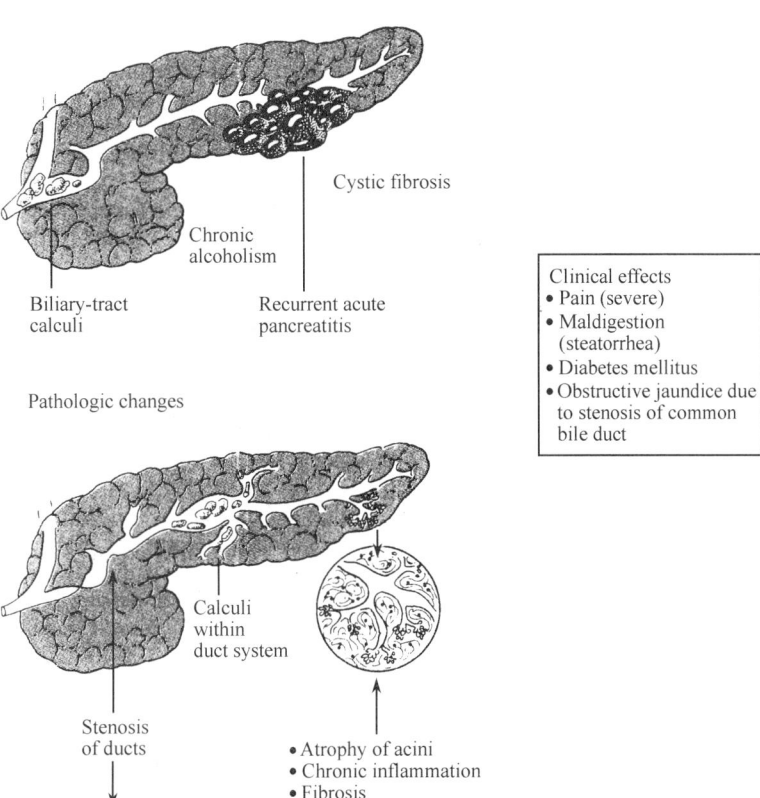

Figure 8-53 Chronic pancreatitis – etiologic factors, pathologic changes, and clinical effects

B. Pathology (Figure 8-53)

Chronic pancreatitis is characterized by shrinkage of the pancreas as a result of fibrosis and atrophy of acinar structures. The changes usually involve the gland diffusely; more rarely, a firm, localized mass forms and that is difficult to distinguish grossly from carcinoma.

The pancreatic ducts show multiple areas of stenosis with irregular dilation distally. Ducts are filled with inspissated secretions that may undergo calcification to form calculi (Figure 8-54). Diffuse calcification imparts a rock-hard consistency to the gland.

Microscopically, there is acinar loss with marked fibrosis. At the end stage there are almost no recognizable acini, and the gland is composed of dilated ducts separated by collagen. Islets tend to withstand destruction better than acini. A variable lymphocytic infiltrate is present.

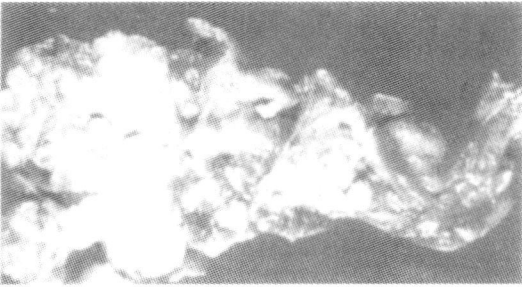

Figure 8-54 Chronic pancreatitis, showing markedly dilated ducts containing calculi. The pancreatic parenchyma between the ducts has undergone marked atro phy and fibrous contraction

C. Clinical Features

Pain is the dominant symptom. It may be constant or intermittent and can be so severe as to lead to narcotic dependence. In many cases, pain is associated with acute exacerbations, and the patients are asymptomatic between relapses. When pain is caused by dilation of the duct system, surgical correction by draining the dilated duct system may provide relief.

Pancreatic exocrine insufficiency due to failure of secretion of pancreatic juice leads to steatorrhea, malabsorption of fat-soluble vitamins, and weight loss. Endocrine insufficiency (diabetes mellitus) occurs in about 30% of cases.

The course is variable. Many patients have recurrent attacks of severe pain, vomiting, and elevation of serum amylase, due probably to repeated acute episodes (chronic relapsing pancreatitis). Acute attacks may be followed by formation of pancreatic pseudocysts.

In about 5% of patients with severe sclerosing chronic pancreatitis affecting the head of the pancreas, obstruction of the common bile duct leads to deep jaundice. This condition is difficult to differentiate from jaundice due to pancreatic carcinoma.

The diagnosis of chronic pancreatitis is made on clinical grounds. There are no specific laboratory tests, but the presence of calcification on x-ray provides supportive evidence. In chronic disease, the amount of residual pancreatic tissue may be insufficient to cause elevation of serum amylase.

D. Treatment and Prognosis

Treatment of chronic pancreatitis consists of management of the pain, malabsorption, and diabetes. When pain can not be controlled by drugs, surgery to drain the pancreatic duct often has good results. Malabsorption and diabetes mellitus can be controlled by dietary supplements and insulin if necessary. The complications of diabetes mellitus represent the main threat to life.

CARCINOMA OF THE PANCREAS

Carcinoma of the pancreas is understood to involve the exocrine pancreas; islet cell neoplasms are classified separately.

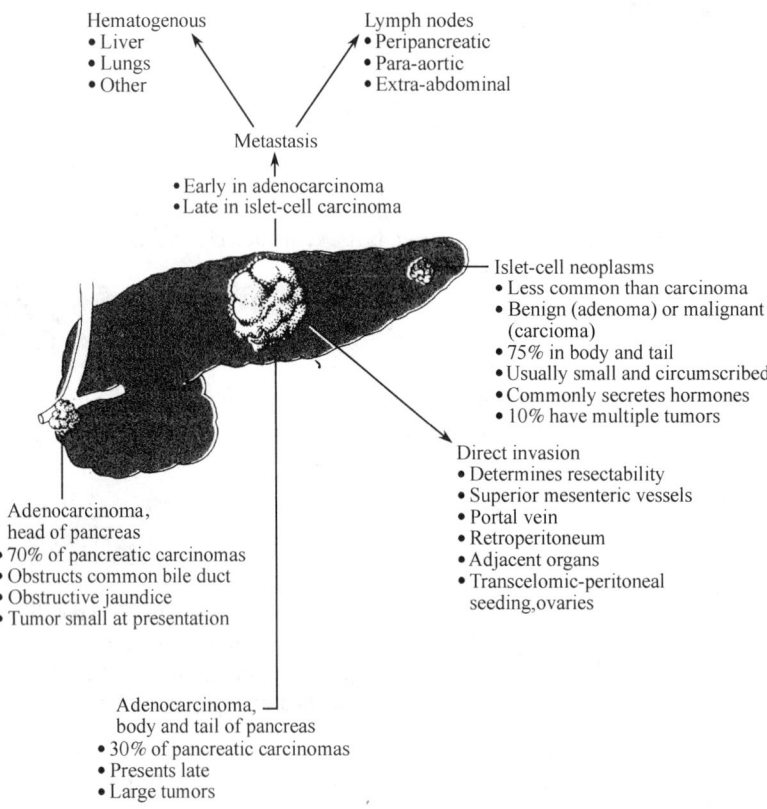

Figure 8-55 Solid pancreatic neoplasms

A. Incidence and Etiology

The incidence of pancreatic carcinoma is not high among digestive system carcinomas. Increasing tendency in the incidence has be seen recently in China. Pancreatic carcinoma occurs mainly after age 50 years.

The etiology is unknown. There is a sixfold increased risk in diabetic women but not in diabetic men. A large number of dietary factors have been proposed, including decaffeinated coffee and high-fat diets. Cigarette smokers show a fivefold increase in incidence. Expression of the K-ras oncogene is present in many pancreatic carcinomas.

B. Pathology (Figure 8-55)

Carcinomas occur throughout the pancreas: 70% in the head, 20% in the body, and 10% in the tail; 99% take origin from the ducts (ductal carcinoma; Figure 8-56) and the remainder from the acini (acinar cell carcinoma).

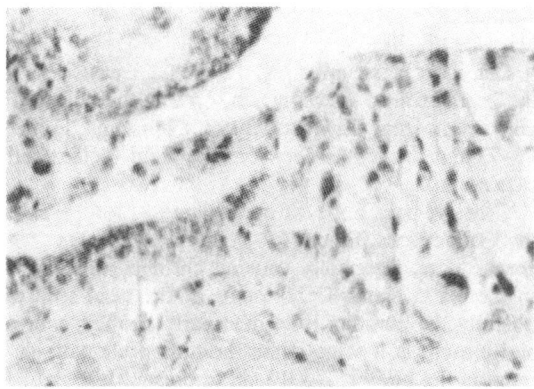

Figure 8-56 Carcinoma of the pancreas, showing the origin from a pancreatic duct. Contrast the normal ductal epithelial cells on the left with the greatly enlarged and pleomorphic carcinoma cells on the right and in the lumen

Grossly, pancreatic carcinoma presents as a hard infiltrative mass (Figure 8-57) that obstructs the pancreatic duct, frequently causing chronic pancreatitis in the distal gland. Carcinomas of the head tend to obstruct the common bile duct early in their course and present at a stage when the tumor is small. Tumors in the body and tail tend to present late and be very large. Pancreatic carcinoma frequently evokes marked fibrosis; it may distort the duodenal loop, producing a typical " inverted 3 " appearance on barium x-ray studies.

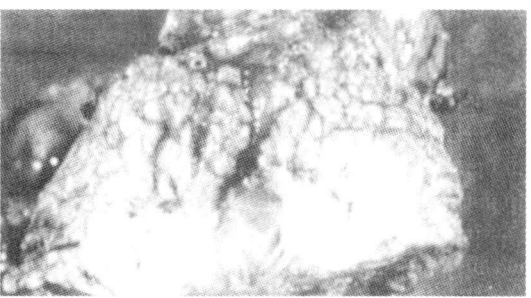

Figure 8-57 Carcinoma of the head of the pancreas, showing the typical hard infiltrative mass

Microscopically, over 90% of cases are well-differentiated adenocarcinomas, associated with marked fibrosis. Perineural invasion is common (Figure 8-58). The remaining 10% include adenosquamous carcinomas, anaplastic carcinomas – which contain spindle cells and pleomorphic giant cell (sarcomatoid and pleomorphic carcinomas)-and acinar cell carcinomas. Rarely, acinar cell carcinomas secrete lipase into the bloodstream and cause fat necrosis in the subcutaneous tissue and bone marrow throughout the body.

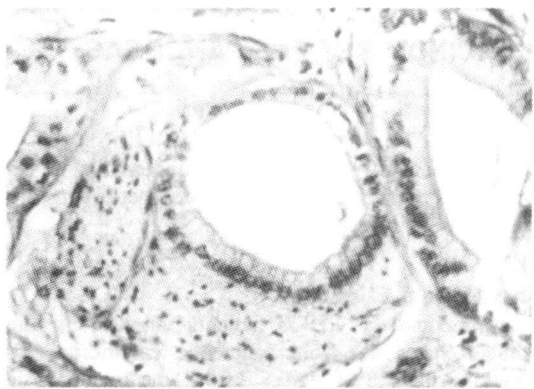

Figure 8-58 Well-differentiated carcinoma of the pancreas, showing perineural invasion (the nerve is at the bottom center of this photograph). The carcinoma cells show minimal cytologic abnormality

C. Spread

The tumor tends to infiltrate into surrounding structures. Spread along the perineural fascial spaces is a typical feature. Lymphatic involvement occurs early, with metastasis to regional lymph nodes. Bloodstream spread also occurs early, with the liver being the most common site of secondary deposits.

D. Clinical Features

Carcinoma of the head of the pancreas presents with common bile duct obstruction. Carcinoma of the body and tail presents at a late stage with an abdominal mass, severe weight loss, and anemia. A high proportion of patients presents with evidence of metastatic disease, most often in the liver. Skin rashes and lytic bone lesions due to fat necrosis may be present in lipase secreting acinar cell carcinomas.

Computerized tomography is effective in establishing the presence of a solid mass. Percutaneous fine-needle aspiration of the mass under radiologic guidance provides tissue for cytologic examination and is an excellent method of making the diagnosis.

E. Treatment and Prognosis

Most pancreatic carcinomas are inoperable at presentation. Small carcinomas confined to the head of the pancreas may be cured by total pancreaticoduodenectomy (Whipple procedure). Chemotherapy could be used in the treatment. The prognosis is dismal: mean survival is 6 months after diagnosis, and the overall 5-year survival rate is less than 5%.

(Zhang Xianghong)

Chapter 9 The Diseases of Hematopoietic and Lymphoid Systems

Zhang Shuhua

CHAPTER CONTENTS
- Structure and Function of Hematopoietic and Lymphoid System
- Infection and Reactive Proliferations
    Nonspecific Reactive Hyperplasia
    Specific Infections of Lymph Nodes
- The Lymphoid Neoplastic
    Classification of Lymphoid Neoplasms
    Precursor B- and T-lymphoblastic
    Mature B-cell Neoplasms
    Mature T- and NK-cell Neoplasms
    Hodgkin's Lymphoma
- Myeloid Neoplasms
    Acute Myeloblastic Leukemias
    Chronic Myelogenous Leukemias
- Histocytic Neoplasms
    Acute Disseminated Langerhans Cell Histocytosis
    Eosinophilic Granuloma

The disorders of the hematopoietic and lymphoid systems encompass a wide range spectrum of diseases. They may primarily affect the red cells, the white cells or the hemostatic mechanisms. Diseases of red cells and white cells include anemia, leukopenias, and thrombocytopenia. In contrast, proliferation may be reactive, such as reactive lymphadenitis, leukocytosis, and thrombocytosis, or neoplasm, such as leukemias and malignant lymphomas. The hematopoietic and lymphoid systems, unlike other organ systems, not confine to a single anatomic site. Therefore, when diseases of hematopoietic and lymphoid are considered, it is important to remember that the hematopoietic and lymphoid cells are spread throughout the body. For example, a patient who is diagnosed, on the bases of a lymph node biopsy, as having a malignant lymphoma, may also have neoplastic lymphocytes in the bone marrow and peripheral blood and be considered to have leukemia. The neoplastic lymphoid cells in the marrow may suppress normal production of red cells and platelets, resulting in anemia and thrombocytopenia, and cause liver and spleen enlargement when they infiltrate them. These apparently diverse manifestations have the same underlying bases. In the following discussion we first briefly introduce the structure and function of hematopoietic and lymphoid, describe some non-neoplastic conditions, and then mainly consider in some detail malignant proliferation of white cells.

STRUCTURE AND FUNCTION OF HEMATOPOIETIC AND LYMPHOID SYSTEM

Hematopoietic and lymphoid system is composed of myeloid tissue (bone marrow) and lymphoid tissues (thymus, spleen, lymph nodes and extranode lymphoid tissues). The thymus and bone marrow are often termed **central lymphoid tissues** in that they are central to the prenatal development of the immune system, but they do not participate in the immune response in the adult. The remaining lymphoid organs are actively involved in the immune response, and constitute the **peripheral lymphoid tissue.**

The lymph nodes are surrounded by a connective tissue capsule, with trabeculasrs that extend into the substance of the node and provide a framework for the contained cellular elements. Beneath the capsule is a slit-like space, the subcapsular sinus. There are three distinct regions recognized within normal lymph nodes. They are: **the cortex**, which contains nodules of B-lymphocytes either primary or as germinal centers; **the paracortex or deep cortex**, which is the T-cell dependent region of the lymph node; and **medullar**, containing the medullary cords and sinuses which drain into the hilum.

The appearance of the follicles varies according to their state of activity. Primary follicles appear as round aggregates of lymphocytes. Secondary follicles appear following antigenic stimulation and are characterized by the presence of germinal centers. The cells present in these formations are B-lymphocytes known as follicles center cells (centroblasts and centrocytes), macrophages and follicle dendritic cells. The germinal center is surrounded by a mantle of small B-lymphocytes.

Within the lymphoid system there are several focal concentrations of immune cells (lymph nodes, spleen, tonsils, etc) wherein lymphocytes, macrophages, and other immune cells are arranged in a manner advantageous to the various interactions that make up the immune response. It is no accident that major accumulations of lymphoid tissue occur at portals of antigen entry: the tonsils (mouth and nose), the respiratory and gastrointestinal submucosa (for inhaled and ingested antigens), the lymph nodes (for lymph drainage of skin and organs), and the spleen (as the blood filter). The histologic appearances of lymphoid tissue are largely dependent upon the degree of antigenic stimulation. Reactive follicles (foci of B-cell proliferation) only appear following exposure to antigen. Likewise, immunoblasts are only present in the face of recent antigenic stimulation, while plasma cells indicate activity of some weeks' duration.

In the embryo, blood formation may occur in a variety of places in the body, such as liver and spleen. Aparr from the fact that lymphocytes and large mononuclear cells continue to be produced throughout life in lymphoid tissue towards the end of foetal life the main centers of hematopoietic activity shift once more and become localized in the red marrow of bones. After birth, the bone marrow is the sole site of production of erythrocytes, granulocytes, and platelets. It also produces blood monocytes, which are part of the macrophage system. At birth, hematopoietic marrow is present in the medullary cavity of all the bones of the body. With increasing age, the hematopoietic marrow is replaced by adipose tissue in the bones of the extremities, and hematopoietic marrow is found only in the axial skeleton.

INFECTION AND REACTIVE PROLIFERATIONS

NONSPECIFIC REACTIVE HYPERPLASIA

Reactive hyperplasia within lymphoid tissue represents the tissue manifestation of the immune response and consists of three interrelated elements: (1) follicular hyperplasia (the B-cell response); (2) paracortical hyperplasia (the T-cell response); and (3) sinus histiocytosis (the histiocyte [macrophage] response). In practice, any one of these may predominate, but most responses represent an admixture of all three.

In B-cell hyperplasia, the reactive follicles are usually large and conspicuous (Figure 9-1), consisting of actively proliferating B-cells among which are scattered variable numbers of histiocytes and dendritic reticulum cells. The reactive follicles develop from small clusters of B-cells (sometimes called **primary follicles**) in the outer part (cortex) of the lymph node. The first phase of follicular formation appears to be the trapping of antigen by dendritic reticulum cells, which then serve to stimulate local B-cell proliferation, leading to development of a collection of actively transforming B-lymphocytes (**the secondary or reactive follicles**).

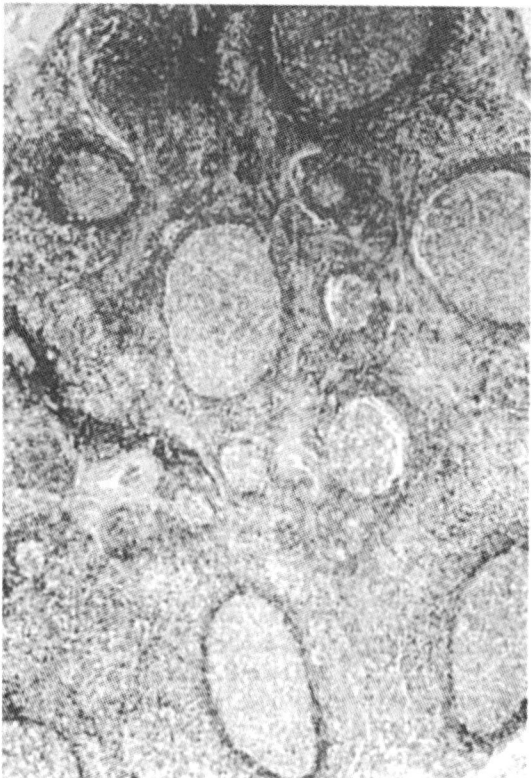

Figure 9-1 Reactive hyperplasia of a lymph node showing features of a predominantly B cell response, characterized by enlarged follicles with prominent reactive centers

A similar reaction occurs among T-cells in the paracortex following trapping of antigen by interdigitating reticulum cells. In some instances, the T-cell response may predominate; follicles may then be inconspicuous. This type of response particularly is seen in viral infections or postvaccination, e. g. in lymph nodes draining the vaccination site.

Lymph nodes draining a malignant neoplasm frequently show reactive hyperplasia, and in many instances, the most prominent component is marked expansion of the sinuses, which are filled with histiocytes (**sinus histiocytosis**).

Many cases of nonspecific reactive hyperplasia are localized in that the antigen source also is confined to a particular region of the body. An example is enlargement of lymph nodes in the neck in conjunction with streptococcal pharyngitis. Generalized reactive hyperplasia may occur with an antigen that is distributed throughout the body, e. g. in the viremic phase of viral infections, of which rubella is an excellent example.

SPECIFIC INFECTIONS OF LYMPH NODES

Infections of the lymph nodes combine: (1) features of the immune response to microbial antigens, (2) features of inflammation, and (3) specific changes that may be produced by the infectious agent. The presence of the specific agent in the lymph nodes often permits diagnosis by culture of the node, which should be requested at the time of biopsy.

Infectious Mononucleosis

Infectious mononucleosis is characterized by a florid T-cell hyperplasia, often so extensive that the follicles are totally obscured. In addition, the number of immunoblasts and T-cells in intermediate stages of transformation is so high that the node may appear to be totally replaced by large cells (Figure 9-2), leading to possible misdiagnosis as malignant lymphoma. These large transformed lymphocytes are the same cells that appear in increased numbers in the peripheral blood (so-called Downey cells).

Infectious mononucleosis is caused by the **Epstein-Barr virus** (EBV), which specifically infects B-cells (which have a receptor for the EBV on their surface). Infected B-cells then express viral antigens on their surfaces to which the T-cells mount a vigorous immune response. The histologic appear-

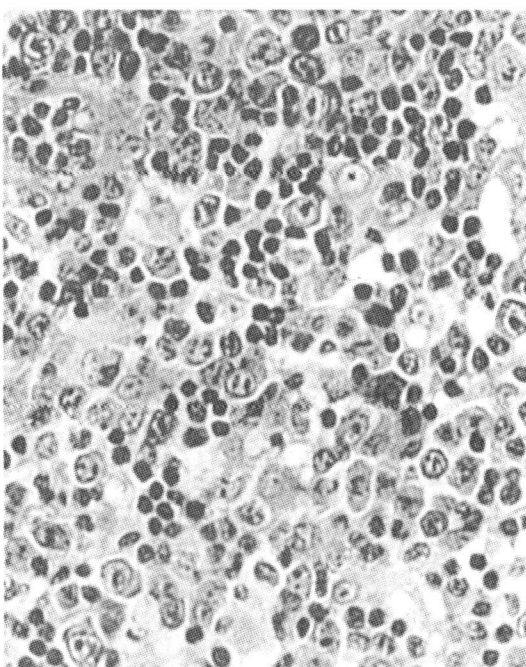

Figure 9-2   Infectious mononucleosis involving a lymph node. This is a high-magnification photograph showing the expanded paracortical region and T-cells in different stages of transformation. Numerous large nuclei with prominent nucleoli scattered throughout the region represent T immunoblasts

ance of infectious mononucleosis may be mimicked closely by other acute viral illnesses, including infection with cytomegalovirus, hepatitis virus, herpes simplex (type 2), rubella, and adenovirus; or by vaccination with attenuated live viruses.

Infectious mononucleosis is more common in children and young adults and is transmitted via the upper respiratory tract (kissing disease). Patients with this disorder present as acute onset of fever, sore throat, lymphadenopathy, and hepatosplenomegaly. Mild liver dysfunction may be present. The disease is often milder in young children and more severe in young adults.

It may be diagnosed by the peripheral blood appearance (lymphocytosis with Downey cells) but should be confirmed serologically as described bellow. Lymphoid biopsy is not necessary in the face of serologic confirmation unless there is continuing enlargement of lymph nodes in the face of clinical resolution of the viral infection.

The traditional serologic test for infectious mononucleosis is the detection of heterophil antibodies by the **Paul-Bunnell test**, of which the **Monospot test** is a well-known example. Heterophil antibodies are cross-reactive with a variety of different tissues in different species and are not specific for infectious mononucleosis. Their detection, however, does provide a useful screening test. Recently, tests for specific antibodies against EBV antigens have become available, and these now represent the most specific tests for infectious mononucleosis. IgM antibody to viral capsid antigen (VCA) appears early in the disease, followed by IgG antibodies that persist over a long period; antibodies to EBV membrane antigen and nuclear antigen appear late but persist for life.

Tuberculosis of Lymph Nodes

See Chapter 14.

Human Immunodeficiency Virus Infection

See Chapter 10.

THE LYMPHOID NEOPLASMS

All lymphoid neoplasms are derived from a single transformed cell and are therefore monoclonal. Lymphoid neoplasms, both malignant lymphomas and lymphocytic leukemias, are a group of tumors that their clinical manifestations and behaviors vary widely. In fact, they are the same disease in different clinic stages, resulting in diverse manifestations. Both lymphomas and lymphocytic leukemias may initially arise from lymphoid tissues or hematopoietic tissue and then involve each other. Some neoplastic cells circulate and frequently are found widely distributed throughout the lymphoid tissues, which process is termed leukemia. If the proliferation dominantly affects the lymphoid tissues or if a tissue mass is the presenting feature, the process is termed lymphoma, usually within lymph nodes and less often in extranodal lymphoid tissues, such as the tonsil, gastrointestinal tract, and spleen. This distinction is arbitrary, and in children the term lymphoma-leukemia is sometimes used for these reasons. The two forms may coexist and lymphoma frequently evolves toward a leukemic state (Figure 9-3). As tumors of immune system, lymphoid neoplasms often disrupt normal immune regular mechanism. Both immunodeficiency and autoimmunity may be seen.

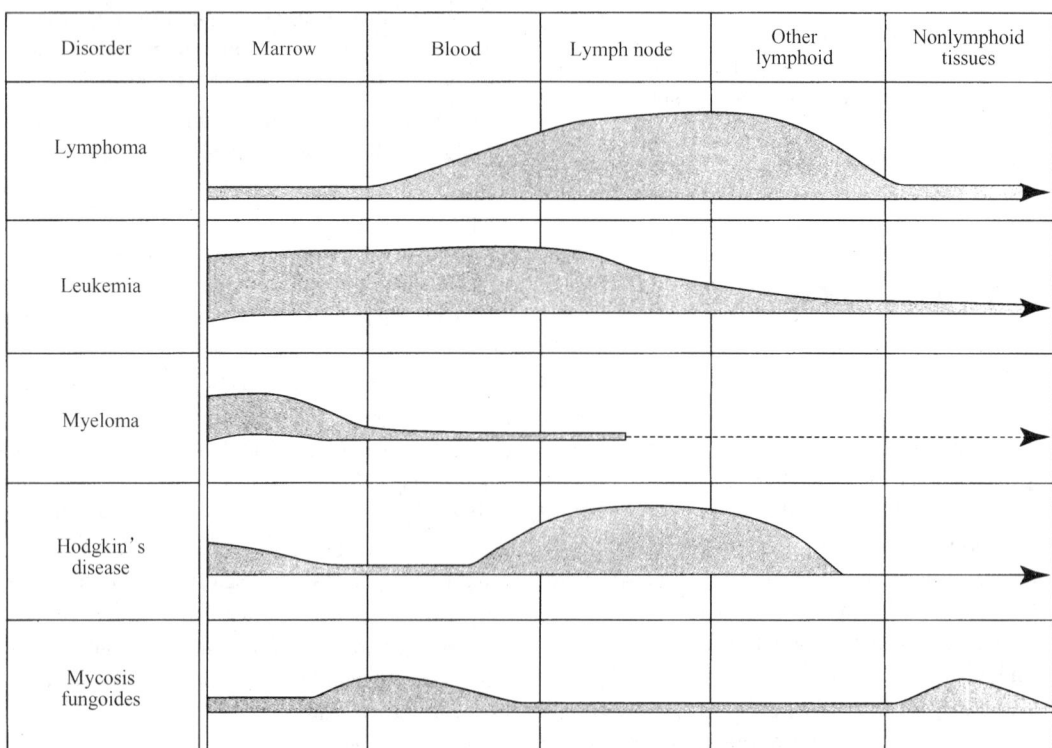

Figure 9-3 Sites of involvement in lymphoma-leukemia

The diagnosis of lymphoid neoplasms usually depends on the biopsy of lymph node or other organs affected. Loss of the normal nodal architecture, particularly if coupled with a lack of the normal admixture of cell types seen in the immune response, is evidence that the lymphoproliferation is neoplastic. Lymphoid neoplasms are usually classified as **non-Hodgkin's lymphomas** (NHLs) and **Hodgkin's lymphomas** based on the features of tumor cells. NHLs account for about 70% to 80% of all malignant lymphomas in our country.

CLASSIFICATION OF LYMPHOID NEOPLASMS

Lymphoid neoplasms show enormous variation in clinical behavior and response to therapy. The aim of classification is to identify homogeneous subgroups that behave in a predictable way. The lymphoid neoplasms, like neoplasms of other tissues, are named according to the normal cell they most closely resemble. Several morphologic stages can be identified in the process of lymphocytes transformation from stem cell to mature cells according to the transformation pattern of lymphocytes proposed by Lennert et al in 1975 (Figure 9-4). These morphologic changes result in the classification of lymphoid neoplasms varied greatly because they could occur at any stage in the process of lymphocyte transformation.

There are several classifications for lymphoid neoplasm in the past decades, such as Rappaport classification (1956), Lukes and Collins classification (1974), an international working group of pathologists, molecular biologists, and clinicians formulated the " Working Formulation of Non-Hodgkin's Lymphomas for Clinical Usage " (1975), the Revised European, American Classification of Lymphoid Neoplasms (abbreviated as REAL, 1994), and so on. REAL classification, considering the morphology, cell of origin, clinical features, and genotype, segregates lymphomas into three major categories: (1) tumors of B-cells, (2) tumors of T-cells and NK-cells, and (3) Hodgkin's lymphoma.

According to the principles of REAL classification WHO formulates a classification of lymphoid neoplasms in 2000 (Table 9-1). The objective of the new WHO classification is to offer pathologists, oncologists and geneticists worldwide a system of classification for lymphoid neoplasms. The present classification is the result of consensus meeting at a nomenclature that is practical and reflects the latest advances in the understanding of the pathogenesis of lymphoid neoplasms.

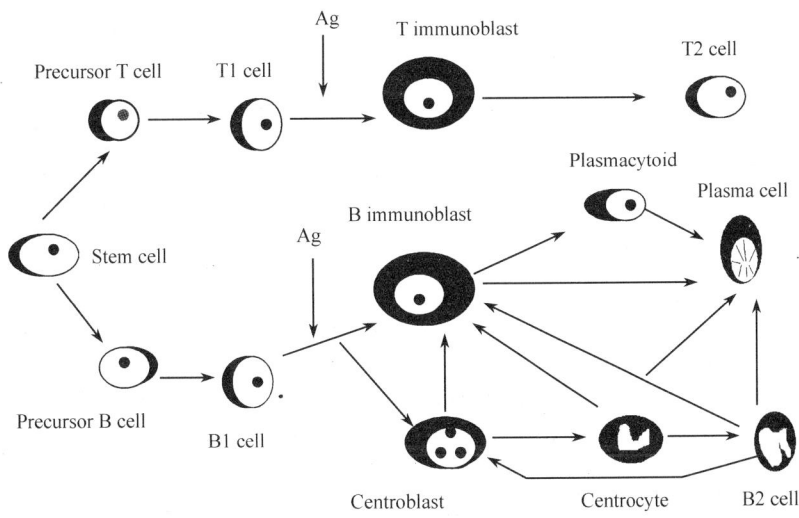

Figure 9-4 The transformation pattern of lymphocytes proposed by Lennert et al in 1975

Table 9-1 WHO classifications of lymphoid neoplasms (2000)

B-cell neoplasms 　**Precursor B-cell neoplasm** 　　Precursor B-lymphoblastic leukemia/ lymphoma 　**Mature B-cell neoplasms** 　　Chronic lymphocytic leukemia/Small lymphocytic lymphoma 　　B-cell prolymphocytic leukemia 　　Lymphoplasmacytic lymphoma 　　Splenic marginal zone lymphoma 　　Hairy cell leukemia 　　Plasma cell myeloma 　　Solitary plasmacytoma of bone 　　Extraosseous plasmacytoma 　　Extra-nodal marginal zone B-cell lymphoma of mucosa-associated lymphoid tissue (MALT) 　　Nodal marginal zone B-cell lymphoma 　　Follicular lymphoma 　　Mantle cell lymphoma 　　Diffuse large B-cell lymphoma 　　Mediastinal (thymic) large B-cell lymphoma 　　Intravascular large B-cell lymphoma 　　Primary effusion lymphoma 　　Burkitt lymphoma/leukemia **T-cell and NK-cell neoplasms** 　**Precursor T-cell neoplasm**	Precursor T-lymphoblastic leukemia 　　Blastic NK-cell lymphoma 　**Mature T-cell and NK-cell neoplasms** 　　T-cell prolymphocytic leukemia 　　T-cell large granular lymphocytic leukemia 　　Aggressive NK-/T-cell leukemia 　　Adult T-cell leukemia/lymphoma 　　Extranodal NK-/T-cell lymphoma, nasal type 　　Enteropathy-type T-cell lymphoma 　　Hepatosplenic T cell lymphoma 　　Subcutaneous panniculitis-like T-cell lymphoma 　　Mycosis fungoides 　　Sézary syndrome 　　Primary cutaneous anaplastic large cell lymphoma 　　Peripheral T-cell lymphoma, unspecified 　　Angioimmunoblastic T-cell lymphoma 　　Anaplastic large cell lymphoma **Hodgkin's lymphoma (Hodgkin's disease)** 　**Nodular lymphocyte predominant Hodgkin's lymphoma** 　**Classical Hodgkin's lymphoma** 　　Nodular sclerosis classical Hodgkin's lymphoma 　　Lymphocyte-rich classical Hodgkin's lymphoma 　　Mixed cellularity classical Hodgkin's lymphoma 　　Lymphocyte-depleted classical Hodgkin's lymphoma

PRECURSOR B- AND T-LYMPHOBLASTIC

Leukemia/Lymphoma

These are high-grade NHLs composed of diffuse sheets of medium-sized lymphoid cells. They may be B-or T-cell lineage. Because the various lymphoblastic tumors are morphologically indistinguishabl and often cause similar signs and symptoms, the pre-B-cell and pre-T-cell neoplasms are discussed here together.

These aggressive tumors affect predominantly in children, accounting for about 80% of childhood leukemia. The pre-B-cell lymphoma mainly affects children, but the pre-T-cell tumors mainly affect adolescent males. Pre-B-cell lymphoblastic tumors characteristically present as leukemias with extensive bone marrow and peripheral blood involvement. Pre-T-lymphoblastic tumors commonly manifest mediastinal masses involving the thymus. Therefore, both pre-B- and pre-T-lymphoblastic tumors usually present clinical appearance of lymphoblastic leukemia (ALL) at some time during their course.

A. Morphology

Microscopically, the lymph nodes affected by neoplastic cells are replaced by small to medium-sized blastcells with scant cytoplasm and inconspicuous nucleoli. Most pre-T-cell lymphomas showing mediastinal masses progress rapidly to a leukemia phage, but other cases present as marrow involvement only. The bone marrow is extensively involved by the lymphoblastic cells, especially pre-B-cell lymphoma. Splenomegaly and hepatomegaly are usually mild at presentation in these diseases. Meningeal infiltration is an important feature. In the blood smear slide, the nuclei of lymphoblasts with Wright-Giemsa staining show somewhat coarse and clumped chromatin and one or two nucleoli; myeloblasts tend to have fine chromatin and more cytoplasm, which may contain granules. It is practically essential to distinguish ALL from AML as the responses of these two neoplastic cells to therapy are different.

B. Blood and Bone Marrow Changes

In peripheral blood the white cell count is usually increased, sometimes to more than $100,000/\mu l$ but in about 50% of cases, it is less than $10,000/\mu l$. The majority of nucleated cells are leukemic blasts

(Figure 9-5). Anemia is almost always present. The platelet count is usually depressed to less than 100,000/μl. The bone cellularity, where the blasts make up 60% to 100% of all the cells, is markedly increased in all cases of acute leukemia. Bone pain and tenderness result from marrow expansion with infiltration of the subperiosteum.

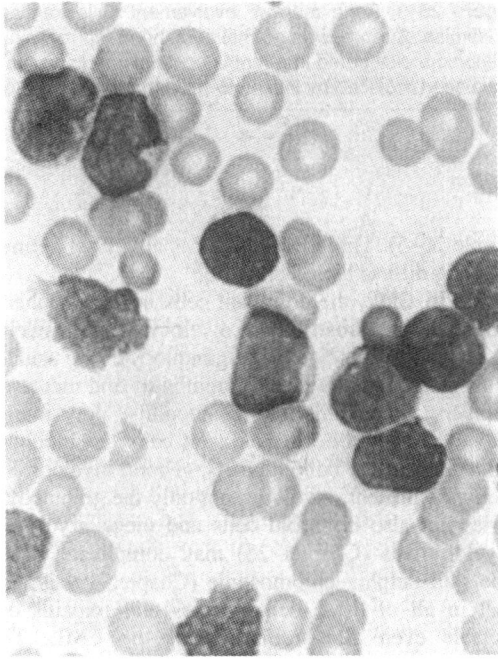

Figure 9-5 Peripheral blood changes in ALL, showing a marked increase in the number of leukocytes. The cells are large, and resemble the lymphoblatsts seen in early stages of lymphocytic differentiation. Note the fragmentation of the fragile leukemic cells, which is a common finding in peripheral blood smears of patients with acute leukemia

C. Other Organs Changes

Generalized lymphadenopathy, splenomegaly, and heptatomegaly indicate dissemination of the leukemic cells, occurring in all acute leukemias but being more marked in these diseases. Central nervous system manifestations include headache, vomiting, and nerve palsies resulting from meningeal spread. These clinical features are more common in children than in adults and are more common than that of AML.

D. Immunophenotype and Karyotype

TdT, a DNA polymerase and a utility marker for these diseases, is present in more than 95% of cases. It is necessary to perform specific immunologic staining to subtype further into pre-B- and pre-T-cell types, such as CD19 (B-cell) and CD2 (T-cell). About 90% of patients with lymphoblastic leukemia/lymphoma have nonrandom karyotypic abnormalities. Hyperdiploidy (>50 chromosomes/cell) is very common in pre-B-cell tumors. This karyotypic change is related to the presence of a cryptic (12; 21) chromosomal translocations involving the TEL1 and AML1 genes. The presence of these abnormalities usually indicates a good outcome, but the translocations involving the ML1 gene on chromosome 11q23 or the Philadelphia (Ph) chromosome in pre-B-cell neoplasms imply a poor outcome. Pre-T-cell tumors have gene rearrangements that entirely different from those found in pre-B-cell tumors, which indicate that they have a distinct molecular pathogenesis.

E. Clinical Features

The manifestations in these diseases are similar to that of AML. They also show anemia, hemorrhage and infection as well as related symptoms, characterized by an acute clinical onset. Combination of chemotherapy, using several anticancer agents simultaneously in various combinations, has improved the prognosis of patients with these tumors dramatically. Recently, acute leukemias have been treated more aggressively with the intention of destroying all the hematopoietic cells in the marrow, including leukemic cells, followed by rescue of the patients by bone marrow transplantation. One of the great success stories in oncology is the treatment of these diseases.

MATURE B-CELL NEOPLASMS

Many tumors of mature B-cells arise from and recapitulate the follicular growth pattern of normal B-cells. Thus, in certain B-cell tumors, the neoplastic cells are clustered into identifiable nodules resembling normal follicles. These tumors are called follicular lymphomas. Other B-cell tumors do not produce nodules; instead they spread diffusely in the lymph nodes. This architecture is referred as diffuse lymphoma. The normal architecture of the lymph node is effaced.

Chronic Lymphocytic Leukemia (CLL)/Small Lymphocytic Lymphoma (SLL)

In fact, small lymphocytic lymphoma and chronic lymphocytic leukemia are the virtually identical tumors. It is a disease of affecting persons older than 50 years of age. Most patients are leukemic at the time of diagnosis. They usually have an insidious onset and a slow rate of progression.

A. Morphology

The lymph nodes are replaced by sheets of mature lymphocytes, which are round, small compact with dark-staining round nuclei, scanty cytoplasm and uniform in shape and size, and scattered ill-defined foci of large cells termed prolymphocytes. The foci of mitotic active prolymphocytes are called proliferation centers, which are useful for CLL/SLL in diagnosis. In addition to lymph nodes, the bone marrow (Figure 9-6), spleen, and liver are involved in almost all cases. The lymphocyte count is between $50,000/\mu l$ and $200,000/\mu l$ (Figure 9-7). The CLL cells tend to fragment and frequently disrupted mechanically during preparation of the blood film, producing specific "smudge cells". Prolymphocytes in variable numbers are also usually found in the blood smear.

B. Immunophenotype and Karyotype

The neoplastic cells express B-cell markers, such as CD19, CD20, and CD23, surface immunoglobulin (e.g. IgM, IgD), and either κ or λ light chain, indicating monoclonality as CLL/SLL are of B-cell origin. They also express T-cell related antigen CD5. There are about 50% of cases with karyotypic abnormalities. Trisomy 12 and deletion of chromosomes 11 and 12 are the most common abnormalities.

A

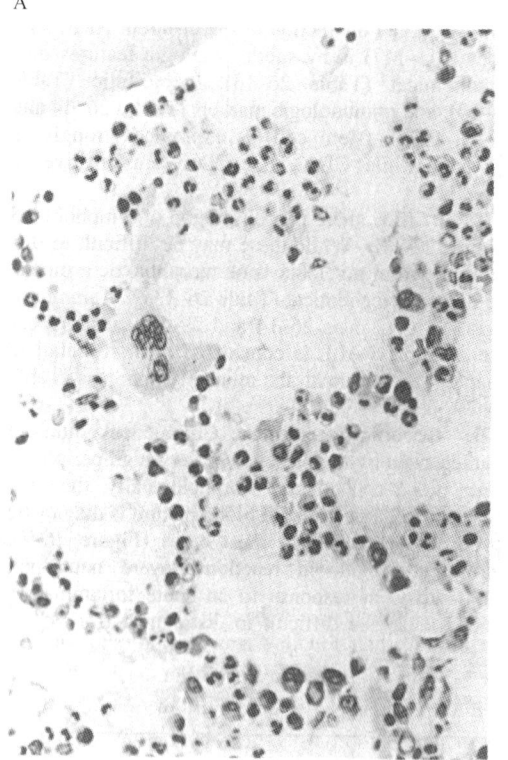

B

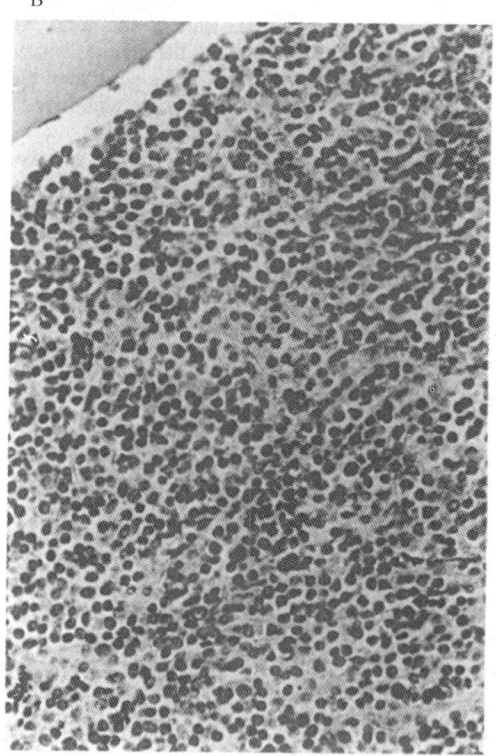

Figure 9-6 Bone marrow involvement in leukemia. A represents normal adult bone marrow, showing multinucleated megakaryocytes and erythroid precursors distributed in a matrix containing adipocytes. B shows that the marrow fat and normal hematopoietic cells have been replaced by leukemic cells. In this example of CLL, the leukemic cells resemble small lymphocytes

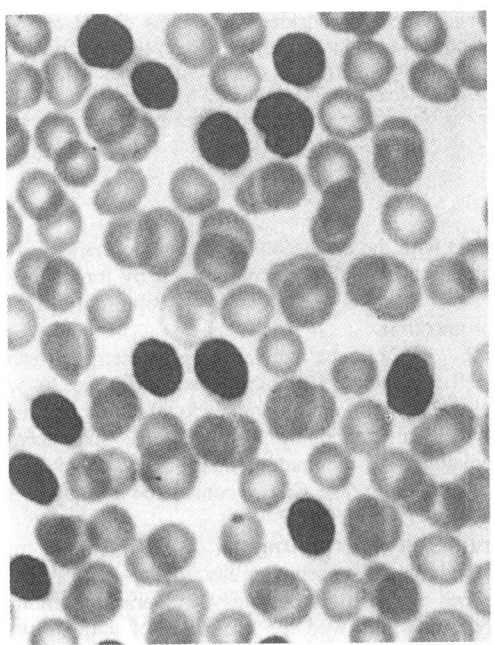

Figure 9-7 Peripheral blood changes in CLL, showing a marked increase in the number of leukocytes. The cells resemble small lymphocytes

C. Clinical Features

CLL/SLL is often asymptomatic. Many cases are diagnosed as a result of routine blood tests or clinical examination for some other reasons. The symptoms are nonspecific, including easy fatigue, weight loss, and anorexia. There is increased susceptibility to bacteria infections because of hypogammaglobulinemia. Generalized lymphadenopathy and hepatosplenomegaly are manifested in about 50% to 60% cases. The prognosis of CLL/SLL is good and the patients with these diseases may survive for 10 years or more from diagnosis and die of an unrelated cause. The median survival time is of 4 to 6 years. Anemia, hemorrhage and infection become life-threatening in the stages. Occasionally, CLL/SLL tends to transform to more aggressive tumors, such as prolymphocytic lymphoma or diffuse large B-cell lymphoma. The prognosis is extremely poor once transformation occurs.

Follicular Lymphoma

Follicular lymphoma is a tumor derived from germinal center B-cells, characterized by a nodular or follicular architecture. It is one of the commonest types of NHLs and is a disease of late adult life with a peak age incidence in the sixth and seventh decades. It accounts for 10% to 40% of all NHLs.

A. Morphology

Microscopically, the closely packed neoplastic cells replace the normal lymph node architectures. Tumor cells resemble normal germinal center B-cells, which may have a purely follicular growth pattern (Figure 9-8) or may have a mixed pattern with follicular and diffuse areas. The predominant neoplastic cells are centrocyte-like, which are slightly larger than resting lymphocytes, with an angular cleaved nuclear contour characterized by prominent indentations and linear infoldings. Nuclear chromatin is coarse and condensed, and nucleoli are indistinct. These small cleaved cells are mixed with variable numbers of larger centroblast-like cells that are three to four times the size of resting lymphocytes. Mitoses are infrequent and single necrotic cell is not found. These indicators are helpful to distinguish neoplastic follicles from reactive germinal centers, in which both mitoses and apoptosis are marked.

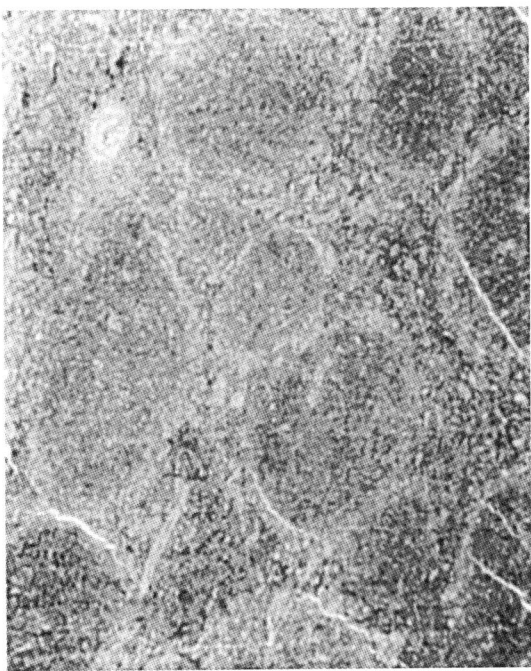

Figure 9-8 Follicular lymphoma. Such a follicular pattern is seen only in B cell lymphomas and is favorable histologic feature

B. Immunophenotype and Karyotype

These neoplastic cells express pan-B-cell markers, such as CD19 and CD20, and many tumor cells are positive for the more restricted B-cell marker CD10. BCL protein is positive in neoplastic cells, but negative in normal germinal center B-cells.

Most of the cases have specific chromosome translocation involving the immunoglobulin heavy chain promoter region on chromosome 14 and the anti-apoptotic gene BCL2 on chromosome 18 (t14;18) (q32; q21). This translocation causes the constitutive overexpression of BCL2 protein, rendering follicular lymphoma cells relatively resistant to apoptosis.

C. Clinical Features

Follicular lymphoma occurs mainly in older persons. Most patients with this disease present painless, slowly progressive lymphadenopathy, which is frequently generalized. Involvement of bone marrow is common in follicular lymphoma at the time of diagnosis. The peripheral blood involvement is uncommon. This disorder is an indolent disease, but it is generally regarded as incurable when disseminated. The median survival time is of 7 to 9 years. It is worth noted that in about 40% of patients the disease will transform into a diffuse large B-cell lymphoma. Their lack of response to chemotherapy may be caused in part by the antiapoptotic effect of BCL2, which may protect the neoplastic cells from the effects of chemotherapeutic agents. Progression is often related to mutation in the TP53 gene.

Diffuse large B-cell Lymphomas

Diffuse large B-cell lymphomas (DLBL) form the commonest type of high-grade NHLs and include several forms of NHLs that share certain features, including a B-cell phenotype, a diffuse growth pattern, and an aggressive clinical history. Therefore, it is the most important type of lymphoma in the adults, accounting for about 50% of all adults NHLs. DLBL occurs mainly in older patients (median age about 60 years), but may occur in childhood, accounting for 15% of childhood lymphoma.

A. Morphology

DLBL is characterized by a diffuse outgrowth of large B-cells, which may display centroblastic or immunblastic cytology. The nuclei of the neoplastic cells are large (at least three to four times the size of resting lymphocytes) and can present a variety of forms. The centroblastic-like cells with round, irregular, or cleaved nuclear contours, dispersed chromatin, and several distinct nucleoli predominate. The cytoplasm tends to be pale and modest in volume. The immunoblastic-like cells have a round or multilobulated large vesicular nucleus with one or two centrally placed prominent nucleoli. The cytoplasm is abundant and can be deeply staining and pyroninophilic or clear.

B. Immunophenotype and Karyotype

DLBL expresses pan-B-cell markers, such as CD19, CD20, CD79a and IgM and/or IgG as well as κ or λ light chain. A variety of cytogenic abnormalities are seen in DLBL. The commonest one is the t(14;18) translocation resulting in the deregulation of the BCL2 gene and about one third of these diseases show rearrangement of the BCL6 gene.

C. Clinical Features

The majority of patients present with rapidly progressive nodal disease, often asymptomatic mass at a single nodal or extranodal site. The involvement of gastrointestinal tract, skin, bone, or brain, which is not common at the time of diagnosis, may be the presenting features. With the progression of the disease, however, any site may be involved, and leukemic picture rarely emerge. The prognosis of the patients with this disease is poor if untreated. With intensive combination chemotherapy, however, complete remission can be achieved in 60% to 80% of the patients, and, of these, about 50% remain free of disease for several years.

Burkitt Lymphoma

Burkitt lymphoma is a distinctive type of B-cell lymphoma, regarded as lymphoblastic in some classification. It is endemic in para-Africa and occurs much less commonly in other regions. The disease is associated with EBV infection and malaria.

A. Morphology

The histological appearances are distinctive, with tightly packed lymphoblasts interspersed with phagocytic macrophages (Figure 9-9). The tumor cells are monotonous, intermediate in size, and have round or oval nuclei containing two to five prominent nucleoli. There is a moderate amount of faintly basophilic or amphophilic cytoplasm, which is intensely pyroninophilic. The mitosis, which is characteristic of this tumor, is very common. As the tumor cell is dead, the numerous tissue macrophages will engulf the dead cell. Because these benign macrophages are often surrounded by a clear space, they create a "starry sky" pattern.

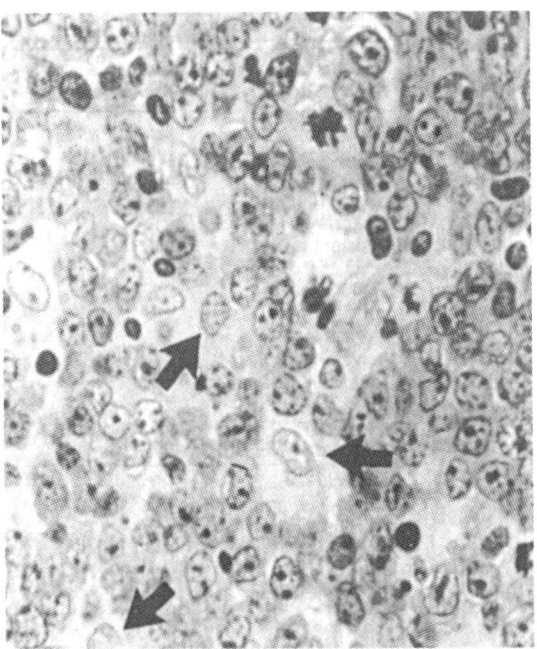

Figure 9-9 Burkitt lymphoma. The cells resemble lymphoblasts and are characterized by small size, round nuclei with prominent nucleoli, a high mitotic rate, and the presence of scattered hitoticytes that give a starry sky appearance. This is a high-grade lymphoma

B. Immunophenotype and Karyotype

The neoplastic cells express surface IgM and pan-B-cell markers, such as CD19 and CD10. The pathogenesis of Burkitt lymphoma is closely related to translocations involving the MYC gene on chromosome 8. Most translocations fuse MYC with the IgH gene on chromosome 14, but variant translocations involving the κ or λ light chain loci on chromosome 2 and 22, respectively, are also found. The results of these translocations are the inappropriate overexpression of the MYC protein, which has potent transforming activity.

C. Clinical Features

Both the endemic and non-African (sporadic cases) cases mainly affect children and adolescents, accounting for about 30% of childhood NHLs. The disease rarely arises in lymph nodes. Involvement of the maxilla or mandible is the common presentation in African, whereas abdominal tumors (bowel, retroperitoneum, ovaries) are more common in North America. Burkitt lymphoma is a high-grade tumor that may be the fastest growing human neoplasm. With very aggressive chemotherapy regiments, however, the majority of patients can be cured.

Extranodal Marginal Zone B-cell Lymphoma of Mucosal-Associated lymphoid Tissue (MALT)

MALT lymphomas are a group of lymphoma that arise from MALT, such as salivary glands, small and large bowels, lungs, and some mucosal sites (e.g. the orbit and breast). They make up at least a quarter of all NHLs. It is now clear that MALT lymphomas are distinctive forms of NHLs.

Histologically, these tumors share common histological and cytological features wherever they occur, characterized by the presence of reactive germinal centers surrounded by a population of neoplastic B-cells which resemble normal B-cells that home to areas of the margins of B-cells follicles. The tumor cells infiltrate the epithelial structure to form the characteristic lesions of MALT lymphomas, i.e. the **lympho-epithelial lesions**. MALT lymphomas are associated with the cytogenetic abnormalities t(1; 14), involving the BCL10 and IgH genes; and t(11; 18), involving the MALT1 and IAP2 genes. These tumors appear to remain localized for long periods and have an indolent natural history, often with a very good prognosis.

MATURE T- AND NK-CELL NEOPLASMS

Peripheral T-cell Lymphoma, Unspecified

T-cell lymphomas are relatively uncommon in America and Europe, accounting for no more than 15% of NHLs cases, but they are relatively common in Asia, accounting for 20% to 30% in our country. This increased disease prevalence is due to the presence of an endemic retrovirus, the human T-cell leukemia/lymphoma virus (HTLV1), which appears to be a causative agent in some forms of T-cell malignance.

The spectrum of T-cell lymphomas seems as broad as that of B-cell tumors. The histological recognition of different subtypes of nodal peripheral T-cell lymphoma is difficult to perform reliable because morphology is not a good indicator of clinical behaviors.

For this reason the majority of these tumors have been categorized as this group. Therefore, within this group of tumors the size and shape of the neoplastic T-cells are varied obviously (a heterogeneous group of tumors). Although the morphology of T-cell lymphomas is variable in size and shape of cells, they share common features, such as the architectures of lymph node replaced by the tumor cells, mainly affected paracortex with vascular proliferation, composed of a group of heterogeneous tumor cells with a number of nonneoplastic reactive cells (such as eosinophils, histiocytes, and plasma cells). The neoplastic cells express T-cell markers, such as CD2, CD3, and CD5.

Mycosis Fungoides(MF)

MF, which is a disease of adult life with a tendency to involve older age groups, is a cutaneous T-cell lymphoma. The neoplastic T-cells usually have a helper cell phenotype (CD4) and form a band-like upper dermal infiltrate with moderate degree of epidermal infiltration, often forming small aggregates of cells within the epidermis (termed Pautrier's microabscesses) usually in association with epidermal Langerhan's cells. The neoplastic T-cells are larger than normal lymphocytes and usually have a markedly irregular profile imparting a cerebriform appearance.

MF is classified into three stages according to its progression in clinic: (1) **the patch stage**, characterized by erythematous macules usually occurring on areas not exposed to sunlight; (2) **the plaque stage**, with elevated scaly plaques which may be pink or red/brown and are often intensely pruritic; (3) **the tumor stage**, with dome-shaped firm tumors which may ulcerate.

With the progression of disease the density of lymphoid infiltrate increases from the patch to the tumor stage. Although MF is initially confined to the skin, lymph node and visceral organs involvement become clinically apparent later in the course of the disease and are particularly common in the tumor stage. The prognosis is poor, with a median survival of only 2.5 years, when the visceral organ involvement, whereas the prognosis of patients with limited extent cutaneous disease is good, mean survival 12 years.

Extranodal NK-/T-cell Lymphomas

These tumors are derived from cytotoxic T-cells or NK-cells and are highly aggressive. About 80% to 100% of cases are EBV DNA or its encoded protein positive. The most common site is the nasal cavities or paranasal sinuses. Other sites may include skin, gastrointestinal tract, testis, kidney, upper respiratory tract and rarely the eye/orbit. Clinical presentation varies depending on the primary sites of involvement. Commonly patients present with a nasal mass with bleeding and local bony destruction. About 10% to 20% of patients presenting with nasal NK-/T-cell lymphoma may also have skin involvement at the same time.

Although extranodal NK-/T-cell lymphomas are found in various places, they often bear very similar histological features throughout. Characteristic features include a prominent but not invariable angiocentric/angiodestructive growth pattern, extensive mucosa ulceration, coagulative necrosis and pseudoepitheliomatous hyperplasia. Often admixed are prominent inflammatory cells including plasma cells, histocytes and often eosinophils. Tumor cells vary greatly in size, but, in most cases, they are composed of medium-sized cells or a mixture of small and large cells. They often have granular or vesicular nuclei with irregular nuclear contour and inconspicuous nucleoli and moderate pale to clear cytoplasm. Mitosis is easily found. The most typical immunophenotypes of extranodal NK-/T-cell lymphoma is: CD2 +, CD3 +, or express NK-cell marker CD56. The prognosis of extranodal NK-/T-cell lymphoma is variable. Some patients respond well to chemotherapy such as CHOP combined with local radiation, achieving complete remission and others die of disseminated disease despite aggressive therapy.

HODGKIN'S LYMPHOMA

Hodgkin's lymphoma (also called Hodgkin's disease) is a primary malignant tumor of lymphoid tissues, which characterized by the presence of **Reed-Sternberg (R-S) cells** in the involved tissues. It arises almost invariably in a single node or chain of nodes and spreads characteristically to the anatomically contiguous nodes. It accounts for 15% of all lymphomas and shows a peak age incidence in the third and fourth decades. The reasons that it separated from the NHLs are as follows: (1) there is morphologically characterized by the presence of distinctive R-S cells admixed with a variable infiltrate of reactive, nonmalignant inflammatory cells; (2) it is often associated with somewhat distinctive clinical features, including systemic manifestations, such as fever; (3) its stereotypic pattern of spread allows it to be treated differently than most other lymphoid neoplasm. Recent molecular studies have clearly demonstrated that it is, in most cases, a tumor of B-lymphocytes. It, therefore, best considered an unusual form of lymphoma.

Morphology

Macroscopically, affected lymph nodes are enlarged with a smooth surface. The cut surface is usually homogeneously pale white, although in some histological subtypes a nodular or fibrotic appearance may be present. Microscopically, affected lymph nodes show a partial or complete destruction of their normal architectures by a mixed infiltrate containing lymphocytes, histiocytes, plasma cells, and eosinophils as well as R-S cells of Hodgkin's lymphoma. These malignant cells are large, have abundant, slight eosinophilic cytoplasm and range from 15 to 45 μm in diameter. They take the form of mononuclear Hodgkin's cells, or of R-S cells that have a large, pale multilobed nucleus and a prominent eosinophlic nucleolus about the size of a RBC. Particularly characteristics are two **mirror-image** nuclei or nuclear lobes (Figure 9-10), each containing a large acidophilic nucleolus surrounded by a distinctive clear zone. The nuclear membrane is distinct.

Although the diagnosis of Hodgkin's lymphoma depends upon the finding of classic R-S cells, these cells show little evidence of nucleic acid synthesis or proliferative activity. Large mononuclear cells (called Hodgkin's cells) that resemble R-S cells are the proliferative cells in Hodgkin's lymphoma.

The histologic picture of Hodgkin's lymphoma is particularly distinctive in that the neoplastic R-S cells are few in number and are admixed with variable numbers of lymphocytes, plasma cells, histiocytes, eosinophils, neutrophils, and fibroblasts, all of which are considered to be reactive (Figure 9-11). Yet the lymph node may be totally destroyed, and an identical process may progress to involve many lymph nodes, spleen, liver, bone marrow, and extralymphatic tissues. This is a contrast with other malignant neoplasms, in which the malignant cells predominate in the involved tissues.

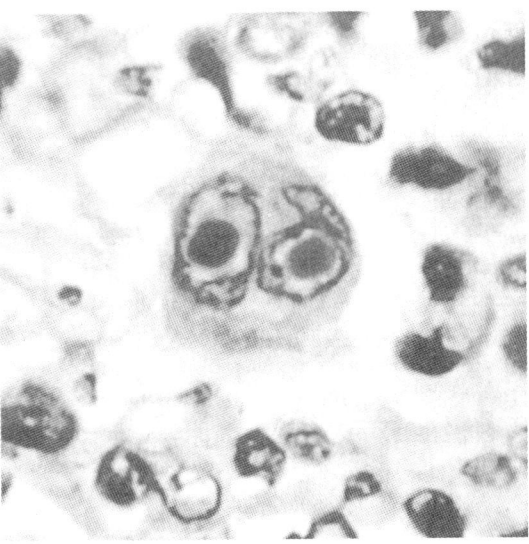

Figure 9-10 Hodgkin's lymphoma. High magnification of a classical Reed-Sternberg cell with two nuclei containing the typical large nucleoli

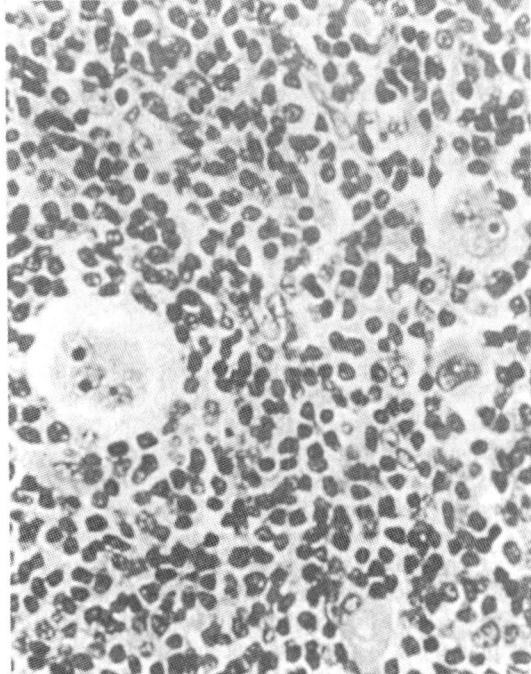

Figure 9-11 Hodgkin's lymphoma, mixed cellularity showing multinucleated Reed-Sternberg cells in background of cells that include lymphocytes, plasma cells, eosinophils, histiocytes and mononuclear Reed-Sternberg cells

Classification of Hodgkin's Lymphoma

Hodgkin's lymphoma is classified based on the appearance of the abnormal cells and the reactive cells under the microscope. The varying relative proportions of R-S cells (and mononuclear variant cells), lymphocytes, histiocytes, and areas of fibrosis have permitted subclassification of Hodgkin's lymphoma into two subtypes, i. e. **nodular lymphocyte predominant Hodgkin's Lymphoma** and **classic Hodgkin's lymphoma** according to the new WHO classification. The later type is further classified into nodular sclerosis type, mixed cellular type, lymphocytes predominance type, and lymphocyte depletion type. They have epidemiologic, prognostic, and therapeutic differences.

A. Nodular Lymphocyte Predominant Hodgkin's Lymphoma

This type (<10%) is characterized by the presence of numerous mature-looking lymphocytes with a variable number of benign histiocytes. Other types of reactive cells, such as eosinophils, neutrophils, and plasma cells, are scanty or absent, and classic R-S cells can be found. It tends to affect young adult males and may include a conspicuous component of reactive histiocytes. There is a nodular growth pattern that suggests it derives from B-cell, but occasionally it is diffuse. It typically presents as stage I or II disease and progresses slowly. This type has an excellent prognosis. Almost all the tumor cells are positive for CD20, CD79a, BCL6 and CD45, and most of the cases are CD75 positive with immunohistologic staining.

B. Classic Hodgkin's Lymphoma

Classic Hodgkin's lymphoma is usually rich in typical R-S cells, especially in mixed cell type. But they are rare in lymphocyte predominant Hodgkin's lymphoma.

- **Nodular sclerosing Hodgkin's lymphoma** (30%-60%) has a good prognosis, usually presenting as early stage disease. Young women are particularly affected, and mediastinal involvement is common. Nodular sclerosis is histologically characterized by broad bands of collagen circumscribing nodules of involved tissue and by the presence of large R-S cell variants that have multilobulated nuclei and abundant pale cytoplasm (**lacunar cells**).
- **Mixed cellular Hodgkin's lymphoma** (20%-40%) has an intermediate histologic appearance with numerous lymphocytes, plasma cells, eosinophils, and R-S cells (Figure 9-10). The prognosis is intermediate between that of lymphocyte predominant and lymphocyte depleted lymphomas. The response to therapy is usually good. It is more common after age 50 years.
- **Lymphocyte predominant Hodgkin's lymphoma** (5%) is characterized by a paucity of typical Hodgkin's and R-S cells and abundant lymphocytes, but scanty or absent of other reactive cells, sometimes admixed with a variety of histiocytes. Typical R-S cells are few but its distinctive variant, which is called the "**popcorn**" cell because of its excessively lobulated nucleus, is rich and characteristic. This kind of cells expresses B-cell marker (CD20). The patients with this disease have an excellent survival.
- **Lymphocyte depleted Hodgkin's Lymphoma** (<2%) has the worst prognosis and typically presents as stage III or stage IV disease in elderly patients. Lymph nodes are replaced by a destructive process containing numerous pleomorphic mononuclear and classic R-S cells, variable amounts of diffuse fibrosis, and very few lymphocytes. This type is often refractory to therapy.

Staging of Hodgkin's Lymphoma

Staging is an important determinant in the treatment and prognosis of patients with Hodgkin's lymphoma. The staging system currently used is that proposed at the Ann Arbor workshop in 1971 (Table 9-2).

Table 9-2 Staging of Hodgkin's and non-Hodgkin's lymphoma

Stage I	Involvement of a single lymph node region (I) or of a single extralymphatic organ or site (Ie)
Stage II	Involvement of two or more lymph node regions on the same side of the diaphragm alone (II) or with involvement of an extralymphatic organ or site and of one or more lymph node regions on the same side of the diaphragm (IIe)
Stage III	Involvement of both sides of the diaphragm (III) which may also be accompanied by localized involvement of an extralymphatic site (IIIe) or the spleen (IIIs) or both (IIIse)
Stage IV	Disseminated involvement of one or more extralymphatic organs such as liver, lung and bone marrow with or without lymph node involvement

Clinical Features of Hodgkin's Lymphoma

Hodgkin's Lymphoma is more common in males and shows a peak incidence in early adulthood. It, like NHLs, usually represents as a painless enlargement of the lymph nodes, most often in the upper half of the body, with involvement of cervical and/or axillary lymph nodes, and spreads to anatomically contiguous nodes. Radiological evidence of mediastinal involvement is present in over 40% of patients and on occasion may be massive. With advantage of the disease, the involvement of spleen, liver, bone marrow, and other organs and tissues may appear. Some patients with this disease have systemic symptoms, such as weight loss, unexplained pyrexia of 39℃, anemia, and drenching night sweats. In spite of intensive research and a wealth of immunologic data, the diagnosis of Hodgkin's lymphoma is still based entirely upon histologic examination-the finding of the classic R-S cell in pathologic tissue is considered essential for diagnosis.

Localized forms of Hodgkin's lymphoma may be treated with either radiation or chemotherapy. Chemotherapy is highly effective when multiple agents are used and may lead to cures even in patients with disseminated (late stage) disease. The 5-year survival rate of patients with stage Ⅰa or Ⅱa diseases is close 100%. Fifty per cent of patients with advanced disease (stage Ⅳa or Ⅳb) can achieve 5-year disease-free survival.

MYELOID NEOPLASMS

Myeloid neoplasms arise from hematopoietic stem cells. There are three types of myeloid neoplasms: (1) acute myeloblastic leukemia, (2) myelodysplastic syndromes, and (3) chronic myeloproliferative disorders. In this section we mainly discuss myelogenous leukemias, which are characterized by diffuse replacement of normal bone marrow by leukemic cells with variable accumulation of abnormal cells in the peripheral blood and infiltration of organs, such as liver, spleen, lymph nodes, menings and gonads by leukemic cells. These changes result in anemia, hemorrhage and infections. Leukemias are very common in the worldwide. The number of new cases of leukemias in the United States is about 25,000 per year, with 15,000 to 20,000 deaths. Death rates have fallen because of increasing effective treatment. The death rates of leukemias are listed in the 6th to 7th place in all malignant tumors in our country, but they take the first place in children and adolescents neoplasms.

ACUTE MYELOBLASTIC LEUKEMIAS (AML)

Acute myeloblastic leukemia is an extremely heterogeneous neoplasm. It primarily affects adults (mean age 50 years). The incidence of this disorder increases steadily with age.

A. Classification of AML

Based on the results of morphologic, histochemical, immunophenotypic, and karyotypic studies (of these tests, karyotypicing is most predictive of outcome) AMLs are classified into eight subgroups by FAB classification.

- **M0** It is a type of minimally differentiated, accounting for 2% to 3% of AML. The blasts lack definitive cytologic AML and cytochemical markers of myeloblasts but express myeloid lineage antigens.
- **M1** It is a type without differentiation, accounting for 20% of AML. Very immature myeloblasts predominate; few granules or Auer rods are found. It has a worsen prognosis.
- **M2** This is a type with differentiation, accounting for 30% to 40% of AML. Myeloblasts and promyelocytes are predominant and Auer rods commonly present. The type presences of t(8;21) translocation related to good prognosis.
- **M3** Acute promyelocytic leukemia accounts for 5% to 10% of AML. It may cause disseminated intravascular coagulation. The presence of t(15;17) translocation is characteristic and responds for retionic acid treatment. Hypergranular promyelocytes are often with many Auer rods per cell and may have reniform or bilobed nuclei.
- **M4** Acute myelomonocytic leukemia accounts for 20% to 30% of AML. Myelocytic and monocytic differentiations are evident. Monocytosis presents in peripheral blood. The presence of inv16 or del16q associates with better prognosis.
- **M5** Acute monocytic leukemia accounts for 10% of AML; monoblasts (peroxidase-negative, esterase-positive) and promonocytes are predominant. It usually occurs in children and young adults. Gum infiltration is common and relates to abnormalities of

chromosome 11q23.

- **M6** Acute erythroleukemia accounts for 5% of AML. Bizarre, multinucleated, megaloblastoid erythoblasts predominate and myeloblasts also present. High blood count and organ infiltration are rare. Persons affected are of advantage age.
- **M7** Acute megakaryocytic leukemia accounts for 1% of AML. Blasts of megakaryocytic lineage predominate. Myelofibrosis or increased bone marrow reticulin are often noted.

B. Morphology

The blasts have delicate chromatin, three to five nucleoli, and fine azurophilic granules in the cytoplasm. Infiltrated myeloblasts can be distinguished from lymphoblasts with routine Wright-Giemsa stains. In some cases there are red-staining rod-like structures (Auer rods) which are more often present in the promyelocytic variant. Therefore, Auer rods, only seen in neoplastic myeloblasts, are a helpful diagnostic indicator when present.

C. Blood and Bone Marrow Changes

In peripheral blood the white cell count is usually increased, but the counts of greater than $100 \times 10^9/L$ are not uncommon. The cellularity of bone marrow is obviously increased. Blast cells constitute at least 30% of nucleated cells present and often greater than 80%.

D. Other Organs Changes

Spleen is often infiltrated with leukemic blast cell, which results in the spleen enlargement, but it is minor in contrast to that in chronic leukemia. The liver is usually mild enlargement. There is a diffuse infiltration with leukemic blasts in the lobule along the sinusoid of liver. Infiltration of the gums and skin is a peculiar feature of the monocytic types of AML (M4). Rarely, a local tissue mass taking place in the bone, orbit, skin, lymph node, gastrointestinal tract, prostate and breast, (chloroma or granulocytic sarcoma) may be the first manifestation of AML.

E. Histochemistry and Immunophenotype

Cases with myelocytic differentiation are typically positive for the enzyme myeloperoxidase. Auer rods are intensely peroxidase positive. Lysosomal nonspecific esterases staining can demonstrate monocytic differentiation.

The labeling of immunology is varied in AML. Most cases express some myeloid-associated antigens, such as CD13, CD14, CD15, or CD64. Because mutipotent stem cells express CD33, myeloid progenitor cells are positive for CD33.

F. Clinical Features

The onset is often very rapid and progression to death from anemia, hemorrhage, or infection occurs within weeks if no treatment is given. Thrombocytopenia is marked. Anemia, often severe and rapidly developing, causes pallor and hypoxic symptoms. Thrombocytopenia may produce abnormal bleeding or purpura. Neutropenia results in infections, fever, and ulceration of mucous membranes. AML is a destructive disease. Patients with karyotypic aberrations ($t[8;21]$, $inv[16]$) have a 50% chance of long-term disease-free survival, but the overall long-term disease-free survival is only 15% to 30% with conventional chemotherapy. Currently, allergenic marrow transplantation seems to be the only method that can lead to cure of the disease.

CHRONIC MYELOGENOUS LEUKEMIAS (CML)

Chronic leukemias (usually including CLL and CML, see page 274) have an insidious onset and a slow rate of progression. Most patients present with slowly development anemia and enlargement of organs infiltrated by leukemia cells.

CML is one of the diseases of chronic myeloproliferation disorders. It accounts for 15% to 20% of all cases of leukemia. The peak incidence is in the fourth and fifth decades of age.

A. Morphology

CML is characterized by the presence of very high peripheral blood cell counts. Leukocytosis is a uniform feature, with occasional cell counts in excess of $300 \times 10^9/L$. The cell pictures in the blood are myelocytes, promyelocytes, myeloblasts and normoblasts present as well as large numbers of band cells and mature polymorphonuclear granulocytes. Platelets are increased, normal or reduced. Normochromic anemia is often present. The leukocytes are abnormal, as exemplified by an absence or severe reduction of their content of alkaline phosphatase, a feature unique to CML and diagnosis value. The bone marrow is hypercellular with marked reduction of fat spaces. The spleen is enlarged, often massively. Hapatomegaly is also frequently present. Liver infiltration with CML leukemic cells is mainly in the sinusoids.

B. Karyotype

In approximately 95% of patients with CML the Ph chromosome can be demonstrated in granulocytic, erythroid, and megekaryocytic precursors, as well as B-cells and, in some cases, T-cell. This cytogenetic change is a reliable marker of the disease. Ph chromosome is a state that part of the chromosome 9, including the Abelson oncogene (c-ABL), is translocated to chromosome 22, with exchange of chromosomal segments between 9 and 22. Interaction of c-ABL with BCR locus genes on chromosome 22 produces a new chimeric gene BCR-ABL (gene fusion). This new gene encodes a fusion protein consisting of portions of BCR and the tyrosine kinase domain of ABL, which possesses an increased, dysregulated tyrosine activity playing a critical role in the pathophysiology of CML.

C. Clinical Features

CML usually has an insidious onset, a slow rate of progression, and the initial symptoms may be nonspecific (e.g. easy fatigability, weakness, and weight loss). Massive splenomegaly and hepatomegaly are common presenting complains in patients with CML. Sometimes the first symptom is a dragging sensation in the abdomen, caused by **the extreme splenomegaly** that is characteristic of this condition. The laboratory findings are critical in making the diagnosis. When a patient with CML has a bone marrow containing more than 5% myeloblasts, that patient is defined as being in the accelerated or blast phase of the disease.

The chronic phase of CML persists for 1 to 10 years (median survival being 3 years even without treatment). Finally, there is an accelerated phase that eventually (50% of cases) enters blast crisis (resembling acute leukemia). In the remaining 50% cases, blast crises occur abruptly, without an intermediated phase.

It is necessary to distinguish CML from a **leukemoid reaction**, which also shows an obviously elevation of granulocyte count in response to infection, stress, chronic inflammation, and certain malignant neoplasms. The peripheral blood picture of leukemoid reaction resembles that of CML but may be distinguished from it by the neutrophil alkaline phosphatase level, which is elevated in the leukemoid reaction and decreased in CML. Examination of the peripheral blood smear provides valuable clues to etiology. Reactive neutrophilias are characterized by the presence of predominantly mature forms. In neoplastic proliferations of granulocytic cells, less mature forms are present in the peripheral blood. Most important for differentiating leukemoid reaction from CML is the presence of the Ph chromosome in CML, which is quite typical of CML, but absent in leukemoid reaction.

HISTOCYTIC NEOPLASMS

The term histiocytosis includes a variety of proliferative disorders of histiocytes or macrophages. Some are malignant tumors, such as very rare histiocytic lymphoma. Others are benign, such as the reactive histiocytic proliferations in lymph nodes. A small cluster of relatively rare condition, which is between these two extremes of the proliferative disorders of histiocytes, is the Langerhan's cell histiocytosis characterized by the clonal proliferation of a special type of cell, the Langerhan's cell. Langerhan's cells are dendritic antigen-presenting cells that are normally distributed in many organs, most obviously the skin.

These disorders, in the past, were regarded as histiocytosis X and subdivided into three categories: Letterer-Siwe syndrome (generalized histiocytosis), Hand-Schüller-Christian disease, and eosinophilic granuloma. Based on the recent studies, these three conditions are believed to represent the different expressions of the same disease. Both human leukocyte antigen DR (HLA-DR) and CD1 antigen are positive in the proliferating Langerhan's cells. HX bodies (Birbeck granules) in the cytoplasm of these cells are characteristic. They are showed to have a pentalaminar, rod-like, tubular structure, with characteristic periodicity and sometimes a dilated terminal end (tennis rocket appearance) under electron microscopy. The proliferating Langerhan's cells have abundant, often vacuolated, cytoplasm, with vesicular nuclei under light microscopy, which is different from their normal dendritic counterparts.

Langerhan's cell histiocytosis is divided into three types: acute disseminated Langerhan's cell histiocytosis, unifocal eosinophilic granuloma, or multifocal granuloma.

ACUTE DISSEMINATED LANGERHANS CELL HISTIOCYTOSIS

Acute disseminated Langerhans cell histiocytosis (also called Letterer-Siwe syndrome) appears to represent the aggressive end of the spectrum, with widespread lesions of bone and lymphoid tissue. The condition is uncommon and occurs usually before 2 years of age. The dominant clinical signs are the development of skin lesions due to infiltration by Langerhans cells. Most of the patients present hepatosplenomegaly, lymphadenopathy, pulmonary lesions, and destructive osteolytic bone lesions. Anemia, thrombocytopenia, and recurrent infections are often noted owing to the extensive infiltration of the marrow. Thus, the clinical signs and symptoms may resemble that of acute leukemia. The prognosis of the patient untreated is poor. Fifty per cent of the patients with intensive chemotherapy survive 5 years.

EOSINOPHILIC GRANULOMA

Both unifocal and multifocal eosinophilic granulomas are characterized by expanding, erosive accumulation of Langerhan's cells, usually within the medullar cavities of bones. The proliferative Langerhan's cells are variably admixed with eosinophils, lymphocytes, plasma cells, and neutrophils. The eosinophilic component ranges from scattered mature cells to sheet-like masses of cells. The calvarium, ribs, and femur are commonly involved.

Unifocal lesion is a relatively benign disease that involves bone, particularly the skull and ribs of children and young adults, although long bones are sometimes involved. It may be asymptomatic or may cause pain and tenderness, and pathologic fracture. Radiologically, it presents as a well-demarcated lytic lesion. This disorder may heal spontaneously or may be cured by local excision or irradiation.

Multifocal lesions have a less favorable prognosis. It usually affects children presenting with fever, diffuse eruptions, particularly on the scalp and in the ear canals; and frequent bouts of otitis media. Lymphadenopathy, hepatomegaly, and splenomegaly present by the infiltrate of Langerhan's cells. The base of the skull is characteristically involved, producing the triad of proptosis, lytic bone lesions in skull, and diabetes insipidus – the last due to destruction of the posterior pituitary. The combination of calvarial bone defects, diabetes insipidus, and exophthalmos is referred to as the Hand-Schüller-Christian triad. Most patients with this disease experience spontaneous regression and others can be treated with chemotherapy.

CDla and S-100 protein are positive of Langerhan's cells with immune techniques. Birbeck bodies can be found with electron microscopy. These indicators are useful for the diagnosis of Langerhan's cell histiocytosis.

Chapter 10 Diseases of Immunity

Wang Yalan

CHAPTER CONTENTS
- The Immune Response
    - Characteristics of the Immune Response
    - Types of the Immune Response
- Immunologic Injury
    - Autoimmune Diseases
        - Lupus Erythematosus
        - Rheumatoid Arthritis
        - Sjögren's Syndrome
        - Polymyositis-Dermatomyositis
        - Scleroderma (Progressive Systemic Sclerosis)
        - Transplant Rejection
- Deficiencies of Immune Response
    - Congenital (Primary) Immunodeficiency
    - Secondary and Acquired Immunodeficiency

THE IMMUNE RESPONSE

The immune response is a complex series of cellular interactions activated by the entry into the body of foreign (nonself) antigenic materials such as infectious agents and a variety of macromolecules. After processing by macrophages, the antigen is presented to lymphocytes, which are the major effector cells of the immune system (Figure 10-1). Lymphocyte activation by antigen results in proliferation and transformation of the lymphocytes, which lead to two main types of immune response: cell-mediated immunity and humoral immunity.

CHARACTERISTICS OF THE IMMUNE RESPONSE

The immune response is characterized by (1) specificity (i. e. reactivity is directed toward and restricted to the inducing agent, termed the antigen); (2) amplification (the ability to develop an enhanced response on repeated exposure to the same antigen); and (3) memory (the ability to recognize and mount an enhanced response against the same antigen on subsequent exposure even if the first and subsequent exposures are widely separated in time). These features distinguish the immune response from other nonspecific host responses such as acute inflammation and nonimmune phagocytosis.

Tolerance to Self Antigens

The concepts of self and nonself (foreignness) are central to immunologic reactivity (Figure 10-2). Many molecules in a host individual are antigenic (i. e. they may induce an immune response) if introduced into another individual but are not recognized as antigens by the host. This failure to respond to self antigens is natural tolerance, and it prevents the immune system from destroying the host's own tissues. Tolerance to self antigens is induced during embryonic development, and it also demonstrates specificity and memory.

Specificity

The specificity of the immune response is dependent on the ability of the immune system to produce an almost unlimited number of antibodies of differing specificity plus an almost equally diverse repertoire of T lymphocytes bearing specific antigen receptors on their surfaces. An antigen evokes a response from a specific B or T lymphocyte that is preprogrammed to react against it (i. e. the lymphocyte bears receptors with appropriate specificity for the antigen). Foreign antigens must be recognized by the immune system before an immune response can develop. An optimal immune response to most antigens occurs only after interaction of the antigen with macrophages, T lymphocytes, and B lymphocytes (Figure 10-1). Macrophage acting in this role is termed an antigen-processing cell. Dendritic re-

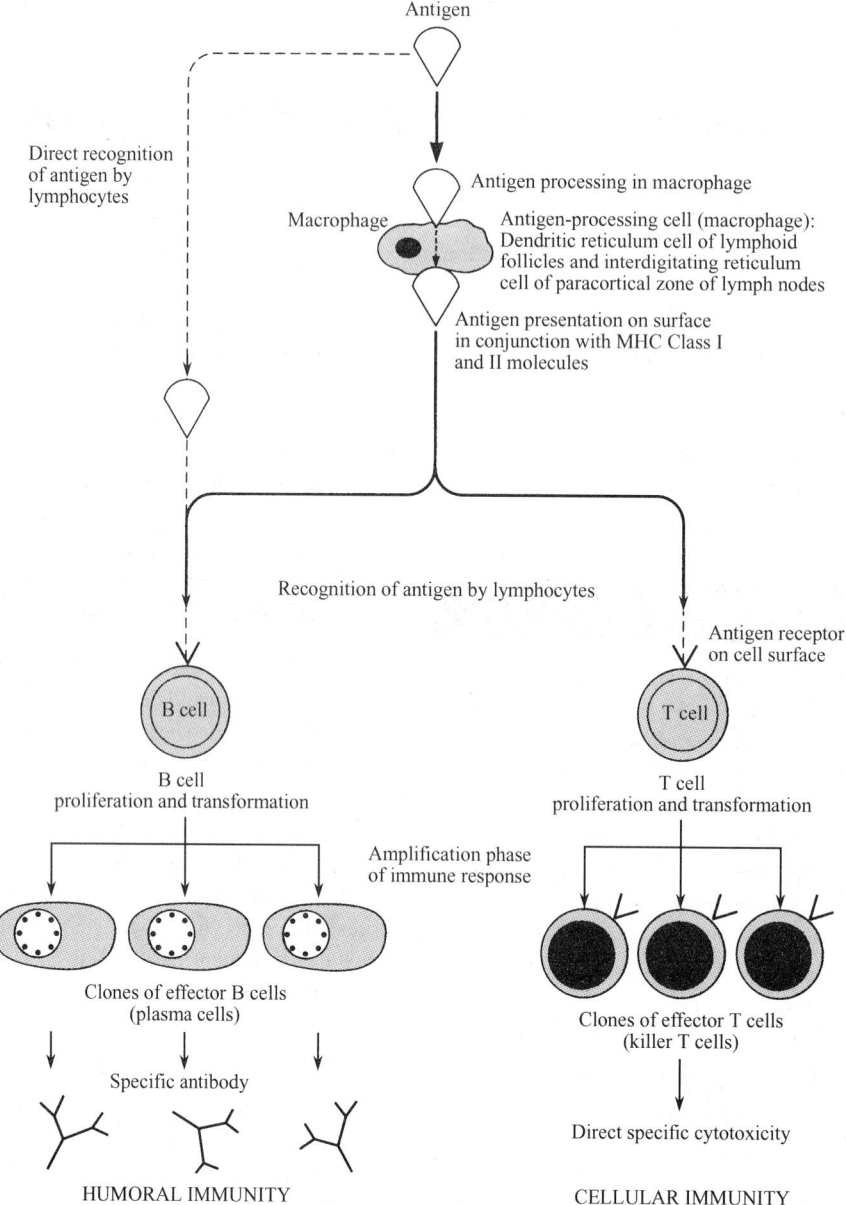

Figure 10-1 Summary of the immune response. Lymphocytes (both B and T) bearing specific antigen receptors are induced to proliferate (amplification phase) after they react with an antigen. The process by which lymphocytes recognize an antigen commonly involves an antigen-processing cell (various types of macrophages). Proliferation produces the effector cells of the immune response. Effector B cell (plasma cells) produce specific antibody, which mediates humoral immunity. Effector T cell exert a direct cytotoxic effect and mediate cellular immunity. Humoral immunity is so called because it can be transferred from an immune individual to a susceptible one by injection of serum containing antibody; cellular immunity can be transferred only by injection of live T cell. (MHC, major histocompatibility complex.)

ticulum cells in lymphoid follicles and interdigitating reticulum cells in the paracortical zone of lymph nodes are believed to be specialized macrophages adapted to process antigens for B and T cell, respectively.

This receptor function on the surface of lymphocytes is performed by immunoglobulin on B cell and by an immunoglobulin-like molecule on T cell. When challenged by an antigen, the specific lymphocyte (B or T) selectively multiplies into a clone of sensitized effector cells that can mount a highly specific response against that antigen: from B cell, plasma cells that in turn produce immunoglobulin; from T cell, cytotoxic T lymphocytes (Figure 10-1). This specific response usually has a net protective effect (immunity); occasionally, adverse reactions develop that cause tissue injury (hypersensitivity).

TYPES OF THE IMMUNE RESPONSE

Memory is an essential component of the immunoresponse because it facilitates an enhanced, more effective response upon second and subsequent exposures to a particular antigen. Based on whether the immune system has been previously exposed to the antigen or not, two types of immune response can be recognized.

The Primary Immune Response

The primary immune response follows the first exposure to a particular antigen. Although antigen is recognized almost as soon as it is introduced into the body, several days elapse before enough immunoglobulin are produced to be detected as an increase in serum immunoglobulin levels. IgM is the first immunoglobulin produced during the primary response; IgG production follows. Immunoglobulin levels typically peak and then decline over several days.

The Secondary Immune Response

The secondary response follows repeated exposure to an antigen. Recognition again occurs immediately, but production of a detectable increase in serum immunoglobulins occurs much more rapidly (2-3 days) than that in the primary response. IgG is the principal immunoglobulin secreted during the secondary response. In addition, peak levels are higher and the decline occurs much more slowly than in the primary response.

Immunologic Memory

The mechanism underlying immunologic memory has not been satisfactorily explained. Following stimulation by antigen, lymphocyte proliferation (clonal

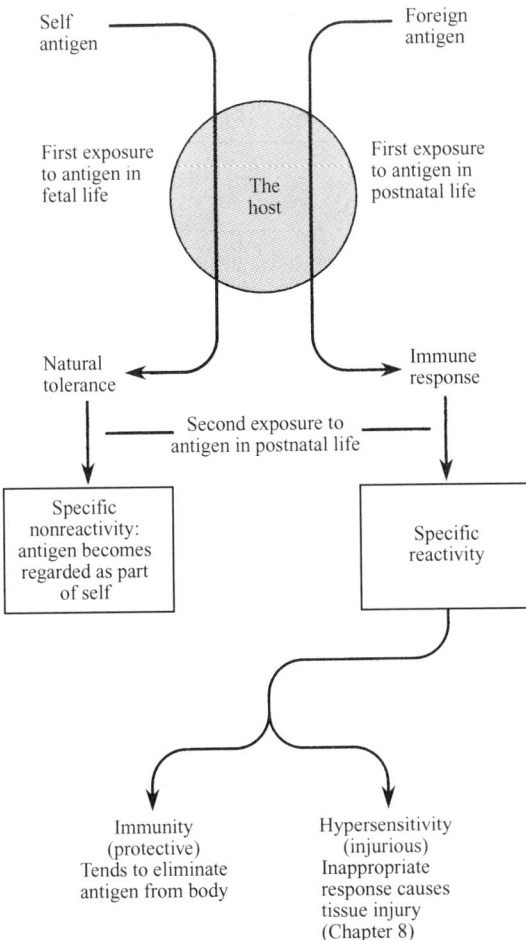

Figure 10-2 Antigens are molecules that induce an immune response in an appropriate recipient (host). From the point of view of an individual organism, antigens can be self (ie, part of the host's own tissues) or foreign. The developing fetal immune system usually encounters only self antigens, to which tolerance occurs. After birth, foreign antigens are encountered and the nature of the host response changes to an immune response (Figure 4-1) designed to neutralize and remove the antigen. Note that if a foreign antigen is presented in fetal life, natural tolerance may result. If a self antigen is hidden from the immune system in fetal life and first presented in postnatal life, an immune response may result. Tolerance, then, is an active decision by the immune system not to mount an immune response to a specific antigen (specific nonreactivity). By contrast, an immune response is an active decision that mobilizes the immune system into a complex response against that antigen (specific reactivity). This immune response usually is protective (immunity) but occasionally may be harmful to the host (hypersensitivity)

expansion) occurs that produces a large number of effector cells (plasma cells in the B cell system; cytotoxic T cell in the T cell system) as well as other small lymphocytes that reenter the cycle and serve to replenish the pool of cells bearing the appropriate receptor. It has been argued that because these cells are the product of antigen-induced proliferation, they are capable of an enhanced response if they encounter the antigen again (i.e. they act as memory cells). In the B cell family, these cells may also have undergone the switch from producing IgM to IgG, and that change may explain the immediate production of IgG during the secondary immune response.

IMMUNOLOGIC INJURY

AUTOIMMUNE DISEASES

Introduction

The immune system recognizes the body's own antigens as self antigens and does not react against them (natural tolerance). Autoimmune diseases occur when a breakdown of this natural tolerance leads to an immune response against a self antigen.

Table 10-1 Autoimmune diseases

Diseases	Autoantibodies[1]
Systemic multiorgan diseases	
Systemic lupus erythematosus	Antinuclear
	Anti-DNA(double-stranded)
	Anti-DNA(single-stranded)
	Anti-Sm
	Antiribonucleoprotein
	Others
Mixed connective tissue disease(MCTD)	Antinuclear
	Antiribonucleoprotein
Progressive systemic sclerosis	Antinuclear
	Anticentromere
Dermatomyositis	Antinuclear
	Antimyoglobin
Rheumatoid arthritis(and Sjögren's syndrome)	Anti-immunoglobulin(rheumatoid factor)
Restricted organ-specific diseases	
Myasthenia gravis	Anti-acetylcholine receptor
Hashimoto's thyroiditis	Antithyroglobulin
Graves'disease(toxic goiter)	Thyroid-stimulating immunoglobulin
Insulin-resistant diabetes mellitus	Anti-insulin receptor
Juvenile insulin-dependent diabetes mellitus	Anti-insulin
	Anti-islet cell
Goodpasture's syndrome	Anti-lung basement membrane
	Anti-glomerular basement membrane
Pernicious anemia	Anti-parietal cell
	Anti-intrinsic factor
Addison's disease	Anti-adrenal cell
Bullous pemphigoid	Anti-skin basement membrane
Pemphigus vulgaris	Anti-skin intercellular matrix
Hypoparathyroidism	Anti-parathyroid cell
Primary biliary cirrhosis	Antimitochondrial

Diseases	Autoantibodies[1]
Chronic active hepatitis	Antinuclear Antihepatocyte Anti-smooth muscle
Vitiligo	Antimelanocyte
Infertility(male)	Antispermatozoal
infertility(female)	Antiovarian(corpus luteum)
Hemolytic anemia	Antierythrocyte
Neutropenia	Antileukocyte
Thrombocytopenia	Antiplatelet

(Continued)

[1] The antibodies named are those typical of each disease state, and not all patients with the disease will demonstrate them. In addition, the presence of these various antibodies is not necessarily limited to a particular disease state(eg, antithyroglobulin antibody is present in Hashimoto's disease [90%], myxedema[70%], Graves'disease[40%], nontoxic goiter and thyroid cancer[30%], pernicious anemia [25%], and normal controls[5%-10%]).

Many diseases are believed to have a basis in autoimmunity(Table 10-1). The antigens involved may be on a specific cell type(organ-specific autoimmune disease) or may be universal cellular components such as nucleic acids and nucleoproteins (systemic, or non-organ-specific autoimmune disease). In some organ-specific autoimmune diseases, circulating antibodies against nonspecific cellular elements are also present (e.g. antimitochondrial antibodies in primary biliary cirrhosis). Some of these are of diagnostic value but do not necessarily play a significant role in the pathogenesis of the disease; formation of autoantibodies may simply reflect release of sequestered antigens as a result of some other type of injury (e.g. 30% of patients with myocardial infarction due to ischemia show circulating antibody to heart muscle after 6 weeks). In normal individuals, formation of such antibodies is suppressed after a few weeks.

Many autoimmune diseases show an increased familial incidence (e.g. systemic lupus erythematosus, Hashimoto's thyroiditis, pernicious anemia), and certain autoimmune diseases also seem to be associated with specific HLA antigens (e.g. HLA-D3 with systemic lupus erythematosus [Table 10-2]). Clarification of the critical role played by MHC class I and class II (HLA) molecules in the antigen recognition phase of the immune response offers a glimmer of understanding. The close spatial relationship of the different HLA genes on chromosome 6 may then help to explain the association of certain HLA types with abnormalities of the immune response.

Table 10-2 Selected HLA antigens and their association with autoimmune disease[1]

HLA Antigen	Associated Diseases
DR2	Multiple sclerosis, Goodpasture's syndrome
DR3	Celiac disease, myasthenia gravis, Graves' disease, systemic lupus erythematosus, insulin-dependent diabetes mellitus
DR4	Rheumatoid arthritis, pemphigus vulgaris, IgA nephropathy
DR5	Hashimoto's thyroiditis, pernicious anemia, juvenile rheumatoid arthritis
B27	Ankylosing spondylitis, Reiter's disease, uveitis

[1] The relative increased risk of disease in patients with the associated antigen variges: for ankylosing spondylitis and HLAB27 it is 90 times higher than in the general population. Expressed another way, among patients with ankylosing spondylitis, 80%-90% have HLA-B27, whereas in the general population 8% have this antigen.

The Mechanism of Autoimmune Diseases

A. Breakdown of Natural Tolerance

1. Immunologic tolerance to self antigens

Natural tolerance to an antigen results when the immune system is presented with that antigen during fetal life. Two principal hypotheses have been proposed to explain the mechanism of natural tolerance.

- Clonal Deletion Hypothesis: According to Burnet's clonal deletion hypothesis, the lymphocyte clones that have receptors for antigens encountered in fetal life (self antigens) are deleted in the deve-loping organism. Adults should therefore lack self-reactive clones. The subsequent development of autoimmunity is explained by the emergence of forbidden clones of lymphocytes that are reacting to self antigens, presumably the result of a new B or T cell gene rearrangement at the stem cell level.
- Specific Cell Suppression Hypothesis: The clonal deletion hypothesis is probably oversimplified because it has been shown that normal individuals do have lymphocytes with receptors for self antigens. These lymphocytes were obviously not deleted but nevertheless have been suppressed or in some way prevented from reacting. The activity of T suppressor cells and the presence of suppressor factors in blood have been proposed as possible mechanisms. The latter may include antibodies that either mask self antigens or, alternatively, bind to the antigen receptors of lymphocytes to preclude the recognition of self antigens. This idea is not too dissimilar from the concept of an anti-idiotype response, in which antibodies produced against immunoglobulin idiotypes serve to down-regulate antibody production.

2. Breakdown of natural tolerance(autoimmunity)

Autoimmunity represents a breakdown of natural tolerance and the subsequent occurrence of a specific humoral or cell-mediated response against the body's own antigens. Cellular injury in autoimmune diseases is caused by both humoral and cell-mediated hypersensitivity (types II, III, and IV). Several different mechanisms have been proposed (Table 10-3).

Table 10-3 Proposed mechanisms of autoimmune diseases

Proposed Mechanism	Antigens Involved in Pathogenesis	Reason for or Cause of Mechanism	Resulting Autoimmune Disease
1. Emergence of sequestered antigen	Thyroglobulin(?)	Antigen sequestered in thyroid follicle	Hashimoto's thyroiditis
	Lens protein	Antigen sequestered from bloodstream	Sympathetic ophthalmitis
	Spermatozoal antigens	Antigen developed in adult life	Infertility(male)
2. Alteration of self antigens	Drugs, viruses, other infections	Attachment of hapten, partial degradation	Hemolytic anemias, systemic lupus(?) erythematosus, rheumatic fever (?)
3. Loss of serum suppressor antibodies	Many types	B cell deficiency; congenital Bruton's agammaglobulinemia	Many types
4. Loss of suppressor T cell	Many types	T cell deficiency; postviral infection	Rare
5. Activation of suppressed lymphocyte clones	Epstein-Barr virus; other viruses(?)	B cell stimulation	Rheumatoid arthritis(?)
6. Emergence of forbidden clones	Many types	Neoplastic transformation of lymphocytes; malignant lymphoma and lymphocytic leukemias	Hemolytic anemia, thrombocytopenia
7. Cross-reactivity between self and foreign antigens	Antistreptococcal antibody and myocardial antigens	Antibody against foreign antigen reacts against self antigen	Rheumatic fever
8. Abnormal immune response genes(Ir genes)	Many types	Loss of control of the immune response due to lack of Ir genes	Many types[1]

[1] Immune response(Ir) genes are closely linked to HLA antigens. Those autoimmune diseases in which Ir gene abnormalities play a part are associated with an increased incidence of certain HLA types(Table10-2)

The mechanisms involved in producing cell injury in autoimmune diseases include types II, III, and IV hypersensitivity. Type II cytotoxic hypersensitivity is the mechanism responsible for many organ-specific diseases such as autoimmune hemolytic anemia and pemphigus vulgaris. Type II hypersensitivity is characterized by an specific antibody, commonly IgG and Ig M, which is produced against the antigen and interacts with it on the surface of cell and forms antigen-antibody that causes the destruction of that cell. In many of these organ-specific autoimmune diseases, type IV hypersensitivity also plays an important role – e. g. in Hashimoto's thyroiditis, T cell-mediated direct cytotoxicity is believed to be the dominant mechanism of cell damage even though antithyroid antibodies are present in the blood and probably contribute to cell necrosis by type II cytotoxic hypersensitivity.

Type III (immune complex) hypersensitivity is responsible for many of the multi-organ autoimmune diseases exemplified by systemic lupus erythematosus. Deposition of immune complexes at various sites in the body activates complement and causes acute inflammation and injury. These are characterized by systemic necrotizing vasculitis.

B. Genetic Factors

Autoimmune Diseases are involved with genetic factors. There are some evidences. Familial clustering can be seen in some human autoimmune diseases such as SLE. Some of autoimmune diseases link with HLA, especially class II antigen. For example, SLE links with HLA DR2 and DR3.

C. Microbial Agents

A variety of microbes, such as bacteria, mycoplasmas and viruses, involve in autoimmune diseases. There are several ways for triggering autoimmune reactions. Some microbes make the structures of antigenic determinant change or share cross-reacting epitopes with self-antigens. So bypassing T-cell tolerance, viruses such as EBV and bacterial products may activate nonspecific polyclonal B cell and thus induce product autoantibodies. Some microbes may result in loss of suppressor T cell function.

Types of Autoimmune Diseases

A. Lupus Erythematosus

Lupus erythematosus is a connective tissue disease that exists in two clinical forms: (1) systemic lupus erythematosus (SLE), which is a progressive and often severe condition involving multiple systems; and (2) discoid lupus erythematosus, in which skin involvement dominates the clinical picture, usually without systemic disease.

1. Incidence

SLE is common in the United States, more so in nonwhites (particularly blacks) than whites. The disease is also common in Western Europe but less so in Asia. Women are affected ten times more frequently than men. The usual age at onset of disease is 20 – 40 years.

2. Etiology and pathogenesis

The cause of lupus erythematosus is unknown (Figure 10-3). There is little doubt that it is mediated by an abnormal immune response associated with the presence of a variety of antibodies and immune complexes in the plasma that are responsible for the pathologic effects seen in lupus erythematosus. The cause of this response is widely believed to be autoimmune, although there is evidence for viral and genetic influences.

a. Autoimmune origin

• Antinuclear antibodies: There is considerable evidence that SLE is a type of autohypersensitivity (autoimmune) disease. The formation of antinuclear antibodies (ANA) is important in pathogenesis. A variety of antinuclear antibodies are present in the serum of all patients with systemic lupus erythematosus and are tested for and characterized by immunologic techniques (Table 10-4). The presence of antibody against double-stranded DNA is highly specific for lupus erythematosus, while antibodies against single-stranded DNA, RNA, and nucleoproteins are also found in other connective tissue diseases.

• Immune complexes: Immune complexes formed between antinuclear antibodies and nuclear antigens are detectable in the serum and at sites of disease activity in the walls of small blood vessels, the skin, and glomerular basement membrane. Deposition of immune complexes in the tissue (Figure 10-3) activates complement and leads to inflammation by a type III hypersensitivity reaction. Serum complement levels are frequently reduced in the active phase of SLE.

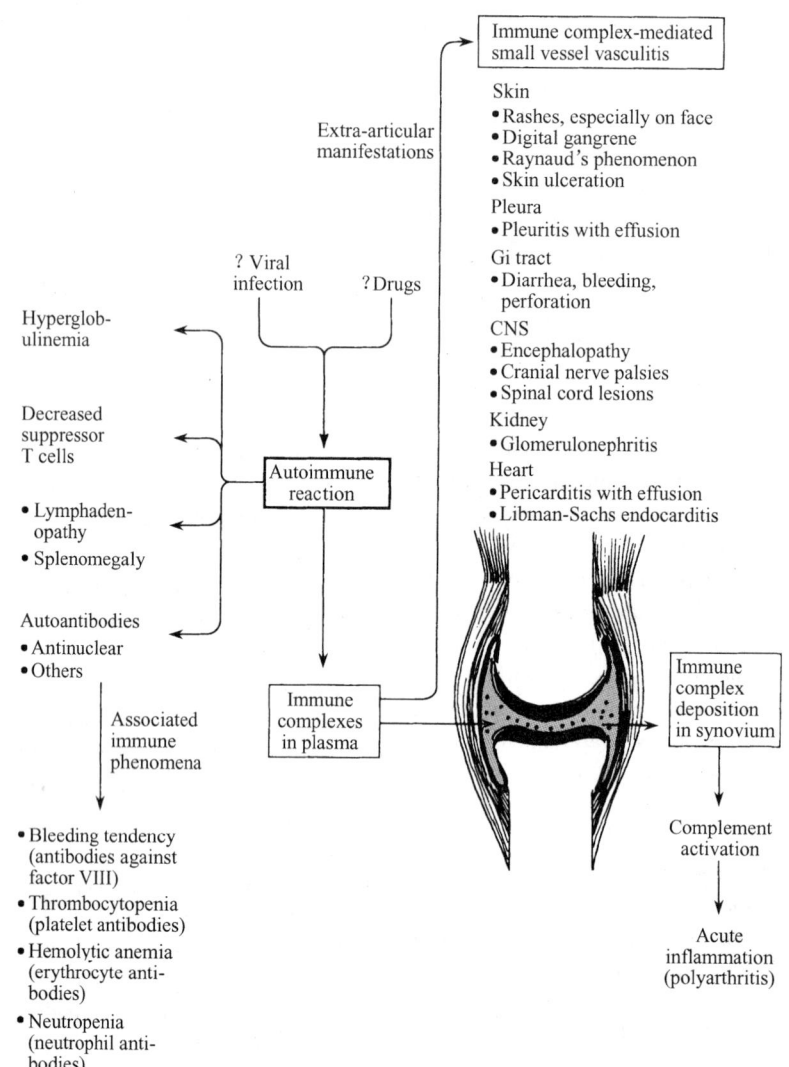

Figure 10-3 Etiologic factors and pathogenesis of systemic lupus erythematosus

Table 10-4 Antibodies in systemic lupus erythematosus (SLE) and other autoimmune connective tissue diseases

Antibody	Incidence	Antigen	Clinical Significance
Antinuclear antibodies[1]			
Anti-DNA	70%	DNA	Anti-double-stranded DNA is specific for SLE; anti-single stranded DNA is not specific
Anti-Sm	30%	Ribonucleoprotein (Smith Ag)	Specific for SLE
Anti-RNP	40%	Ribonucleoprotein	High titer in mixed connective tissue disease
Anti-histone	70%	Histones	Positive in 95% of cases of drug-induced SLE
Anti-Ro (SS-A)	30%	Ribonucleoprotein	Associated with Sjögren's syndrome and nephritis
Anti-La (SS-B)	10%	Ribonucleoprotein	Associated with Sjögren's syndrome

Antibody	Incidence	Antigen	Clinical Significance
Anti-centromere	<5%	Centromere	Associated with CREST syndrome
Anti-Sci 70	<5%	DNA topoisomerase	Associated with systemic sclerosis
Anti-Jo 1	<5%	tRNA synthetase	Associated with polymyositis
Other antibodies			
Anticardiolipin	50%	Phospholipid	Associated with thrombosis, spontaneous abortion; lupus anticoagulant; false-positive VDRL
Antierythrocyte	60%	RBC surface Ag	Hemolysis (rare)
Antiplatelet	?	Platelet surface Ag	Thrombocytopenia
Antilymphocyte	70%	Lymph surface Ag	(?) T cell dysfunction
Antineuronal	60%	Neuron surface Ag	(?) Central nervous system lupus

[1] Negative test for antinuclear antibodies makes diagnosis of SLE very unlikely because it is positive in 95% of patients.

- Numerous autoantibodies other than antinuclear antibodies are also found in SLE. These include (1) rheumatoid factor (20%–30%); (2) antibodies that give a false-positive reaction in serologic tests for syphilis; (3) antibodies against plasma coagulation proteins, most commonly factor VIII, producing bleeding diathesis; and (4) antibodies against antigens on erythrocytes, leukocytes, and platelets, which may lead to immune destruction of these cells in the peripheral circulation.

b. Genetic factors

Genetic predisposition to SLE has been suggested because of the high concordance of clinical SLE in monozygotic twins and the increased frequency of the disease in first-degree relatives. HLA-DR2 is more common in SLE, leading to the suggestion that the presence of the corresponding immune response gene may predispose to the development of autoreactivity against nuclear antigens. The occurrence of SLE in patients with inherited deficiency of early complement factors (C1, C2, and C4) is also of interest because the genes for C2 and C4 are known to be closely linked to the HLA-DR region.

c. Others

SLE is known to be precipitated by drugs such as hydralazine (an antihypertensive) and procainamide (used to control cardiac arrhythmias). Drug-induced disease may be similar to idiopathic SLE, including the presence of antinuclear antibodies, but renal disease is rare. Withdrawal of the drug often causes reversal of the disease and gradual disappearance of the antinuclear antibodies. Infectious agents-mainly viruses-have been suggested as causing lupus erythematosus, but no infectious agent has been isolated consistently from patients' tissues. Sex hormone and UV have also been suggested as causes.

The tissue injury of viscera is mainly mediated by immune complexes (type III hypersensitivity), especially the deposition of DNA-anti-DNA complex in small blood vessel walls and near the glomerular basement membrane. Specific anti-red cells, anti-white cells and platelets antibody damage hemocytes mediated by type II hypersensitivity. Antinuclear antibodies are not cytotoxic, but can react with nuclei of damaged cells and make the cells become homogeneous to produce so-called LE (lupus erythematosus) bodies or hematoxylin bodies. It is valuable to SLE diagnosis. Neutrophils or macrophages having engulfed the LE bodies are called LE (lupus erythematosus) cells.

3. Pathology and clinical feature

Pathologic and clinical features of the disease are dependent on which antibodies and immune complexes are present and what their target tissues are. Sites of immune complex deposition show evidence of complement-mediated tissue necrosis and acute inflammation. The presenting features are quite diverse (Table 10-5).

Table 10-5 Clinical features of systemic lupus erythematosus (SLE)

	Presenting Feature[1] (%)	Prevalence (%)
Arthritis	50	90
Skin rashes	25	70
Fever[2]	20	80
Pleurisy or pericarditis	10	25
Renal disease[3]	5	65
Neurologic symptoms	5	25
Raynaud's phenomenon	2	10
Others: lymphadenopathy, malaise, weakness, weight loss, anemia, thrombocytopenia, neutropenia		

[1] Note that in many patients, more than one of these features are present, eg, skin rash and arthritis.

[2] Fever is the only feature at presentation in 20% of patients. It is present in a larger number of cases in association with other features.

[3] Although not the most common presenting feature renal disease occurs later and is the most common direct cause of death in SLE.

- Small vessel vasculitis: immune complex injury of arterioles is typical, with fibrinoid necrosis of the media and infiltration of the wall and perivascular tissue by neutrophils, lymphocytes, and plasma cells. Thrombosis is common and may lead to ischemia and tissue necrosis. In the skin, there may be digital gangrene and ulceration; and in the gastrointestinal tract, diarrhea, bleeding, intestinal obstruction, and perforation. These vascular changes progress to intimal fibrosis, with a characteristic laminated (onion skin) appearance.
- Hyperplasia of the lymphoid system: Enlargement of lymph nodes or spleen occurs in 50% of patients with SLE. This is due to nonspecific follicular and paracortical lymphocytic proliferation.
- Skin: Immune complex deposition occurs in the basement membrane of the skin, where it can be perceived as lumpy deposits by electron microscopic and immunologic techniques. The resulting complement activation and inflammation lead to a skin rash, typically over the malar regions of the face (butterfly rash). Skin biopsy of lesions shows epidermal atrophy, hyperkeratosis, vacuolar degeneration of the basal layer, and a patchy dermal perivascular lymphocytic infiltrate. Skin rash occurs some time in the course of the disease in 70% of cases.

In patients with discoid lupus erythematosus, the skin lesion is the sole abnormality. In discoid lupus, immune complex deposition is restricted to the area of the rash; in systemic lupus, immune complex deposition is widespread even in clinically normal skin.

- Joints: Joint inflammation (arthritis) or pain (arthralgia) occurs in 90% of patients with SLE. Both large and small joints may be involved, and initial involvement may resemble rheumatoid arthritis. Joint involvement in SLE is usually mild.
- Heart: The heart is involved in 10%–20% of cases of SLE. The immune complex-mediated injury may involve any layer of the heart. Cardiac lesions in patients with systemic lupus erythematosus include pericarditis which is fibrinous with effusion, myocarditis, and Libman-Sachs endocarditis. These complications are usually not serious.

Libman-Sachs endocarditis: It is the most characteristic cardiac lesion of SLE. It is characterized by nonbacterial verucous endcarditis. Multiple, small, flat vegetations occur on the mitral and tricuspid valves. Both chordae tendineae, and the mural endocardium are involved. SLE valvulitis is rarely severe enough to cause valve dysfunction.

- Nervous System: Clinical manifestations due to central nervous system vasculitis and ischemia occur in 25% of patients. Convulsions, mental disorders (emotional lability, dementia, psychosis), cranial nerve palsies, and spinal cord dysfunction may result. The cerebrospinal fluid in such patients often shows moderately increased protein levels and a mild increase in lymphocytes.
- Kidneys: Renal involvement occurs in approximately two thirds of patients and represents the most common mode of death in SLE. Clinical manifestations include proteinuria, microscopic hematuria, nephrotic syndrome, acute nephritic syndrome, and renal failure. During the phase of active disease, serum complement levels are decreased.

Renal lesions are due to immune complex deposition.

Light microscopy shows a variety of changes (Table 10-6). Focal and diffuse proliferation of capillary endothelial cells is the most serious microscopic abnormality. Mesangial hypercellularity is more common but less ominous. Diffuse or segmental basement membrane thickening produces the typical wire loop lesions (Figure 10-4) of SLE. Small, ill-defined basophilic bodies (hematoxyphil bodies) may rarely be found in areas of glomerular damage and are specific for SLE. Immunofluorescence shows lumpy IgG and C3 in the glomerular basement membrane and mesangium. Electron microscopy shows large immune complexes in the subendothelial, mesangial, and subepithelial regions. Wire loop lesions correspond with the presence of large subendothelial deposition of immune complexes and can be distinguished from membranous glomerulonephritis of SLE, in which there are subepithelial deposits.

Table 10-6 World Health Organization categories of glomerular disease in systemic lupus erythematosus

Class	Pathologic Change	% With Glomerulonephritis	Clinical Features
I	No change		Mild disease with microscopic hematuria or proteinuria; slow progression
II	Mesangial glomerulonephritis	10%	
III	Focal proliferative glomerulonephritis	30%	Severe disease with rapid progression to renal failure
IV	Diffuse proliferative glomerulonephritis	50%	
V	Diffuse membranous glomerulonephritis	10%	Nephrotic syndrome; slow progression to renal failure

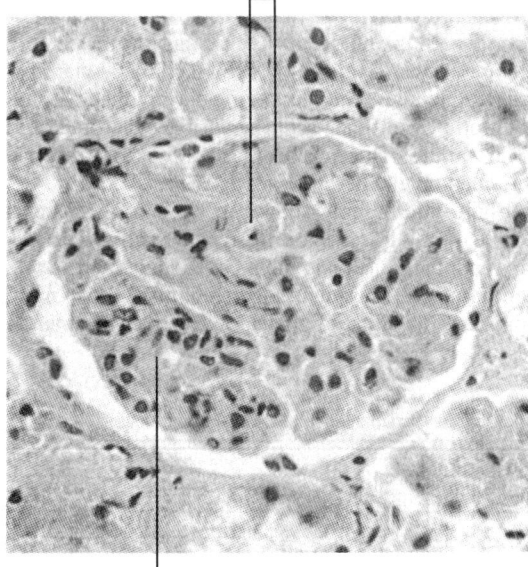

Figure 10-4 Systemic lupus erythematosus, showing focal mesangial cell proliferation and diffuse thickening of basement membrane

The clinical features and prognosis depend on the histologic class of disease (Table 10-6). Eventually, many patients with SLE glomerular disease progress to chronic renal failure.

4. Diagnosis

The diagnosis of lupus erythematosus is based on its clinical features and confirmed by demonstration of serum antinuclear antibodies (ANA), particularly anti-double-stranded DNA. The absence of ANA virtually rules out a diagnosis of SLE because less than 5% of patients with SLE are ANA-negative (Table 10-4). Histologic examination of tissues such as the skin and kidney does not provide specific evidence of the disease but in combination with clinical features often leads to the diagnosis.

5. Course and prognosis

The course of SLE is variable. Rarely, patients have a severe acute illness that is refractory to treatment. Most patients pursue a chronic course, with repeated exacerbations and remissions. Corticosteroid therapy is usually effective in controlling exacerbations, and with such therapy the survival rate is approximately 90% at 10 years.

Most deaths are due to renal failure followed by central nervous system disease. The complications of immunosuppressive drug therapy also account for significant morbidity and many deaths.

Patients with discoid lupus erythematosus have a chronic skin disorder. There is little danger of death unless systemic symptoms supervene (about 10% of patients develop SLE).

B. Rheumatoid Arthritis

Rheumatoid Arthritis is a chronic disease of unknown cause characterized by progressive and potentially deforming arthritis.

1. Incidence

Rheumatoid arthritis is common in the United States and Western Europe, affecting 1%–2% of the population. Females are affected three to five times more frequently than males. The highest age incidence is between 25 and 55 years. Rheumatoid arthritis is less common in tropical countries.

2. Etiology and pathogenesis

The exact cause of rheumatoid arthritis is unknown (Figure 10-5). A genetic predisposition is suggested by an increased incidence in families, a 30% concordance rate in identical twins compared with 5% in fraternal twins, and an association with HLA-DR4 in affected white patients. Rheumatoid factor-an autoantibody (usually IgG) - is present in the plasma of about 90% of patients with rheumatoid arthritis, but its presence is not specific for the disorder because it is present in other autoimmune diseases and in 5% of healthy persons. Immune complexes composed of rheumatoid factor and IgG have been found in the synovial fluid of some patients with rheumatoid arthritis. Complement levels are also frequently decreased in active disease, suggesting that complement activation by deposited immune complexes may play a role.

3. Pathology

a. Articular manifestations: Rheumatoid arthritis typically presents with symmetric involvement of the small joints of the hands and feet, classically, the proximal interphalangeal joints (Figure 10-6). Involvement of larger joints is the initial manifestation in a minority of patients.

The synovial membrane of affected joints becomes swollen, congested, and thickened due to vasodilation and hyperplasia of lining synovial cells. This is followed by proliferation of granulation tissue containing numerous lymphocytes and plasma cells (this fleshy tissue is termed pannus). T helper lymphocytes represent the dominant cell type. Local production of interleukins, tumor necrosis factor, and other cytokines accounts for many features of synovi-

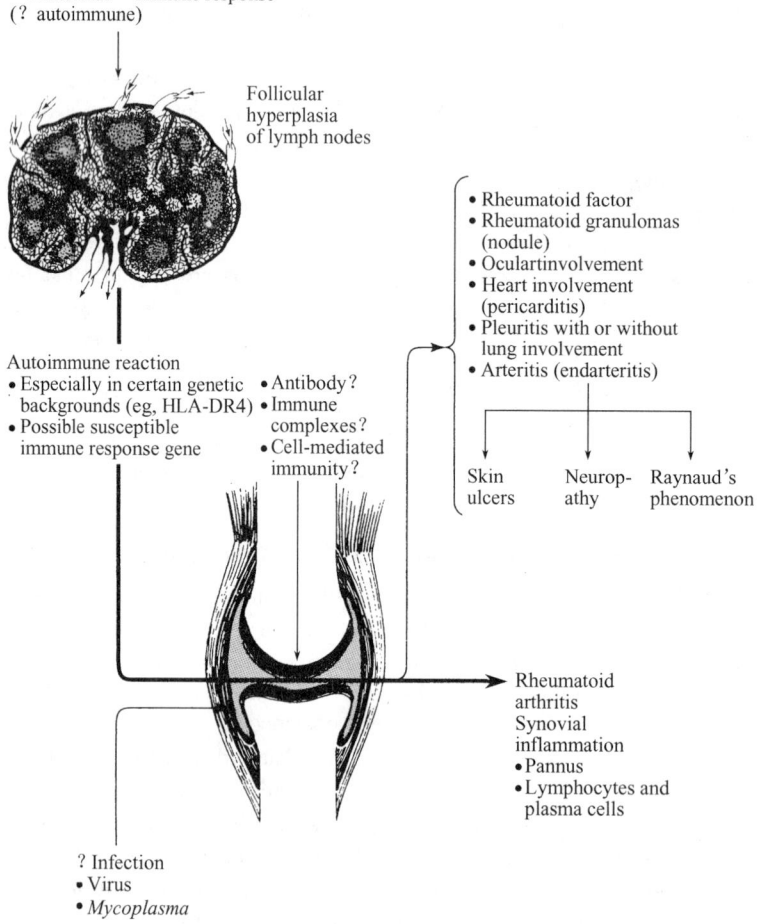

Figure 10-5 Proposed etiologic factors and pathologic effects of rheumatoid arthritis

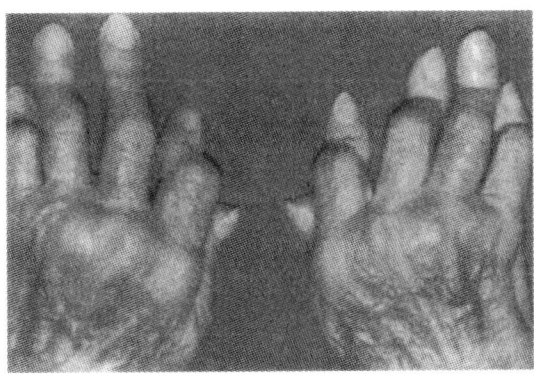

Figure 10-6 Rheumatoid arthritis (chronic phase, severe disease), showing symmetric involvement and severe deformity. Note dominant involvement of the proximal interphalangeal joints

tis. Neutrophils are scarce in the synovial tissue but abundant in synovial fluid.

The pannus eventually erodes articular cartilage, subchondral bone, and periarticular ligaments and tendons. Progressive destruction of the joint follows, with fibrosis, increasing deformity, and restriction of movement. The mechanism of destruction of cartilage and bone is not known but is probably related to synthesis of collagenase and other proteases in the pannus.

b. Extra-articular manifestations: Rheumatoid arthritis is a systemic disorder. In a minority of patients, tissues other than joints show significant pathologic change (Table 10-7). Subcutaneous rheumatoid nodules are granulomas 1-2 cm in diameter seen commonly around the elbow, usually in patients with severe disease. They are characterized microscopically by an area of fibrinoid necrosis of collagen surrounded by palisading histiocytes (Figure 10-7).

Table 10-7 Rheumatoid arthritis: Systemic manifestations and laboratory findings

Systemic Manifestations	Description
Pyrexia, malaise	Interleukin-1, tumor necrosis factor
Rheumatoid nodules	Subcutaneous granulomas with a central area of fibrinoid necrosis of connective tissue; tender 1-to 2-cm nodules at elbow and wrist particularly (see Figure 10-7)
Vasculitis	Particularly endarteritis; may lead to skin ulcers (ischemia), Raynaud's phenomenon, and peripheral neuropathy
Cardiac lesions	The myocardium is rarely involved (arrhythmias); pericarditis occurs in 10%
Lung lesions	Pleuritis, pleural effusions; large necrotizing rheumatoid nodules in lung; diffuse pulmonary fibrosis; nodular fibrosis of lung (in miners exposed to coal duat: Caplan's syndrome)
Neurologic lesions	Peripheral neuropathy (due to arteritis); mononeuropathy due to spinal nerve compression; carpal tunnel syndrome (median nerve compression); cervical cord compression (atlantoaxial joint involvement)
Ocular lesions	Keratitis, scleritis, granulomas, uveitis (iris inflamed); rare
Amyloidosis	Primary pattern of distribution
Lymphadenopathy, splenomegaly	In up to 25% of cases, especially in juvenile form (Still's disease) and Felty's syndrome
Laboratory findings Positive rheumatoid factor (90% of classic adult cases but <20% of childhood cases) Leukocytosis common (leukopenia in Felty's syndrome) Raised erythrocyte sedimentation rate Polyclonal hypergammaglobulinemia (in 50%) Positive ANA (antinuclear antibody), usually in low titer (10%-40%)	

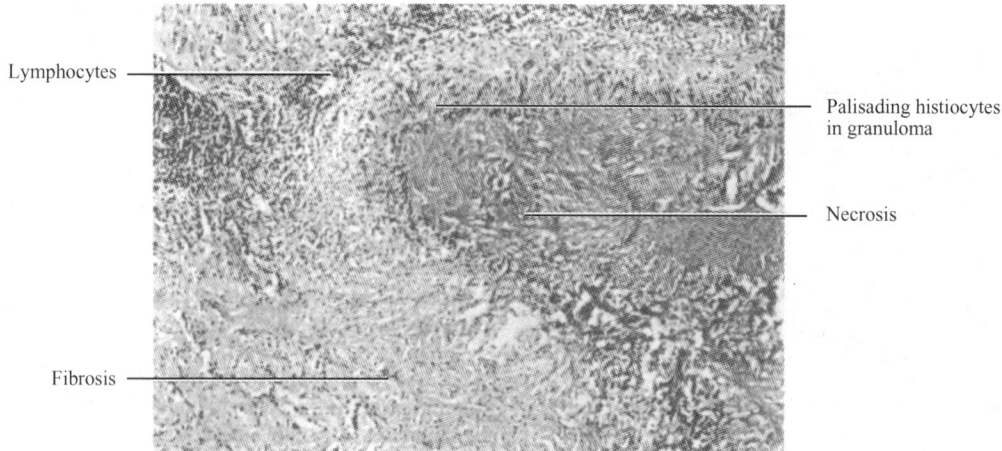

Figure 10-7 Subcutaneous rheumatoid nodule, showing a central area of necrosis of collagen surrounded by palisading histiocytes

4. Clinical features

Involved joints are swollen, painful, and stiff. Stiffness is maximal in the morning after the joint has been inactive during the night. The swollen joints are warm and tender, and movement is restricted. Swelling of the proximal interphalangeal joints of the fingers produces a typical spindled appearance of the fingers. Many patients have systemic symptoms such as tow-grade fever, weakness, and malaise.

Joint deformity occurs early in severe cases. Restriction of movement may cause rapid disuse atrophy of muscles around the joint.

5. Course and prognosis

Rheumatoid arthritis is usually slowly progressive. In 10%–20% of patients, the disease remits completely after the first attack. Most other patients develop a chronic disease characterized by relapses and remissions, with slowly progressive disability from joint destruction. After 10 years of disease, about 10% of patients are severely disabled while about 50% are still fully employed.

Poor prognostic factors include a classic pattern of disease with high levels of rheumatoid factor in the serum, the presence of rheumatoid nodules, and onset of disease before age 30 years. In such patients, progress may be rapid.

6. Variants of rheumatoid arthritis

• Felty's syndrome: Felty's syndrome occurs in older individuals with long-standing rheumatoid arthritis and high titers of rheumatoid factor. It is characterized by splenic enlargement and neutropenia. Anemia and thrombocytopenia may also occur.

• Juvenile rheumatoid arthritis (Still's disease): Still's disease is rheumatoid arthritis in a patient under 16 years of age. It is characterized by acute onset with high fever, leukocytosis, splenomegaly, arthritis, and skin rash. There may also be pericarditis and inflammation of the iris (uveitis). Rheumatoid factor is usually not present.

Patients with Still's disease commonly have monarticular involvement, frequently of a large joint. Growth abnormalities may occur if the disease strikes before the age of epiphysial closure.

Fifty percent of patients with Still's disease undergo complete remission. Others progress to severe joint disease with extra-articular manifestations.

C. Sjögren's Syndrome

Sjögren's syndrome is an autoimmune disease in which there is immune-mediated destruction of the lacrimal and salivary glands. It is manifested clinically as dry eyes (keratoconjunctivitis sicca) and dry mouth (xerostomia) due to failure of gland secretion. It is commonly associated with other autoimmune diseases, notably rheumatoid arthritis. Patients with Sjögren's syndrome have an increased incidence of malignant lymphomas in the salivary gland.

About 75% of patients have rheumatoid factor in the blood, and 70% have antinuclear antibodies. Specific autoantibodies directed against ribonucleoproteins designated anti-Ro (SS-A) and anti-La (SS-B) have been identified in the serum of 60% of patients with Sjögren's syndrome.

Histologically, the lacrimal and salivary glands show marked lymphocytic and plasma cell infiltration with destruction of the glandular epithelium and fibrosis.

The diagnosis can be made by clinical tests to demonstrate absence of secretion of tears and by lip biopsy, which shows the typical histologic changes in the mucus glands of the lip (Figure 10-8).

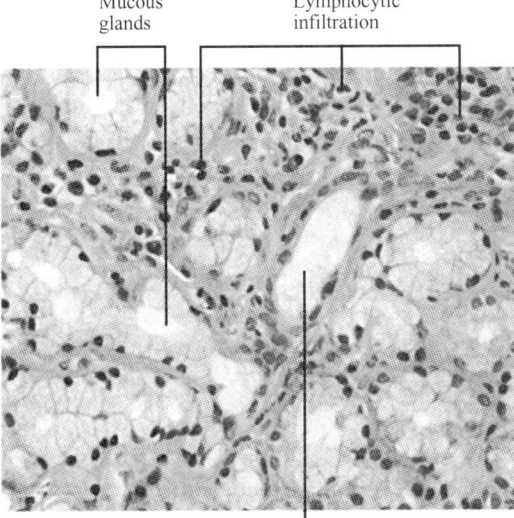

Figure 10-8 Lip biopsy in Sjögren's syndrome, showing infiltration by lymphocytes and plasma cells of minor salivary glands

D. Polymyositis-Dermatomyositis

Polymyositis-dermatomyositis is an uncommon connective tissue disease affecting women twice as frequently as men. Onset of disease is maximal between the ages of 40 and 60 years.

The cause is unknown. An immunologic basis is likely, although the exact mechanism is not clear. Antinuclear antibodies occur in the serum of most patients, and immune complex deposition with complement activation can be demonstrated in many cases of dermatomyositis. Cell-mediated autohypersensitivity has also been implicated.

Patients with polymyositis-dermatomyositis -particularly those over 60 years of age-are at increased risk for malignant neoplasms. Carcinoma of the lung is the most common, but carcinoma of the breast, kidney, stomach, and uterus also occur. The incidence of cancer in patients with dermatomyositis is around 8%.

The basis of the relationship between polymyositis-dermatomyositis and malignant neoplasms is unknown.

1. Pathology and clinical features

Polymyositis-dermatomyositis is a chronic disease that affects skeletal muscle in all cases and skin in 50% of cases. Visceral involvement is uncommon.
- Myositis: Skeletal muscle is involved in all cases. The proximal muscles of the limb girdles are commonly the first affected, with involvement of pharyngeal and respiratory muscles in severe cases.

In the acute phase, affected muscles show edema, lymphocytic infiltration, myofibrillary necrosis, and phagocytosis of dead muscle. This is followed by muscle atrophy and fibrosis. Clinically, there is muscle weakness associated with pain and tenderness, with the latter feature useful in distinguishing polymyositis from muscular dystrophies. During the acute phase, serum creatine kinase and aldolase levels are greatly elevated, and creatinuria may be present when there is severe muscle necrosis.

Muscle biopsy, demonstrating inflammatory changes, permits distinction from muscular dystrophy and other causes of myositis.
- Skin changes: (50% of cases) Skin changes are caused by vasculitis and typically take the form of a violaceous edematous rash (heliotrope rash) involving the upper eyelids, sometimes extending to the malar region of the face and neck. Dermal atrophy and calcification occur in the later stages. In 30% of patients, skin changes are associated with Raynaud's phenomenon.

2. Course

Polymyositis-dermatomyositis has a chronic course characterized by increasing disability from muscle wasting. The main danger of the disease is from the associated malignant neoplasms.

E. Scleroderma (Progressive Systemic Sclerosis)

Scleroderma (called progressive systemic sclerosis) is an uncommon connective tissue disease characterized by vasculitis affecting small vessels and widespread deposition of collagen. The tissue damage not only involves to skin, but also to multiple viscera. So it is usually called progressive systemic sclerosis now.

Progressive systemic sclerosis occurs more commonly in females and has its onset most frequently in the ages from 20 to 50 years.

1. Etiology

Progressive systemic sclerosis is probably an autoimmune disorder and is closely related to SLE. Antinuclear antibodies are usually present in the serum. The most characteristic antinuclear antibody for progressive systemic sclerosis has specificity against nucleolar RNA. Deposition of immune complexes in tissues has been demonstrated in renal and vascular lesions.

The mechanism underlying the excessive fibrosis is unknown.

2. Pathology and clinical features

The pathologic changes in affected tissue include vasculitis, which is identical histologically with that seen in systemic lupus erythematosus ; it tends to be more chronic . Marked fibrosis dominates the histologic appearance.

Progressive systemic sclerosis usually has an insidious onset. Systemic symptoms are uncommon. In many patients, the disease is restricted to the skin for many years before visceral involvement occurs.

- Skin: (Affected in 90% of cases.) The skin of the fingers and face is the most common first site of disease. Initially, the skin is edematous, with vasculitis and often petechial hemorrhages. Progressive fibrosis follows, involving the entire dermis and extending to the subcutaneous tissue. The epidermis becomes thin, and all adnexal structures (hair, sweat glands, etc) undergo atrophy. Enlarged vessels are frequently present and visible as telangiectases. Trophic ulceration of the skin is common, and dystrophic calcification may occur.

Severe skin changes lead to claw-like contracted hands and restriction of facial movements (Figure10-9).

- Gastrointestinal Tract: (60% of cases.) The entire gastrointestinal tract may be affected, with the esophagus and small intestine showing maximal disease. Dysphagia, deficient peristalsis, and matabsorption follow. CREST syndrome is a variant of progressive systemic sclerosis consisting of calcinosis, Raynaud's phenomenon, esophageal dysmotility, sclerodactyly (involvement of the fingers), and telangiectasia. An autoantibody to centromeres is commonly present.

- Kidneys: (60% of cases.) Glomerular changes result from immune complex deposition and include basement membrane thickening and mesangial hypercellularity. Small arterioles in the kidney freq-

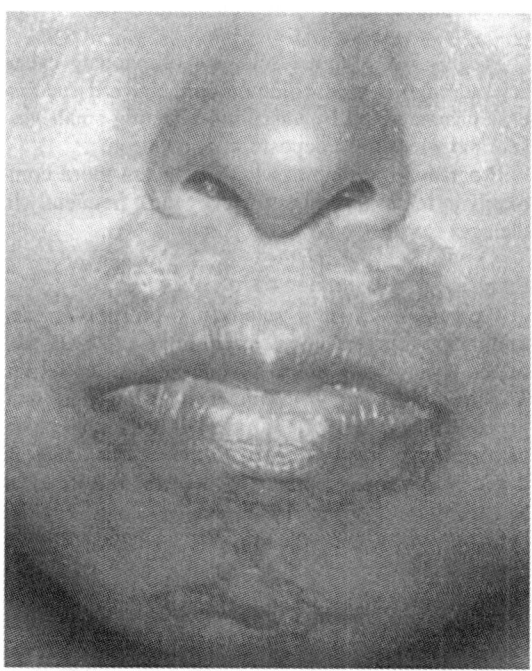

Figure 10-9 Progressive systemic sclerosis, showing scarring and stretching of the skin of the upper lip. Numerous small telangiectatic vessels are also present

uently show intimal fibrosis, leading to glomerular ischemia, decreased glomerular filtration rate, and renal failure.

- Lungs: (20% of cases.) Pulmonary involvement in progressive systemic sclerosis takes the form of a diffuse interstitial pneumonitis and fibrosis identical to that seen in idiopathic pulmonary fibrosis. The end stage is a honeycomb lung with respiratory failure.

3. Course

The clinical course is usually chronic. The occurrence of symptomatic visceral disease (especially renal disease) is an ominous sign. Treatment with immunosuppressive drugs is of limited value.

TRANSPLANT REJECTION

Introduction

The frequency of tissue (organ) transplantation has increased dramatically in clinical practice since the early 1970s. Corneal, skin, and bone grafts are routinely performed. Renal transplantation is performed with a high success rate in most large medical centers. Heart, lung, liver, and bone marrow transplants are being performed more often and with increasing success.

The only absolute limitations upon tissue transplantation are the immunologic reactions against the transplanted cells and the availability of appropriate donor organs. Autografting-transplantation of the host's own tissues as autologous grafts from one part of the body to another (e. g. skin, bone, venous grafts)-does not cause immunologic rejection reactions (Figure 10-10). Exchange of tissue between genetically identical (monozygotic) twins (isografts) does not evoke an immune response because the tissue is perceived as self.

Before an immune response can occur, antigens must be exposed to the immune cells in the circulation. Certain avascular grafts (e. g. corneal) can thus be performed between different individuals without immunologic rejection because the absence of a blood circulation prevents immune cells from reaching the graft.

Autograft
(autologous graft)
self to self, accepted

Isograft
Identical twin to twin,
accepted

Allograft
Person to person
(not identical twins),
variable degree of rejection

Xenograft
(heterologous graft)
species to species,
strong rejection

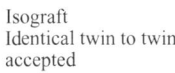
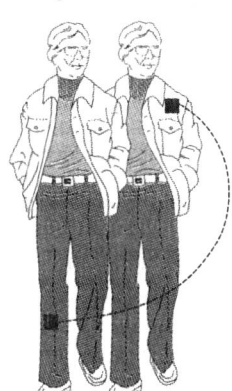
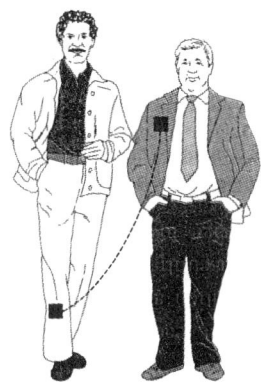
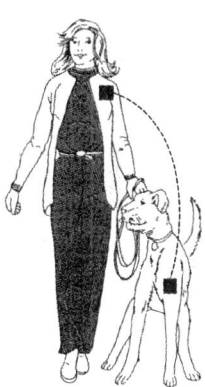

Figure 10-10 Different types of tissue transplants (grafts)

Transplantation of tissue between genetically dissimilar hosts evokes an immunologic response that may lead to rejection; the severity of the rejection reaction increases as the genetic differences between host and recipient increase. Currently, almost all organ transplants performed in humans use organs derived from humans. A transplant between genetically dissimilar members of the same species is called an allograft (allotransplant). Xenografts (heterologous grafts) are transplants obtained from a species different from the recipient (e. g. experimental baboon transplants done on an emergency basis); such grafts evoke a severe immunologic reaction and are almost never used.

Mechanisms of Transplant Rejection(Table 10-8)

A. Host Versus Graft Reaction (HVGR)

Host immunologic reactivity against transplanted cells may be directed against many antigens on the surface membrane of cells. These are called host versus graft reaction (HVGR). These include antigens on erythrocytes, antigens on the surface of nucleated cells. Human leukocyte antigen (HLA) is the most important antigen in transplant rejection.

The antigens of the HLA (human leukocyte antigen) complex are histocompatibility antigens (i. e. genetically determined isoantigens that elicit an immune response when grafted onto the tissues of an individual with a different genetic makeup). In humans, the major histocompatibility complex (MHC) are divided into three class: Ⅰ, Ⅱ and Ⅲ.

Class Ⅰ molecules includes HLA-A, HLA-B, and HLA-C. Class Ⅰ antigens, although first recognized on leukocytes (hence the term HLA), are expressed on almost all tissues. Class Ⅰ molecules play a critical role in antigen recognition by cytotoxic T cell.

Class Ⅱ includes HLA-DR, HLA-DP, and HLA-DO. Class Ⅱ antigens have a restricted tissue distribution, principally on B cell, macrophages, antigen-

Table 10-8 Immunologic mechanisms involved in transplant rejection

Active Immunologic Factor in Recipient	Type of Hypersensitivity	Target Sites in Transplant	Pathologic Effect	Type of Clinical Rejection
Preformed antibody against donor transplantation antigens	Type II cytotoxic	Small blood vessels in donor tissue	Fibrinoid necrosis and thrombosis of small vessels; ischemic necrosis of parenchymal cells	Hyperacute rejection
	Type III immune complex formation (local, Arthus-type)			
Circulating antibody formed due to humoral immune response against donor transplantation antigens	Type II cytotoxic	Parenchymal cells	Acute necrosis of parenchymal cells	Acute rejection
	Type III immune complex formation (local, Arthus-type)	Small blood vessels	Fibrinoid necrosis and thrombosis in acute phase; intimal fibrosis and narrowing in chronic phase	Acute rejection, chronic rejection
Activated T cell elicited by cellular immune response against donor transplantation antigens	Type IV	Parenchymal cells	Progressive, slow loss of parenchymal cells	Chronic rejection

processing cells, and activated T cell; they participate in antigen recognition by CD4 (helper) T cell.

Both humoral and cell-mediated mechanisms play a role in transplant rejection. Although transplant rejection is sometimes considered a hypersensitivity phenomenon because cell injury occurs, it is actually a normal immune response that constitutes an appropriate reaction to foreign antigens.

1. Humoral mechanisms

Humoral mechanisms are mediated by antibodies that may be present in the recipient's serum before transplantation or may develop after the foreign tissue is transplanted. Preoperative testing for preformed antibody against transplanted cells is accomplished by the direct tissue cross-match, which involves an in vitro reaction between donor cells (blood lymphocytes) and recipient serum. Humoral factors injure transplanted tissue through reactions that are equivalent to type II and III hypersensitivity reactions. Antibody-antigen interaction on the surface of transplanted cells result in cell necrosis, and immune complex deposition in blood vessels activates complement, producing acute necrotizing vasculitis (Figure 10-11) or chronic intimal fibrosis with narrowing of the vessels. Immunoglobulin and complement in these lesions can be detected by immunologic techniques.

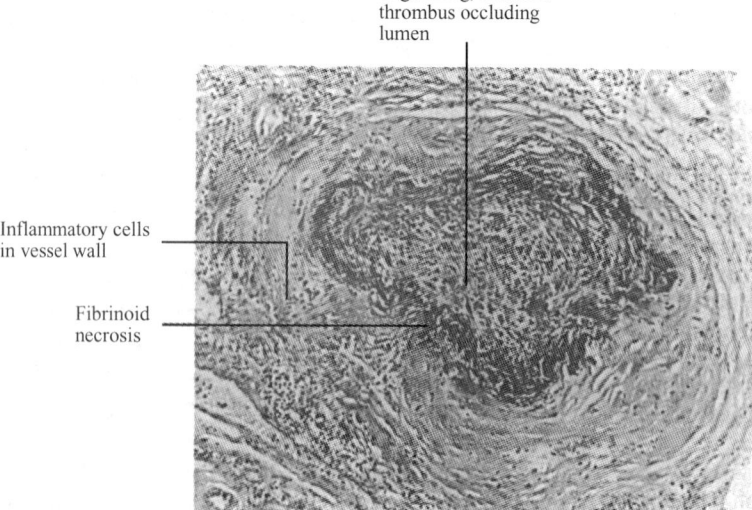

Figure 10-11 Acute rejection of a transplanted kidney showing the effects of immune complex injury in a medium-sized artery. Note the fibrinoid necrosis, vasculitis, and occlusion of the lumen by organizing thrombus

2. Cell-mediated mechanisms

Cell-mediated mechanisms involve T lymphocytes that become sensitized to transplanted antigens. These lymphocytes cause cell injury through direct cytotoxicity and secretion of lymphokines. Cell-mediated injury is characterized by acute (Figure 10-12) and chronic (Figure 10-13) necrosis of parenchymal cells accompanied by lymphocytic infiltration and fibrosis (Figure 10-13). Cellular mechanisms are more important than humoral mechanisms in the rejection process.

B. Graft-Versus-Host Disease (GVHD)

Graft-versus-host disease is a risk in severely T cell-deficient patients who receive viable foreign immunocompetent cell in blood transfusions and bone marrow transplants.

Graft-versus-host disease may occur in any situation where significant numbers of HLA-incompatible and viable lymphocytes are introduced into an immunodeficient host, as in transplantation of allogeneic bone marrow or gut or, less often, following transfusion of lymphocytes in blood. The absence of host T cell immunity prevents destruction of these foreign cells, which can then react against the host. It is usually fatal.

Graft-versus-host disease was first elucidated in inbred strains of mice, in which bone marrow trans-

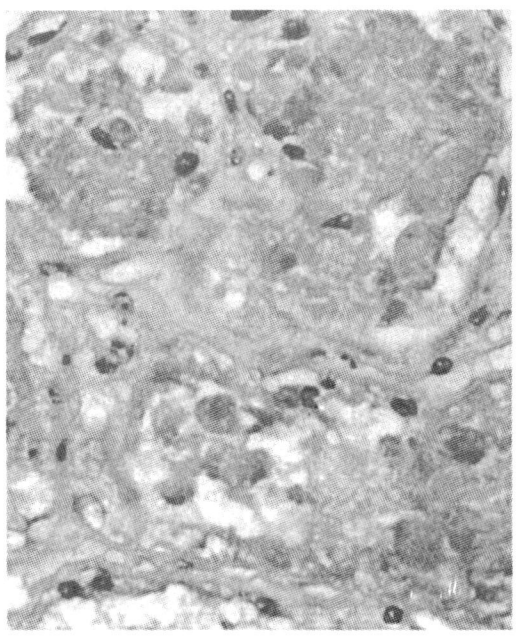

Figure 10-12 Acute renal tubular necrosis in a trans-planted kidney 1 week after transplantation. The kidney also showed extensive necrotizing vasculitis that may have contributed to necrosis by causing ischemia. Note that the renal tubular outlines are intact. This patient recovered with aggressive immunosuppressive therapy; the renal tubular epithelium regenerated rapidly

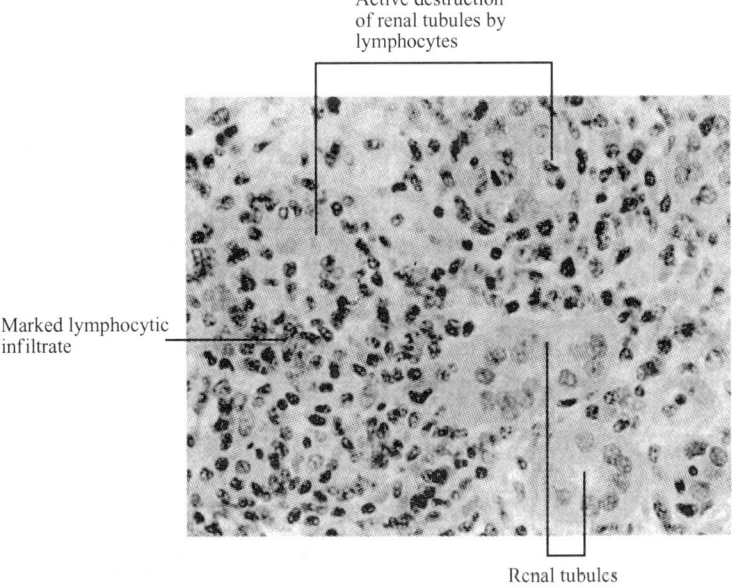

Figure 10-13 Rejection of a transplanted kidney, showing direct T cell-mediated cytotoxicity. The kidney is diffusely infiltrated by lymphocytes that are actively destroying renal tubular cells. Scattered residual renal tubular cells are present

plants from parents to first-generation hybrid offspring produced a fatal wasting condition known as runt disease, (In this experimental situation, parental lymphocytes see the offspring as foreign, but not vice versa.) The process was shown to be mediated by T lymphocytes reacting against foreign MHC antigens.

It was proposed by Starzl et al that there is exchange of migratory leukcytes between graft ctransplanted organ and recipient. So, both HVGR and GVHD may occur in solid organ transplantation and bone marrow transplantation. This form of cell migration between graft and recipient may be the basis of tolerance.

Clinical Types of Transplant Rejection

Transplant rejection takes a variety of forms, ranging from a dramatic reaction occurring within minutes after transplantation to one that occurs so slowly that evidence of transplant failure only becomes apparent years after the transplant. The mechanisms involved in these different types of rejection are also different.

A. Hyperacute Rejection

Hyperacute rejection is a fulminant reaction occurring within minutes after transplantation and characterized by severe necrotizing vasculitis (Figure 10-11) with diffuse ischemic damage to the transplanted organ. Deposition of immune complexes and complement activation in the wall of involved vessels can be demonstrated by immunologic techniques.

Hyperacute rejection is due to the presence in the recipient's serum of high levels of preformed antibodies against antigens on the transplanted cells. The antigen-antibody reaction produces an Arthus-type immune complex injury in the vessels of the transplant. Since development of direct tissue cross-matching, hyperacute rejection has become rare.

B. Acute Rejection

Acute rejection is common and may occur within days to months after transplantation. It is acute because even though its expression may be delayed until several months after transplantation, it progresses rapidly once it has begun. It is characterized by cellular destruction and organ failure (e. g. acute myocardial necrosis and failure in a heart transplant).

Both humoral and cell-mediated mechanisms operate in acute rejection. Immune complexes are deposited in the small vessels of the transplant and cause acute vasculitis, leading to ischemic changes. Cell-mediated immune rejection is characterized by parenchymal cell necrosis and lymphocytic infiltration of the tissue (Figure 10-13). In renal transplants, acute rejection is manifested as acute renal failure with renal tubular necrosis and marked interstitial lymphocytic infiltration (Figure 10-12). Acute rejection can often be successfully treated with immunosuppressive drugs such as corticosteroids (e. g. prednisone) and cyclosporine or with antilymphocyte serum to ablate the patient's T cell.

C. Chronic Rejection

Chronic rejection is present in most transplanted tissues and causes progressive changes with slow deterioration of organ function over a period of months or years. The patient often has a history of episodes of acute rejection controlled by immune suppressive therapy.

Treatment of chronic rejection attempts to achieve a balance between the rate of transplant destruction and the severity of the toxic effects of immunosuppressive drugs used to prevent rejection.

D. GVHD

The pathologic features show much in common with the multi-organ autoimmune diseases. Chronic cases (onset later than 100 days) tend to develop widespread fibrosis with lymphocyte infiltration, reminiscent of systemic sclerosis. More acute cases (onset sooner than 100 days) show focal epithelial cell necrosis in skin, intestinal crypts, bile ducts, and hepatic parenchymal cells. Skin rashes, diarrhea, and liver failure may result. Involvement of the bone marrow leads to anemia, neutropenia, and deepening immunosuppression.

DEFICIENCIES OF IMMUNE RESPONSE

The nonspecific inflammatory response and the immune response act synergistically in defense against infection. Deficits in either process often result in increased susceptibility to attack by pathogenic microorganisms, manifested clinically as recurrent or intractable infection or as an opportunistic infection, i.e. infection by a pathogen of low virulence that does not cause disease in a normal host.

The development of infections depends on the specific immunodeficiency. T cell deficiency predisposes to infections with viruses, mycobacteria, fungi, and other intracellular organisms such as Pneumocystis carinit and Toxoplasma gondii, B cell deficiency predisposes to pyogenic bacterial infections. These infections reflect the relative importance of cell-mediated and humoral responses in the defense against different microbial agents. The diseases caused by immunodeficiency are called as immunodeficiency disease. They include two types: congenital (primary) immunodeficiency and secondary immunodeficiency.

CONGENITAL (PRIMARY) IMMUNODEFICIENCY

All types of congenital immunodeficiency are rare. It occurs more commonly in infant and associated with inheritance. It results in recurrent infections. A few of the more common syndromes will be summarized in Table 10-9.

Table 10-9 Primary immunodeficiency diseases

	Peripheral Blood Lymphocytes	Peripheral Blood T Cells	Peripheral Blood B Cells	Tissue Lymphoid Cells	Serum Immunoglobulin	Other Features
Bruton's congenital agammaglobulinemia	N	N	↓	Absence of follicles and plasma cells	↓↓	Neutropenia
Selective IgA deficiency	N	N	N	N	↓ (IgA only)	Common (1 : 1000 general population)
Variable immunodeficiency	N	N	N or ↓	Decrease in plasma cells	↓	Associated autoimmune disease
DiGeorge syndrome (Thymic hypoplasia)	↓	↓↓	N	T cells depleted in thymus-dependent areas	N	Parathyroids absent
Nezelof's syndrome (T lymphopenia)	↓	↓	N	T cells depleted in thymus-dependent areas	N or ↓	Heterogeneous group
Severe combined immunodeficiency	↓↓	↓↓	↓↓	Absent	↓↓	Lack of adenosine deaminase
Wiskott-Aldrich syndrome	N or ↓	N or ↓	N	N	↓ (Especially IgA)	Involuted thymus, thrombocytopenia, eczema
Ataxia-telangiectasia	↓	N or ↓	N	Variable	↓ (Especially IgA)	Embryonic type thymus; lymphomas common

SECONDARY AND ACQUIRED IMMUNODEFICIENCY

Immunoparesis of varying degree is fairly common. It occurs most often as a secondary phenomenon in various diseases (Table 10-10) and is rarely a primary disease.

Table 10-10 Acquired immunodeficiency

	Mechanism
Primary disease	Rare; usually manifested as hypogammaglobulinemia in adults. Due to increased numbers of suppressor T cells
Secondary to other diseases	
Protein-calorie malnutrition	Hypogammaglobulinemia
Iron deficiency	Impaired T cell function
Postinfectious (measles, leprosy)	Often lymphopenia; usually transient
Hodgkin's disease	Impaired T cell function
Multiple myeloma	Impaired immunoglobulin production
Lymphoma or lymphocytic leukemia	Decreased number of normal lymphocytes
Advanced cancer	Depressed T cell function, other unknown mechanisms
Thymic neoplasms	Hypogammaglobulinemia
Chronic renal failure	Unknown
Diabetes mellitus	Unknown
Aging	Decreased number of T cells in some people
Drug-induced immunodeficiency	Common; caused by corticosteroids, anticancer drugs, radiotherapy, or deliberately induced immunosuppression in transplant patients
Human immunodeficiency virus (HIV) infection (AIDS)	Reduced number of T cell, mainly helper T cell

Acquired Immune Deficiency Syndrome (AIDS) (Figure 10-14)

A. Incidence

AIDS has become the most common immunodeficiency disease in the United States since it was first recognized in 1981 in Los Angeles. Subsequent retrospective studies indicate that cases may have occurred around the world as long ago as 1960. It is believed that more than 33 million persons, many of whom are infants, are infected with HIV (human immunodeficiency virus). Internationally, the disease is most common in Southeast Asia and sub-Saharan Africa. More than 4 million persons are infected with HIV in China.

B. Definition

AIDS was initially defined on the basis of the occurrence of certain opportunistic infections and cancer indicative of impaired mediated immunity. The definition has been revised (most recently in January 1993) to incorporate the results of HIV antibody testing and CD4 (helper T cell) levels (Table 10-11). A presumptive diagnosis of AIDS-based on the presence of certain strong indicator diseases-may still be made in the absence of a positive HIV antibody test.

Table 10-11 Definition and diagnosis of AIDS: Simplified criteria[1]

A. **Positive HIV antibody test plus:**
(1) CD4 count
 $\geqslant 500/\mu L$ HIV infected, asymptomatic
 $200-499/\mu L$ Pre-ALDS, ARC (ALDS-related complex)
 $<200/\mu L$ AIDS (definitive)
  or
(2) **Presence of certain indicator diseases (see below)**
 = AIDS (definitive)

B. **HIV antibody test indeterminate or not performed, plus:**
 CD4 $< 200/\mu L$, or indicator disease = presumptive AIDS[2]

C. **HIV antibody test negative, with:** Absence of any other known cause of immunodeficiency, plus CD4 $< 200/\mu L$, or indicator disease[2] = presumptive AIDS

Indicator Diseases for Diagnosis of AIDS

- **Opportunistic infections**
  (a) **Strong indicator diseases:** Candidiasis, cryptococcosis, cryptosporidiosis (diarrhea), CMV, herpes simplex, *M avium* intracellulare complex infection, *P carinii* infection, toxoplasmosis (brain)
  (b) **Recurrent bacterial infections** (excluding otitis media and skin infections), coccidioidomycosis, histoplasmosis, isosporiasis (diarrhea), tuberculosis, *Salmonella* septicemia

(Continued)

- **Malignancies**:
  - (a) **Strong indicator diseases**: Kaposi's sarcoma or lymphoma or brain (<60 years of age)
  - (b) Kaposi's sarcoma or lymphoma of brain (>60 years of age), or other lymphoma or invasive carcinoma of cervix
- **Other indicator diseases**: HIV encephalopathy, HIV wasting syndrome

[1] The information here is simplified. Current full criteria are exceedingly complex, as much for political or legal reasons as for medical need. The CDC Revised 1993 Classification may be found in MMWR Morbid Mortal Wkly Rep 1992;41(RR17):1.

[2] The presence of strong indicator diseases such as persistence of certain opportunistic infections - group (a) - in unusual sites or characteristic malignancies in patients under 60 years of age-group (a) - allows a definitive diagnosis of AIDS even in the absence of a positive HIV antibody test.

C. Etiology and Pathogenesis

AIDS is caused by an RNA retrovirus called human immunodeficiency virus (HIV) - previously called human T cell lymphotropic virus type III (HTLV III) and lymphadenopathy-associated virus (LAV). There are two types in HIV: HIV-1 and HIV-2. HIV-1 include 9 subtypes (A to H and O subtypes). Different strains of HIV are beginning to appear, with definition based on the env (envelope) protein. HIV-2 has recently been described in Africa with cases also reported elsewhere, including the United States and China. HIV-2 produces a very similar disease. The primary targets of viral attack are helper (CD4-positive) T lymphocytes. The virus uses the cell surface CD4 receptor molecules for its entry. Other cell types that share common epitopes with the T lymphocyte receptor e. g. macrophages and cells in the central nervous system are also susceptible to infection with HIV.

The entry of HIV into T lymphocytes may result in (1) acute destruction of the cell, which contributes to a progressive depletion of CD4 cells at a rate of approximately 80,000/μL/yr; or (2) latent infection, with insertion of the proviral genome into the host DNA. Infection of humans with HIV is almost invariably associated with the appearance of anti-HIV antibodies in the serum, usually within 6 months after infection. These antibodies are not protective, and HIV viremia persists despite their pre-sence. Detection of anti-HIV antibodies and viral isolation from the blood or infected cells are important diagnostic tools.

D. Transmission

Patients and persons who are asymptomatic HIV positive are the sources of infectivity. (1) HIV infection is essentially a sexually transmitted disease. Transmission of HIV during sexual contact occurs at a rate lower than that of gonorrhea or hepatitis B; estimates of the risk associated with a single heterosexual encounter with an HIV-infected partner range from 5% to 15% - compared with 30% in the case of gonorrhea. Estimates of transmission rates between regular (repeat) sexual partners vary: female → male, 10% - 20%; male → female, 20% - 50%; male → male, > 50%. The risk is increased by the coexistence of other venereal diseases associated with open genital sores. The use of condoms has been recommended as a means of decreasing HIV transmission during sexual contact. (2) Transmission also occurs through direct injection into the blood by intravenous drug users or less often by transfusion of blood products (Figure 10-14). Transmission of HIV by blood transfusion and blood products is highly efficient, with the result that more than 90% of individuals transfused with infected blood become infected. (3) The risk of transmission by other body fluids such as saliva and tears is very low despite the presence of HIV in such fluids. (4) The risk of infection of health care workers is also low, although a few cases of HIV infection have been reported after accidental blood spills and needle sticks. The risk of infection by casual contact with an infected person is almost nill. (5) The transmission rate from infected mother to infant is in the order of 10% - 20%.

HIV infection occurs in several high-risk groups: (1) Male homosexuals and bisexuals account for over 60% of cases of AIDS in the United States. (2) Intravenous drug abusers account for about 15% of cases. (3) Heterosexual female contacts of male bisexuals and intravenous drug abusers account for less than 10% of cases in the United States, but the proportion is rising rapidly (almost 50% of all new cases in some areas). (4) Patients transfused with blood products - most importantly hemophiliacs and infants - represent an estimated 2% of cases.

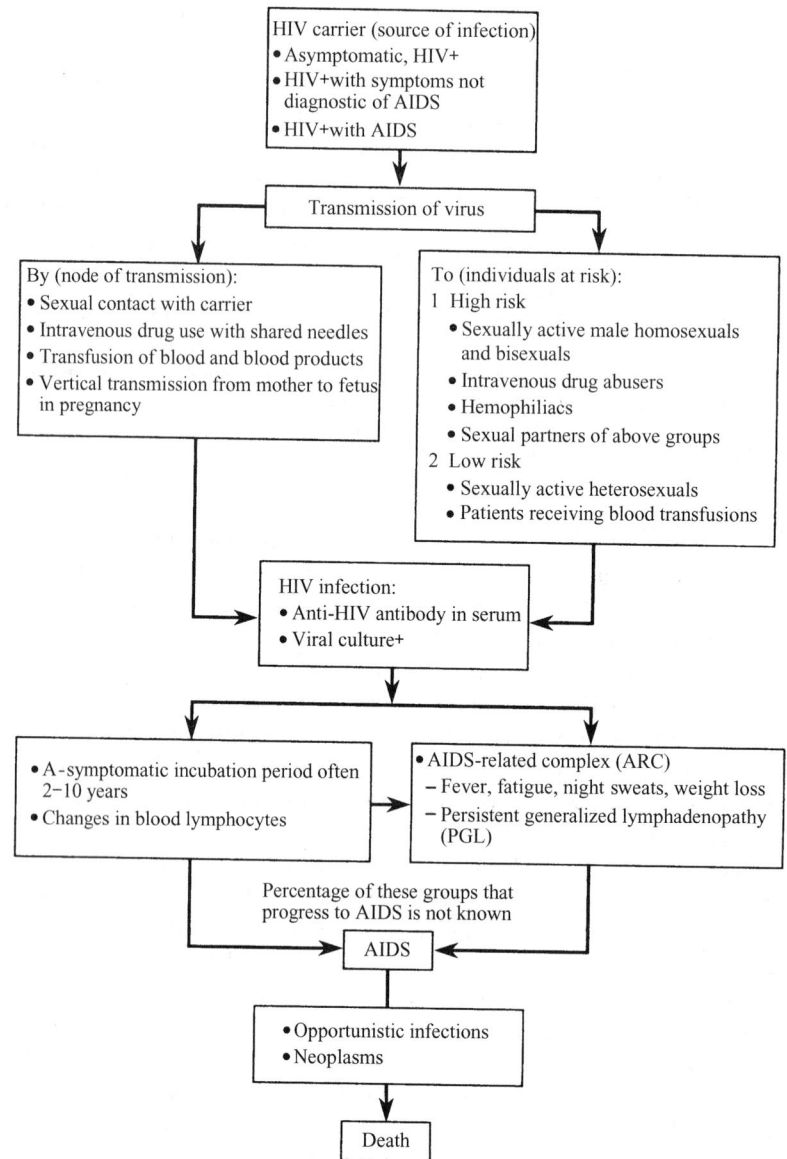

Figure 10-14 Summary of infection with human immunodeficiency virus (HIV) in humans. Percentages quoted are for the United States

E. Manifestations and Stages of HIV Infection

1. Incubation period

The incubation period between HIV infection and development of AIDS has been calculated in patients infected by blood transfusion - a documented date of inoculation - to be a median of about 4.5 years. In sexually transmitted disease, it appears to be longer, i.e. 8 - 10 years. The incubation period is shorter in young children than in adults. During the incubation period, individuals are positive for HIV antibody and may show changes in the periphe-ral blood lymphocytes, but they are asymptomatic. The percentage of asymptomatic HIV-positive individuals who go on to develop AIDS is unknown, but it is thought to be high.

2. Changes in the immune system

HIV infection leads to a decrease in the number of

helper inducer (CD4-positive) T cell in the peripheral blood. This may be accompanied by an increase in the number of suppressor/cytotoxic (CD8-positive) T cell, resulting in a decreased CD4:CD8 ratio. These changes in the immune system lead to functional immunodeficiency. The decreased CD4:CD8 ratio is not diagnostic of HIV infection and may occur in several other immunodeficiency states.

3. AIDS-Related complex (ARC)

Patients with ARC are HIV-positive and symptomatic but have none of the indicator diseases that are used to define AIDS. ARC patients complain of fatigue, weight loss, night sweats, and diarrhea and have superficial fungal infections of the mouth, fingernails, and toenails.

4. Pathology

Pathologic changes include changes of lymph nodes, opportunistic infections and malignant neoplasms.

- Changes of lymph nodes: Changes of lymph nodes are the lymph node abnormalities. In the early stages, infected lymph nodes show marked reactive follicular hyperplasia with characteristic histologic features - a condition called persistent generalized lymphadenopathy (PGL). Histologically, the lymph nodes show follicular and paracotical hyperplasia, with very large conspicuous follicles in the early stages. Irregular loss or fragmentation of the mantle zone (the rim of small lymphocytes around the follicle) is characteristic. The helper: suppressor ratio typically is reversed in the lymph nodes. (In other forms of reactive hyperplasia, T helper cells predominate in the lymph node.) In later stages, there is progressive depletion of lymphocyte in lymph nodes, and 10% develop aggressive B cell lymphomas. HIV can be isolated from the lymph nodes of patients with PGL.
- Opportunistic infections: Among the opportunistic infections, the following are the most common: P carinii pneumonia, esophageal candidiasis, cytomegalovirus infections, atypical mycobacterial infections, toxoplasmosis of the brain, cryptosporidiosis of the intestine, herpes simplex infections, and papova virus infection of the brain (progressive multi focal leukoencephalopathy).
- Malignant neoplasms: Kaposi's sarcoma and malignant B cell lymphomas are the most common malignant neoplasms that develop in AIDS. The occurrence of malignant neoplasms may be related to the role of the immune response in removing developing malignanT cell that arise in the body (failure of immune surveillance), or it may be due to sustained immune stimulation of an inadequate immune system in which the usual controls of cellular proliferation are lacking (e.g. leading to B cell lymphoma).

Kaposi's sarcoma is a malignant vascular cancer that affects the skin (Figure 10-15) and many internal organs. It is the cancer whose suddenly increased incidence and appearance in a much younger age group caused AIDS to be first recognized in 1981. Since that year, these patients have been shown also to have an increased incidence of high-grade non-Hodgkin's malignant B cell lymphomas, particularly of the central nervous system.

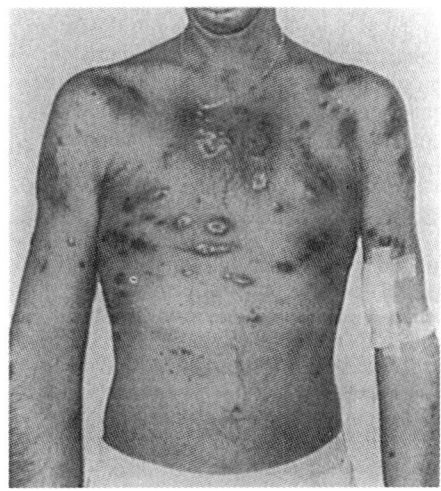

Figure 10-15 Kaposi's sarcoma, disseminated, in a patient with AIDS. Note the presence of multiple elevated dark purple skin lesions

F. The Prospects for Prevention

The main method of prevention of AIDS currently available is public education about the methods of transmission of HIV. The use of condoms and safe sex practices has been recommended as ways to decrease the risk of infection.

Screening of blood donors for HIV antibody has markedly decreased the incidence of AIDS transmitted by transfusion of blood products. Health care workers, policemen, and firemen routinely take precautions to decrease the risk of becoming infected. The use of gloves, fluid-proof gowns, masks, and safe needle disposal methods should be routine safety precautions for health care workers and others at risk.

The two main directions of research in AIDS are aimed at developing a vaccine that will prevent infection or a drug that will be effective in treatment. Both a vaccine and an effective drug are not apparent in the immediate future.

G. Course and Treatment of AIDS

AIDS is a disease that relentlessly and invariably progresses to death. Almost all patients are dead 5 years after diagnosis, but many die much sooner. Treated patients continue to develop additional opportunistic infections. Combination therapy with reverse transcriptase inhibitors and protease inhibitors has shown improved survival.

Chapter 11   Diseases of the Urinary System

Deng Hong

CHAPTER CONTENTS
- Structure and Function of the Kidneys
    - Structure of the Kidneys
    - Renal Function
    - Clinical Manifestations of Renal Disease
    - Methods of Evaluating Renal Structure and Function
- Glomerular Diseases
    - Pathologic Changes
    - Pathogenesis of Glomerular Disease
    - Classification of Glomerulonephritis
    - Acute Diffuse Proliferative Glomerulonephritis
    - Rapidly Progressive Glomerulonephritis
    - Membranous Glomerulonephritis
    - Minimal Change Glomerulonephritis
    - Focal Segmental Glomerulosclerosis
    - Membranoproliferative Glomerulonephritis
    - Mesangial Proliferative Glomerulonephritis
    - IgA Nephropathy
    - Chronic Glomerulonephritis
- Tubulointerstitial Diseases
    - Infectious Diseases
    - Toxic Tubulointerstitial Diseases
- Neoplasms of the Kidney and the Urinary Bladder
    - Renal Cell Carcinoma
    - Nephroblastoma
    - Urothelial Neoplasms of the Urinary Bladder

STRUCTURE AND FUNCTION OF THE KIDNEYS

STRUCTURE OF THE KIDNEYS

The kidneys are located in the retroperitoneum and weigh 130 - 150 g each. The surface is smooth and invested in a capsule, which in turn is surrounded by perinephric fat and Gerota's fascia.

The anatomic unit of the kidney is the nephron, which is composed of the glomerulus, proximal convoluted tubule, loop of Henle, distal convoluted tubule and collecting tublule. Each kidney contains approximately 1 million nephrons.

Glomerular diseases constitute some of the major problems encountered in nephrology, while the structural and functional changes of glomerulus are of significance in the renal disorder.

The glomerulus (Figure 11-1) is composed of (1) an afferent and efferent arteriole; (2) intervening capillaries lined by endothelial cells (glomerular tuft); (3) the outer surface of the capillaries, which is covered by epithelial cells (podocytes), continuous with the epithelium of Bowman's space and the proximal tubule; (4) the mesangium, composed of mesangial cells and matrix; and (5) the basement mambrane. The many anionic moieties present within the capillary wall, including the acidic proteoglycans of the glomerular basement membrane and the sialoglycoproteins of epithelial and endothelial cell coats.

The following structures have been noticed especially:
- The glomerular endothelial cells are fenestrated in the cytoplasm, each fenestra being 70 to 100 nm in diameter.
- The glomerular basement membrane (GBM) is with a thick, electron-dense central larger, the lamina densa, and thinner, electron-lucent peripheral layer, the lamina rara interna and lamina rara externa. The GBM is composed of collagen (mostly type Ⅳ), laminin, polyanionic proteoglycans, fibronectin and several other glycoproteins.
- Podocytes possess interdigitating processes embedded in and adherent to the lamina rara externa of the basement membrane. Adjacent foot processes are separated by 20-to 30-nm-wide filtration slits, which

are bridged by a thin diaphragm composed of nephrin. Nephrin is one of the members of the immunoglobulin superfamily, expresses specifically in glomerulus and is critical to maintenance of the selective glomerular permeability.

- The mesangium is lying between the capillaries. The mesangial cells are contractile and are capable of proliferation, of producing both matrix and collagen, and of secreting a number of biologically active mediators.

RENAL FUNCTION

Glomerular Filtration

Ultrafiltration of plasma occurs in the glomerular capillaries, driven by the hydrostatic pressure head in the arteriolar end of the capillary (Table 11-1). The normal glomerular filtration membrane forms a barrier to molecules in the plasma that is based largely on (1) capillary endothelial cell junctional fenestrations, which normally restrict the passage of molecules with molecular weights greater than 70,000 (Figure 11-1); (2) basement membrane polyanions such as acidic proteoglycans, which impart a negative charge that selectively prevents the filtration of anionic particles such as albumin; and (3) the epithelial cell, which acts as a physical barrier.

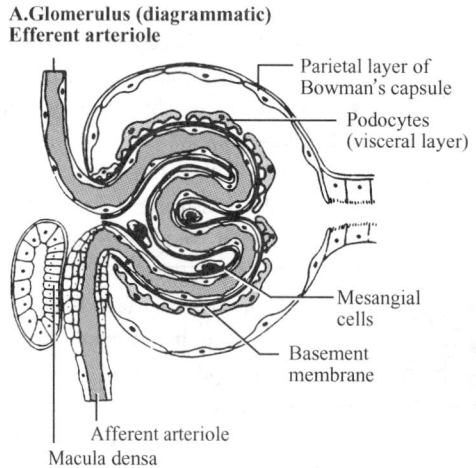

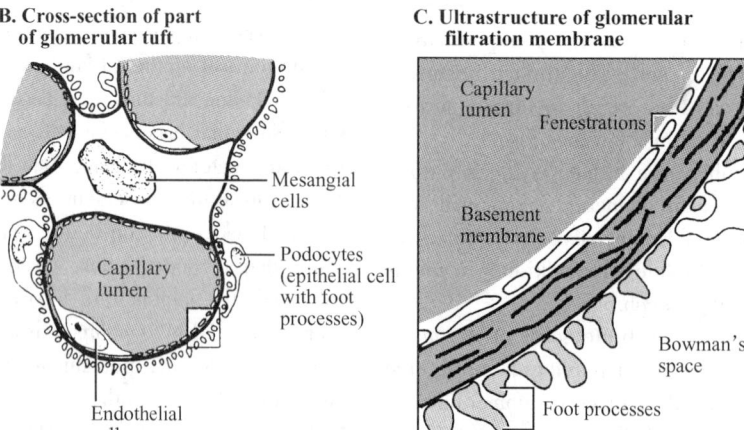

Figure 11-1 Detailed structure of glomerulus and glomerular filtration membrane composed of endothelial cell, basement membrane, and podocyte

The glomerular filtration rate (GFR) is normally about 120mL/min. It may be measured accurately by the clearance of exogenous inulin (inulin clearance test) or endogenous creatinine (creatinine clearance test).

Tubular Reabsorption (Table 11-1)

Eighty percent of the glomerular ultrafiltrate volume is absorbed actively in the proximal tubule. Potassium, glucose, and amino acids are completely reabsorbed.

Approximately 30 mL/min of isotonic fluid is delivered to the loop of Henle. The loop of Henle passes down into the medulla and establishes a countercurrent exchange mechanism that causes a progressive increase in tonicity from the corticomedullary junction to the tip of the papillae. Establishment of the countercurrent exchange mechanism depends on active secretion of sodium into the interstitium by cells in the ascending loop of Henle. There is otherwise little fluid or electrolyte exchange in the loop of Henle.

Table 11-1 Functional anatomy of the nephron

Juxtaglomerular apparatus	Renin production
Glomerulus	Produces ultrafiltrate of plasma (glomerular filtration rate 120mL/min)
Proximal convoluted tubule	Resorption of: Water (80%) Glucose (100%) K^+ (100%) Amino acids (100%)
Loop of Henle and vasa recta	Countercurrent exchange and multiplier mechanisms
Distal convoluted tubule and collecting duct	Resorption of: Water (antidiuretic hormone-controlled) Na^+ (in exchange for K^+ and H^+, controlled by aldosterone) Acidification

The following changes in the tubular fluid occur in the distal convoluted and collecting tubules:

- **Water reabsorption** occurs under the influence of antidiuretic hormone. Medullary hypertonicity produced by the countercurrent exchange and multiplier mechanisms is vital to the urine concentration mechanism. Of the 120 mL filtered at the glomerulus, only 1–2 mL normally passes through as urine.
- **Sodium reabsorption** occurs under the influence of aldosterone in exchange for potassium and hydrogen ions.
- **Acidification** of urine occurs. The total acid excreted per day by the kidney is only about 1% of that excreted by the lungs as CO_2. Nonetheless, failure of this mechanism will, after several days, result in metabolic acidosis.

Excreted urine contains precisely regulated quantities of sodium, potassium, water, chloride, bicarbonate, phosphate, and ammonium ions. Normal urine contains only a trace amount of protein, derived mainly from tubular secretion (Tamm-Horsfall protein) and no glucose or amino acids. It has a high concentration of excretory products: urea, uric acid, and creatinine.

CLINICAL MANIFESTATIONS OF RENAL DISEASE

Hematuria

Many renal diseases are characterized by the passage of blood in the urine (hematuria). There may or may not be pain. When bleeding is severe, hematuria is recognized by red discoloration of urine. When bleeding is slow, hematuria does not produce any visible change but can be diagnosed by the presence of erythrocytes in a sample of urinary sediment (microscopic hematuria). Hematuria has many causes (Table 11-2).

Proteinuria

Proteinuria is a common finding in many renal diseases, and testing for it is a useful screening test for renal disease. The trace amount of protein normally present in urine does not give a positive reaction with the usual screening tests. In a few individuals, orthostatic (postural) or exercise proteinuria occurs following recumbency or vigorous physical activity; the condition has no clinical significance.

Urinary casts are formed when protein and other organic matter in the renal tubules solidifies. Casts are elongated cylindric structures with a diameter equal to that of the renal tubule. The presence of casts in urine is indicative of disease of the nephron. Casts may contain protein only (hyaline casts) or may include erythrocytes (red cell casts), leukocytes (white cell casts), and tubular cells (epithelial casts).

Table 11-2 Causes of hematuria

Renal diseases
  Acute and chronic glomerulonephritis
  Primary types, usually proliferative glomerulonephritis (including Goodpasture's syndrome and IgA nephropathy)
  Secondary to systemic lupus erythematosus, polyarteritis nodosa, Henoch-Schönlein purpura
  Acute and chronic pyelonephritis
  Neoplasms
  Calculi
  Trauma
  Drug or chemical toxicity
  Papillary necrosis
  Polycystic disease

Diseases of bladder, ureters, urethra
  Cystitis
  Urethritis
  Neoplasms
  Calculi
  Trauma

Systemic disease causing bleeding from genitourinary tract
  Malignant hypertension
  Systemic embolism in infective endocarditis
  Bleeding diathesis or anticoagulant therapy
  Osler-Weber-Rendu disease

Nephrotic Syndrome

Nephrotic Syndrome is characterized by massive proteinuria (>3.5 g protein/1.73 m^2 surface area/d), hypoproteinemia, generalized edema and hyperlipidemia (Table 11-3). Nephrotic syndrome may result from any condition that causes increased glomerular capillary permeability to proteins (Table 11-4). The prognosis varies according to the underlying disease.

Acute Nephritic Syndrome

Acute nephritic syndrome is a clinical syndrome characterized by decreased urinary volume (oliguria), hematuria, mild proteinuria, elevation of serum urea and creatinine (azotemia or uremia), hypertension, and mild edema. Acute glomerular disease associated with a decreased glomerular filtration rate is the major cause. Again, the prognosis depends upon the cause.

Acute Renal Failure

Acute renal failure is defined as marked diminution of urine output to less than 400 mL/d (oliguria; anuria would be complete absence of urine output). If persistent, it leads to elevation of serum creatinine and urea plus hypertension due to retention of sodium and water. There are many causes. In acute tubular necrosis, in some cases of glomerulonephritis, and in pre- and postrenal causes, the process is reversible and the patient may be expected to recover after treatment. Acute cortical necrosis and severe forms of glomerulonephritis are irreversible and often require long-term dialysis or renal transplantation.

Table 11-3 Major differential features of the principal clinical renal diseases

	Nephrotic Syndrome	Acute Nephritic Syndrome (Acute Nephritis)	Acute Renal Failure	Chronic Renal Failure	Acute Pyelonephritis
Urine output	N or ↓	↓	↓↓ or 0	↑ (cannot concentrate)	N (rarely ↓)
Proteinuria	+++	+ to +++	+ to ++	+ to ++	++
Hematuria	− (rarely +)	+	±	±	− (rarely +)
Edema	++	+	±	±	−
Serum albumin	↓↓	N	N	N	N
Serum urea or creatinine	N (until late)	↑	↑↑	↑	N
Blood pressure	N	↑	↑	↑	N
Other	↑ Serum cholesterol, casts	Hyperkalemia	Hyperkalemia, acidosis	Isosthenuria	White cells in urine (often purulent), frequency, dysuria, culture positive

Table 11-4 Common causes of nephrotic syndrome

Primary glomerular diseases
    Minimal change disease
    Membranous glomerulonephritis
    Mesangial proliferative glomerulonephritis
    Focal glomerulosclerosis
Secondary to other diseases
    Hereditary: Alport's syndrome; congenital nephritic syndrome
    Diabetic nephropathy
    Infections: Poststreptococcal glomerulonephritis, hepatitis B, HIV infection, malaria
    Drugs and Toxins: Gold; heroin; poison ivy; insect stings
    Systemic lupus erythematosus
    Amyloidosis
    Henoch-Schönlein purpura
    Renal vein thrombosis
    Multiple myeloma

Chronic Renal Failure

Chronic renal failure (chronic uremia) is characterized by a variety of abnormalities (Figure 11-2) resulting from a decrease in the total number of nephrons. The kidneys normally have a total of 2 million nephrons. Chronic renal failure appears only when the number of nephrons is reduced to about 25% of this number. Again, there are many causes, which are discussed in this chapter (Table 11-6).

The manifestations of chronic renal failure are numerous and affect virtually every organ in the body.

A. Uremia and Azotemia

Failure of renal excretory function resulting in increased serum urea and creatinine occurs only when failure is advanced. A much more sensitive assessment of chronic renal failure is the creatinine clearance test, which is an estimate of the glomerular filtration rate. Decreased glomerular filtration is proportionate to nephron loss. Serum urea and creatinine become elevated only when creatinine clearance decreases to about 30%–40% of normal.

B. Inability to Concentrate Urine

This is one of the early clinical manifestations of chronic renal failure. It leads to polyuria (increased urine output), nocturia (excessive passage of urine at night), and isosthenuria (passage of a urine that varies little from a specific gravity of 1.010). Polyuria frequently causes dehydration.

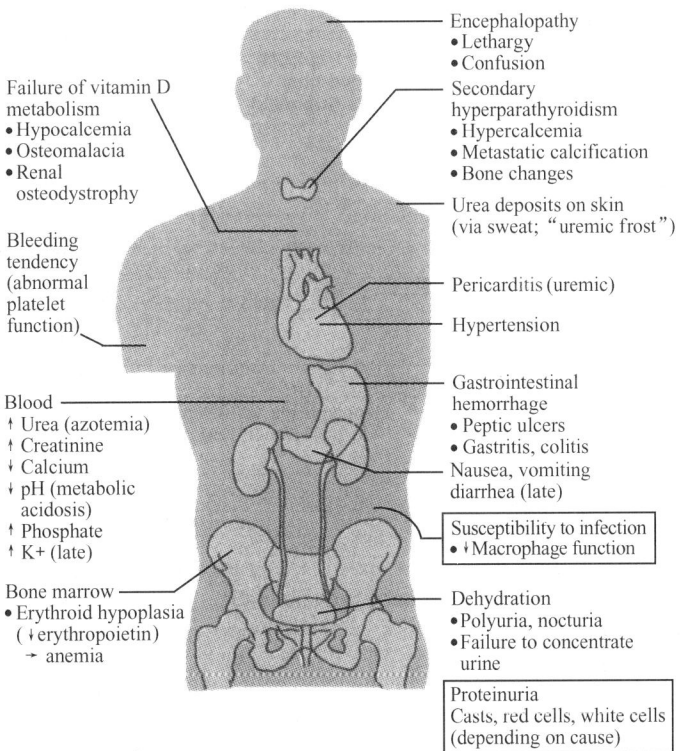

Figure 11-2 Clinical sequelae of chronic renal failure

C. Metabolic Acidosis

Failure of hydrogen ion excretion results in accumulation of acid in the blood (the body produces excess acid during cell metabolism), leading to metabolic acidosis.

D. Secondary Hyperparathyroidism and Renal Osteodystrophy

Failure of renal activation of vitamin D in chronic renal failure leads to defective intestinal absorption of calcium and hypocalcemia. The low plasma calcium causes compensatory parathyroid hyperplasia and increased parathyroid hormone secretion (secondary hyperparathyroidism). Abnormal calcium and phosphate metabolism leads to bone changes (renal osteodystrophy) and metastatic calcification. Renal osteodystrophy is a complex combination of osteomalacia and the effects of hyperparathyroidism (osteitis fibrosa cystica). Metastatic calcification in the walls of small vessels may cause ischemia changes in affected tissues.

E. Hematologic Disorders

Decreased erythropoietin production by the kidney leads to normochromic normocytic anemia. Platelet function is abnormal, causing a bleeding tendency. Gastrointestinal hemorrhage is a common clinical manifestation of chronic uremia.

F. Cardiovascular Disorders

Chronic renal failure is frequently associated with hypertension, caused by sodium and water retention in the kidneys. In most cases, plasma renin levels are normal; in a few, they are elevated and contribute to the hypertension. Renal failure in an advanced stage may also cause acute fibrinous or hemorrhagic pericarditis by an unknown mechanism.

G. Encephalopathy

Chronic renal failure is often associated with abnormalities in cerebral function, causing disturbances in the level of consciousness. Uremic encephalopathy is presumed to be due to retention of unknown end products of protein metabolism.

Hypertension

Hypertension occurs in both acute and chronic renal failure and may be the presenting feature of renal disease; the principal mechanism is retention of sodium and water as a result of decreased glomerular filtration. In a few patients with renal disease – most commonly renal artery stenosis-increased renin secretion contributes to hypertension.

METHODS OF EVALUATING RENAL STRUCTURE AND FUNCTION

The diagnosis of renal disease generally occurs in two steps: (1) Recognition of the major clinical syndrome being manifested (Table 11-3). Each syndrome has its differential diagnosis (Tables 11-2, 11-4 and 11-5); (2) Identification of the specific renal disease responsible. Common examination methods include physical examination, radiologic examination, examination of urine and blood, and renal biopsy.

Table 11-5 Causes of chronic renal failure

Diabetic nephropathy (28%)
Hypertensive renal disease (25%)
Chronic glomerulonephritis (21%)
Polycystic disease (4%)
Other causes (22%)
Chronic glomerulonephritis
Obstructive nephropathy
Amyloidosis
Multiple myeloma
Analgesic nephropathy
Nephrolithiasis
Hypercalcemia

Examination of Urine

Routine urine examination should be part of every complete physical examination (Table 11-6). Most of the chemical tests and microscopic examination of the sediment can be easily performed by the physician in an office or ward laboratory. The availability of dipsticks has made chemical urine testing relatively easy. Abnormalities detected by these means should be confirmed by formal testing in the pathology department.

Renal Biopsy

Percutaneous renal biopsy is a safe procedure that provides a cylindric core of renal tissue for histologic examination. Samples are also processed for electron microscopy and immunofluorescence. These studies have provided an objective method of diagnosis of renal disease and have increased our understanding of many pathologic processes. Before biopsy is undertaken, it is necessary to demonstrate that both kidneys are present and that there is no bleeding abnormality.

Table 11-6 Examination of urine

Physical evaluation	
Color	
Colorless	Polyuria; normal
Cloudy	Phosphates, carbonates, urates, white blood cells, lipid; may be normal
Dark	Bilirubin, blood
Red, red-brown	Blood, hemoglobin, porphyrins
Black	Homogentisic acid, melanin
Various	Drugs, food dyes
Odor	
Foul, ammoniacal	Probable infection with urea-splitting bacteria
Various unusual odors	Possible metabolic disorders such as phenylketonuria (mousy) or isovaleric acidemia (sweaty)
Volume (especially 24-hour)	Polyuria, oliguria; normal range is about 600 – 2000 mL /24 h for an adult. Nocturia: >400 mL at night
Specific gravity	Normal range is 1.005 – 1.025; consistent value of 1.010 is isosthenuria and indicates inability to concentrate urine, as in chronic renal failure
pH	Dietary factors, renal tubular disorders, chronic renal failure, acidosis, alkalosis
Chemical evaluation	
Protein	Normally, traces only. Numerous causes – must exclude renal failure
Blood	Chemical test may detect myoglobinuria and hemoglobinuria also. Microscopy should always be used to confirm hematuria
Glucose	Glycosuria strongly suggests diabetes mellitus. Other causes rare
Bilirubin	Obstructive jaundice, liver diseases
Ketones	Starvation, diabetic ketotic coma
Urobilinogen	Increased in hemolytic or hepatocellular jaundice; absent in obstructive jaundice
Prophobilinogen	Positive in porphyrias. Salicylates and other drugs may cause positive tests
Examination of sediment (microscopic evaluation)	
Red blood cells	See Table 11-3
Casts: red cell, white cell, granular, epithelial	Many renal diseases
White blood cells	Pyelonephritis, cystitis, other renal disease
Malignant cells by cytologic examination	Cancer, especially of the bladder
Crystals	Various types often present. Little diagnostic significance
Bacteriologic examination (culture)	Specific organisms, pyelonephritis, cystitis, urethritis

GLOMERULAR DISEASES

This group of renal disease is characterized by primary abnormalities of the glomerulus, both structural (inflammation, cellular proliferation, basement membrane thickening, fibrosis, epithelial cell changes) and functional (increased permeability causing proteinuria or hemorrhage of glomerular origin). Glomerular diseases may be congenital or acquired. Congenital glomerular diseases (the most common being Alport's syndrome, in which nephritis is associated with nerve deafness and cataract) are very rare. This chapter deals with acquired glomerular diseases.

PATHOLOGIC CHANGES

Glomerular diseases may be **focal**, showing abnormality in some but not all the glomeruli; or **diffuse**, where all glomeruli are affected. In **segmental** glomerular involvement, only a portion of each individual glomerulus is affected, in contrast to a **global** change, which involves entire glomeruli. Combinations of these terms are commonly used; eg, in focal segmental involvement the abnormality is present in some but not all glomeruli and the affected glomeruli are only partially involved.

Identification of exact morphologic changes in the glomerulus in renal biopsy specimens is important in the differential diagnosis of glomerular diseases. Some knowledge of these changes is necessary because different glomerular diseases show varying combinations of these same basic features.

A. Proliferation of Cells in the Glomerulus

Any of the different cell types in the glomerulus may undergo proliferation in different diseases.
- **Mesangial cell proliferation** is recognized by the presence of increased numbers of nuclei (in excess of three) in the central part of a glomerular lobule. Mesangial cells are part of the phagocytic mechanism of the glomerulus.
- **Endothelial cell proliferation** causes obliteration of the capillary lumen.
- **Epithelial cell proliferation**, when extensive, leads to formation of a crescent-shaped mass of cellular or collagenized tissue that obliterates Bowman's space. Epithelial cell proliferation is believed to be stimulated by fibrin deposition in Bowman's space.

B. Infiltration of the Glomerulus by Inflammatory Cells

Infiltration with neutrophils, lymphocytes, and macrophages is present in many cases of acute glomerulonephritis. Acute inflammation is accompanied by fluid exudation and swelling of the glomerulus (exudative glomerulonephritis).

C. Capillary Basement Membrane Thickening

Increased amounts of basement membrane material may be detected by light microscopy as a thickened capillary wall. The basement membrane can be specially stained with silver stains and seen by electron microscopy. Basement membrane thickening is commonly associated with deposition of immune complexes, immunoglobulins, and complement. Such deposition may be subepithelial, intramembranous, or subendothelial and is seen only by immunofluoresence and electron microscopy. Regardless of its cause, basement membrane thickening typically causes increased glomerular capillary permeability to proteins, leading to nephrotic syndrome.

D. Increased Mesangial Matrix Material

This pathologic picture is commonly due to deposition of immunoglobulins and complement in the mesangium (positive staining on immunofluorescence and visible on electron microscopy).

E. Epithelial Foot Process Fusion

This feature can be seen only by electron microscopy. It is a nonspecific change that is believed to result whenever there is increased leakage of protein from the glomerular capillaries.

F. Fibrosis

Fibrosis (sclerosis) can affect part of the glomerulus (mesangium, Bowman's space) or may be global. Global sclerosis produces an obsolescent nonfunctional glomerulus and is followed by atrophy and fibrosis of the corresponding nephron (tubules). It may follow most of the changes described above or may be the primary abnormality (Figure 11-3).

PATHOGENESIS OF GLOMERULAR DISEASE

Most forms of primary glomerular disease are caused by two principal humoral immunologic mechanisms (Figure 11-4). Evidence for cell-mediated reactions exists in minimal change glomerular disease.

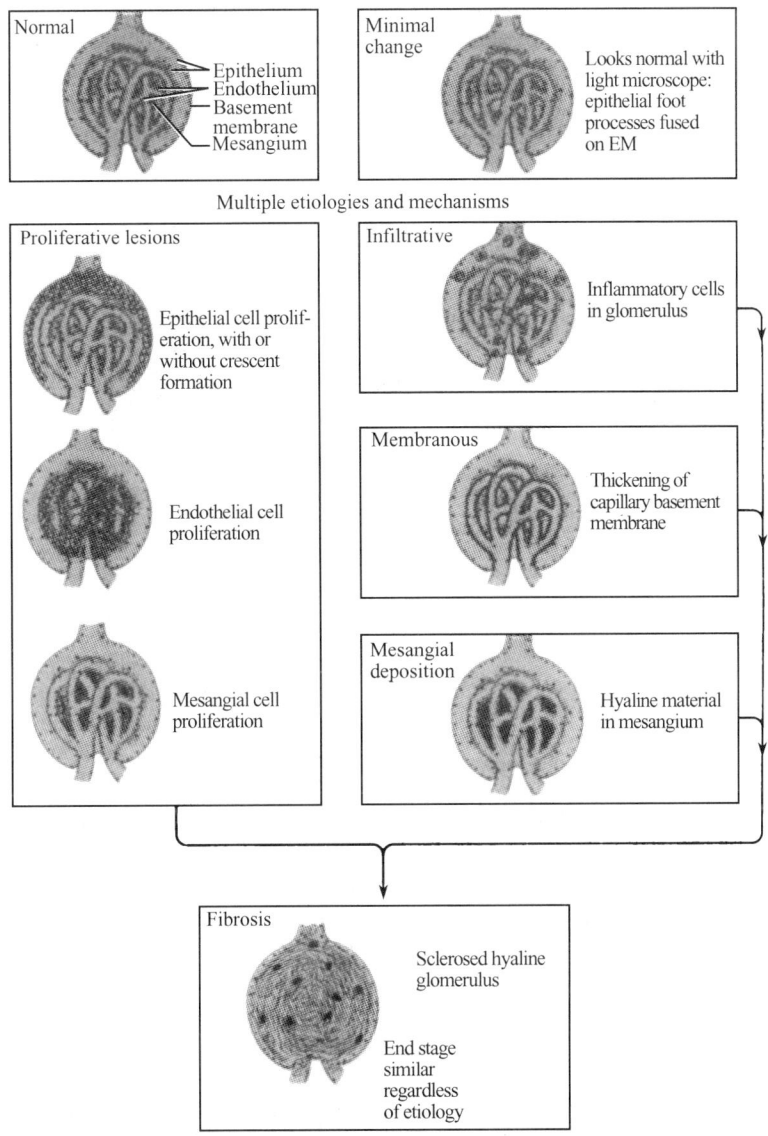

Figure 11-3 Basic pathologic changes that occur in glomerular diseases

A. Immune Complex Disease (Type III Hypersensitivity)

Immune complex disease is the most common cause of glomerular injury. Circulating immune complexs are deposited on the glomerular filtration membrane or in the mesangium (Figure 11-4); complement fixation and inflammation follow.

Immune complex deposition may produce most or all of the pathologic features described above, with one or the other predominating in different diseases. Immunoglobulin and complement are demonstrable by immunofluorescence. This staining pattern on immunofluorescence is "lumpy-bumpy" (i.e. granular), corresponding to irregular deposition of the immune complexes. Immune complexes are visible with the electron microscope as electron-dense deposits.

B. Antibody Reaction Against Antigens on the Glomerular Filtration Membrane

1. Anti-glomerular basement membrane antibody

Deposition of anti-glomerular basement membrane

(GBM) antibodies directed against epitopes on the type IV collagen molecules of the basement membrane leads to complement fixation (Figure 11-4), with glomerular lesions that by light microscopy are identical to those seen in immune complex disease. Immunofluorescence, however, shows linear deposition of immunoglobulin and complement in the base ment membrane. Linear deposition of antibody depends on the fact that the antigenic epitope is part of a repeating subunit uniformly expressed in the basement membrane.

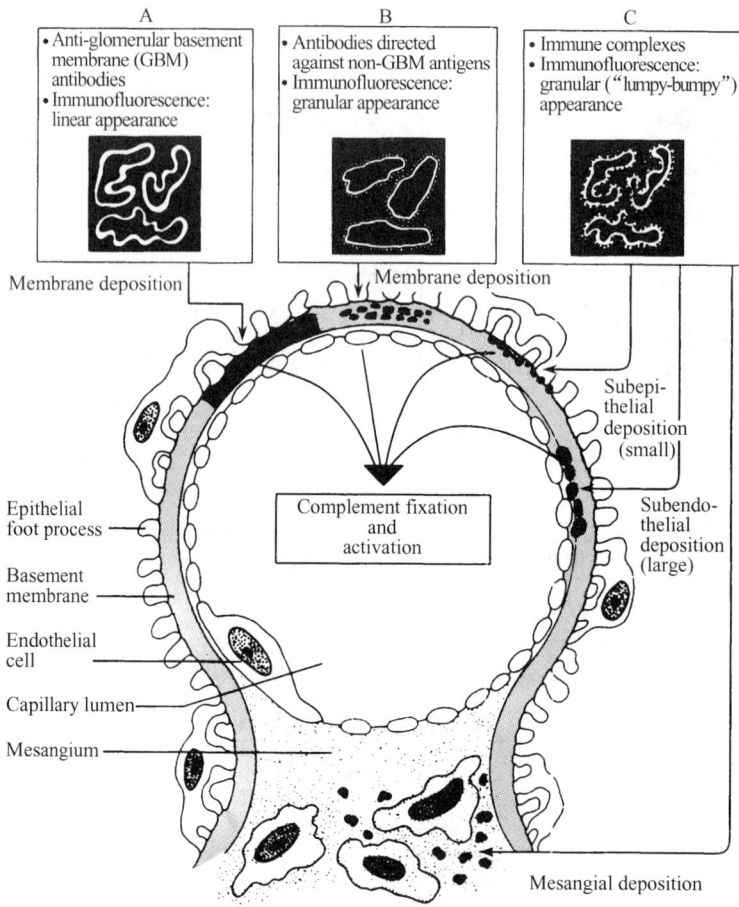

Figure. 11-4 Basic types of glomerular injury. A: Injury caused by anti – GBM antibody, which produces a linear pattern on immunofluorescence. B: Injury caused by antibodies directed against non – GBM antigens, which produces a granular pattern. C: Injury caused by immune complex deposition, which also produces a granular pattern. In most cases, glomerular damage results from complement activation due to (at left) the action of anti – glomerular basement membrane antibody, and (at right) immune complex deposition. In both instances, complement activation results in damage. These two types of injury can be distinguished by their different staining patterns on immunofluorescence

2. Antibodies against non-GBM antigens

The glomerular filtration membrane harbors other kinds of antigens against which antibodies may be directed. These non-GBM antigens are not uniformly distributed in the membrane, and antibody deposition may produce a granular rather than linear pattern on immunofluorescence, resembling immune complex injury. Two such antigen types are recognized: (1) An intrinsic antigen, which is a component of the endocytotic clathrin-coated pits of the epithelial cell is believed to be the antibody target in experimental Heymann's nephritis in rats. A similar antigen may be involved in human membranous glomerulonephritis; and (2) extrinsic antigens (derived from drugs, plant lectins, aggregated protein molecules, and products of infectious agents) may become planted on the filtration membrane and become the target for an antibody reaction.

In all these humoral immunologic reactions, complement activation occurs and represents the final common pathway for producing glomerular injury. In some cases, this is associated with inflammation and entry of neutrophils. In others, as in membranous glomerulonephritis, it leads to increased basement membrane permeability without inflammation.

CLASSIFICATION OF GLOMERULONEPHRITIS

The classification of glomerulonephritis uses a combination of clinical (congenital or acquired; acute or chronic), morphologic (proliferative, membranous, minimal change), and immunologic criteria (Table 11-7).

Table 11-7 Classification of glomerular diseases

Congenital glomerulonephritis
Hereditary nephritis (includes Alport's syndrome)
Congenital nephrotic syndrome
Primary acquired glomerulonephritis
Diffuse proliferative glomerulonephritis
Crescentic glomerulonephritis
Membranous glomerulonephritis
Minimal change glomerular disease
Focal segmental glomerulosclerosis
Membranoproliferative (mesangiocapillary) glomerulonephritis
IgA nephropathy
Chronic glomerulonephritis
Secondary acquired glomerulonephritis
Systemic lupus erythematosus
Diabetes mellitus
Amyloidosis
Goodpasture syndrome
Polyarteritis nodosa
Wegener granulomatosis
Henoch-Schöenlein purpura
Bacterial endocarditis

ACUTE DIFFUSE PROLIFERATIVE GLOMERULONEPHRITIS (ACUTE POSTSTREPTOCOCCAL GLOMERULONEPHRITIS)

Acute diffuse proliferative glomerulonephritis is one of the most common renal diseases in childhood. It is less common in adults. Occurrence is worldwide, at times in epidemic distribution.

A group A beta-hemolytic streptococcal infection of the pharynx or skin precedes the glomerulonephritis by 1 – 3 weeks. Not all streptococcal infections are associated with the risk of glomerulonephritis. Certain streptococcal M types-especially types 1, 4, 12, and 49-are "nephritogenic."

Organisms other than beta-hemolytic streptococci may cause glomerulonephritis (nonstreptococcal acute glomeruloephritis). Convincing data exist to incriminate *Staphylococcus aureus*, *Streptococcus pneumoniae*, *Neisseria meningitidis*, the plasmodia of malaria, *Toxoplasma gondii*, and some viruses.

Immune complexes formed between antigens in the organism and host antibody are deposited in the glomerular filtration membrane, fix complement, and lead to inflammation. The specific streptococcal antigen involved in forming circulating immune complexes is not known.

Pathology

Grossly, the kidneys are slightly enlarged and have a smooth surface. In severe cases there are scattered petechial hemorrhages. Light microscopic examination shows diffuse glomerulonephritis. The glomeruli are enlarged, edematous, and hypercellular (Figure 11-5; see also Table 11-8). The increased cellularity is due to proliferation of endothelial and mesangial cells plus infiltration with neutrophils and a few eosinophils. Epithelial proliferation producing crescents may be present in a few glomeruli. Rarely, crescent formation is extensive and results in rapidly progressive renal failure. Marked edema and endothelial swelling causes a narrowing of capillary lumens.

The immune complexes may be seen on light microscopy as characteristic humps, particularly in trichrome-stained sections. These correspond to large, dome-shaped electron-dense deposits on the epithelial side of the basement membrane (subepithelial humps) on electron microscopy (Figure 11-5). Deposits in other locations such as the mesangium and the subendothelial and intramembranous regions are frequently present.

Immunofluorescence shows a granular (lumpy-bumpy) deposition of IgG and C3 along the glomerular basement membrane and in the mesangium (Figure 11-5).

Clinical Features

Most patients with acute diffuse proliferative glomerulonephritis present with an abrupt onset of the acute nephritic syndrome, characterized by mild periorbital edema, hypertension, and elevated serum urea and creatinine. A few patients present with nephrotic syndrome.

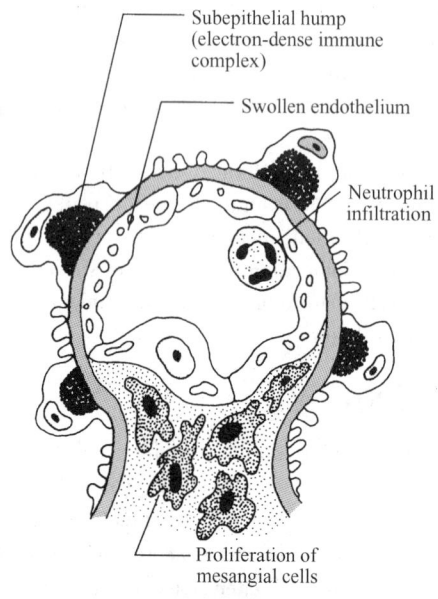

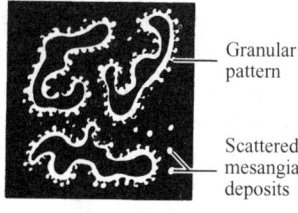

Immunofluorescence

Figure 11-5 Acute diffuse proliferative glomerulonephritis, characterized by the deposition of electron–dense immune complexes in the subepithelial and mesangial regions. Complement activation leads to proliferation of cells and inflammation

Throat and skin cultures are usually negative because the streptococcal infection has usually resolved. Serum levels of antistreptococcal antibodies such as antistreptolysin O and antihyaluronidase are often elevated. A transient reduction in serum C3 component of complement, with return to normal within 8 weeks, is common. Tests for circulating immune complexes are often positive.

Treatment and Prognosis

Treatment is supportive. The short-term prognosis is excellent, within 95% of patients making a clinical recovery within 6 weeks and returning to normal renal function within a year. Abnormalities in urinary sediment may persist for several years. A small number of patients progress rapidly to renal failure within 1–2 years. These cases are associated with the presence of numerous epithelial crescents (crescentic glomerulonephritis – see below).

The long-term prognosis is controversial. Most studies indicate that children with poststreptococcal glomerulonephritis do not suffer progressive renal disease; however, a few studies report an increased incidence of chronic renal failure after initial resolution.

The prognosis is much worse (1) in adults, in whom chronic disease occurs in 30%–50% of cases; (2) in patients who have an atypical clinical presentation; and (3) in patients who have persistent heavy proteinuria.

RAPIDLY PROGRESSIVE GLOMERULONEPHRITIS (CRESCENTIC GLOMERULONEPHRITIS)

Rapidly progressive glomerulonephritis (RPGN) is a rare disease defined by two criteria: (1) The presence of crescents in more than 70% of the glomeruli. Crescents are produced in part by proliferation of the parietal epithelial ceello in Bowman's space and in part by infiltration of monocytes. (Figure 11-6). Crescents represent irreversible damage that always causes severe residual scarring of the affected glomerulus. Fibrin can be demonstrated in the crescent and is thought to induce its formation. (2) The occurrence of rapidly progressive renal failure, with end-stage disease occurring within months after onset.

Rapidly progressive glomerulonephritis is a heterogeneous condition that probably represents the end results of severe glomerular damage occurring in many diseases (Table 11-9). So that RPGN is a clinical syndrome and not a specific etiologic form of GN. Poststreptococcal glomerulonephritis and Goodpasture's syndrome accout for many of the cases.

After these known diseases have been rules out, there remain a group of patients classified as having idiopathic rapidly progressive glomerulonephritis. In this group, approximately 20% have anti-glomerular basement membrane antibody in serum and a linear pattern on immunofluorescence (type I), and 30% have features of immune complex disease (type II). In the remaining 50%, immunofluorescece shows minimal activity (pauci-immune, or type III).

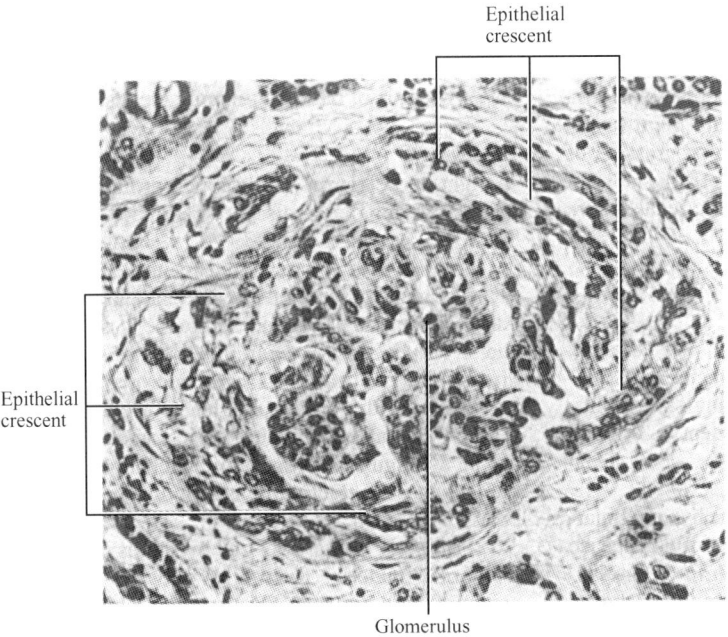

Figure 11-6 Glomerulus, showing an epithelial crescent

Pathology

Most of glomeruli (more than 70% usually) must show crescent formation for this diagnosis to be made because scattered crescents are present in many glomerular diseases. Immunofluoresence studies show variable findings depending upon the cause. Electron microscopy shows varying destructive changes in the glomeruli.

Treatment and Prognosis

Treatment is unsatisfactory, and the prognosis is very poor without dialysis or transplantation. A few cases of occurrence of the disease in transplanted kidneys have been reported.

MEMBRANOUS GLOMERULONE-PHRITIS

Membranous glomerulonephritis is an important and common cause of nephrotic syndrome in adults (mean age 35 years). It is rare in children.

Eighty-five percent of cases of membranous glomerulonephritis are idiopathic. A few cases are associated with (1) systemic infections, including hepatitis B, malaria, schistosomiasis, syphilis, and leprosy; (2) drugs such as penicillamine, captopril, and heroin, (3) toxic metals such as gold and mercury; (4) neoplasms, including carcinomas, malignant lymphomas, and Hodgkin's lymphoma; (5) collagen diseases such as systemic sclerosis, and mixed connective tissue disease; and (6) miscellaneous conditions including renal vein thrombosis and sickle cell disease.

Idiopathic membranous glomerulonephritis is characterized by the presence of IgG and complement as granular deposits in the subepithelial region indicative of a chronic antigen-antibody reaction. Circulating immune complexes are rarely present. It has been suggested that the mechanism of injury is via antibodies produced against non-GBM antigens in the basement membrane-either intrinsic (in the idiopathic form, which resembles Heymann's nephritis in experimental rats) or extrinsic planted antigens (in the secondary forms of the disease).

The mechanism whereby the antigen-antibody reaction causes injury is also unknown. Complement fixation occurs but does not cause inflammation. Rather, it increases membrane permeability, probably by action of the toxic C_{56789} complex, and stimulates synthesis of basement membrane material.

Pathology

Light and electron microscopy permit recognition of four stages of the disease (Figure 11-7; see also Table 11-8:

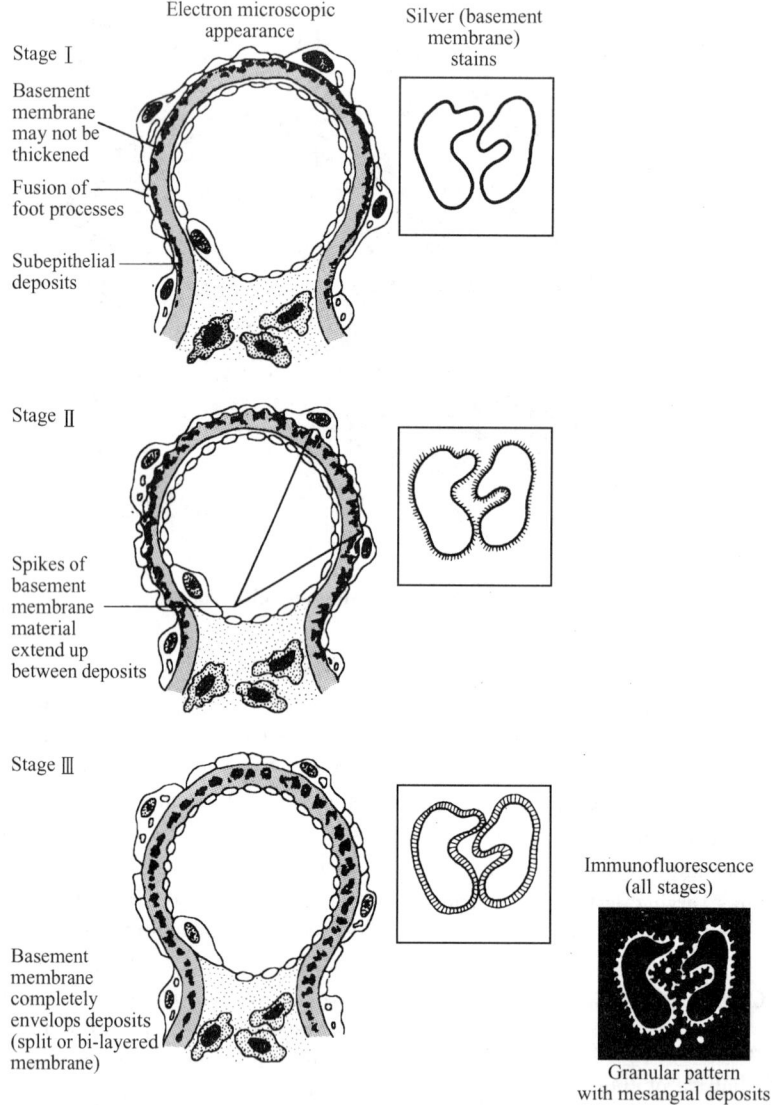

Figure 11-7 Membranous glomerulonephritis. In stage I disease, light microscopy resembles minimal change disease but can be differentiated on electron microscopy and immunofluorescence because of the presence in membranous glomerulonephritis of immune complexes. In later stages of the disease, protrusion of basement membrane material around the immune complexes produces spikes (stage II), a chain-link appearance (stage III) and irregular thicken of basement membrane (stage IV), when the basement membrane is stained with silver stains. Light microscopy shows thickened basement membrane in these later stages

Table 11-8 Differential features of glomerular disease

Disease	Usual clinical Findings	Proliferative	Membranous	Immunofluorescence Pattern	Ig	Complement	Fibrin	Electron Microscope	Diffuse/Focal	Mechanism
Acute diffuse proliferative glomerulonephritis	Acute nephritic syndrome, Nephritic syndrome	+ Crescents (occasionally)	−	Granular	IgG	+	−	Subepithelial humps	Diffuse	Immune complex
Rapidly progressive glomerulonephritis	Acute nephritic Syndrome, rapidly progressive	+ Crescents	−	Granular, linear, or pauci-immune	IgG/IgA	+	+	Variable deposits	Diffuse	Immune complex or basement membrane antibody
Membranous glomerulonephritis	Proteinuria, nephrotic syndrome, chronic renal failure	−	+	Granular	IgG	±	−	Subepithelial deposits, spikes, split basement membrane	Diffuse	Immune complex formed in situ
Minimal change glomerular disease	Nephrotic syndrome	−	−	−	−	−	−	Foot process fusion	Diffuse	T-cell mediated
Focal segmental glomerulosclerosis	Proteinuria, nephrotic syndrome	+ Focal	±	Granular	IgM, IgA	+	+	Foot process fusion	Focal plus segmental	Immune complex
Membranoproliferative Glomerulonephritis I	Acute nephritic Syndrome, nephrotic syndrome	+ Endothelial, mesangial	+	Granular	IgG	+	−	Subendothelial deposits, split basement membrane	Diffuse	Immune complex
II	Nephrotic syndrome, chronic renal failure			Granular	−	+	−	Thick basement membrane, dense deposits	Diffuse	Immune complex; probably alternative pathway
Mesangial proliferative glomerulonephritis	Nephrotic syndrome, asymptomatic proteinuria and/or hematuria, chronic nephritic syndrome	+ Mesangial	−	Mesangial	IgG/IgM	+	−	Mesangial deposits	Diffuse	unknown
IgA nephropathy	Nephrotic syndrome, proteinuria, hematuria, acute nephritic syndrome	+ Mesangial	−	Mesangial	IgA	+	−	Mesangial deposits	Diffuse	Immune complex
Chronic glomerulonephritis	Chronic renal failure	Any of above		Granular, linear; variable				Variable	Diffuse	Immune complex/antibasement membrane antibody

Table 11-9 Causes of rapidly progressive (crescentic) glomerulonephritis

Postinfectious
  Poststreptococcal glomerulonephritis
  Nonstreptococcal glomerulonephritis
  Infective endocarditis
Multisystem diseases
  Goodpasture's syndrome
  Systemic lupus erythematosus
  Henoch-Schönlein purpura
  Berger's disease (IgA nephropathy)
  Polyarteritis nodosa
  Wegener's granulomatosis
  Membranoproliferative glomerulonephritis
Drugs: Pennicillamine
Idiopathic
  Type I : with anti-GBM antibodies (20%)
  Type II : with immune complexes (30%)
  Type III : pauci-immune (50%)

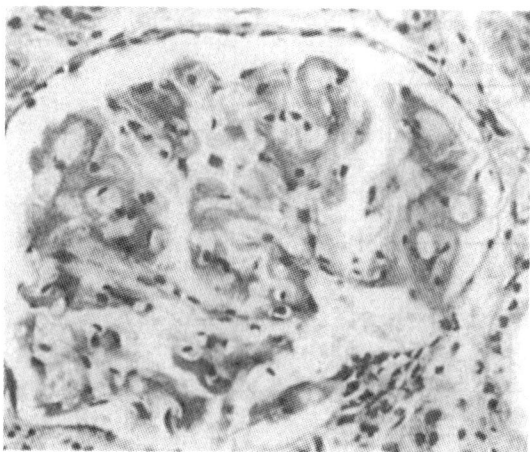

Figure 11-8 Membranous nephropathy, showing diffuse thickening of the glomerular basement membrane. Cellularity is normal

- **Stage I** is characterized by the deposition of dome-shaped subepithelial electron-dense deposits. At this stage, the basement membrane is near normal, and a misdiagnosis of minimal change glomerular disease may be made on light microscopy. Protein leakage from the glomerulus leads to epithelial foot process fusion, but membranous glomerulonephritis can be distinguished from minimal change disease by the presence of electron-dense immune complex deposits.
- **Stage II** is characterized by spikes of basement membrane material protruding outward toward the epithelial side between the deposits, which are now larger. These basement membrane spikes are seen on light microscopy with silver stains (deposits are not stained).
- **In stage III**, the spikes enlarge and fuse on the epithelial side of the deposits; on silver stains, the basement membrane now appears to be split, connected by the spikes (giving an appearance on silver stain that has been likened to a chain with the unstained immune complex deposits appearing as bubbles or holes between the links of the chain). At this stage, basement membrane thickening can be detected on routine light microscopy (Figure 11-8).
- **Stage IV** is the later stage which characterized by irregular thicken of basement membrane.

There is no hypercellularity of the glomerulus in pure membranous glomerulonephritis. With progression, increasing thickness of the basement membrane converts the glomerulus into a hyaline mass. The changes of idiopathic membranous glomerulonephritis are identical to those of secondary disease.

Immunofluorescence shows granular deposits of IgG and C3 corresponding to the subepithelial deposits.

Clinically, patients with membranous glomerulonephritis present with either the nephrotic syndrome or asymptomatic proteinuria. The proteinuria is nonselective. Hematuria is absent in the early stage of the idiopathic disease.

Most patients have a slow progression to chronic renal failure. Recent evidence suggests that 70% of patients are alive at 10 years. The prognosis is better in females and much better in children.

MINIMAL CHANGE GLOMERULO-NEPHRITIS

Minimal change glomerulonepritis disease occurs most often in young children and is relatively uncommon in adults. It accounts for 80% of cases of nephrotic syndrome in children under 8 years of age.

Etiology and Pathogenesis

The basic change in minimal change glomerulonepritis appears to be related to loss of basement membrane polyanions (mainly heparan sulfate proteoglycan), which reduces the negative charge in the membrane. This decreases the filtration barrier to anionic molecules in the plasma - such as albumin - which are permitted to pass through, often in large amounts. Selective loss of albumin among all the plasma proteins is a typical feature of minimal change glomerulonepritis. The fusion of foot processes of the epithelial cell is believed to be a nonspecific reaction to increased protein filtration.

The cause of the chemical change in the basement membrane is unknown. An immunologic basis is strongly suggested by (1) its association with infections, immunizations, and atopic disorders such as hay fever and eczema; and (2) its excellent response to immunosuppressive drugs such as corticosteroids. Its association with Hodgkin's disease (where T lymphocyte abnormalities are common) and the finding that T lymphocytes of patients with minimal change glomerulonepritis produce lymphokines when cultured with renal tissue suggest that minimal change glomerulonepritis may be a cell-mediated immunologic disease.

Pathology

Light microscopy shows no abnormality (hence the term minimal change). Immunofluorescence shows absence of immunoglobulin or complement deposition. Electron microscopy shows fusion of the foot processes of the epithelial cells (epithelial cell disease) (Figure 11-9; see also Table 11-9). These changes disappear during remission.

Clinical Features

Minimal change glomerulonephritis causes nephrotic syndrome. The proteinuria is almost always highly selective, with loss of only low-molecular-weight anionic proteins. Selectivity of proteinuria is assessed by the ratio of transferrin (low-MW) to IgG (high-MW) concentrations in urine. In highly selective proteinuria, the value is high; in nonselective proteinuria, it approaches 1. Hematuria, hypertension, and azotemia are absent.

Treatment and Prognosis

High-dosage corticosteroid therapy causes a dramatic decrease in proteinuria, with most patients showing complete remission within 8 weeks. After withdrawal of steroids, about 50% of patients relapse intermittently for up to 10 years. Those who undergo relapses are steroid-sensitive, that is, each relapse responds well to steroid therapy.

Resistance to steroids or development of renal failure is rare and should prompt a search for some other diagnosis, usually focal glomerulosclerosis or membranoproliferative glomerulonephritis. The prognosis for life and renal function for patients with minimal change glomerulonephritis is almost the same as that of the general population.

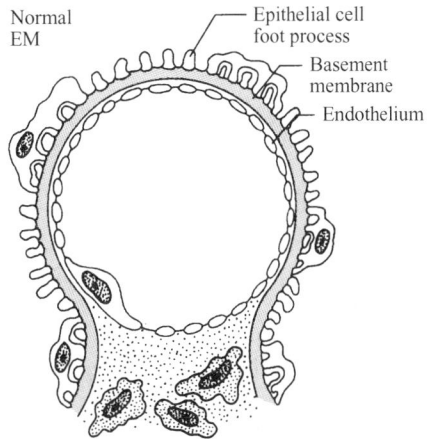

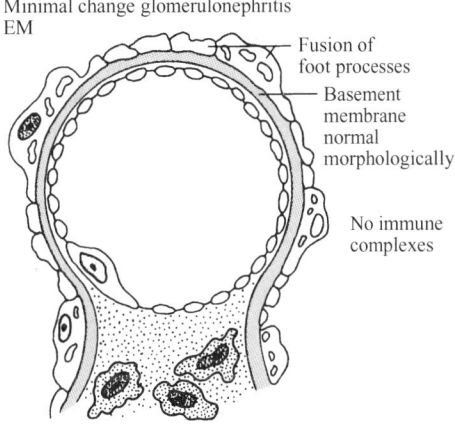

Figure 11-9 Minimal change glomerulonephritis. The only abnormality is fusion of epithelial foot processes, which is visible only by electron microscopy. Note that fusion of foot processes is not a specific abnormality

FOCAL SEGMENTAL GLOMERULO-SCLEROSIS

Focal segmental glomerulosclerosis is an uncommon disease that accounts for 10% of cases of nephrotic syndrome in children and young adults. The cause is unknown. In a few patients, focal segmental glomerulosclerosis is associated with intravenous heroin abuse, and a few cases have been described in HIV-positive patients, in whom the virus is present in glomerular and tubular epithelial cells.

Pathology

Focal segmental glomerulosclerosis is characterized by the presence of a focal segmental sclerotic area (pink hyaline material) in the peripheral part of the glomerulus, frequently near the hilum. Lipid droplets are often present as vacuoles in the sclerotic area. The glomeruli affected first are in the juxtamedullary (deep cortical) region, and a superficial renal biopsy may easily miss the involved glomeruli, leading to a diagnosis of minimal change glomerulonephritis. (Many cases of steroid-resistant minimal change glomerulonephritis prove to be focal segmental glomerulosclerosis.)

Immunofluorescence shows granular IgM, C3, and sometimes IgA, and fibrinogen deposition in the affected glomeruli. Electron microscopy shows an increase in the amount of mesangial matrix and collapse of the glomerular capillaries in areas of glomerulosclerosis. Epithelial cell foot processes are fused. In some areas, there is a loss of epithelial cells. Epithelial cell damage is believed important in pathogenesis.

Clinical Features

Focal segmental glomerulosclerosis is associated with nephrotic syndrome or asymptomatic proteinuria. The proteinuria is nonselective. Prognosis is poor, with slow progression to chronic renal failure. Focal glomerulosclerosis associated with HIV infection has a much worse prognosis, with renal failure developing 6–12 months from onset. There is no response to corticosteroid therapy. A few patients have disease recurring in the allografts after renal transplantation.

MEMBRANOPROLIFERATIVE GLOMERULONEPHRITIS (MESANGIO CAPILLARY GLOMERULONEPHRITIS)

Membranoproliferative glomerulonephritis (MPGN) is characterized by the presence of a combination of thickening of the capillary wall and proliferation of mesangial cells. Two distinct patterns are recognized (Figure 11-10).

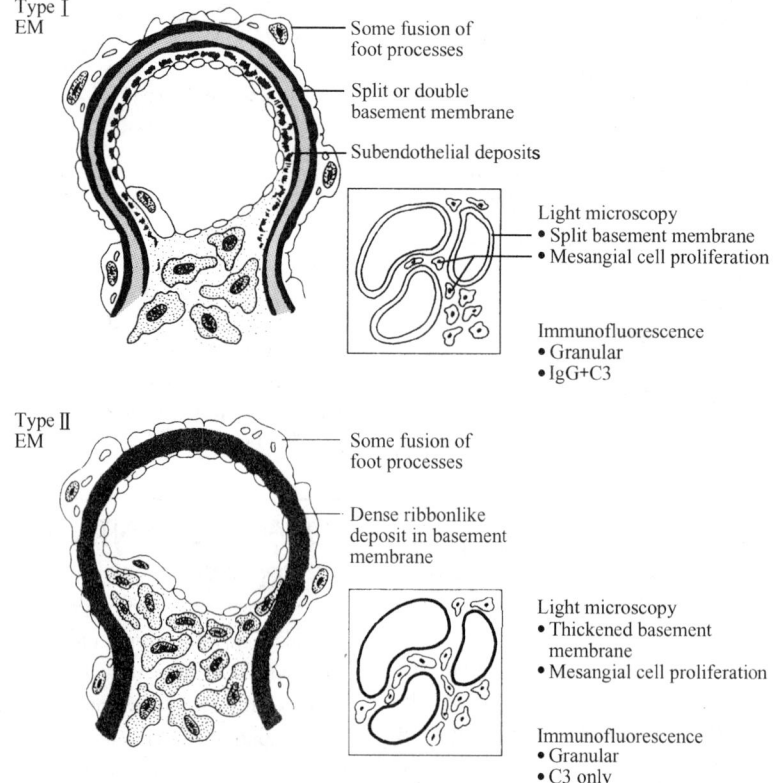

Figure 11-10 Membranoproliferative glomerulonephritis. Type I disease is characterized by subendothelial immune complexes, a split (tram track) basement membrane, and deposition of IgG and C3. Type II is characterized by a densely thickened, ribbon-like basement membrane and the presence of C3 only on immunofluorescence

Membranoproliferative Glomerulonephritis Type I(With Subendothelial Deposits)

Type I membranoproliferative glomerulonephritis accounts for 65% of cases. It is characterized by deposition of subendothelial immune complexes in the glomerular capillary. Most cases have no known cause.

Light microscopy shows diffuse thickening of capillary walls and proliferation of mesangial cells. The basement membrane appears to be split (double-contour, or tram-track, appearance). Immunofluorescence shows granular deposition of IgG and C3 in the capillary wall. Electron microscopy shows the diagnostic subendothelial deposits.

Clinically, type I is a disease of children and young adults who present with nephrotic syndrome or a mixed nephrotic-nephritic pattern. Serum C3 levels are decreased in the majority of cases. Progression is variable, but the overall prognosis is poor.

Membranoproliferative Glomerulonephritis Type II (Dense Deposit Disease)

Type II membranoproliferative glomerulonephritis accounts for the remaining 35% of cases. It is characterized by a dense intramembranous ribbon-like deposit on electron microscopy, leading to basement membrane thickening.

Light microscopy shows an eosinophilic, refractile, uniformly thickened basement membrane. Mesangial proliferation is less prominent than in type I. Immunofluorescence shows granular deposition of C3 in the capillary wall and mesangium. Immunoglobulins are not found.

Clinically, children and young adults tend to be affected most frequently. Presentation is identical to that of type I. Serum C3 levels are low, but C1q, C2, and C4 levels is normal, suggesting C3 activation by the alternative pathway. Almost all patients have C3 nephritogenic factor in the serum. C3 nephritogenic factor is an IgG autoantibody that binds to alternative pathway C3 convertase. The mechanism by which this is related to glomerular injury is unknown. The prognosis is poor.

MESANGIAL PROLIFERATIVE GLOMERULONEPHRITIS

Proliferation of mesangial cells as the only abnormality in a renal biopsy specimen is a nonspecific finding. Mesangial proliferative glomerulonephritis is best classified according to the predominant type of immunoglobulin present in the glomerulus.

IgG deposition is common and may occur as an isolated finding or in the healing phase of postinfectious glomerulonephritis. The pathogenesis is unknown in the most cases.

The light microscopy shows increased numbers of mesangial cells in the glomeruli (more than the normal three nuclei; see Figure 11-3). The mesangial matrix material is increased. Immunofluorescence shows the presence of IgG or IgM and C3 in the mesangium. Electron microscopy shows the presence of mesangial electron-dense deposits in some cases.

Clinically, children and young adults tend to be affected most frequently. The symptom is associated with nephrotic syndrome or asymptomatic proteinuria and/or hemaurine. Prognosis is various, some good, but recurrent; some poor, with slow progression to chronic renal failure.

IgA NEPHROPATHY (BERGER's DISEASE)

IgA nephropathy accounts for 10% of cases of nephrotic syndrome in both adults and children. It is most common in the age group from 10 - 30 years and has a male predominance. The etiology is unknown.

On light microscopy, there is mesangial hypercellularity and increased matrix material. Sclerosis is common with progressive disease. Immunofluorescence shows IgA deposits in the mesangium as confluent masses or discrete granules. C3 is frequently present. Electron microscopy shows mesangial hypercellularity, sclerosis, and electron-dense deposits.

Clinically, patients present with hematuria, often at the time of an upper respiratory infection. Hematuria is frequently recurrent. Proteinuria and microscopic hematuria commonly persist. Though progression of the disease is very slow, the ultimate prognosis is not good. Most patients progress to chronic renal failure after a mean interval of 6 years.

CHRONIC GLOMERULONEPHRITIS

Chronic glomerulonephritis is a common pathologic lesion in the kidney that probably represents the end stage of many diseases affecting glomeruli (Figure 11-3). Most patients give a past history suggestive of glomerular disease. In 20% of patients, the first presentation is at the end stage with chronic renal failure.

Grossly, the kidneys are greatly reduced in size, and the cortex shows a finely irregular surface (granular contracted kidney; Figure 11-11). The cortex is narrowed, corticomedullary demarcation is obscured, and the arteries stand out because of thickened walls.

Microscopically, the narrowed cortex shows a great decrease in the number of nephrons. Glomeruli show diffuse sclerosis, with many converted to hyaline balls (Figure 11-12). There is atrophy of intervening tubules, and residual tubules often show dilation and are filled with pink proteinaceous material (thyroidization). Interstitial fibrosis is present and may be severe.

Immunofluorescence and electron microscopy show variable changes. Less fibrotic glomeruli may show evidence of electron-dense deposits containing IgG, IgA, and C3. These are important in distinguishing chronic glomerulonephritis from other conditions such as hypertensive nephrosclerosis and chronic pyelonephritis that may result in sclerosis of glomeruli, granular contraction of the kidneys, and chronic renal failure. Immunoglobulin and complement deposition are not present in chronic pyelonephritis and hypertensive nephrosclerosis.

Clinically, patients show chronic renal failure and hypertension and frequently have microscopic hematuria, proteinuria, and sometimes nephrotic syndrome.

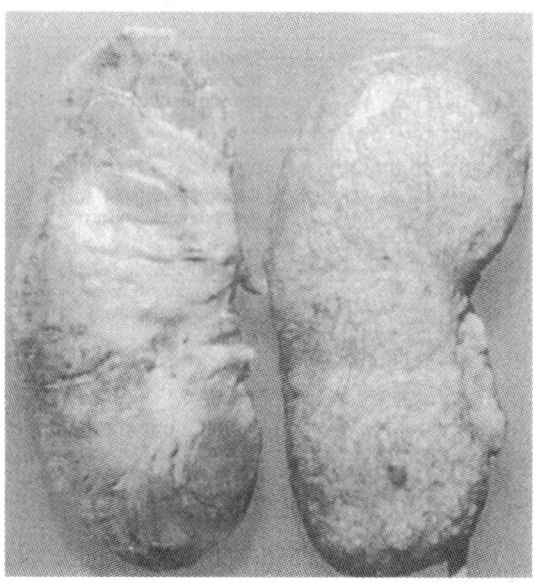

Figure 11-11 Chronic glomerulonephritis, showing a granular surface of the kidney. The cut surface shows a greatly thinned cortex and poor demarcation between cortex and medulla

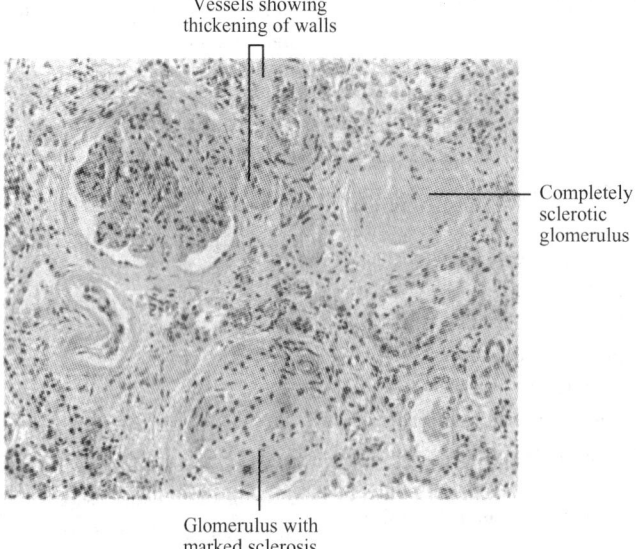

Figure 11-12 Chronic glomerulonephritis, showing three glomeruli with varying degrees of fibrosis

TUBULOINTERSTITIAL DISEASES

Tubulointerstitial Diseases are a group of renal disorders characterized by primary abnormalities in the renal tubules or interstitium. There are four principal causes: infectious, toxic, metabolic, and immunologic.

The morphologic changes in tubulointerstitial disease include the following:
• Acute tubular necrosis, which if widespread causes acute renal failure.
• Atrophy of tubules, with fibrosis of the interstitium associated with nephron loss and chronic renal failure.
• Interstitial inflammation, either acute, with numerous neutrophils in the tubules and interstitium (acute interstitial nephritis); or chronic, with lymphocytes, plasma cells, macrophages, and fibroblasts (chronic interstitial nephritis)
• Tubular basement membrane thickening, as occurs in diabetes, amyloidosis, and transplant rejection.
• Deposition of abnormal substances such as calcium, amyloid, urate, myeloma proteins, and oxalate in the tubules and interstitium.

INFECTIOUS DISEASES

Acute Pyelonephritis

A. Incidence

Acute pyelonephritis is extremely common - more so in females than in male (10:1). Acute pyelonephritis occurs at all ages, with highest frequency during early sexual activity and during pregnancy.

B. Etiology

Acute pyelonephritis is a bacterial infection, usually ascending from the lower urinary tract. Ascent of infection from the bladder is facilitated when vesicoureteral reflux is present. This is more important in children but occurs also in adults. Bacteria spread from the renal pelvis to the tubules by intrarenal reflux. Reflux from the pelvis into the tubules is common: over 60% of normal kidneys have reflux into at least one papilla. Hematogenous infection of the kidney is uncommon. Factors important in etiology are as follows (Figure 11-13):
• A short urethra, as in females.
• Stasis of urine from any cause. The high incide-

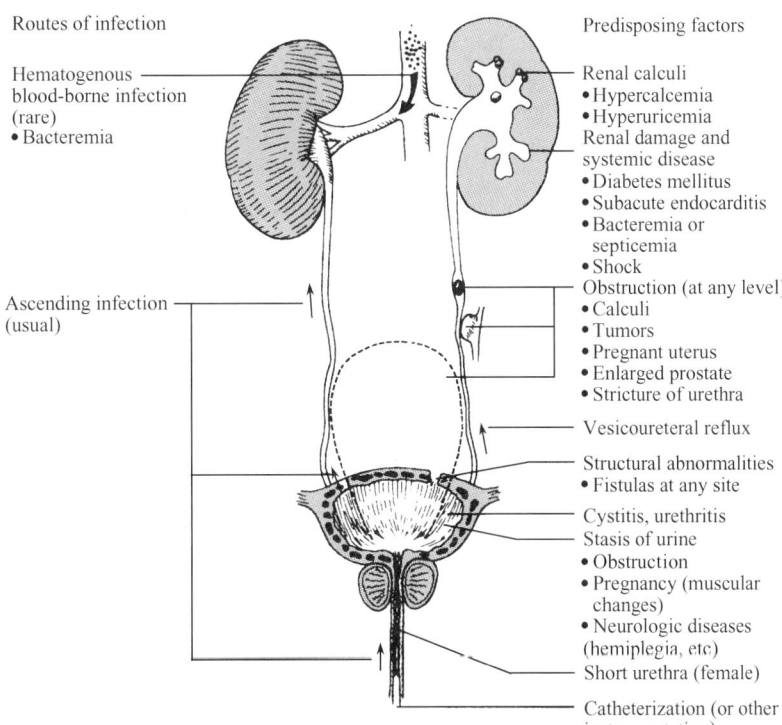

Figure 11-13 Etiologic factors associated with acute pyelonephritis

nce of urinary infections during pregnancy is believed to be the result of increased serum levels of progesterone, which decreases activity of the urinary tract smooth muscle, promoting stasis of urine.
- Structural abnormalities in the urinary tract that promote stasis of urine or establish a communication between the urinary tract and an infected site, such as fistulous tracts between the urinary tract and intestine, skin, or vagina.
- Vesicoureteral reflux of urine. Fifty percent of infants and young children with pyelonephritis show evidence of reflux, which is often familial and is due to an abnormality in the way the ureters enter the bladder.
- Catheterization of bladder. Strict aseptic precautions must be taken, and even then an indwelling urinary catheter is almost invariably associated with infection.
- Diabetes mellitus.

C. Bacteriology

Seventy-five percent of cases of acute pyelonephritis are causes by *Escherichia coli*. When infections occur secondary to obstruction or catheterization, other organisms occur more often: *Klebsiella*, *Proteus*, *Enterococcus faecalis*, and *Pseudomonas aeruginosa*.

Postpubertal females have a significant incidence (5%) of asymptomatic bacteriuria (usually *E coli*), increasing to nearly 20% in pregnancy. The relationship of asymptomatic bacteriuria to acute pyelonephritis is not clearly established.

D. Pathology

Grossly, acute pyelonephritis may be unilateral or bilateral. The kidney is enlarged and shows areas of suppuration (abscesses) in the cortex with radial yellow streaks traversing the medulla (Figure 11-14). The renal pelvis is erythematous and frequently covered with exudates. Extension to the perinephric space with formation of a perinephric abscess is not uncommon.

Microscopically, there is an acute suppurative inflammation beginning in the renal tubules, which show infiltration by neutrophils and hyperemia (Figure 11-15). Liquefactive necrosis of the tubules (suppuration) follows. Involvement is characteristically patchy.

E. Clinical Features

Onset is with high fever, chills, rigors, and flank pain. Dysuria and increased frequency are present in most cases.

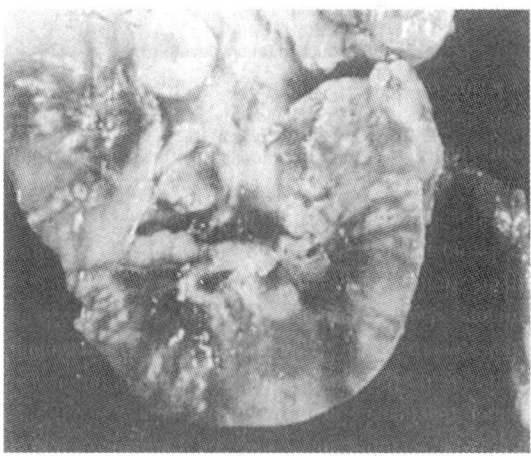

Figure 11-14 Acute pyelonephritis, showing diffuse hyperemia of the parenchyma and opened renal pelvis and multiple radially oriented suppurative streaks

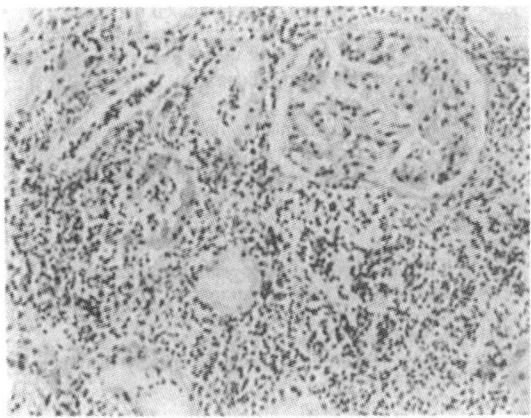

Figure 11-15 Acute pyelonephritis, showing replacement of renal tubules by acute inflammatory cells in the large part of the picture. An exudate with neutrophils is present in the lumens of some of the residual tubules

The urine shows mild proteinuria, with neutrophils, white cell casts, and bacteria in the sediment. The diagnosis is made by quantitative urine culture (colony count). A positive culture with over 100,000 organisms/mL is diagnostic.

F. Treatment and Prognosis

Treatment with antibiotics is effective. In an uncomplicated case, an antibiotic is selected that has activity against *E coli* (e.g. ampicillin or trimethoprim-sulfamethoxazole). When culture and antibiotic sensitivity results are available, the antibiotic may be changed accordingly.

The prognosis is excellent. Most patients recover completely, and there are no long-term sequelae from a single episode. Recurrent attacks are associated with increasing fibrosis and may lead to chronic pyelonephritis.

G. Complications

1. Gram-negative sepsis with shock

Blood culture is frequently positive in patients with acute pyelonephritis. In a few cases, bacteremia is severe and causes Gram-negative shock. The mortality rate is then high.

2. Pyonephrosis

When infection supervenes in an obstructed, hydronephrotic kidney, the dilated pelvicaliceal system becomes filled with pus. This is called pyonephrosis.

3. Perinephric abscess

Extension of infection through the renal capsule leads to abscess formation in the perinephric fat.

4. Renal papillary necrosis

Patients with diabetes mellitus who develop acute pyelonephritis tend to have more severe disease characterized by renal papillary necrosis (extreme inflammation of the papillae, which become necrotic and slough into the calices).

5. Emphysematous pyelonephritis

This disorder, characterized by anaerobic bacterial fermentation of glucose with gas formation in the renal parenchyma, occurs rarely in diabetic patients. Radiologic visualization of gas in the renal parenchyma is the basis for clinical diagnosis. Emphysematous pyelonephritis is a severe infection, often complicated by gram-negative shock and death. It is an indication for emergency nephrectomy.

Chronic Pyelonephritis

A. Incidence and Etiology

Infectious chronic pyelonephritis accounts for 15% - 20% of cases of chronic renal failure. Several different etiologic factors are recognized (Figure 11-16).

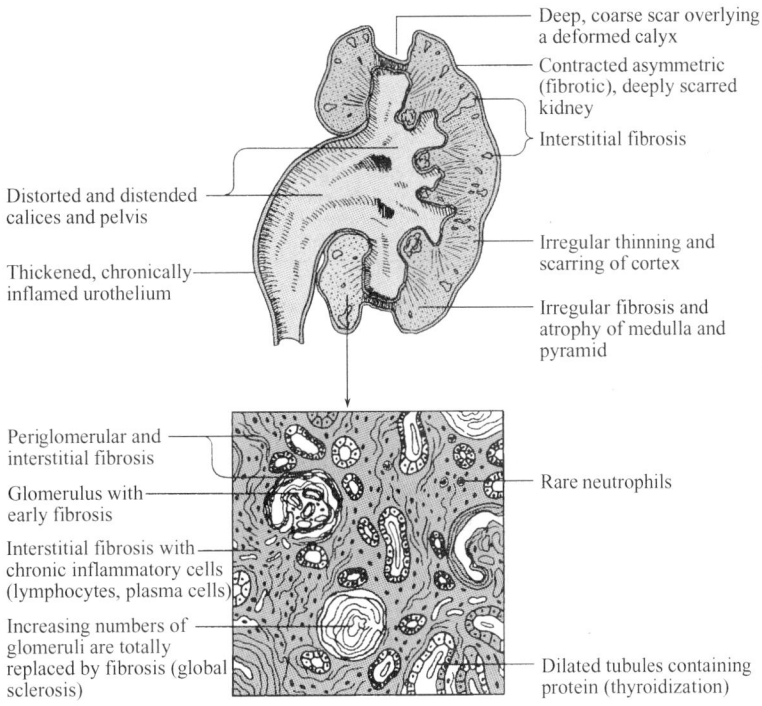

Figure 11-16 Pathologic features of chronic pyelonephritis

1. Chronic obstructive pyelonephritis

Chronic obstructive pyelonephritis is common and occurs at all ages in both sexes. Obstruction may be mechanical (e.g. calculi, prostatic hyperplasia, tumors, congenital anomalies, retroperitoneal fibrosis) or paralytic (neurogenic [neuropathic] bladder). About 50% of patients give a history of a previous episode of acute pyelonephritis.

2. Chronic pyelonephritis associated with vesicoureteral reflux

About 50% of children with vesicoureteral reflux develop chronic pyelonephritis; regurgitation of urine from the renal pelvis into the collecting tubules may be etiologically important. Early diagnosis of childhood vesicoureteral reflux (by voiding cystography) permits treatment to prevent chronic pyelonephritis.

B. Pathology (Figure 11-16)

Kidneys involved by chronic pyelonephritis usually show asymmetric involvement, with irregular scarring and contraction. Deep cortical pits due to scarring over a deformed calix are typical. Deformity of the pelvicaliceal system is common. Hydronephrosis and suppuration may be present in cases due to obstruction (chronic suppurative pyelonephritis).

Chronic pyelonephritis may be distinguished grossly from chronic glomerulonephritis by the asymmetry of renal involvement and the larger size of the cortical scars (pitted scarred kidney) in the former.

Microscopically, there is marked patchy inflammation and fibrosis of the interstitium. The inflammatory cells are lymphocytes and plasma cells with scattered neutrophils. Periglomerular fibrosis later progresses to global sclerosis. Hypertrophy and dilation of surviving tubules may be present (called thyroidization because the numerous packed, dilated tubules superficially resemble thyroid follicles). Immunofluorescence and electron microscopy do not show immune complex deposition in the glomeruli (Table 11-10).

Cases in which lipid-laden foamy histiocytes are conspicuous are sometimes classified as xanthogranulomatous pyelonephritis. Xanthogranulomatous inflammation is associated with enlargement of the kidney and the presence of caliceal staghorn calculi. The inflammatory process frequently extends into the perinephric tissues and may involve adjacent organs (e. g. colon, skin of the back, diaphragm, and pleura). Rarely, fistulas form between the renal pelvis and these organs.

Table 11-10 Differential diagnosis of a granular, contracted kidney

	Chronic Glomerulonephritis	Chronic Pyelonephritis	Benign Nephrosclerosis (Hypertension)
Renal involvement	Symmetric	Asymmetric	Symmetric
Granularity of surface	Fine	Coarse	Fine
Glomeruli	Global sclerosis	Periglomerular fibrosis	Global sclerosis
Interstitial inflammation	Mild or absent	Present	Mild od absent
Vascular changes	Present	Present	Present, marked
Ig, C3, immune complexes	Present	Absent	Absent
Bacterial culture	Negative	May be positive	Negative

C. Clinical Features

Chronic pyelonephritis usually manifests as hypertension or chronic renal failure. Pyuria (neutrophils in urine), mild proteinuria, and bacteriuria are present. In end-stage pyelonephritis, bacteriuria may be absent, and differentiation from chronic glomerulonephritis then becomes difficult.

TOXIC TUBULOINTERSTITIAL DISEASES

Analgesic Nephropathy

Excessive use of analgesics is a relatively common cause of chronic renal disease in Australia and Europe but is rare in the United States. Analgesic nephropathy was first described following the use of analgesic powders containing phenacetin, aspirin, and caffeine. Phenacetin is believed to be the main offender.

Pathologically, analgesic nephropathy is characterized by necrosis of the apices of the renal papillae (renal papillary necrosis), which may be shed in the urine, causing ureteral colic. Interstitial medullary fibrosis and calcification may also occur. The mechanism of necrosis of renal papillae is unknown.

Clinically, there is hematuria, ureteral colic, hypertension, and progressive renal failure. The diagnosis may be suspected radiologically by the presence of calcification in the renal papillary region.

In some cases, the shed necrotic renal papillary tissue may be identified in a sample of urine.

Drug-induced Nephrotoxicity

A. Acute Interstitial Nephritis

Several drugs cause acute interstitial nephritis. Methicillin, other penicillin derivatives, sulfonamides, and various diuretics have been incriminated. Many cases show features of an immune hypersensitivity reaction. Immunofluorescence shows linear deposition of IgG, C3, and part of the methicillin molecule in the tubular basement membrane in methicillin-induced cases.

Pathologically, there is tubular degeneration and necrosis and marked inflammation of the interstitium with lymphocytes, plasma cells, and eosinophils.

Clinically, patients develop renal symptoms about 2 weeks after exposure to the drug. Fever, hematuria, proteinuria, skin rash, and eosinophilia are common. Acute renal failure develops in 50% of cases.

Recovery usually occurs when the drug is withdrawn.

B. Acute Renal Tubular Necrosis

Drug-induced acute renal tubular necrosis has been reported as result of exposure to (1) aminoglycosides (gentamicin, kanamycin); (2) amphotericin B, an antifungal agent; (3) cephaloridine; and (4) methoxyflurane, an anesthetic agent.

NEOPLASMS OF THE KIDNEY AND THE URINARY BLADDER

RENAL CELL CARCINOMA

Renal cell carcinoma is the most common malignant neoplasm of the kidney (Table 11-11) and accounts for 2%-3% of all cancers in adults. It occurs most frequently in the sixth decade but is not rare in younger patients. It is believed to be derived from proximal tubular epithelial cells. No strong etiologic factors have been identified; 60% of patients with von Hippel-Lindau syndrome and 10% with dialysis cystic disease of the kidney develop renal cell carcinoma. Tumors are frequently multiple and bilateral in these cases. Many renal cell carcinomas are associated with deletions in chromosome 3, suggesting that absence of a recessive gene that encodes a tumor suppressor substance may be involved in the pathogenesis. Familial forms of renal carcinoma are associated with 3;8 and 3;11 translocations.

Table 11-11 Malignant renal neoplasms; Risk factors

	Renal Cell Carcinoma	Transition Carcinoma of Renal Pelvis	Nephroblastoma
Age	50 +	50 +	0 - 10 years
Sex	M > F	M > F	M = F
Frequency	90% of adults renal cancers	10% of adult renal cancers	99% of childhood renal cancer
Genetic factors	Rare familial cases; deletion involving chromosome 3	None known	Deletion of part of chromosome 11 in some case
Associated conditions	Von Hippel-Lindau syndrome (rare); dialysis cystic disease	Other urothelial neoplasms	Aniridia
Identified etiologic factors	Thorotrast (rare); smoking (slight effect)	smoking (marked influence), calculi, aniline dyes	None

Pathology

Grossly, renal cell carcinoma varies in size from small to massive. Commonly solid (Figure 11-17), it may contain cystic areas or may be predominantly cystic (Figure 11-18). The cut surface is variegated, with yellow-orange areas mottled with hemorrhagic (red-black) and fibrous (gray) areas (Figure 11-17). Calcification is common. The yellow color of the neoplasm is caused by the high lipid content of the neoplastic cells.

Renal cell carcinomas may infiltrate locally through the capsule of the kidney and rarely through the fascia around the perinephric fat to infiltrate surrounding organs (Figure 11-19). Invasion into renal vein is common; occasionally, tumor extends along the lumen of the inferior vena cava - rarely, all the way into the right atrium.

·340· **TEXTBOOK OF PATHOLOGY**

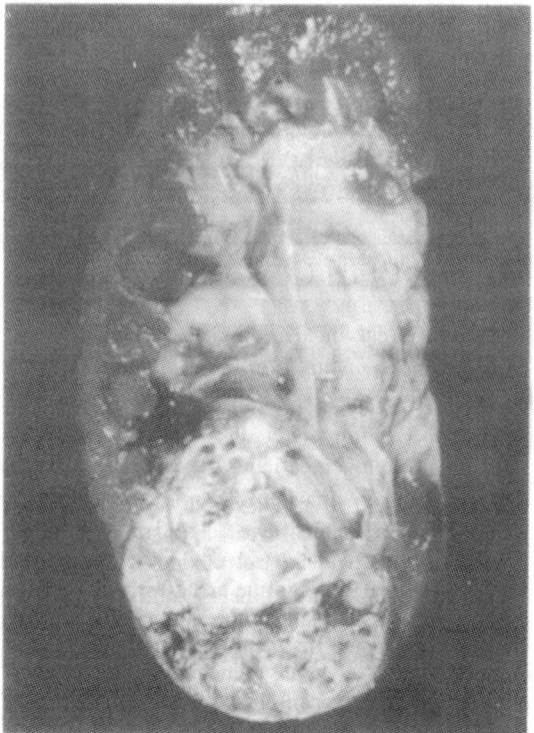

Figure 11-17 Renal cell carcinoma. Typical appearance, showing a solid mass with a variegated cut surface. The tumor is confined to the kidney in this example

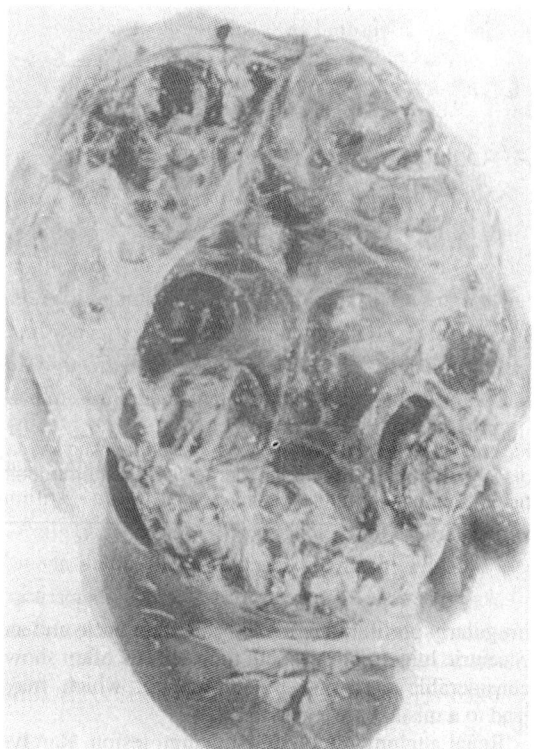

Figure 11-18 Renal cell carcinoma, predominantly cystic. Solid foci are seen at the bottom and on the left side of the mass

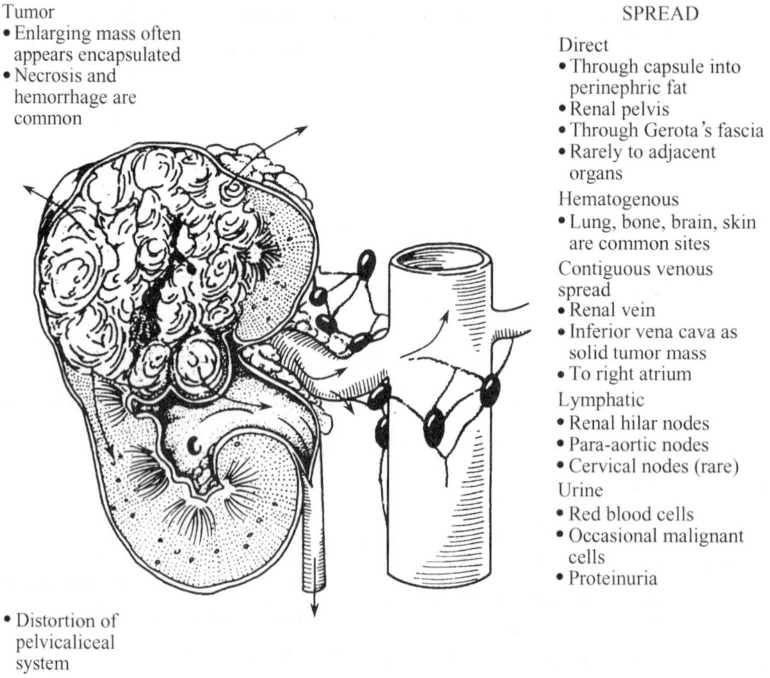

Tumor
- Enlarging mass often appears encapsulated
- Necrosis and hemorrhage are common

- Distortion of pelvicaliceal system

SPREAD

Direct
- Through capsule into perinephric fat
- Renal pelvis
- Through Gerota's fascia
- Rarely to adjacent organs

Hematogenous
- Lung, bone, brain, skin are common sites

Contiguous venous spread
- Renal vein
- Inferior vena cava as solid tumor mass
- To right atrium

Lymphatic
- Renal hilar nodes
- Para-aortic nodes
- Cervical nodes (rare)

Urine
- Red blood cells
- Occasional malignant cells
- Proteinuria

Figure 11-19 Pathologic features and spread of renal cell carcinoma

Microscopically, based on the molecular origins of the tumor, renal cell carcinomas are classified as three most common forms: clear cell carcinomas, papillary renal cell carcinomas and chromophobe renal carcinomas. The cells of clear cell renal carcinoma are composed of a mixture of clear cells and granular oncocytic cells. The clear cells are large, with small nuclei and abundant clear cytoplasm rich in lipid and glycogen (Figure 11-20). There is little cytologic atypia. The granular cells present pink granular cytoplasm, with small round, regular nuclei. Necrosis, cystic change, calcification, the cells are arranged in glandular papillary and tubular formations separated by a highly vascular stroma and hemorrhage are commonly present.

Papillary renal cell carcinoma exhibit varying degrees of papilla formation separated by a highly vascular stroma. The cells can have clear or pink cytoplasm. Chromophobe type renal cell carcinoma cells usually present clear, flocculent cytoplasm with very prominent, distinct cell membranes. The nuclei are surrounded by halos of cleared cytoplasm.

A histologic grading system ranging from grade I (well-differentiated) to grade IV (anaplastic) has been shown to correlate with prognosis. The nuclear size and appearance form the basis for histologic grading.

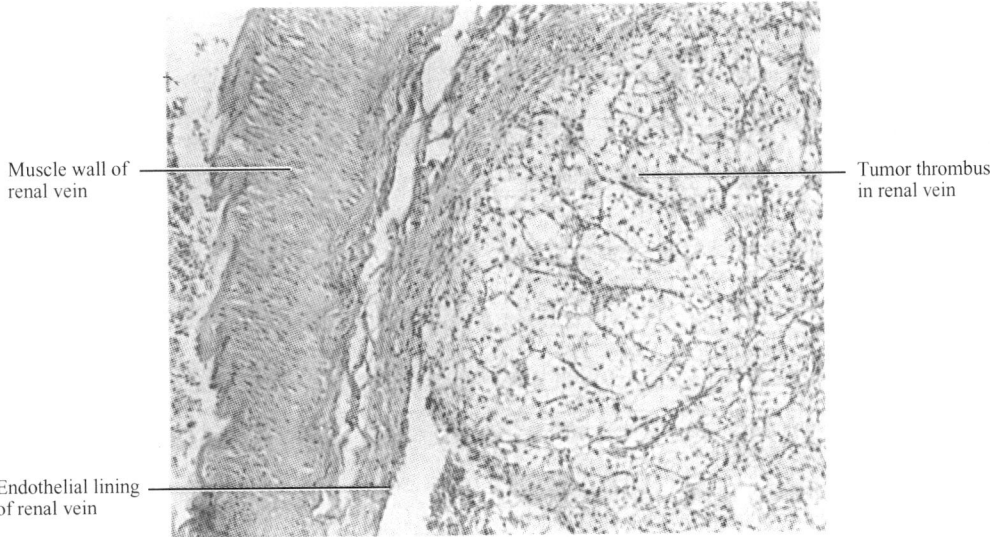

Figure 11-20 Renal cell carcinoma, clear cell type, showing tumor in the renal vein at the hilum

Clinical Features

The usual presentation is with hematuria (Table 11-12). A renal mass may be palpable when the tumor reaches a large size. Metastases occur early and may be the reason for clinical presentation when they occur with relatively small asymptomatic tumors. Common metastatic sites are lungs, bone, liver, brain, and skin.

Extension of the neoplasm into the renal vein on the left side may obstruct the testicular vein, which drains into it, causing a scrotal varicocele. Extension into the renal vein may also very rarely cause venous infarction of the kidney. Extension into the inferior vena cava may occlude it, leading to edema in the lower extremities.

A few renal cell carcinomas secrete hormones, including (1) parathyroid hormone-like substances that cause hypercalcemia, low serum phosphate, and a clinical syndrome resembling primary hyperparathyroidism; (2) erythropoietin, causing polycythemia; and (3) other hormones such as prolactin (causing galactorrhea), renin (causing hypertension), prostaglandins, and gonadotropins.

The diagnosis is made by intravenous pyelography, CT scan, or angiography, which show the presence of a renal mass. These radiologic studies are important in identifying the extent of invasion, such as involvement of a renal vein or inferior vena cava, which may require special handling at surgery.

Table 11-12 Clinical presentation of renal cell carcinoma

Hematuria	70%
Flank mass	50%
Flank pain	50%
Fever	5%
Metastatic disease	5%
Left scrotal varicocele Inferior vena caval obstruction Polycythemia (erythropoietin production) Hypercalcemia (parathyroid hormone-like molecule) Hypertension (renin production) Cushing's syndrome (adrenocorticotropic hormone-like molecule) Galactorrhea (prolactin production)	Rare

Treatment and Prognosis

Treatment of renal cell carcinoma is surgical removal, which is very successful in clinical stage I carcinomas. The prognosis correlates well with clinical stage (Table 11-13). Histologic grade is a relatively minor prognostic indicator.

Renal cell carcinoma is unpredictable in its biologic behavior. It has been known in rare cases to regress spontaneously, and it is not uncommon for metastases to regress, at least temporarily, after removal of the primary neoplasm. Renal cell carcinoma may also remain dormant for long periods, and cases have been recorded in which a metastatic lesion has occurred up to 30 years after treatment of the primary tumor.

Table 11-13 Renal cell carcinoma; commonly used staging system in the United States. The TNM system uses different criteria and probably replace this system ultimately

Stage	Criteria	5-year Survival Rate[1]
I	Confined to kidney; no capsular invasion	70%
II	Invades perinephric fat	30%
III	Involvement of renal vein[2] or regional nodes	<10%
IV	Extension beyond perinephric fat (Gerota's fascia) or distant metastases	<5%

[1] Five-year survival rate following aggressive surgery, with radio- and chemotherapy where appropriate.

[2] Recent evidence suggests that survival rates in patients with renal vein involvement, including cases where the tumor thrombus extends into the inferior vena cava, are much high than 10% if patients are treated with radical surgery. Reevaluation of renal vein involvement as a criterion for stage III disease is necessary.

NEPHROBLASTOMA (WILMS' TUMOR)

Nephroblastoma is the most likely common of renal cancers in childhood. Most cases occur between 1 and 7 years of age. Adult nephroblastoma occurs rarely.

Nephroblastoma is believed to arise from primitive blastema cells that may persist in the outer part of the kidney in the first few months of life. A virus is known to cause nephroblastoma in birds. An antigen (W antigen) has been found in some human tumors and may be a clue to a viral origin of this neoplasm.

Genetic Features

All bilateral and approximately one-third of unilateral nephroblastomas are hereditary. Many patients have deletions in the short arm of chromosome 11, including loss of the cancer suppressor gene WT-1. Loss of both normal alleles is required for the development of Wilm's tumor. In the inherited form of the disease, one allele is inherited in a defective form so that only one acquired mutation is required. Hereditary Wilms' tumor is associated with aniridia.

Pathology

Grossly, nephroblastoma is commonly a large, firm tumor that is usually soft but may undergo cystic change (Figure 11-21). Bilateral nephroblastoma occurs in about 8% of cases. Microscopically, the most primitive nephroblastomas resembles renal blastema, which is the primitive mesodermal tissue of the embryonic renal anlage and is composed of small, somewhat spindle-shaped cells with hyperchromatic nuclei and scant cytoplasm. Undifferentiated neoplasms may display anaplasia, necrosis, and a high rate of mitotic figures. Differentiation may occur into epithelial tubular structures, primitive glomerular structures

(Figure 11-22), and a variety of mesenchymal tissues such as cartilage, smooth muscle, striated muscle, and bone. Rarely, tumors of childhood resembling Wilms' tumor are composed of cells showing primitive skeletal muscle-like differentiation (rhabdoid sarcoma) or clear cells (clear cell sarcoma). These histologic subtypes have a more aggressive behavior than the usual Wilms' tumor and represent tumors that respond poorly to treatment and are associated with high mortality rates.

According to the degree of differentiation, three histologic grades are recognized. Grade I (differeti-

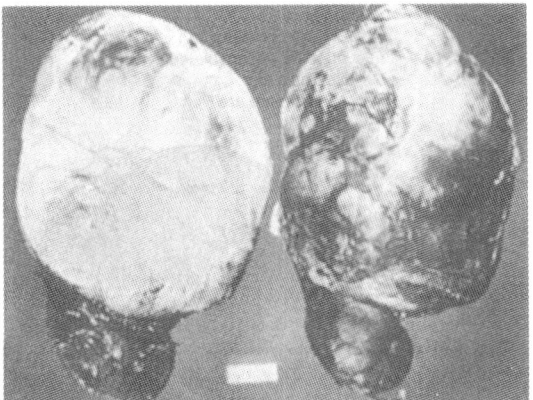

Figure 11-21 Nephroblastoma (Wilms' tumor). The cut surface (left) has a fleshy homogeneous appearance with focal hemorrhage. The kidney is greatly enlarged

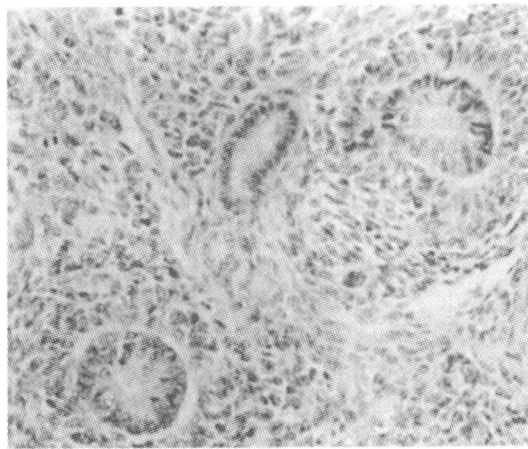

Figure 11-22 Nephroblastoma, showing primitive oval cells resembling renal blastema with focal differentiation into tubules

ated) neoplasms have the best prognosis. Grade III (anaplastic) neoplasms have the worst prognosis.

Clinical Features and Treatment

Most patients with nephroblastoma present with a large abdominal mass that is usually felt by a parent. Nephroblastoma is staged clinically according to the size of tumor, the presence of tumor on either side of the midline, and distant spread. Treatment combines surgery, radiation, and chemotherapy. The prognosis has improved dramatically with introduction of more effective chemotherapeutic agents (e.g. dactinomycin, vincristine). Currently, the 5-year survival rate exceeds 80% even when metastases are present. For tumors confined to the kidney and resected surgically, the 5-year survival rate exceeds 90%.

UROTHELIAL NEOPLASMS OF THE URINARY BLADDER

Bladder cancer is fairly common, and it is responsible for about 3% of cancer deaths in the United States and Europe. The incidence is 40,000 per year in the United States and the death rate is 10,000 per year. The disease has a marked geographic variation. In Japan, the incidence is extremely low, while in Egypt it accounts for 40% of cancers (because of the high incidence of schistosomiasis)

Etiology

Bladder cancer has been related to several chemical carcinogens such as aniline dyes containing benzidine and 2α-naphthylamine, which were responsible for bladder cancer in workers in the dye, rubber, and insulating cable industries. The latent period may be many years.

Probably the most important etiologic factor in the genesis of human bladder cancer in the United States is cigarette smoking. Smoking increases the risk to two to four times that of nonsmokers. The mechanism by which smoking causes bladder cancer is unknown. In Egypt, schistosomiasis is important, producing squamous metaplasia, dysplasia, and squamous carcinoma.

Abnormalities in chromosomes 9 and 17 have been reported in the cells of urothelial neoplasms.

Pathology

A. Overt Urothelial Neoplasms

Urothelial neoplasms may occur anywhere in the

bladder mucosa. The most common locations are near the trigone or in a diverticulum. Large tumors may involve a large area of the mucosal surface and cause obstruction of the ureteral orifices (Figure 11-23).

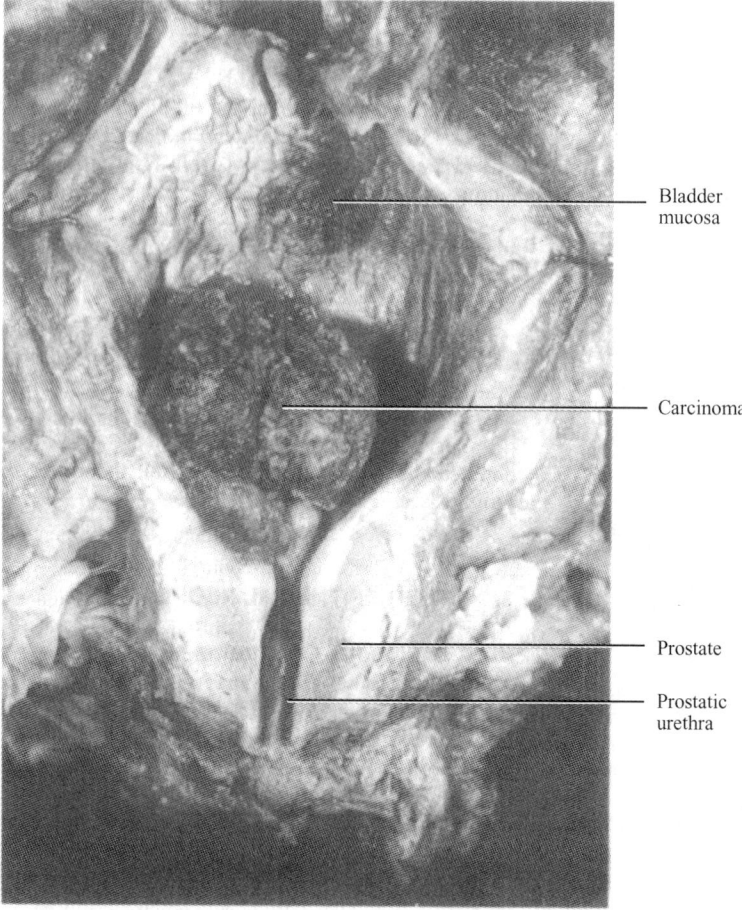

Figure 11-23   Bladder carcinoma, showing a large neoplasm almost filling the lower half of the bladder

The better-differentiated urothelial neoplasms commonly project into the lumen and have a delicate papillary appearance. In contrast, poorly differentiated neoplasms are solid ulcerative lesions that frequently show evidence of infiltration of the bladder wall.

Microscopically, over 90% are transitional cell carcinomas. Squamous or glandular differentiation commonly occurs in transitional cell carcinomas.

The international (WHO) histologic grading system for urothelial neoplasms recognizes four histologic grades.

- **Transitional cell papilloma** is a well-differentiated noninvasive papillary neoplasm that has seven or fewer layers of cytologically normal transitional cells lining the papillary fronds. This tumor is rare and benign but tends to be multifocal, often recurring after surgery.
- **Grade I transitional cell carcinoma** shows well-formed papillary structures lined by an epithelium that is cytologically normal but thicker than seven layers. Invasion is uncommon.
- **Grade II transitional cell carcinoma** has papillary and solid areas. The cells show mild to moderate cytologic atypia and have a greater degree of pleomorphism (Figure 11-24). Invasion may occur.
- **Grade III transitional cell carcinoma** has a predominantly solid invasive growth pattern with or without a papillary structure and shows cytologic anaplasia and a high rate of mitotic figures. It may be difficult to recognize its transitional cell nature. Some authorities recognize a grade IV carcinoma, which represents a more anaplastic variant of grade III with evidence of cell necrosis.

The critical distinction in terms of behavior and treatment is between grade I or II (well-differentiated) and grade III (poorly differentiated) carcinomas.

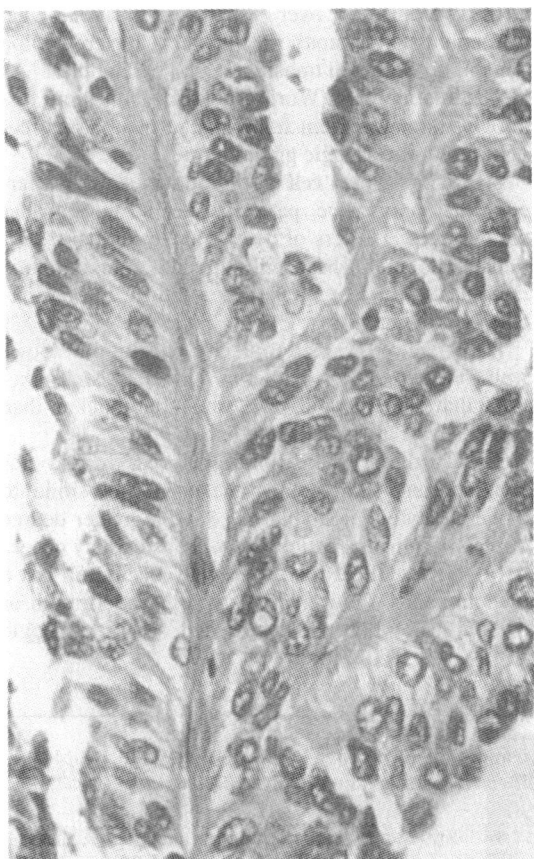

Figure 11-24 Transitional cell carcinoma of the bladder, showing papillary fronds lined by atypical transitional epithelium

Grade III carcinomas are frequently associated with carcinoma in situ of the adjacent mucosa (see below).

Infiltration of the tumor must be assessed independently of histologic grade. Infiltration of lamina propria, muscle wall, or blood vessels has adverse prognostic significance.

B. Dysplasia and Carcinoma in Situ

In high-grade bladder carcinomas, the urothelium is believed to progress through dysplasia to carcinoma in situ before it invades the basement membrane. Carcinoma in situ usually occurs in men over 40 years of age and causes no symptoms or gross changes in the bladder mucosa. Random bladder biopsy or cytologic examination of urine is necessary for diagnosis. Microscopically, the epithelium shows disturbed maturation and cytologic abnormalities such as an increased nuclear: cytoplasmic ratio, disturbed chromatin pattern, and hyperchromasia. Cytologic examination of urine shows maliganant transitional cells.

Carcinoma in situ is frequently multifocal and may extend into the urethra and ureters. The prognosis is bad, with many patients developing high-grade invasive carcinoma.

Clinical Features

Painless hematuria is the most common presenting symptom of bladder carcinoma. Involvement of the trigone may cause frequency and dysuria. Involvement of the ureteral orifice may lead to hydronephrosis and infection. Rarely, invasion of adjacent organs (colon, vagina) (Figure 11-25) leads to fistulous tracts. Dysplaisa and carcinoma in situ are asymptomatic.

The diagnosis is made by cytoscopy and biopsy.

Clinical Staging

Clinical staging depends on the degree of invasion by the neoplasm and the presence of lymph node and distant metastases (Table 11-14).

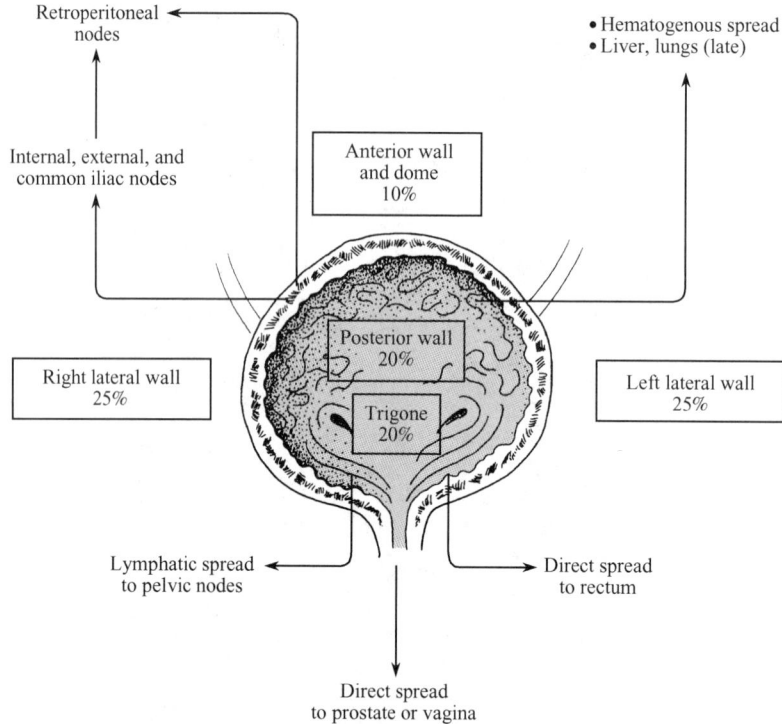

Figure 11-25 Mode of dissemination of urothelial neoplasms of the bladder. The percentages refer to the distribution of cancers in different parts of the bladder

Table 11-14 Staging of transitional cell carcinoma of the bladder[1]

Stage 0	PIS	Carcinoma in situ
	PA	Papillary neoplasm without invasion
Stage A	P1	Invasion of lamina propria
Stage B1	P2	Invasion of superficial half of the muscle wall
Stage B2	P3a	Invasion of deep half of the muscle wall
Stage C	P3b	Invasion through bladder wall into perivesical fat
Stage D1	P4a	Invasion of prostate, vagina, or uterus
	P4b	Tumor fixed to pelvic or abdominal wall
	N1-3	Pelvic nodes involved
Stage D2	M1	Distant metastases
	N4	Involvement of lymph nodes above the aortic bifurcation

[1] These designations are based on the TNM staging system, which is being used more frequently. In this system, P = characteristics of the primary tumor based on pathologic examination; N = node status; M = metastatic status.

Treatment and Proganosis

The mainstay of treatment of bladder cancer is surgery. Radical cystectomy is indicated for poorly differentiated carcinomas and well differentiated carcinomas in which there is muscle invasion. Local resection or partial cystectomy suffices for better-differentiated noninvasive neoplasma. Immunotherapy with intravesical BCG has proved effective for dysplasia and carcinoma in situ.

The prognosis depends both ion clinical stage and histologic grade. With appropriate surgical resection, 50% - 80% of patients with stage II neoplasms survive 5 years. With local extension outside the bladder, the 5-year survival rate drops to 20% - 30%. The better differentiated the neoplasm (lower grade), the better the prognosis.

Chapter 12 Diseases of the Genital System and Breast

Yao Junxia, Li Lianhong, Song Bo

CHAPTER CONTENTS
- The Uterus
    Structure and Function
- Diseases of Cervix
    Chronic Cervicitis
    Neoplasms of the cervix
- Diseases of Body of Uterus
    Endometriosis
    Endometrial Hyperplasia
    Neoplasms of Body of Uterus
- Gestational Trophoblastic Diseases
    Hydatidiform Mole
    Invasive Mole
    Choriocarcinoma
    Placental Site Trophoblastic Tumor
- Ovarian Tumors
    Normal Structure of Ovary
    Classification
    Epithelial Tumors
    Germ Cell Neoplasms
    Gonadal Stromal Neoplasms
- Diseases of the Prostate
    Structure and Function
    Benign Prostatic Hyperplasia
    Carcinoma of the Prostate
- Neoplasms of the Testis and Penis
    Testicular Neoplasms
    Seminoma
    Carcinoma of the Penis
- Diseases of the Breast
    Structure and Function
    Proliferative Changes of the Breast
    Neoplasms of the Breast
    Diseases of the Male Breast

THE UTERUS (BODY AND ENDOMETRIUM)

STRUCTURE AND FUNCTION

The uterus is a pear-shaped muscular organ situated in the pelvis between the bladder anteriorly and the rectum posteriorly. It is partially covered by the peritoneum of the pelvic floor.

The uterus is customarily divided into the body and the cervix. The body is lined by the endometrium, whose thickness varies at different ages and stages of the menstrual cycle. The endometrium is composed of endometrial glands and mesenchymal stromal cells, both of which are very sensitive to the action of female sex hormones. At the internal os, the endometrium becomes continuous with the endocervical canal, which is lined by columnar epithelium and contains mucous glands. The epithelium changes again at the junction of the endocervix and ectocervix, where it becomes stratified squamous epithelium.

The normal endometrium shows cyclic changes caused by corresponding changes in ovarian hormone production. The endometrial cycle is divided into a preovulatory proliferative phase that is the result of estrogenic stimulation(Figure 12-1) and a postovulatory secretory phase that is directed by progesterone secretion by the corpus luteum. Day 1 of the cycle is the onset of menstruation. Menstruation is the result of a sudden decrease in estrogen and progesterone due to degeneration of the corpus luteum.

DISEASES OF CERVIX

CHRONIC CERVICITIS

Moderate numbers of lymphocytes, plasma cells, and histiocytes are present in the cervix in all females. Chronic cervicitis is therefore difficult to de-

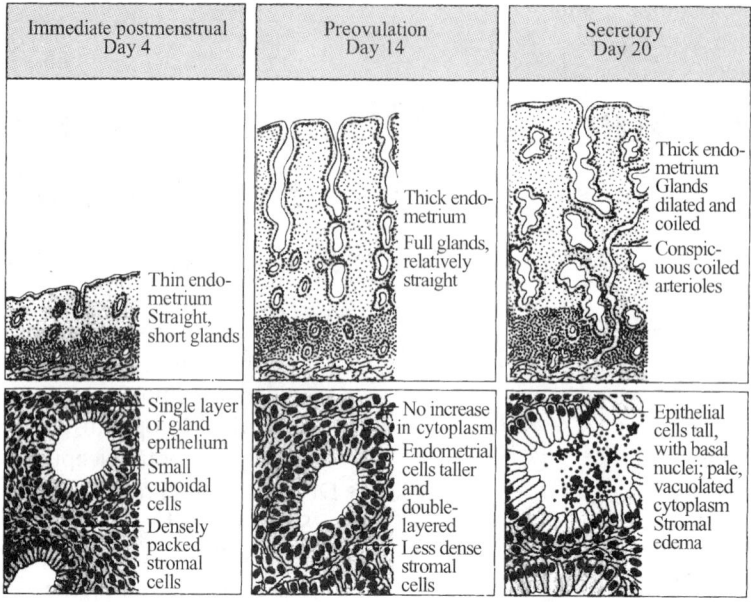

Figure 12-1 Endometrial changes during the menstrual cycle

fine pathologically. The presence of detectable cervical abnormalities such as granularity and thickening along with increased numbers of chronic inflammatory cells in a biopsy specimen is considered necessary to warrant a diagnosis of chronic cervicitis.

Chronic cervicitis is most commonly seen at the external os and endocervical canal. In most young women, there is downgrowth of the columnar epithelium below the exocervical os – ectropion; thus, the squamocolumnar junction comes to lie below the exocervix. This "exposed" columnar epithelium may appear reddened and moist and has been called cervical "erosion". This term is misleading however, nothing is really being eroded and the condition is entirely normal. These cervical changes are a natural response to the female hormone.

Remodeling occurs continuously with regeneration of both squamous and columnar epithelium. Frequently, overgrowth of the regenerating squamous epithelium blocks the orifices of endocervical glands to produce retention (nabothian) cysts. Chronic cervicitis may be associated with fibrous stenosis of gland ducts leading to nabothian cysts, too.

Squamous metaplasia of the endocervical epithelium is common, probably representing a response to irritation.

Polyps are common lesions of the endocervical canal, usually occurring at about the time of menopause. When large, a polyp may protrude out of the external os. Microscopically, endoceryvical polyps contain hyperplastic endocervical glands and a highly vascular stroma and may show marked chronic inflammation. The surface epithelium of a polyp commonly shows squamous metaplasia. Endocervical polyps are benign, with no increased incidence of neoplasia.

Clinically, chronic cervicitis is often an incidental finding. However, it may produce a mucopurulent to purulent vaginal discharge, and in a few cases associated fibrosis of the endocervical canal may cause stenosis, leading to infertility.

NEOPLASMS OF THE CERVIX

Squamous Carcinoma

Cervical carcinoma was once the most frequent form of cancer in women around the world. The mortality rate from cervical carcinoma has been falling, partly due to early detection of premalignant epithelial dysplasia by routine cytologic screening of cervical smears; many cases are detected and treated in the preinvasive stage.

A. Etiology

Considerable evidence suggests that carcinoma of the cervix is caused by a sexually transmitted carcinogenic agent, probably viral. The risk of developing carcinoma increases with early onset of sexual activity, frequency of coitus, greater number of sexual partners, and stimulation of the human male smegma. It is common in multiparous women who have married early and in prostitutes.

Two viruses are suspected of having an etiologic role in cancer of the cervix.

1. Herpes simplex virus type 2 (HSV-2)

It is thought to play only a minor promoting role.

2. Human papillomavirus

Particularly serologic types 16 and 18, which cause atypical flat condyloma acuminatum – has been found in both squamous carcinoma and dysplastic lesions of the cervix. This is presently considered to be an important etiologic agent.

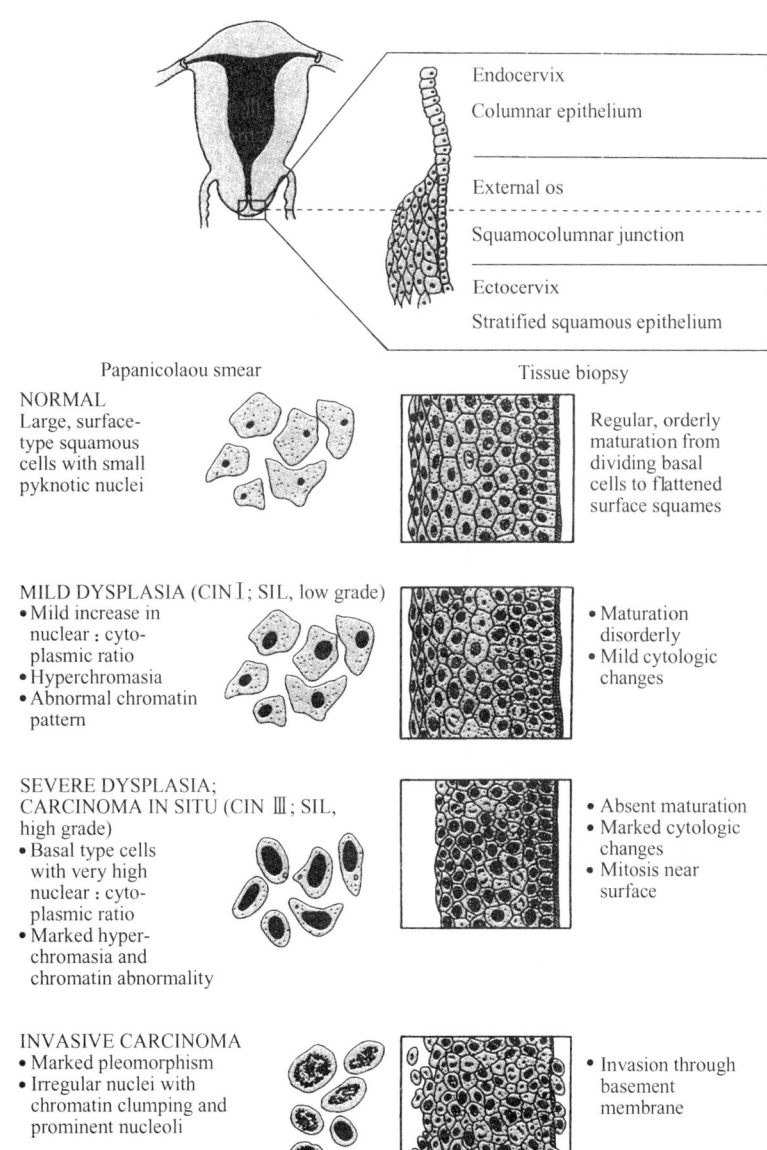

Figure 12-2 Squamous epithelial dysplasia and carcinoma of the cervix, showing criteria used to grade dysplasia. Dysplasia commonly occurs at the squamocolumnar junction. CIN = cervical intraepithelial neoplasia; SIL = squamous intraepithelial lesion

B. Dysplasia of the Cervix (Cervical Intraepithelial Neoplasia, CIN) (Figure 12-2)

Most cervical carcinomas arise in a stratified squamous epithelium that shows precancerous change dysplasia. Dysplasia commonly involves the region of the squamocolumnar junction and the endocervical canal that has undergone squamous metaplasia. Dysplasia is recognized by the presence of cytologic abnormalities in a cervical smear and confirmed by cervical biopsy (Figure 12-3). The cytologic changes include increased nuclear size, increased nuclear:cytoplasmic ratio, hyperchromatism, abnormal chromatin distribution, and nuclear membrane abnormalities. The extent of these changes permits classification (in order of increasing severity) as mild, moderate, or severe dysplasia and carcinoma in situ (Figure 12-2). These cytologic changes on a Pap smear correlate accurately with the degree of abnormal maturation of the epithelium in a subsequent cervical biopsy specimen. In carcinoma in situ, biopsy reveals that maturation is totally lacking, and most of the cytologic changes of carcinoma are present except invasion through the basement membrane.

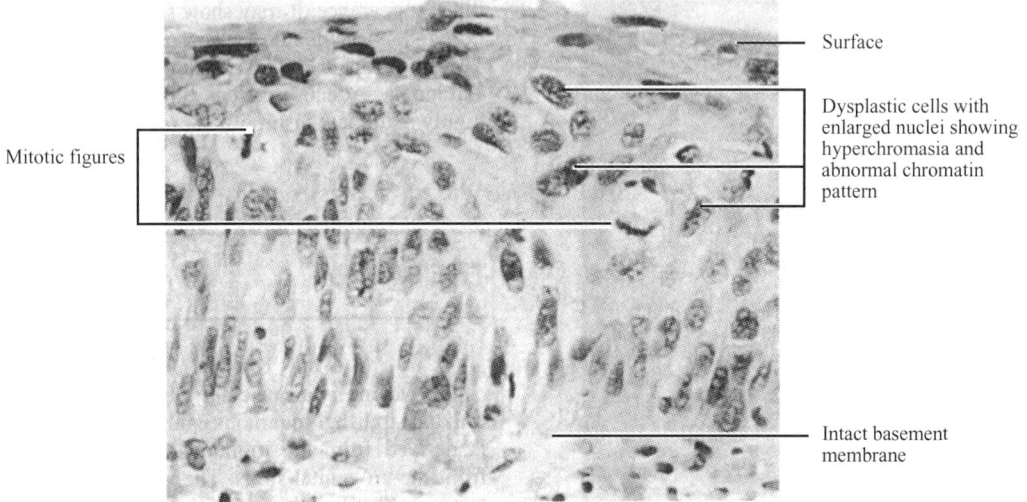

Figure 12-3 Moderate to severe dysplasia (CIN III, high-grade SIL) of the cervical squamous epithelium, showing disordered maturation, increased nuclear:cytoplasmic ratio, hyperchromasia, chromatin clumping, and mitotic figures in the upper part of the epithelium

Dysplasias are reversible lesions, but the more severe the degree of dysplasia the less the tendency to reverse. The time span for progression of dysplasia is variable. The median time for carcinoma to develop is 7 years for mild dysplasia and 1 year for severe dysplasia.

The term cervical intraepithelial neoplasia (CIN) has the same denotation as dysplasia. CIN I is equivalent to minimal dysplasia, CIN II to moderate dysplasia, and CIN III includes severe dysplasia and carcinoma in situ. More recently, dysplasias are classified as low-and high-grade squamous intraepithelial lesions (SIL). LSIL is equivalent to minimal dysplasia or CIN I, HSIL to moderate and severe dysplasia and carcinoma in situ, or CIN II and CIN III.

Dysplasia affects cervical surface epithelium as well as extending down into endocervical glands (gland duct involvement). The significance of gland duct involvement is the same as that of dysplasia of the surface epithelium.

Dysplasia and carcinoma in situ produce no symptoms. The Schiller test, which consists of painting the cervix with aqueous iodine, is helpful in locating areas of dysplasia, since dysplastic epithelium lacks glycogen and will appear as a pale area whereas normal epithelium stains dark brown with iodine.

The treatment of dysplasia is local and conservative. Cryosurgery, electrocoagulation, laser coagulation, and conization-removal of a cone of cervical tissue are all effective.

C. Microinvasive Carcinoma

Microinvasive carcinoma of the cervix is defined as cervical carcinoma in which the total depth of invasion is less than 5mm from the basement membrane (Table 12-1). Microinvasive carcinoma so defined is rarely associated with metastases, and local surgical excision is curative. It should be recognized that the submucosa of the cervix within this 5 mm zone below the basement membrane does contain lymphatics and blood vessels, and metastases are a hypothetical possibility. Nonetheless, the rarity of metastases is a statistical fact.

Table 12-1 Clinical staging of cervical carcinoma

Stage	
Stage 0	Carcinoma in situ (100%)[2]
Stage IA	Microinvasive carcinoma; invasion to a depth < 5 mm from the basement membrane (>95%)
Stage IB	Invasive carcinoma, infiltrating to a depth >5 mm but confined to the cervix (90%)
Stage II	Extension of tumor beyond the cervix to involve the endometrium, vagina (but not the lower third), or paracervical soft tissue (but has not extended to the pelvic side wall) (75%)
Stage III	Extension to the pelvic side wall or involvement of the lower third of the vagina or the presence of hydronephrosis from ureteral involvement (35%)
Stage IV	Extension beyond the pelvis or clinical involvement of bladder or rectal mucosa (10%)

[1] Adapted from American Joint Committee for Cancer Staging and End-Results Reporting; Task Force on Gynecologic Sites; Staging System for Cancer at Gynecologic Sites, 1979.

[2] Figures in parentheses represent 5-year survival rates for the stage.

D. Invasive Squamous Carcinoma (Stage 1B and More Extensive)

Invasive carcinoma is defined as carcinoma infiltrating to a depth of greater than 5 mm from the basement membrane. It occurs most frequently in the age group from 30 to 50 years.

Invasive carcinoma may present grossly as an exophytic, fungating, necrotic mass (Figure 12-4), the most common appearance; as a malignant ulcer; or as a diffusely infiltrative lesion with only minimal surface ulceration or nodularity (uncommon). Microscopically, there are three different types: (1) large cell, nonkeratinizing squamous carcinoma - the most common type, with the best prognosis; (2) keratinizing squamous carcinoma - next most common, with an intermediate prognosis; and (3) small cell carcinoma - rare, with a poor prognosis.

Invasive cervical carcinoma is manifested as abnormal uterine bleeding (commonly irregular and excessive menstrual bleeding or postmenopausal bleeding) or vaginal discharge. Obstruction of the cervical canal may cause blood to accumulate in the uterine cavity and result in infection (pyometron). Colposcopy permits direct visualization and biopsy to make a definitive histologic diagnosis. Cervical carcinoma is staged according to the degree of spread (Table 12-1).

Treatment is a combination of surgery and radiation therapy, depending on the extent of disease. The prognosis depends primarily on the clinical stage of the disease.

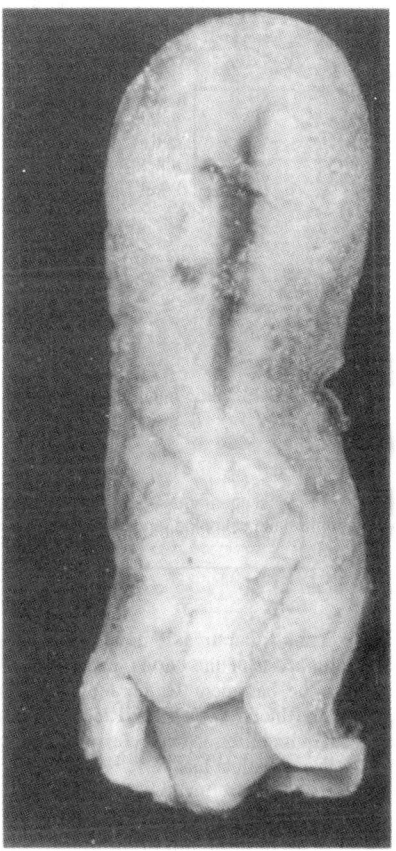

Figure 12-4 Squamous carcinoma of the cervix involving the squamocolumnar junction and most of the endocervical canal. The tumor is mainly to the left of the displaced endocervical canal in this figure

Endocervical Adenocarcinoma

Endocervical adenocarcinoma accounts for 10% – 15% of cervical cancers. It arises in the endocervical glands, presenting as a mass in the endocervical canal. It frequently obstructs the endocervical canal, predisposing to pyometron.

Microscopically, endocervical adenocarcinoma is usually a well-differentiated lesion, often with a papillary appearance. It may show squamous differentiation (a denoacanthoma, adenosquamous carcinoma). The prognosis is less favorable than that of squamous carcinoma. Adenosquamous carcinoma behaves in a highly malignant fashion.

DISEASES OF BODY OF UTERUS

ENDOMETRIOSIS

Endometriosis is the occurrence of endometrial tissue at a site other than the lining of the uterine cavity (Figure 12-5). The "ectopic" endometrial tissue is usually composed of both epithelial and stromal cells and responds to ovarian hormones somewhat like the uterine endometrium.

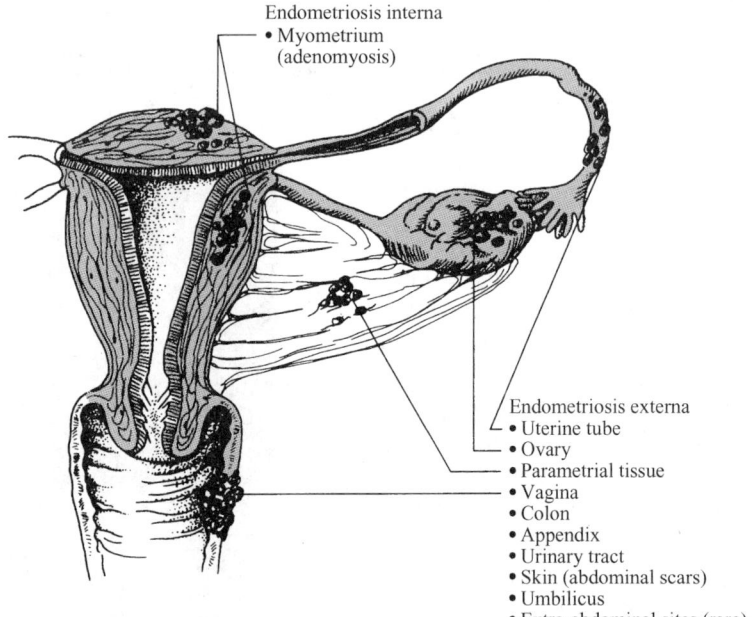

Figure 12-5   Endometriosis, showing sites of involvement

Pathology

There appear to be two types of endometriosis with different pathogenetic mechanisms.

A. Adenomyosis (*Endometriosis Interna*)

Adenomyosis is defined as the presence of endometrial glands and stroma abnormally situated deep in the myometrium (at a depth of more than 3 mm – one low-power field – form the base of the endometrium) (Figure 12-5).

Adenomyosis is common in older women (over 40 years of age) and is documented in about 10% of uteri at autopsy. In about half of cases, adenomyosis is restricted to the inner third of the myometrium. In the remainder, it extends more deeply, not infrequently reaching serosa.

Two distinct forms are recognized: (1) Diffuse adenomyosis, involving much or all of the uterus; and (2) focal adenomyosis, forming a nodular mass that resembles a leiomyoma (sometimes called an adenomyoma).

Adenomyosis responds cyclically to ovarian hormones, leading to hemorrhage with hemosiderin deposition at sites of disease.

B. Extrauterine Endometriosis (*Endometriosis Externa*)

Endometriosis occurring outside the uterus is pathogenetically unrelated to adenomyosis. In order of decreasing frequency, endometriosis externa is found in (1) an ovary; (2) the wall of a uterine tube; (3) parametrial soft tissue; (4) the serosa of the intestine, most commonly the sigmoid colon and appendix; (5) the umbilicus; (6) the urinary tract; (7) the skin at the site of laparotomy scars, usually after surgery on the uterus and most commonly after cesarean section; and (8) extra-abdominal sites such as the lungs, pleura, and bones.

Pathologically, foci of endometriosis appear as cysts that contain areas of new and old hemorrhage (**chocolate cysts**), due to cyclic bleeding that occurs during menstruation. Microscopically, foci are characterized by the presence of endometrial glands surrounded by stroma (Figure 12-6). Evidence of hemorrhage, hemosiderin deposition, and fibrosis are common. Endometriosis of the uterine tube is a common cause of infertility because of luminal obliteration by fibrosis.

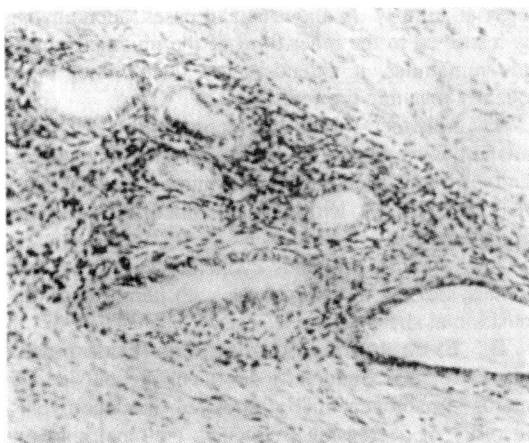

Figure 12-6 Endometriosis, showing endometrial glands surrounded by stroma. This was taken from a nodule on the serosal aspect of the sigmoid colon

Pathogenesis

A. Adenomyosis

Adenomyosis (endometriosis interna) is believed to be the result of abnormal downgrowth of the endometrium into the myometrium, with entrapment of foci of endometrium deep in the uterine muscle.

B. Endometriosis Externa

Two main hypotheses have been advanced. The first is that endometriosis results form metaplasia (differentiation) of the celomic epithelium into endometrial tissue. A hypothesis more favored in current opinion is that endometriosis results form transport of fragments of normal menstrual endometrium from the uterus, through the uterine tubes, and into the peritoneal cavity.

Clinical Features

Clinically, endometriosis may be asymptomatic. The most common symptoms of adenomyosis are dysmenorrhea, menorrhagia, and infertility. With extrauterine endometriosis involving the umbilicus, surgical scars, urinary tract (cyclic hematuria), or colon (rectal bleeding) - or occult, producing cyclic abdominal pain.

ENDOMETRIAL HYPERPLASIA

Endometrial hyperplasia is a premalignant lesion that is caused by unopposed estrogen stimulation. It usually occurs around or after menopause and is associated with excessive and irregular uterine bleeding. The risk of malignancy correlates with the severity of the hyperplasia, which is classified as follows:

Simple hyperplasia (mild hyperplasia) is characterized by an increased number of proliferative glands without cytologic atypia. The glands, although crowded, are separated by densely cellular stroma and are of varying sizes. In some cases, cystically dilated glands predominate (cystic hyperplasia). The risk of endometrial carcinoma is very low.

Complex hyperplasia without atypia (moderate hyperplasia; adenomatous hyperplasia) shows a greater increase in gland number with crowding (Figure 12-7). The epithelial lining is stratified and shows numerous mitotic figures. The lining cells maintain normal polarity and do not show pleomorphism or cytologic atypia. Densely cellular stroma is still present between glands.

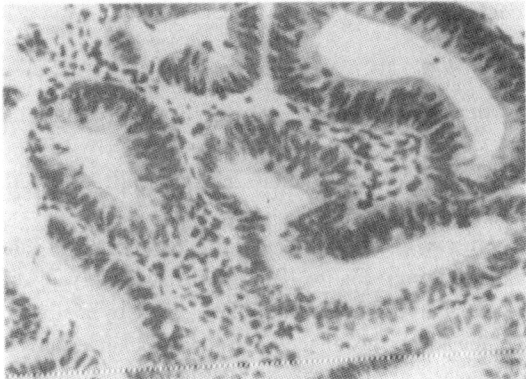

Figure 12-7 Moderate endometrial hyperplasia, showing crowded endometrial glands lined by stratified, cytologically atypical cells

Complex hyperplasia with atypia (severe hyperplasia; atypical adenomatous hyperplasia) is characterized by gland crowding with back-to-back glands and marked cytologic atypia characterized by pleomorphism, hyperchromatism, and abnormal nuclear chromatin pattern. Complex hyperplasia with atypia merges with adenocarcinoma in situ of the endometrium and carries a high risk of endometrial carcinoma.

The changes of endometrial hyperplasia — even the most severe form — are reversible with progesterone therapy.

NEOPLASMS OF BODY OF UTERUS

Endometrial Carcinoma

Endometrial adenocarcinoma is common, accounting for about 10% of cancers in women, and the incidence is increasing in many countries. Ninety percent of cases occur in postmenopausal women, the most common age being 55–65 years.

A. Etiology

Prolonged unopposed estrogen stimulation of the endometrium is believed to be the major etiologic factor. Endometrial hyperplasia precedes cancer in most cases.

Endometrial carcinoma is associated with obesity, diabetes mellitus, and hypertension. The mechanism of this association is unknown. Pregnancy appears to have a protective effect in endometrial carcinoma, probably by opposing estrogenic stimulation; there is a decreased incidence in multiparous as compared with nulliparous women.

B. Pathology

Most endometrial carcinomas present as polypoid, fungating masses in the endometrial cavity (Figure 12-8). The uterus is often asymmetrically enlarged. Invasion into the myometrium occurs early.

Microscopically, endometrial carcinoma is an **adenocarcinoma** (Figure 12-9), and most are well-differentiated, with irregular glands lined by malignant columnar epithelial cells. Endometrial carcinomas are graded according to their degree of histologic differentiation. Well-differentiated carcinomas are grade 1. The presence of large solid areas (grade 2) and poor differentiation (grade 3) implies a worse prognosis. A variant histologic type is papillary serous adenocarcinoma. This resembles ovarian serous carcinoma and has a worse prognosis than the usual endometrial adenocarcinoma.

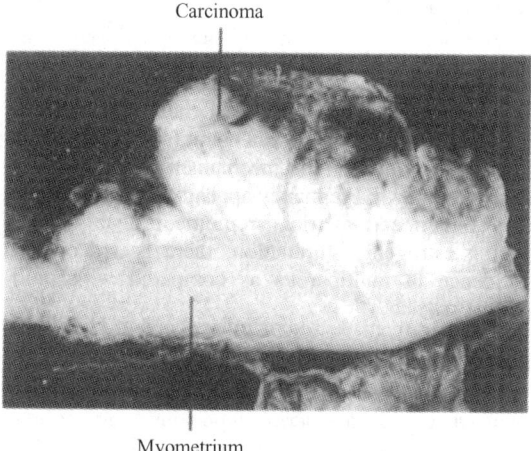

Figure 12-8 Endometrial carcinoma, showing a bulky mass projecting into the uterine cavity. There is invasion of the inner third of the myometrium

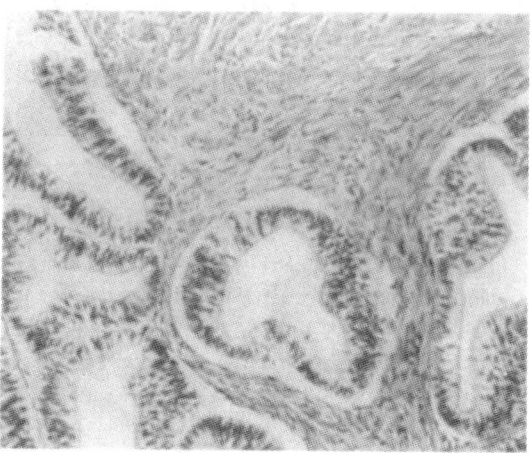

Figure 12-9 Microscopic section from previous figure showing a well-differentiated endometrial carcinoma infiltrating the myometrium

Areas of squamous differentiation are common, and if this feature is prominent the neoplasm is called an **adenoacanthoma**. When the squamous areas are poorly differentiated and show cytologic features of malignancy, the term **adenosquamous carcinoma** is used.

The pathologic stage of the neoplasm, determined by the degree of spread (Figure 12-10), is the most important prognostic factor.

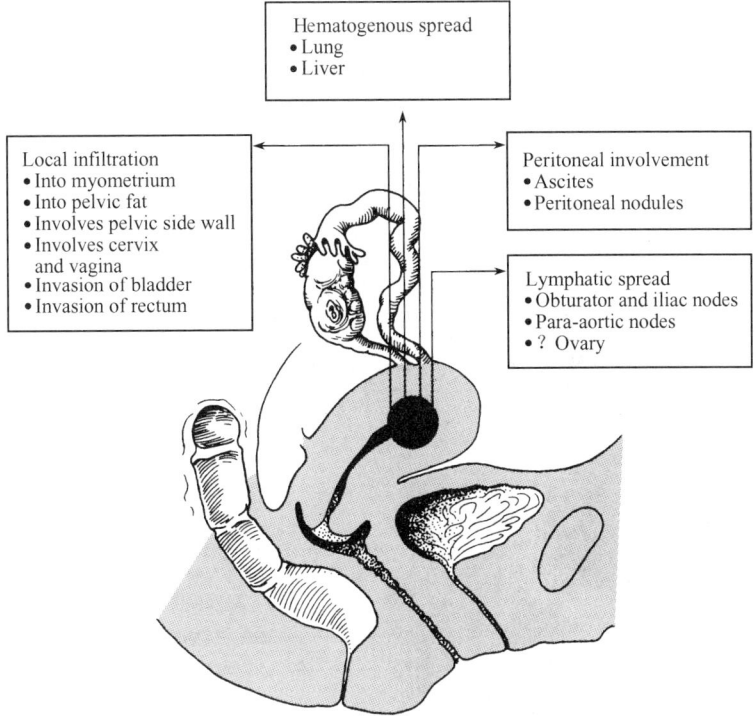

Figure 12-10   Spread of endometrial carcinoma

C. Clinical Features

Abnormal uterine bleeding is the earliest symptom. At the usual age at which endometrial cancer occurs, it is **postmenopausal bleeding.** Endometrial biopsy or curettage is usually diagnostic.

D. Prognosis

The prognosis of patients with endometrial carcinoma depends mainly on the stage of disease (Table 12-2). The histologic grade of the neoplasm is of secondary importance. With treatment, 90% of patients with stage I disease, 40% with stage II, and 10%–20% with more advanced disease will survive 5 years.

Table 12-2   Staging of endometrial carcinoma

Stage	
Stage I	Tumor confined to the corpus uteri
Stage II	Tumor involves the cervix but does not extend beyond the uterus
Stage III	Tumor extends beyond the uterus but does not extend outside the true pelvis
Stage IVa	Tumor invades the mucosa of bladder or rectum or extends beyond the true pelvis
Stage IVb	Distant metastasis

Leiomyoma

Leiomyoma is a benign neoplasm of uterine smooth muscle. It is one of the most common neoplasms in females. Leiomyomas are most common between 20 and 40 years of age. Growth appears to be dependent on estrogens.

Leiomyomas may be solitary or multiple and may be located anywhere in the uterine smooth muscle (Figure 12-11). They often reach large size. Grossly, leiomyomas are circumscribed (Figure 12-12), firm, grayish-white masses with a characteristic whorled appearance on cut section. Histologically, they are composed of a uniform proliferation of spindle-shaped smooth muscle cells (Figure 12-13). Cytologic atypia is sometimes present, particularly in areas of hyalinization, but mitotic figures are scarce. Collagen is present in varying amounts.

Degenerative changes occur frequently: (1) Red degeneration (necrobiosis) is typically seen during pregnancy, when the neoplasm undergoes necrosis and develops a beefy-red color. This change is associated with acute abdominal pain. (2) Cystic degeneration is common and usually does not cause

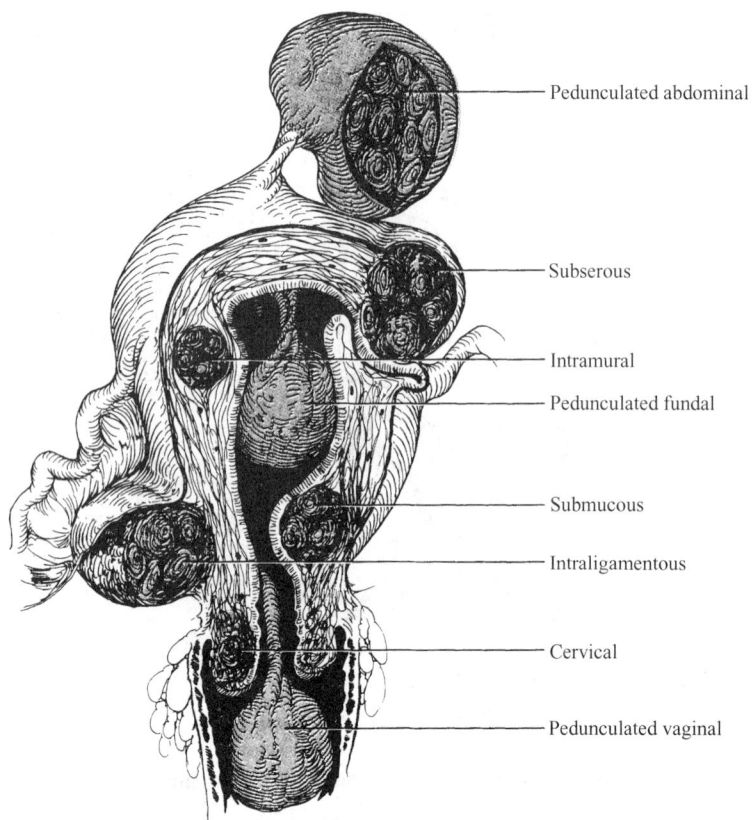

Figure 12-11   Leiomyomas of the uterus, showing different locations where these neoplasms are found in the uterus

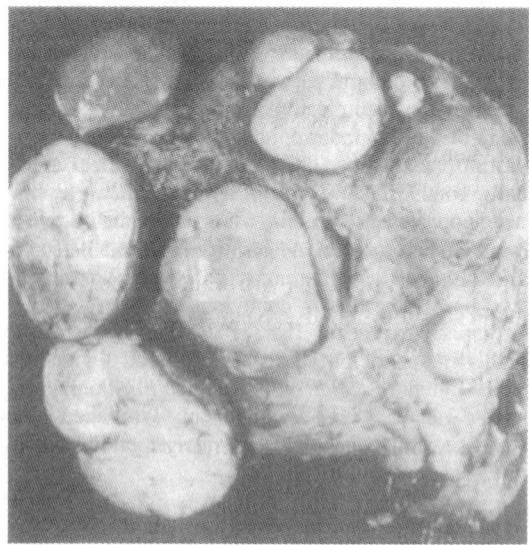

Figure 12-12   Uterine leiomyomas, showing multiple well-circumscribed nodules of varying size with the typical whorled appearance on cut surface

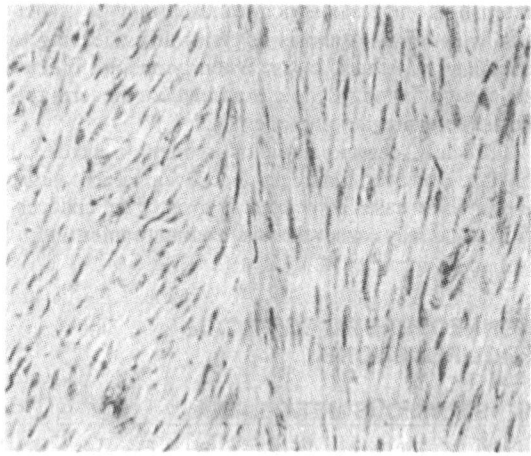

Figure 12-13   Uterine leiomyoma, showing interlacing fascicles of cytologically uniform smooth muscle cells

symptoms. (3) Hyalinization, with broad bands of collagen appearing in the tumor, may be associated with marked cytologic atypia (bizarre leiomyoma) but is still benign, with the cytologic atypia probably representing a degenerative phenomenon. (4) Calcification may rarely be so extensive that the tumor appears as a radiopaque mass on plain x-ray.

(5) Leiomyomas very rarely undergo malignant change.

Leiomyomas are a common cause of excessive uterine bleeding (menorrhagia) and an important cause of infertility. However, most patients are asymptomatic.

Leiomyosarcoma

Leiomyosarcoma is a rare uterine neoplasm. It is nonetheless the most common uterine sarcoma. It arises from smooth muscle of the myometrium, usually de novo rather than from a preexisting leiomyoma.

Leiomyosarcomas appear as bulky, fleshy masses that show hemorrhage and necrosis. Marked cytologic pleomorphism and atypia are usually present. The most important diagnostic criterion is a high rate of mitotic figures (over 10 mitoses per 10 high-power fields).

Leiomyosarcoma is most common in older women, presenting as postmenopausal bleeding or a uterine mass. Local recurrence and hematogenous metastases are frequent. The 5-year survival rate is about 40%.

GESTATIONAL TROPHOBLASTIC DISEASES

HYDATIDIFORM MOLE (MOLAR PREGNANCY)

The incidence of hydatidiform mole varies greatly in different parts of the world. It occurs in one in every 1000 pregnancies in the United States but has a much higher frequency (1:150) in our country.

Etiology

Two distinct types of hydatidifrom mole are recognized:

A. Complete Mole

This results from fertilization by one or two sperms of an ovum that has lost all its chromosomes. In complete moles, all the chromosomal material is derived from sperms. In 90% of cases, a single sperm is involved, and the molar karyotype is 46, XX. In 10%, the karyotype includes Y chromosomes. In complete mole, early embryonic death is the rule, and no fetal parts are seen.

B. Partial Mole

This results from fertilization of an ovum by two sperms: one 23, X and the other 23, Y. Partial moles are therefore triploid (69, XXY). The embryo may develop for a few weeks, and fetal parts may be present when the mole is evacuated.

Pathology

A. Complete Mole

The uterus is usually enlarged. The uterine cavity is filled with a mass of grape-like structures – thin-walled, translucent, cystic, and grayish-white. This represents the hydatidiform mole. No normal fetal parts are identified.

Microscopically, the cysts are composed of hydropic chorionic villi, the interior being filled with an avascular, loose myxoid stroma. Trophoblastic proliferation produces sheets of cytotrophoblastic and syncytiotrophoblastic cells (Figure 12-14). Cytologic atypia may be present.

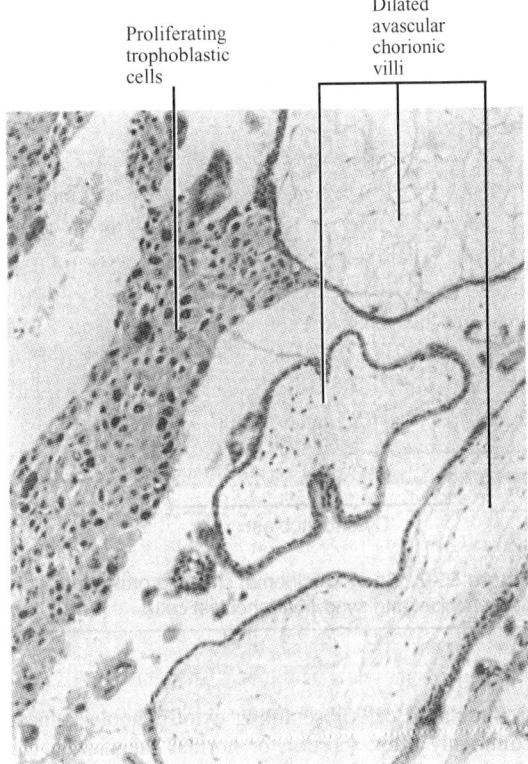

Figure 12-14 Hydatidiform mole, showing dilated, avascular chorionic villi lined by proliferative trophoblastic tissue

Complete mole is associated with greatly elevated levels of chorionic gonadotropin.

B. Partial Mole

The uterus may not be enlarged. The enlargement and edema involves only a proportion of villi, and many normal villi coexist. Fetal parts may be present. The degree of trophoblastic proliferation is mild, and the serum level of chorionic gonadotropin is often only slightly elevated.

Clinical Features

The initial features are those of early pregnancy, including amenorrhea, vomiting of pregnancy – often severe – and a positive pregnancy test. Uterine enlargement is usually greater than in the case of normal pregnancy. Vaginal bleeding usually begins in the third to fourth month. Passage of grape-like clusters admixed with blood may also be observed. Diagnosis is confirmed by the greatly elevated levels of βhCG in the serum.

Hydatidiform mole is treated surgically, with evacuation of the mole from the uterine cavity by curettage. After evacuation, the serum βhCG level falls rapidly to normal; failure to do so indicates residual mole.

Complications

About 2.5% of complete moles are complicated by choriocarcinoma; 10% develop into invasive moles. Partial moles have a minimal risk. In patients who develop invasive mole, the βhCG level does not return to normal after the mole is evacuated. If the βhCG level returns to normal after the mole is evacuated and becomes elevated at a later time, choriocarcinoma should be considered.

INVASIVE MOLE

Invasive mole is a hydatidiform mole that shows extensive penetration of the villi and trophoblast into the myometrium, and extension often reaches the serosal surface.

Invasive mole is associated with necrosis and hemorrhage in the myometrium (Figure 12-15), and uterine rupture may occur. Microscopically, the epithelium of the villi is marked by hyperplastic and atypical changes, with proliferation of both cuboidal and syncytial components.

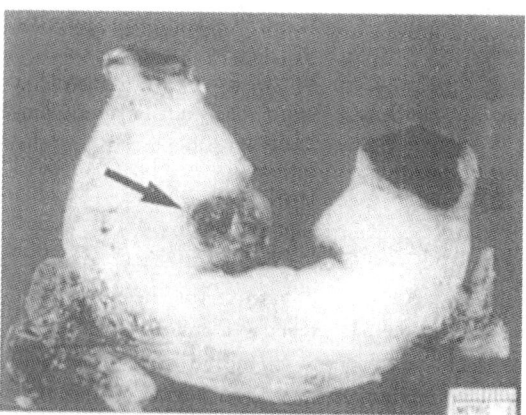

Figure 12-15 Invasive mole (chorioadenoma destruens), showing hemorrhagic mass invading the myometrium (arrow)

In invasive mole, local spread to the broad ligament and vagina may also occur. Hydropic villi may embolize to distant organs, such as the lungs or brain, but these emboli do not constitute true metastases and may actually regress spontaneously. Invasive mole is associated with persistent elevation of βhCG levels after evacuation of the uterine cavity. Without treatment, the mortality rate from hemorrhage or uterine rupture is about 10%. Treatment with chemotherapy is effective.

CHORIOCARCINOMA

Choriocarcinoma of the uterus is a malignant neoplasm of trophoblast. About half follow a hydatidiform mole; others occur after abortion (25%), normal pregnancy (20%), or ectopic pregnancy (5%).

Choriocarcinoma has a relatively high incidence in some parts of Asia and Africa. Histologically, choriocarcinoma arising from a pregnancy is identical to ovarian (or testicular) choriocarcinoma having a germ cell origin.

Pathology

Choriocarcinoma presents grossly as a friable hemorrhagic mass in the uterine cavity. It infiltrates the myometrium extensively, and vascular invasion occurs early, with widespread metastases in lungs, brain, liver, and bone marrow. Microscopically, choriocarcinoma is composed of cytologically malignant sheets of cytotrophobastic and syncytiotrophoblastic cells associated with necrosis and hemorrhage (Figure 12-16). Formed chorionic villi are absent. βhCG can often be demonstrated in the tumor cells.

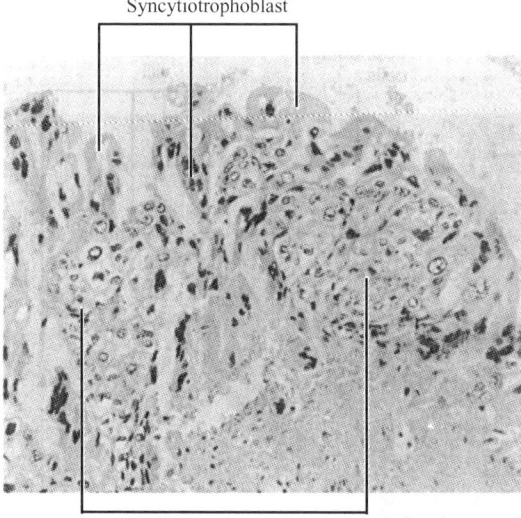

Figure 12-16 Choriocarcinoma, showing proliferating cytotrophoblast and syncytiotrophoblast cells

Clinical Features and Treatment

Patients with choriocarcinoma present with abnormal uterine bleeding, commonly occurring within a few months after normal pregnancy, abortion, or hydatidiform mole. Many patients have metastatic lesions at the time of diagnosis.

With aggressive combined chemotherapy, the 5-year survival rate has improved to over 90% even in patients with widespread metastases at presentation. Serum βhCG levels are extremely useful in monitoring treatment. Elevated βhCG levels in serum indicate persistence of viable trophoblastic tissue.

PLACENTAL SITE TROPHOBLASTIC TUMOR (PSTT)

This is a rare lesion characterized by the diffuse proliferation in the uterus of sheets of intermediate trophoblastic cells resembling cytotrophoblast, most commonly after abortion or normal pregnancy. No chorionic villi or fetal parts are identified. The proliferating cells may show considerable cytologic abnormalities, which results in a resemblance of this lesion to choriocarcinoma. The neoplastic cells contain human placental lactogen, demonstrable by immunoperoxidase techniques. Unlike choriocarcinoma, PSTT shows only a slight elevation of βhCG and no syncytiotrophoblastic cells. The biologic behavior of PSTT is usually benign. Most cases are cured by curettage. A few cases have demonstrated a more aggressive biologic behavior, and rare cases with metastases have been reported.

(Yan Junxia)

OVARIAN TUMORS

NORMAL STRUCTURE OF OVARY

The ovaries are paired ovoid structures, weighing 5-8 g and measuring about 4 cm × 2.5 cm × 1.5 cm in dimension, each situated in the retrouterine space in relation to the lateral part of the uterine tube on each side. The free surface of the ovary is covered by germinal epithelium, which is continuous with the peritoneum. Both of these two types of surface epithelium are derived from the embryonic coelom.

The ovary is divided into a cortex and a medulla. The cortex consists of dense mesenchymal ovarian stromal cells plus germinal follicles and, after puberty, corpora lutea at various stages of maturation. The exact appearance of the ovary depends on the age of the patient and the phase of the menstrual cycle. If the patient is closer to menarche, there are more primordial follicles; if she is closer to menopause, there are more regressed, hyalinized corpora lutea (corpora albicantia). The medulla consists of lose connective tissue, blood vessels, lymphatic vessels and smooth muscle. Scattered embryonic epithelial remnants and hilar cells are often present; hilar cells possess abundant lipid filled cytoplasm and are believed to be analogous to the testicular interstitial cells of Leydig (Figure 12-17). The ovary is a common site of metastasis.

CLASSIFICATION

Ovarian neoplasms arise from one of three ovarian components: the surface celomic epithelium, the germ cells and stroma (Table 12-3).

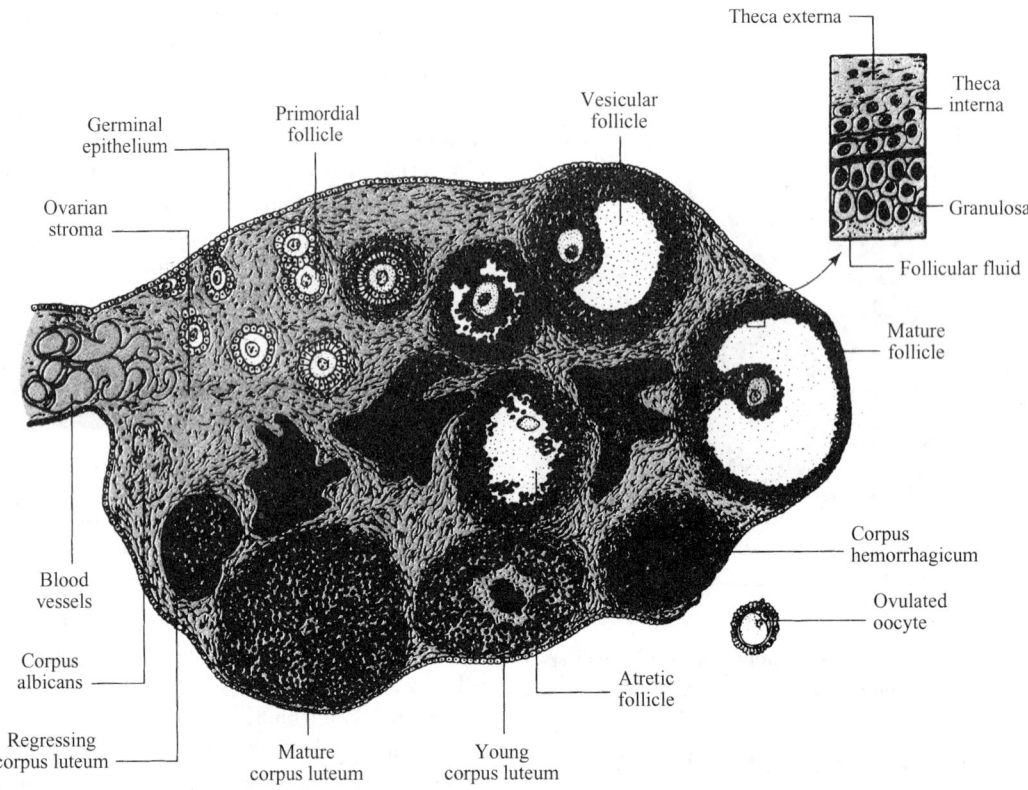

Figure 12-17 Diagram of mammalian ovary, showing the sequential development of a follicle and the formation of the corpus luteum. An atretic follicle is shown in the center, and the structure of the mature follicle is detailed at the upper right

Table 12-3 Classification of ovarian neoplasms

Origin	Tumor	
	Types	Subtypes
Epithelium	Serous	Benign, borderline or malignant
	Mucinous	
	Endometrioid	
	Transitional cell	
Germ cells	Dysgerminoma	
	Teratoma	Mature cystic, immature solid
	Extraembryonic	Yolk sac tumor (endodermal sinus tumor), choriocarcinoma
	Embryonal carcinoma	
	Monodermal (e.g. carcinoid, struma ovarii)	
Sex-cord stroma	Thecoma	
	Granulosa cell tumor	
	Sertoli-Leydig cell tumor	
	Mixed germ cell stromal tumor (gonadoblastoma)	
	Steroid cell tumor	
Malignant, not otherwise specified		
Metastatic cancer		

EPITHELIAL TUMORS

The surface coelomic epithelium of ovary, as a part of mesothelia cells, embryologically gives rise to Mullerian differentiation. Thus, differentiation of epithelial tumors of ovary may take place to resemble tubal mucosa (serous tumors), endocervical mucosa (mucinous tumors) or endometrium (endometrioid tumors). Each of these tumors may be clearly benign, malignant, or borderline. The borderline tumors show some of the features associated with malignancy, such as irregular architecture, nuclear stratification and pleomorphism and mitotic activity, but lack the most important criterion of invasion.

A. Serous Tumors

Serous tumors account for 40% of ovarian neoplasms, and occur in the age group from 15 to 50 years. Benign neoplasms tend to occur in younger women than malignant ones. Serous tumors are frequently bilateral.

1. Benign serous cystadenoma

Grossly, benign serous tumors vary in size from small cysts in the ovary (germinal inclusion cysts; serous cystomas) to large multilocular cystic neoplasms, occasionally up to 40 cm in diameter. The cystic spaces are usually filled with a clear serum fluid, although a considerable amount of mucus may also be present. They have a smooth external surface and a smooth or papillary internal lining. Histologically, the benign form is characterized by a single layer of cuboidal or columnar epithelium which lines the cyst or cysts. A variant of serous cystadenoma containing, in addition, a mass of proliferating fibrous connective tissue between the cystic spaces is known as serous cystadenofibroma.

2. Serous tumor of low malignant potential

Serous tumors of low malignant potential (also called borderline serous tumors) are distinguished from benign serous cystadenomas in having increasing amount of papillary projections and from serous cystadenocarcinoma by the lack of infiltration of the stroma or capsule of the neoplasm. Histologically, the neoplastic cells lining the papillae are taller than those lining benign neoplasms, with stratification (up to three cell layers) and mild cytologic atypia. Calcification in the form of round, laminated psammoma bodies is commonly present.

Serous tumors of low malignant potential may metastasize to the peritoneal cavity and rarely to the lungs. They have a good prognosis (5-year survival rate of 95%) even in the presence of peritoneal metastases.

3. Serous cystadenocarcinoma

Grossly, serous cystadenocarcinomas show irregular solid and cystic areas. The outer surface may be irregular due to infiltrating tumor. Histologically, The cyst epithelial lining has a highly complex papillary pattern with cell stratification, marked cytologic atypia, and stromal or capsular invasion. Calcification in the form of round, laminated psammoma bodies is commonly present. High-grade serous cystadenocarcinoma loses its papillary appearance and becomes indistinguishable from undifferentiated carcinoma in many areas.

Serous cystadenocarcinoma is a highly malignant neoplasm, infiltrating and metastasizing early in its course. Local spread to the peritoneum and omentum occurs early. Lymph node involvement also occurs early, with metastases in pelvic and pare-aortic lymph nodes. Distant metastases occur late, with lung and liver the main sites. The 5-year survival rate is about 20%.

B. Mucinous Tumors

Mucinous tumors account for 25% of ovarian neoplasms, and occur most often in the age group from 15 to 50 years. Most are benign. Mucinous cystadenocarcinoma accounts for 10% of ovarian cancers. Mucinous tumors are less frequently bilateral than serous tumors.

1. Benign mucinous cystadenoma

Grossly, mucinous cystadenoma tends to be larger than serous cystadenoma and typically is a cystic multiloculated neoplasm filled with thick mucoid fluid. The inner lining is smooth, histologically, being composed of uniform tall columnar cells with flattened basal nuclei, and distended with mucin.

2. Mucinous tumors of low malignant potential

Mucinous tumors of low malignant potential (borderline mucinous tumors) are distinguished from benign tumors by the presence of complex papillary projections, cell stratification, and mild cytologic atypia of the epithelial lining; and from carcinoma by the lesser degree of stratification and cytologic atypia and the absence of stromal and capsular invasion.

Mucinous tumors of low malignant potential grow slowly and may spread to the peritoneum, producing multiple mucoid masses with extensive adhesions, called pseudomyxoma peritonei, which is usually associated with mucinous tumors that are lined with epithelium demonstrating intestinal-type features; goblet cells are seen often. Distant metastases are rare. The 5-year survival rate is approximately 90%, but the overall long-term prognosis is poor when there is extensive peritoneal disease.

3. Mucinous cystadenocarcinoma

Grossly, mucinous cystadenocarcinoma may be recognized by the presence of solid areas and evidence of invasion. Histologically, there is marked cytologic anaplasia and extensive infiltration. This highly malignant neoplasm may metastasize to the peritoneal cavity, lymph nodes, and distant organs in a manner similar to serous cystadenocarcinoma. Prognosis is poor.

C. Endometrioid Carcinoma

Endometrioid carcinoma accounts for 20% of malignant ovarian neoplasms. Forty percent of cases are bilateral. It is defined by its microscopic resemblance to endometrial carcinoma. Associated endometriosis is found in about 25% of cases. In some cases concurrent endometrial carcinoma is present, raising the question of whether the ovarian neoplasm is metastatic or a second independent primary. Some endometrioid carcinomas may originate from endometriosis, but in most cases, the tumor is believed to represent endometrioid differentiation of a neoplasm derived from the celomic epithelium.

Endometrioid carcinomas grossly appear as solid and cystic masses that frequently show areas of hemorrhage and necrosis. Microscopically, the cells resemble endometrial epithelial type (Figure 12-18). Squamous metaplasia is seen in 50% of cases.

Endometriod carcinoma has the best prognosis among ovarian carcinomas, with a 5-year survival rate of 50%. Endometrioid tumors of low malignant potential (borderline endometrioid tumors) have been described but are rare.

GERM CELL NEOPLASMS

Germ cell tumors of the ovary are similar in derivation to their counterparts in the testis. Mature teratoma of the ovary is biologically benign at all ages, and is responsible for 80% of all germ cell tumors of

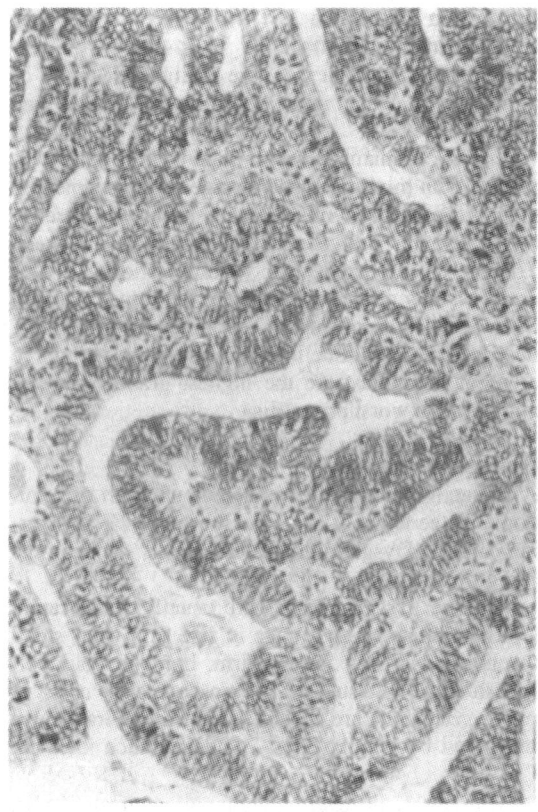

Figure 12-18 Endometrioid carcinoma, showing glandular spaces lined by tall, stratified carcinoma cells resembling the pattern of endometrial carcinoma

the ovary. Immature teratoma of the ovary occurs mainly in the age group under 20 years and is a highly malignant neoplasm. Dysgerminoma and yolk sac carcinoma are similar to their testicular counterparts. Embryonal carcinoma and choriocarcinoma are extremely rare in the ovary.

A. Teratoma

1. Benign cystic teratoma (dermoid cyst)

Benign cystic teratoma accounts for about 15% of ovarian neoplasms. It is bilateral in 10% of cases and occurs in all age groups, most commonly between 20 and 30 years of age.

Benign teratoma (Figure 12-19) appears grossly as a cyst containing thick sebaceous material and hair, so it is sometimes called dermoid cyst. The internal lining is mostly smooth but frequently has a knob-like nodular protrusion in one area (the umbo), in which cartilage, bone, and well-formed teeth may be present. Microscopically, skin elements dominate, including dermal appendages such as hair follicles and sebaceous glands. In most cases, however, structures of endodermal (respiratory and gastrointestinal epithelia) and mesodermal (muscle, fat, cartilage) origin are present, satisfying the definition of teratoma. Glial elements are also commonly present. Rare ovarian teratomas are composed almost entirely of thyroid tissue (struma ovarii) or tissue resembling carcinoid tumor.

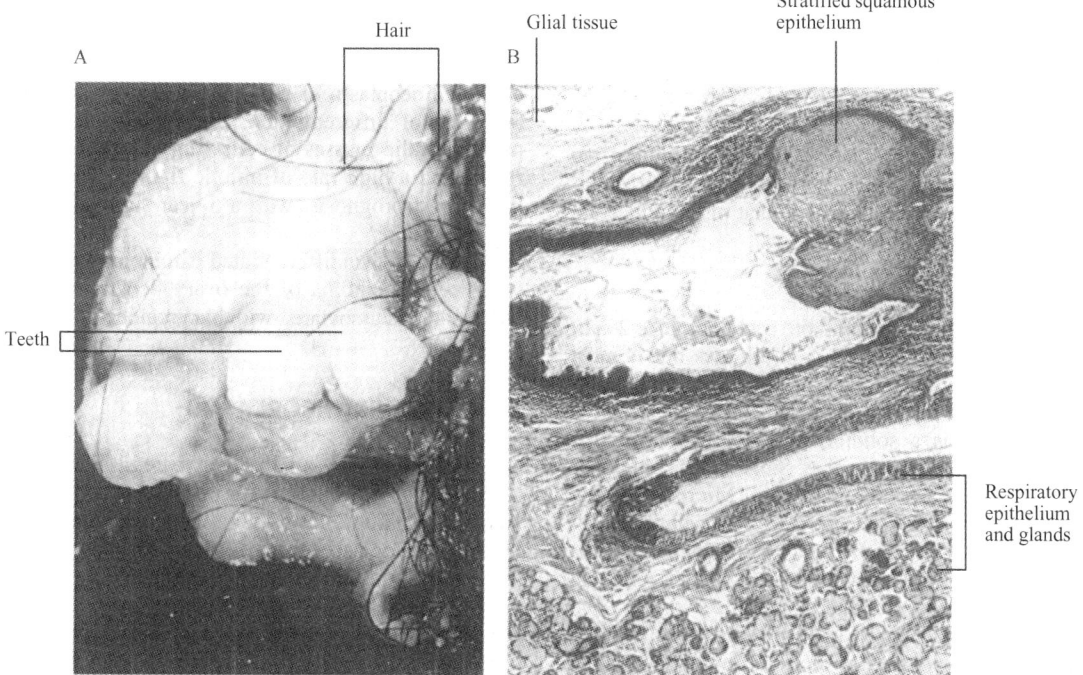

Figure 12-19 A: A portion of a benign cystic teratoma (dermoid cyst) containing teeth and hair. B: Microscopic features of cystic teratoma, showing stratified squamous epithelium, pseudostratified columnar epithelium with adjacent peribronchial glands, and glial tissue

2. Immature teratoma (malignant teratoma)

Immature teratoma is a rare malignant variant of teratoma that occurs mainly in patients younger than 20 years of age.

Immature teratomas are usually solid neoplasms with minimal cystic change, being composed of immature (poorly differentiated) elements derived from all three germ layers. Primitive neuroectodermal (neuroblastic) elements are especially common. Immature tetatoma is graded histologically according to the amount of primitive neuroectodermal tissue it contains; tumors with large areas of neuroblast are the highest grade (grade 3) and have the worst prognosis.

B. Dysgerminoma

Dysgerminoma (Figure 12-20) is the ovarian counterpart of seminoma of the testis. It accounts for about 2% of ovarian cancers, commonly occurring in the age group from 10 to 30 years.

Grossly, dysgerminomas are usually solid, rarely

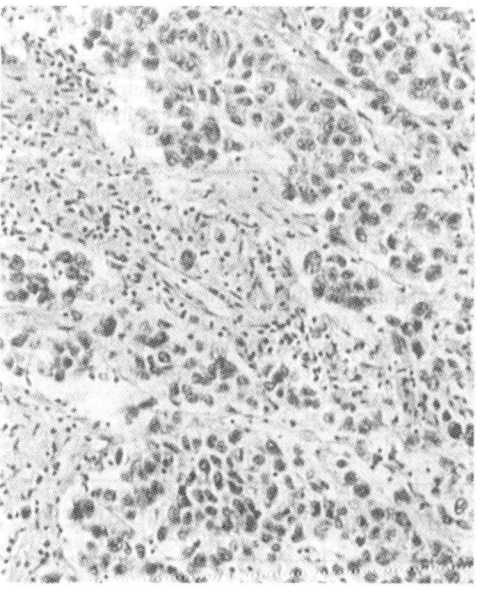

Figure 12-20 Dysgerminoma, showing nests of round germ cells separated by fibrous trabeculae infiltrated by lymphocytes

(5%–10%) bilateral, and range in size from very small to enormous. They have a firm, homogeneous yellowish-white cut surface. Microscopically, most are quite distinctive, having nests and aggregates of large vesicular cells with cleared cytoplasm and centrally placed nuclei separated by trabeculae that have a lymphocytic infiltrate and occasionally, syncytial-type giant cells and granuloma formations. Oct-4 is a sensitive and specific marker in the identification of dysgerminoma (seminoma) and embryonal carcinoma. Although potentially malignant, small dysgerminomas confined to the ovary are usually cured by simple resection. The overall prognosis is good, with a 5-year survival rate of 80%.

C. Embryonal Carcinoma

This rare tumor is analogous anatomically to its counterparts in the testis. The tumor is often with uncircumscription, gray or brownish in transection with hemorrhage and necrosis, and consists mainly of glandulo-duct-like structures with, sometimes, a few "embryo-like bodies". Besides these, there are often structures of dysgerminoma, choriocarcinoma or teratoma etc. in the tumor.

D. Yolk Sac Tumor (Endodermal Sinus Tumor)

Yolk sac tumors are rare, accounting for 1% of ovarian cancers. They occur mainly in females under 30 years of age. Grossly, the neoplasms are solid with areas of necrosis and hemorrhage. Histologically, yolk sac tumors of the ovary are identical to their testicular counterpart, being composed of a lace-like arrangement of primitive cells, sometimes, with structures resembling immature glomeruli (glomeruloid or Schiller-Duval bodies). They are highly malignant neoplasms with a bad prognosis. Alpha-fetoprotein can be detected in the cytoplasm as well as in the serum.

GONADAL STROMAL NEOPLASMS

Gonadal stromal neoplasms account for 5% of ovarian neoplasms. They may be composed of variable mixtures of granulosa cells, theca cells, stromal fibroblasts, and cells resembling testicular Sertoli cells and Leydig cells. They are derived from the ovarian stroma, which in turn is derived from the sex cords of the embryoma gonad.

A. Granulosa-theca Cell Tumors

Granulosa-theca cell tumors account for 2%–5% of ovarian neoplasms, and may occur at any age but are most frequently seen in postmenopausal women. A variant – juvenile granulosa cell tumor – occurs in young women. About 5% are bilateral.

Grossly, granulosa-theca cell tumors are solid yellowish fleshy masses that frequently show extensive hemorrhage and cystic change. Microscopically, they are composed of a variable mixture of granulosa and theca cells (Figure 12-21). The granulosa cells appear as small, uniform cuboidal to polygonal cells, arranged in anastomosing cord, sheets, or strands, with follicular pattern. The formation of small spaces filled with eosinophilic fluid, recapitulating the normal structure of the graafian follicle (Call-Exner bodies), is characteristic. The more elongated theca cells tend to surround the granulosa cell masses.

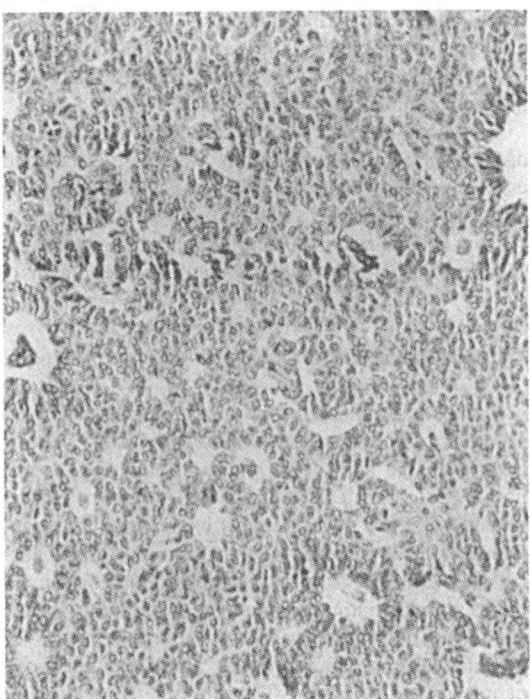

Figure 12-21 Granulosa cell tumor, showing solid sheet-like arrangement of granulosa cells with multiple spaces representing Call-Exner bodies

Granulosa-theca cell tumors typically secrete estrogens, which produce hyperplasia of the endometrium and predispose to endometrial adenocarcinoma.

The biologic behavior of these tumors cannot be predicted on the basis of their histologic features. About 25% behave in a locally aggressive manner. Distant metastases occur in about 10%–15% of cases. The 5-year survival rate for patients with granulosatheca cell tumors is 85%.

B. Thecoma-fibroma

These benign neoplasms arise in the ovarian mesenchymal stroma. They account for 3% of ovarian neoplasms and about 5% are bilateral.

Grossly, the tumors form encapsulated gray-white or somewhat yellw masses, usually less than 20 cm in diameter. Microscopically, many tumors contain a mixture of fibroblasts and theca cells, most being composed principally of fibroblasts. Approximated 20%–40% are associated with marked ascites, and a small proportion also show pleural effusions (Meigs' syndrome).

C. Sertoli-leydig Cell Tumor (Androblastoma; Arrhenoblastoma)

Sertoli-Leydig cell tumors are rare. They occur at all ages, most commonly in the 10 to 30 year age group. Less than 5% are bilateral. They are solid grayish-white neoplasms with areas of hemorrhage, necrosis, and cystic degeneration, and are composed of large cells with abundant eosinophilic cytoplasm arranged in nests or tubules. Sertoli-Leydig cell tumors commonly produce androgens and cause virilization. Rarely, they secrete estrogens. The 5-year survival rate is 90%. Malignant behavior is associated with the less well-differentiated neoplasms.

DISEASES OF THE PROSTATE

(Li Lianhong, Song Bo)

STRUCTURE AND FUNCTION

The prostate gland weighs approximately 20 g encircling the neck of the bladder and upper urethra (Figure 12-22). It is composed of several regions, including one central zone, one peripheral zone, one transitional zone, and one periurethal zone. When prostatic hyperplasia occurs, the periurethal zone is commonly involved, leading to the obstruction of urinary outflow. Whereas majority of prostatic carcinoma occur in the peripheral zone. Histologically, the prostate is a compound tubuloalveolar gland with a stroma composed of smooth muscle and fibrous tissue. Prostatic secretion produced by the epithelial cells is the major volume component of seminal fluid. It is rich in acid phosphatase. The prostate is closely related to the rectum, so permitting digital palpation of its posterior aspect in rectal examination.

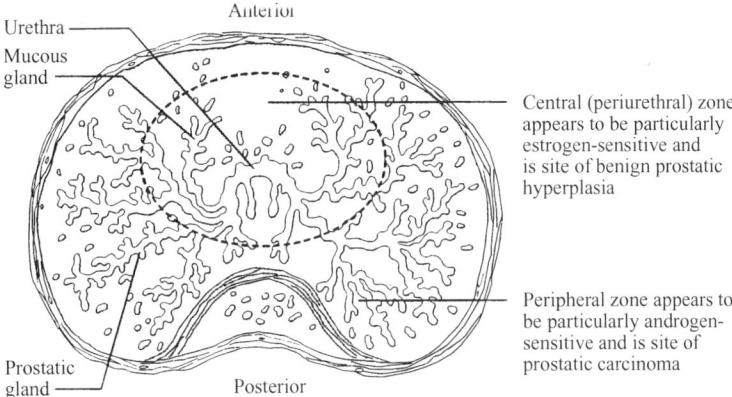

Figure 12-22 Structure of the prostate as seen in a transverse section through the gland

BENIGN PROSTATIC HYPERPLASIA (BPH)

Benign prostatic hyperplasia, also called benign nodular hyperplasia, occurs commonly after the age of 50 years. There is a progressive increase in incidence with age.

The cause of prostatic hyperplasia is unknown. Declining levels of androgens relative to estrogen levels are believed to stimulate glandular and stromal hyperplasia.

Grossly, the periurethral part of the gland is most commonly involved because this area is sensitive to the estrogen. Overall, the gland is enlarged, weighing between 60 and 100 g, uncommonly up to 200 g, and has a firm, soft consistency. The cut surface shows multiple circumscribed solid nodules with small cysts. The urethra appears slit-like and compressed. Microscopically, the nodules are composed of a variable mixture of hyperplastic glandular elements and hyperplastic fibromuscular stroma. The glands are larger than normal and lined by tall epithelium that is frequently with papillary projections. Some glands are dilated, forming smaller to larger cysts. Small areas of infarction and foci of squamous metaplasia are found frequently. Benign prostatic hyperplasia is not considered to be premalignant.

Symptoms of BPH relate to compression of the urethra with obstruction to urinary outflow, and in turn incomplete emptying of the bladder leads to chronic retention of urine and frequency.

CARCINOMA OF THE PROSTATE

Carcinoma of the prostate arises in the prostatic epithelium. It is the most common form of cancer in white men. Ninety-nine percent of cases occur in men over 50 years of age. In China, the incidence of prostatic carcinoma appears as rising tendency in recent years.

A. Etiology

The etiology of prostatic carcinoma is unknown. The low incidence in Japanese men increases to approach that of American whites when they emigrate to the United States, suggesting an important role for environmental factors. Moreover, it is probable that the decreasing androgen levels associating with involutionary changes in the outer part (peripheral zone) of the prostate is involved in the growth of prostatic carcinoma, in which most tumors arise.

B. Pathology

Over 75% of prostatic carcinomas occur in the peripheral zone of the gland - classically in the posterior part. The neoplasm is hard, irregular, ill-defined, and gray or grayish-yellow in color, and the size varies from microscopic to massive.

Histologically, most of prostatic carcinomas are adenocarcinoma that may be well differentiated, forming small or large glands (Figure 12-23A), lined by a single layer of cells. In poorly differentiated carcinomas the tumor cells tend to grow in cords, nests, or sheets and extensively invade the stroma. Perineural invasion (Figure 12-23B) is a common feature of prostatic adenocarcinoma.

In approximately 80% of cases, precancerous lesion (prostatic intraepithelial neoplasia, or PIN) coexists with the carcinoma tissue. High-grade PIN is characterized by the following nuclear changes in a gland: nuclear stratification, enlargement, and hyperchromasia with the presence of large nucleoli, but PIN has no stomal infiltration, and in the outside of the dysplastic cells there is a layer of basal

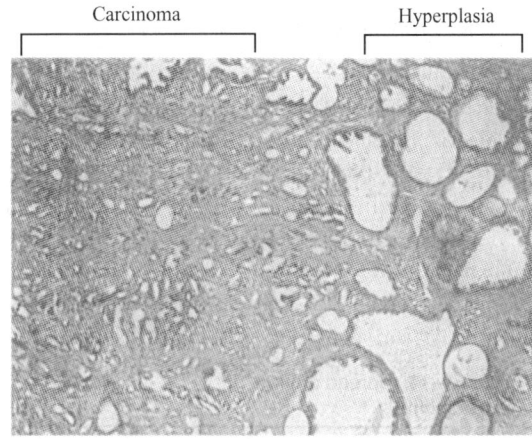

A

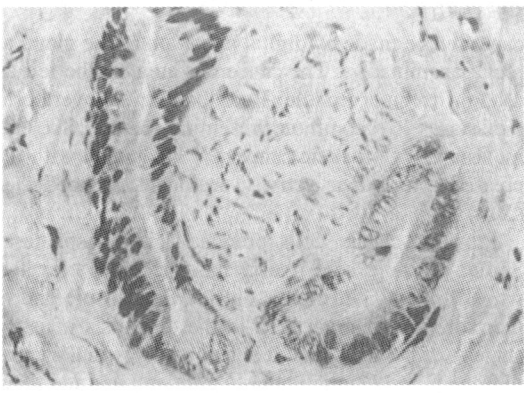

B

Figure 12-23 A: Prostatic carcinoma, low magnification, showing disorganized mass of small carcinomatous glands contrasting with the more regular glands of benign hyperplasia. B: High magnification, showing perineural invasion

cells and the integral basement membrane.

C. Spread

Local extension through the prostatic capsule into pelvic fat occurs early. Local structures such as the seminal vesicles, the base of the bladder, and the ureters are commonly involved. The rectum is rarely invaded, probably because of the presence of the rectovesical fascia.

Lymphatic spread to the regional lymph nodes (iliac, para-aortic, inguinal) is common. Hematogenous spread to the lumbosacral spine occurs early, via communications that exist between the prostatic and vertebral venous plexuses. Systemic hematogenous spread occurs late in the course of prostatic cancer and is more common in high-grade lesions.

D. Clinical Features

Urinary symptoms such as altered flow, hematuria, and frequency occur late because of the usual peripheral posterior location of the tumor. Back pain due to vertebral metastases is a common presenting feature.

The diagnosis can often be made by: digital rectal examination, revealing a hard, irregular nodule. Marked elevation of the serum acid phosphatase and prostate-specific antigen (PSA) are useful for the diagnosis of the cancer. Needle biopsy using a thin needle and ultrasound guidance provides tissue from suspicious areas for histologic diagnosis.

NEOPLASMS OF THE TESTIS AND PENIS

(Li Lianhong, Song Bo)

TESTICULAR NEOPLASMS

Neoplasms of the testis are classified into two main groups on a histogenetic basis: germ cell tumors and nongerminal tumors. Germ cell neoplasms, arising from germ cells, account for over 95% of testicular tumors, and all should be considered malignant. Most of the remaining 5% originate from the stroma or sex cord. The similar types of tumors in the ovary could occur in the testis except cystadenoma, which arises seldom from the testis, and the gross and histological appearances, and biologic characteristics in that of the testis and ovary have no obvious differences. Here we will consider only one of the germ cell tumors: seminoma.

SEMINOMA

It arises in the seminiferous epithelium, and is the commonest type of testicular neoplasms. The peak incidence is 30 – 50 years. Seminomas are divided into three histological variants: typical, anaplastic, and spermatocytic. Grossly, seminomas are firm, solid, and often better circumscribed. The classic seminoma consists of nests of uniform large round cells that have distinct cell membranes, centrally placed nuclei, prominent nucleoli, and clear cytoplasm containing abundant glycogen. The nests of cells are separated by fibrous trabeculae infiltrated by numerous lymphocytes, which is a favorable prognostic feature. Granulomatous inflammation with giant cells and necrosis is present in about 50% of cases, which correlates with a better prognosis. Clinically, seminoma usually presents as a painless mass in the testis. Seminomas are low malignant and extremely radiosensitive, and have a better prognosis.

CARCINOMA OF THE PENIS

The incidence of penile squamous cell carcinoma is low in the circumcised male. It is almost nonexistent in Jews, in whom circumcision is performed at birth, and is seen very infrequently in Moslems, in whom circumcision is performed in the early teens. Penile carcinoma is common in Asian populations, accounting for as much as 10% of male cancers in some Asian countries. It occurs in the age group from 40 to 70 years.

Squamous cell carcinoma of the penis usually begins on the glans and inner surface of the prepuce near the coronal sulcus. The early lesion is commonly an area of epithelial thickening (leukoplakia) followed by formation of papillary lesions or an elevated white papule. Ulceration follows, producing the characteristic indurated, painless ulcer with raised, everted edges (Figure 12-24).

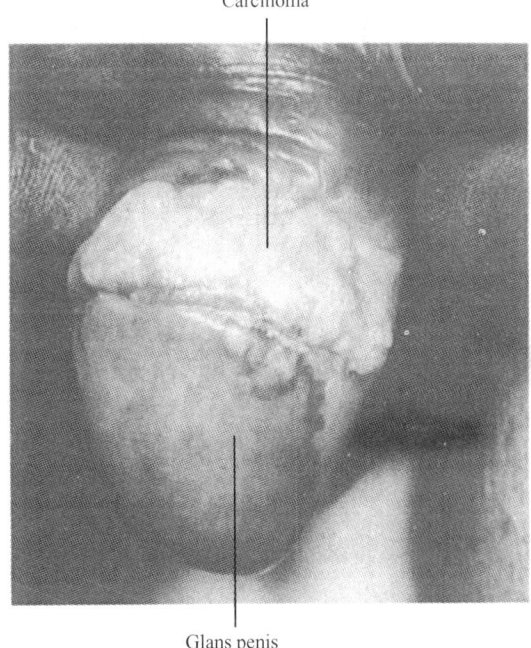

Figure 12-24 Carcinoma of the penis, showing an ulcerated mass at the base of the glans penis

Penile carcinoma commonly appears as a well-differentiated carcinoma. Penile carcinoma with a wart-like appearance similar to condyloma acuminatum, and minimal invasion, rare metastasis, and cytologic abnormality is called verrucous carcinoma. Histologically, verrucous carcinoma is a well-differentiated squamous carcinoma. Just like condyloma acuminatum, human papillomavirus (subtypes 6 and 11) are involved in the causation of verrucous carcinoma, and koilocytosis is also evident in the surface of the tumor. But in contrast to condyloma acuminatum, verrucous carcinoma could invade the underlying tissues.

Penile carcinoma shows slow infiltrative growth locally. At the time of presentation, some patients have regional (inguinal) lymph node involvement. Distant metastases occur only at a late stage.

With adequate surgical removal of the primary, which frequently entails partial or total penectomy and excision of regional inguinal lymph nodes, the overall 5-year survival rate approaches 50%. Radiation therapy is useful in controlling recurrent disease.

DISEASES OF THE BREAST

(Li Lianhong, Song Bo)

STRUCTURE AND FUNCTION

Each breast develops from the epidermal milk line, an embryonic ridge of tissue, in the thoracic region. The adult female restine mammary gland consists of five to ten duct systems, each draining at the nipple by a separate lactiferous duct (Figure 12-25). At puberty, under the influence of female sex hormones, the terminal ducts of each system proliferates distally, giving rise to lobules consisting of a cluster of 10 to 20 ductules or acini. Each terminal duct and its acini compose the terminal duct lobular unit (TDLU).

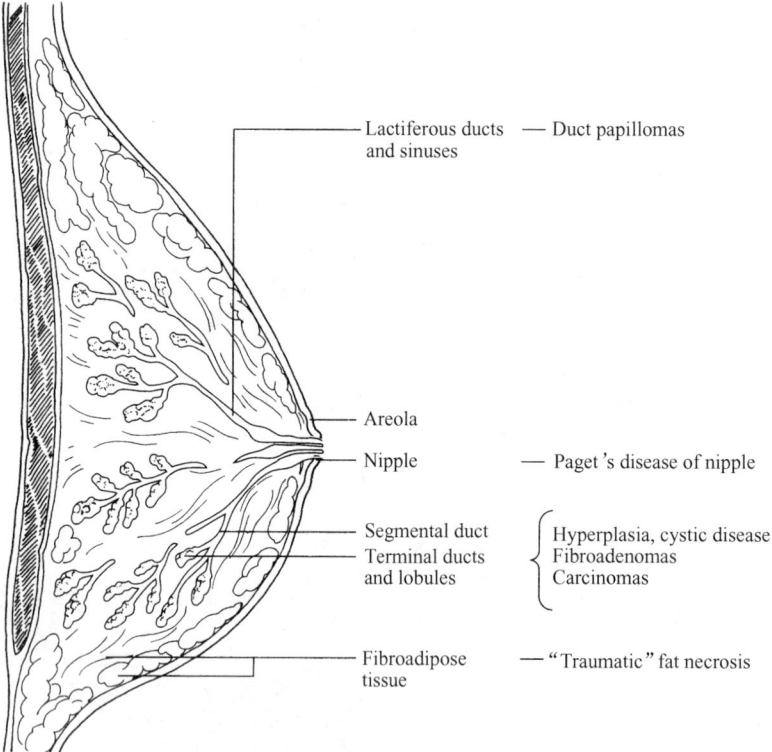

Figure 12-25 Structure of the breast and sites in which common pathologic lesions originate

The breast responds cyclically to menstruation. During the preovulatory phase, estrogen causes the glands and ducts to undergo mild dilation and hypertrophy. During the postovulatory phase, progesterone causes stromal proliferation and edema. These changes may result in mild enlargement of the breast toward the end of the cycle.

During pregnancy, there is marked hyperplasia of the glands that displace the fibroadipose stroma of the breast. Secretion of colostrums, the first milk, begins in the third trimester of pregnancy. The lactating breast is composed of closely packed dilated glands with little intervening stroma. After lactation, the glands atrophy to a level that approaches the prepregnant state.

After menopause, glands, ducts and adipose tissues atrophy further, causing progressive shrinkage in breast size.

PROLIFERATIVE CHANGES OF THE BREAST

Fibrocystic Changes (Fibrocystic Disease; Cystic Mastopathy)

Alterations termed fibrocystic disease of the breast are present in many women and are often of no symptoms, suggesting that they may be physiologic variations rather than disease, but some of the histological changes of fibrocystic disease are associated with an increased risk of breast carcinoma. Fibrocystic changes in the breast are believed to result from response of the breast to cyclic changes in levels of female sex hormones, mainly estrogens. No constant endocrine abnormality has been identified.

A. Changes not Associated with Increased Risk of Breast Carcinoma (Figure 12-26)

• **Fibrosis.** An increase in stromal fibrous tissue is common; when fibrosis predominates, the term fibrous mastopathy is used. Fibrosis is sometimes associated with ductal hyperplasia to form a localized benign lesion called a radial scar, mimicking a small carcinoma when visualized by mammography.

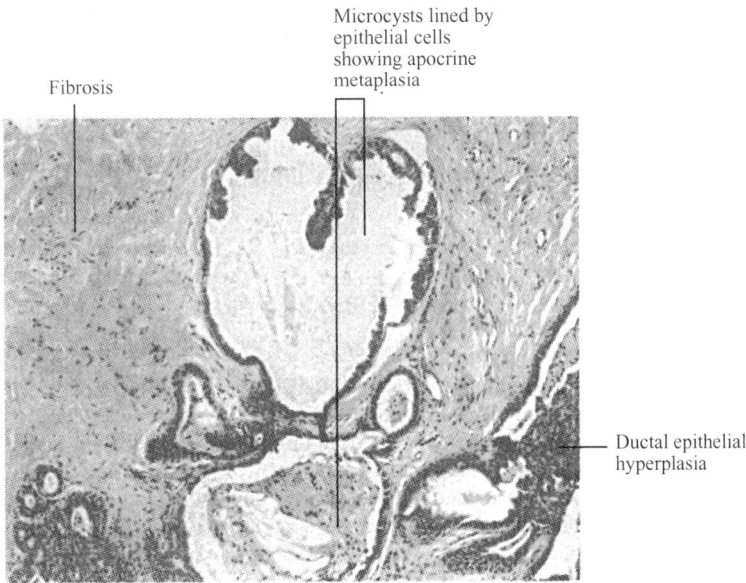

Figure 12-26 Fibrocystic change, showing fibrosis, formation of microcysts, apocrine metaplasia, and focal ductal epithelial hyperplasia

• **Cyst formation.** Cysts with size from small (microcysts) to several centimeters in diameter, occur commonly, probably as the result of duct obstruction. The cysts are lined by flattened or apocrine epithelium and contain a glairy, turbid fluid. On gross examination, many have a bluish color and for that reason are sometimes called blue-domed cysts.
• **Inflammation.** Chronic inflammation, with lymphocyte and plasma cell infiltration, is commonly present. Such lesions are also called "chronic cystic mastitis".
• **Mild ductal or lobular hyperplasia.** Mild hyperplasia of lobules or ductal epithelium is very common, and may be accompanied by sclerosis (fibrosis), leading to marked distortion of the normal lobular pattern, histologically mimicking carcinoma.
• **Apocrine metaplasia.** Metaplasia of the ductal epithelium to an apocrine type (large cells with

abundant pink cytoplasm and decapitation type secretion) is very common.

B. Changes Associated with Increased Risk of Carcinoma

- **Atypical lobular hyperplasia.** Marked proliferation of lobular epithelium is considered to carry a fourfold to fivefold increased risk of carcinoma. The proliferating cells distend the lobule and show cytologic atypia but do not satisfy the histologic criteria of carcinoma in situ.
- **Usual ductal hyperplasia (UDH).** UDH shows moderate to severe hyperplasia of the ductal epithelium. The most important feature of UDH is the presence of an admixture of two or more cell types (epithelial, myoepithelial and/or metaplastic apocrine cells). The cells show indistinct cell margins. The nuclei are unevenly distributed. Usually necrosis is absent.
- **Atypical ductal hyperplasia (ADH).** ADH is characterized by the proliferation of evenly distributed, monomorphic cells with generally ovoid to rounded nuclei. The cells may grow in micropapillae, tufts, fronds, arcades, rigid bridges, solid and cribriform patterns. Nearly 90% of ADH is negative for high molecular weight CK 1/5/10/14, an important feature in differentiating ADH from UDH.

The histological differentiation of atypical ductal hyperplasia from intraductal carcinoma may sometimes be difficult.

Sclerosing Adenosis

This variant is characterized histologically by marked intralobular fibrosis and increased numbers of distorted and compressed acini, and of great clinical important because its clinical and morphologic features may be similar to carcinoma. This disorder affects women, roughly between ages 35 and 45 years.

Sclerosing adenosis is usually, but not invariably, unilateral and tends to affect the upper outer quadrant of the breast. Grossly, the circumscribed lesion has a hard, rubbery consistency, similar to that of breast cancer. Histologically, the number of acini per terminal duct is increased to at least twofold the number in uninvolved lobules. The acini are compressed and distorted in the central portions of the lesion, and usually lined by biphasic layering of epithelial and myoepithelial cells. In some cases, the proliferative element is largely myoepithelial. Always accompanying the adenosis is marked stromal fibrosis. In some cases, this overgrowth of fibrous tissue completely compresses the lumens of the acini and ducts so that they appear as solid cords of cells. This pattern then may be difficult to distinguish histologically from an invasive scirrhous carcinoma.

Besides sclerosing adenosis, there are other types of epithelia proliferation of acini or terminal ducts. The simplest form is called adenosis. It is a frequent, benign, proliferative process, affecting mainly the acinar component of the breast parenchyma. It can be accompanied by fibrosis. Blunt duct adenosis is an organoid microscopic form of hypertrophy and hyperplasia probably of the terminal ducts, giving rise to distended ducts lined by epithelial and myoepithelial cells. Characteristically when an entire lobule is affected, a pattern is produced in which the individual epithelial units are embedded in an abundant fibrous stroma and have blunt lateral margins as well as blunt endings. Other variants include microglandular adenosis and adenomyoepithelial adenosis.

NEOPLASMS OF THE BREAST

Fibroadenoma of the Breast

Fibroadenoma is the most common benign breast neoplasm. The highest incidence is in young women. It presents as a discrete, firm, freely movable nodule in the breast. Multiple fibroadenomas occur in 10% of cases. Grossly, fibroadenomas are encapsulated, firm, and uniformly grayish-white. Fibroadenomas are usually 1–5 cm in diameter but may be larger (giant fibroadenoma). Rarely, fibroadenomas occur in adolescents as rapidly growing mass lesions with evidence of proliferative activity in both glandular and stromal elements. These tumors, called juvenile fibroadenomas, are benign.

Histologically, the tumor is composed of both glandular and fibrous elements. The relative amount of each component varies from case to case. The glands may be surrounded by stromal "pericanalicular fibroadenoma" or compressed and distorted by the latter "intracanalicular fibroadenoma".

Carcinoma of the Breast

Breast carcinoma is the most common cancer in women. There is a marked geographic influence in the incidence of breast carcinoma. The incidence rates of breast cancer in the United States and Europe are four to seven times higher than those in other countries. It is especially common in North America and Western Europe but rare in Japan.

Breast carcinoma incidence rates are associated with female age. It has been estimated that one of every eight American women living to age 90 years will develop breast carcinoma. Breast carcinoma is rare before 25 years of age and uncommon before 30 years; the incidence increases sharply after 40 to 60 years, with a mean and median age of 64 years at diagnosis. Male breast carcinoma is rare, accounting for approximately 1% of all breast carcinoma.

Breast carcinoma is common in the left breast, especially in the outer upper quadrant. It is also situated in other sites, such as in inner upper, inner lower, or bilateral and so on.

A. Etiology

The cause of breast carcinoma is unknown but is probably multifactorial. There are many risk factors for the development of breast carcinoma, identified by epidemiologic studies. Suspected factors are age, diet, geography, breast biopsies and radiation exposure etc., but the major risk factors are hormonal and genetic factors.

1. Genetic factors

Genetic factors are suggested by the strong familial tendency. There is no inheritance pattern, suggesting that the familial incidence is due either to the action of multiple genes or to similar environmental factors acting on members of the same family. Mutation of the BRCA-1 gene is believed to account for 45% of families with a high incidence of breast carcinoma. BRCA-2 has also been reported as important in familial breast carcinoma.

BRCA-1 gene is located on chromosome 17q, BRCA-2 on chromosome 13q. Mutation of BRCA1 can increases the risk of developing ovarian carcinoma, which is as high as 20% to 40%. Mutation of BRCA-2 confers a smaller risk for ovarian carcinoma (10% to 20%) but is often associated with male breast cancer. BRCA-2 and BRCA-2 carriers are also susceptible to other cancers, such as prostate, colon, and pancreas.

BRCA-1 and BRCA-2 are not sequent homology, but they act in similar pathways and interact with the same multiprotein complexes. BRCA-1 and BRCA-2 are all the tumor suppressors. Both arise the risk of malignancy, as they have a loss of function. These protein have a variety of functions, including transcriptional regulation, cell-cycle control, ubiquitin-mediated protein degradation pathways, and chromatin remodeling. A key function for both appears to be their role in protecting the genome from damage by halting the cell cycle and promoting DNA damage repair in a complex process. BRCA-1 is phosphorylated in response to damage and may transduce DNA damage signals from checkpoint kinases to effect proteins. BRCA-1 is also bound with BRCA-2 DNA repair. BRCA-2 can bind directly to DNA and functions in homologous recombination for the error-free repair of double-strand DNA breaks. BRCA-1, but not BRCA-2, interacts with the ER and is involved in X chromosome inactivation. Male breast cancers are markedly increased only in families carrying mutation of BRCA-2.

2. Hormones

Estrogen has been the most extensively studied hormone because of the epidemiologic evidence that prolonged estrogen exposure (early menarche, late menopause, nulliparity, and delayed pregnancy) increases the risk of breast cancer.

Some breast cancers are hormone dependent, being related to the presence of estrogen, progesterone, and other steroid hormone receptors in the nuclei of breast carcinoma cells. Estrogen is believed to exert its effect by causing the cancer cells to secrete growth factors (e. g. epidermal growth factor, EGF) that promote tumor progression. In neoplasia that possess such receptors, hormone (antiestrogen) therapy may slow the growth or cause regression of the tumor.

Postmenopausal hormone replacement therapy slightly increases the risk of breast carcinoma in current users but might not increase the risk of death. Estrogen and progesterone together increase the risk more than does estrogen alone. Invasive lobular carcinomas and other estrogen receptor (ER)-positive carcinomas are reported to be increased in this group does. Oral contraceptives are unlikely to increase the risk of breast carcinoma and can decrease the risk of other malignancies such as ovarian carcinoma. Reducing endogenous estrogens by oophorectomy decreases the risk of developing breast carcinoma by up to 75%.

3. Environmental factors

The importance of environmental factors in the etiology of breast carcinoma has been pointed out by the geographic distribution of this cancer. There is concern that environmental contaminants (organochlorine pesticides) have estrogenic effects on humans. The possible effect of environmental factors on breast carcinoma risk has been investigated. So far specific substances associated with an increased risk of malignancy have not definitively found.

B. Pathology

Based upon histological criteria, several different types of breast carcinoma are recognized, subclassified according to differentiation. (lobular versus ductal) or invasiveness (in situ versus infiltrating)

1. In situ (noninvasive) carcinoma

• **Lobular carcinoma in situ (LCIS)** (Figure 12-27). LCIS is a neoplastic proliferation of lobular epithelial cells that fill and distend all the acini of at least one complete lobular unit, obliterating their lumens. The abnormal cells of atypical lobular hyperplasia (ALH), LCIS, and invasive lobular carcinoma are identical and consist of small cells that have oval or round nuclei with small nucleoli that do not adhere to one another. Signet-ring cells containing mucin are present commonly. LCIS rarely distorts the underlying architecture, and the involved acini remain recognizable as lobules. LCIS almost always expresses estrogen and progesterone receptors, and overexpression of HER2/neu is not observed. The basement membrane is intact; there is no risk of disseminated change as long as the tumor remains in situ. LCIS tends to be multifocal and bilateral.

LCIS does not produce a palpable lesion and is not apparent on mammography. It is usually an incidental pathologic finding in a patient who has had breast tissue removed for some other reason.

The presence of LCIS increases the risk of future development of breast carcinoma tenfold to twelvefold. Both breasts are at risk, with the ipsilateral slightly more so than the contralateral breast. Infiltrating carcinomas associated with LCIS may be eigher ductal or lobular.

The management of a patient with LCIS is highly controversial, and recommended treatment ranges from careful follow-up to bilateral simple mastectomy, because of the increased risk of infiltrating breast carcinoma.

• **Ductal carcinoma in situ (DCIS)** (Figure 12-28). DCIS is characterized by increased proliferation of ductal epithelial cells confined within the basement membrane and subtle to marked cellular atypia, and an inherent but not necessarily obligate tendency for progression to invasive carcinoma. DCIS is frequently multifocal, and commonly associated with infiltrating ductal carcinoma. It is bilateral in 15%–20% of cases.

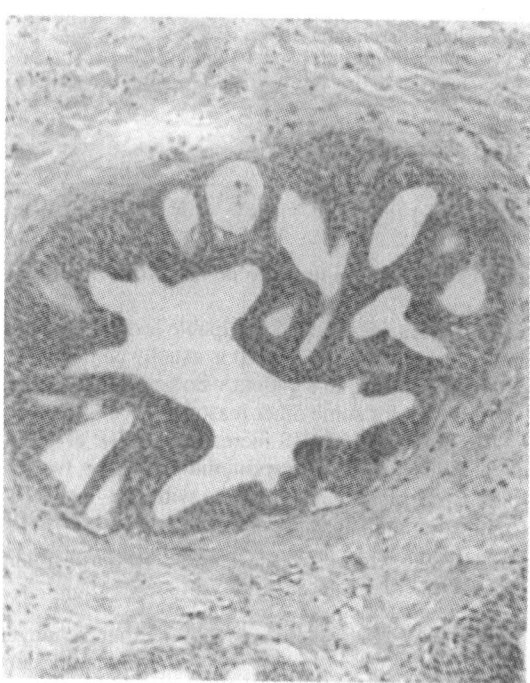

Figure 12-28 Ductal carcinoma in situ, cribriform type. The duct is distended by a uniform population of cells. The basement membrane is intact

Grossly, DCIS may produce a hard mass composed of thickened cord-like structures from which necrotic material can sometimes be expressed. Calcification is a common feature; consequently, DCIS is detectable by mammography. In some cases, however, DCIS is neither palpable nor visualized by

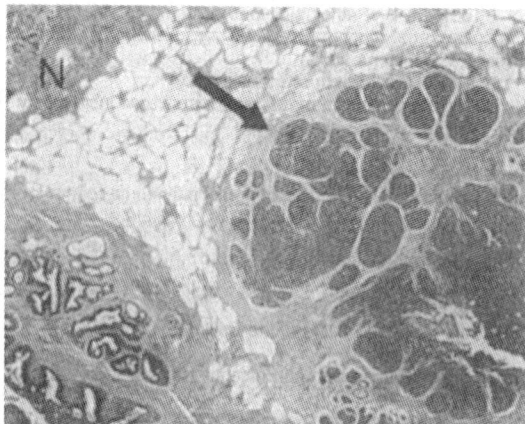

Figure 12-27 Lobular carcinoma in situ. The involved lobule (arrow) shows complete filling and distention of all constituent acini by small round cells. Compare with normal breast lobule at top left(labeled N)

mammography (microscopic DCIS).

Histologically, the DCIS may be classified as low, intermediate and high grade. Low grade DCIS is composed of small monomorphic round cells with subtle increase in nulear-cytoplasmic ratio and inconspicuous nucleoli. The proliferated cells grow in arcades, micropapillae, cribriform or solid patterns. Mitotic figures are rare. Intermediate grade DCIS are often composed of cells cytologically similar to those of low grade DCIS, but with some ducts containing intraluminal necrosis. Others display nuclei of intermediate grade with occasional nucleoli and coarse chromatin. Necrosis may or may not be present. High grade DCIS is composed of highly atypical cells. Nuclei are high grade, markedly pleomorphic, poorly polarized, with coarse, clumped chromatin and prominent nucleoli. Mitotic figures are usually common.

The treatment of DCIS varies with the size of the lesion. For microscopic and small (< 2.5 cm) lesions, local complete excision (lumpectomy) is the usual treatment. For larger lesions, mastectomy is usually done. Axillary lymph node dissection is not indicated if there is no invasion, particularly in lesions smaller than 2.5 cm.

2. Infiltrating (invasive) ductal carcinoma

- **Invasive ductal carcinoma**. Invasive ductal carcinoma is the most common type of breast cancer, comprising 75% of all cases. Grossly, it forms a gritty, rock-hard, grayish-white infiltrative mass. Yellowish-white chalk streaks are characteristic and correspond to a peculiar deposition of elastic tissue (elastosis) around ducts in the area of involvement. Fibrosis may be extensive. Microscopically, highly pleomorphic ductal epithelial cells infiltrate the fibrous stroma. Lymphatic invasion is common.

Paget's disease of the nipple: Paget's disease presents clinically as an eczematous change in the nipple and surrounding skin. It is characterized microscopically by the presence of carcinoma cells in the epidermis. These cells are believed to spread within the epidermis. The cells are large, with abundant cytoplasm that stains positively for mucin and resembles the cells of ductal carcinoma of the breast. In most cases, the underlying breast shows the presence of a ductal carcinoma.

When Paget's disease occurs in a patient without a palpable mass or in one with only intraductal carcinoma, it is an early manifestation of cancer, and the prognosis is good.

- **Infiltrating lobular carcinomas**. Infiltrating lobular carcinomas constitute 5% - 10% of all breast carcinomas. They are similar to infiltrating ductal carcinomas except for (1) a different histological pattern of infiltration, with a tendency to form single rows of cells and concentric arrangement of cells around ducts (targetoid appearance); (2) a slightly higher incidence of bilaterality; and (3) a greater frequency of estrogen receptor positivity.

- **Morphologic variants of breast carcinoma**. Variant forms of breast carcinoma have been recognized. Some of them-like medullary carcinoma, mucinous (colloid) carcinoma, and tubular carcinoma-are important to recognize because they have a better prognosis than the usual infiltrating ductal carcinoma. Medullary carcinomas tend to be large, soft, and very well circumscribed, consisting of sheets of large polygonal cells associated with a marked lymphocytic infiltrate (which may contribute to the good prognosis). Mucinous carcinomas form gelatinous lakes of mucoid material in which cancer cells are suspended. Tubular carcinoma is composed of small, irregular infiltrative cancerous glands.

C. Mode of Spread

Direct spread occurs along the ductal system at an early stage, resulting in involvement of multiple ducts and lobules, often before invasion has occurred. Extension to the nipple in this manner results in Paget's disease. Local invasion may also occur into the breast stroma and then into overlying skin and underlying pectoralis major. Chest wall muscle involvement has a poor prognosis.

Lymphatic spread follows predictable routes according to the site of the primary lesion. The axillary lymph nodes are the primary node group affected. The nodes along the internal mammary artery may be involved in carcinomas located in the medial half of the breast. Spread beyond the axillary node into supraclavicular and cervical nodes is evidence of advanced disease. Local dermal lymphatic obstruction, most commonly due to extensive axillary node involvement, causes edema of the skin (peaud' orange).

Bloodstream spread, with metastatic deposits in bone, liver, and lungs, occurs in the later stages in almost all cases not cured by initial treatment. Entry of cancer cells into the bloodstream probably occurs early in the course of invasive breast carcinoma, but most of these cells are either killed by the immune system or remain dormant in distant organs. Spread via the pleural or peritoneal cavity occurs when the pleura or peritoneum is secondarily involved by the breast cancer. The mechanisms underlying dormancy of metastatic cancer cells and the reasons for their later activation to cause clinically detectable tumor masses are unknown. Dormancy and activation of cancer cells are necessary to explain the occurrence of metastases many years after treatment of the primary tumor.

D. Diagnosis

1. Histologic examination

Histologic examination of a biopsy of the mass is the definitive diagnostic method. Excisional, incisional, or needle biopsies may be performed. Immediate diagnosis of a biopsy specimen by frozen section examination has a high degree of accuracy in experienced hands.

A complete pathologic diagnosis of breast carcinoma should provide the following information: (1) the histological type of carcinoma; (2) the size of the tumor; (3) the stage of disease (Table 12-4); and (4) the estrogen and progesterone receptor status.

2. Receptor status

Receptor status is currently established by bioassay, for which a specimen from the tumor must be freezing diagnosed by the pathologist immediately after excision. Delay in preservation greatly interferes with the results of receptor assay. Immunohistochemical techniques are available for receptor determination on fixed tissue.

3. Cytologic diagnosis

Cytologic diagnosis utilizing a specimen obtained by fine-needle aspiration is increasing in popularity because it is rapid and cost-effective. Cytologic diagnosis is capable only of identifying carcinoma cells. Definitive diagnosis of the histological type of carcinoma still requires histological examination of tissue sections.

E. Treatment

1. Surgery

Surgery has been the mainstay of treatment of breast cancer for the past several decades. The standard treatment was radical mastectomy, which involves removal of the breast along with the pectoral muscles and axillary contents. The realization that this type of surgery may be too extensive led to new approaches. Presently, two forms of treatment are recognized as being equally effective in treating all but very large (>4 cm) lesions. These are (1) modified radical mastectomy, which includes axillary node dissection but preserves the pectoralis muscle; and (2) complete excision with clear margins (lumpectomy), with axillary node dissection followed by radiation. There is a trend toward breast-conserving surgery for treatment of breast carcinoma.

2. Radiotherapy

Breast carcinoma is a moderately radiosensitive tumor. Radiotherapy is indicated when breast-conserving surgery has been performed and in patients who develop locally recurrent disease in the chest wall.

3. Chemotherapy

Chemotherapy has increased the disease-free survival periods in breast carcinoma but is not curative. The rationale for chemotherapy after successful surgical treatment (adjuvant chemotherapy) is that it removes microscopic foci of neoplastic cells in distant sites, thus complementing the role of surgery. Adjuvant chemotherapy is indicated in all but small, well-differentiated, node-negative cancers with no adverse prognostic indicators.

4. Hormonal therapy

Hormonal manipulation – usually antiestrogen therapy – is most effective in patients with estrogen or progesterone receptor – positive carcinomas. (Sixty to 80% of such patients respond; only 10% of receptor-negative patients respond). Removal of estrogens may be achieved surgically (removal of ovaries and adrenal glands) or by antiestrogenic drugs such as tamoxifen. Antiprogesterone agents (RU 486; mifepristone) have recently become available and are in trial.

F. Prognosis

Infiltrating carcinoma of the breast has a 5-year survival rate of about 70%. About 20% of patients who survive 5 years will develop late recurrences. Recurrences of breast carcinoma have been recorded as late as 25 years after the primary tumor was successfully treated. There are most of factors affecting prognosis such as the clinicopathologic stage, the histological type, histological grade, steroid hormone receptors and others.

Staging is the most important predictor of prognosis. Relation between staging and prognosis is as following:
- **Stage 0**: DCIS or LCIS has 5-year survival rate of 92%.

- **Stage I**: Invasive carcinoma of 2 cm or less in diameter including carcinoma in situ with microinvasion without nodal involvement or only metastases but tumor <0.02 cm in diameter has 5-year survival rate of 87%.
- **Stage II**: Invasive carcinoma of 5 cm or less in diameter with up to three involved axillary nodes or invasive carcinoma greater than 5 cm without nodal involvement has 5-year survival rate of 75%.
- **Stage III**: Invasive carcinoma of 5 cm or less in diameter with four or more involved axillary nodes; invasive carcinoma greater than 5 cm in diameter with nodal involvement; invasive carcinoma with 10 or more involved axillary nodes; invasive carcinoma with involvement of the ipsilateral internal mammary lymph nodes; or invasive carcinoma with skin involvement such as ulceration, or satellite skin nodules and so on, chest wall fixation, or clinical inflammatory carcinoma has 5-year survival rate of 46%.
- **Stage IV**: Any breast cancer with distant metastases has 5-year survival rate of 13%.

DISEASES OF THE MALE BREAST

Gynecomastia

Enlargement of the male breast, gynecomastia, is uncommon and may be unilateral or bilateral; it usually presents as a nodule or plaque of firm tissue under the nipple and may be painful. In a few cases, a cause can be identified, such as: testicular atrophy or destruction, as in cirrhosis of the liver, and lepromatous leprosy, conditions associated with increased estrogen levels, as an estrogen-secreting tumor of the testis or adrenal, increased gonadotropin levels, as in choriocarcinoma of the testis, increased prolactin levels, as in diseases of the hypothalamopituitary axis, and drugs, most commonly digoxin.

Gynecomastia is characterized by proliferation of the ducts of the breast, which become surrounded by proliferating edematous stroma. A moderate degree of epithelial hyperplasia is common. Lobular units are absent in most cases.

Carcinoma of the Male Breast

Carcinoma of the male breast is extremely rare. Histological features are identical to those of infiltrating ductal carcinomas in the female. In spite of the small bulk of the breast in men, the diagnosis of male breast carcinoma is usually delayed; 50% of patients have axillary lymph node metastases at the time of diagnosis. As a result, male breast cancer has a worse overall prognosis than female breast cancer.

Table 12-4 Staging of breast carcinoma using the TNM system

Primary tumor (T)	
Tis	Carcinoma in situ. Includes LCIS, DCIS, Paget's disease of the nipple with no underlying tumor
T1	Tumor 2 cm or less in greatest dimension
T2	Tumor >2 cm but not greater than 5 cm in greatest dimension
T3	Tumor >5 cm in greatest dimension
T4	Tumor of any size with extension to chest wall or skin. Includes inflammatory carcinoma
Lymph node (N)	
N0	No regional lymph node metastasis
N1	Metastasis to movable ipsilateral axillary lymph nodes
N2	Metastasis in ipsilateral axillary lymph nodes fixed to one another or other structures
N3	Metastasis to ipsilateral internal mammary lymph nodes
Distant metastasis (M)	
M0	No distant metastasis
M1	Distant metastasis present. (Note: Supraclavicular lymph node metastasis counts as distant metastasis.)
Clinical staging based on above criteria	
Stage 0	Tis N0 M0
Stage I	T1 N0 M0
Stage II A	T1 N1 M0 or T2 N0 M0
Stage II B	T2 N1 M0 or T3 N0 M0
Stage III A	T1 N2 M0, T2 N2 M0, T3 N1 M0, T3 N2 M0
Stage III B	T4 Any N M0 or Any T N3 M0
Stage IV	Any T Any N M1

(Li Lianhong, Song Bo)

Chapter 13 Diseases of the Endocrine System

Song Wenjing

CHAPTER CONTENTS
- Introduction
- Diseases of the Pituitary Gland
    Normal Structure and Function
    Hypothalamus-Posterior Pituitary Disease
    Hypersecretion and Hyposecretion of Anterior Pituitary Hormones
    Pituitary Neoplasms-Adenoma and Carcinoma
- Diseases of the Thyroid Gland
    Normal Structure and Function
    Diffuse Nontoxic and Multinodular Goiter
    Disorders of Thyroid Secretion
    Inflammatory Thyroid Diseases
    Thyroid Neoplasms
    Summary
- Diseases of the Parathyroid Gland
    Normal Structure and Function
    Excessive Secretion of PTH
    Decreased Secretion of PTH
- Diseases of the Adrenal Gland
    Normal Structure and Function
    Excessive Secretion of Adrenocortical Hormones
    Decreased Secretion of Adrenocortical Hormones
    The Adrenal Gland Neoplasms
- The Endocrine Pancreas Diseases
    Normal Structure and Function
    Diabetes Mellitus
    Islet Cell Neoplasms
- * Supplement: Multiple Endocrine Neoplasia Syndromes

This section discusses the main endocrine glands, which include the pituitary, thyroid, parathyroid, adrenal glands and the pancreas (islets of Langerhans). Other organs in the body such as the ovaries (granulosa cells and luteal cells), testes (interstitial cells of Leydig), gastrointestinal tract (pyloric antral G cells), and placenta (chorionic gonadotropin) have endocrine components that are discussed in those chapters.

INTRODUCTION

The pituitary secrets tropic hormones that control the function of the thyroid, the cortisol-producing zones of the adrenal cortex, and the gonads. The pituitary in turn is controlled by releasing and inhibiting hormones secreted by the hypothalamus.

Hormones usually bind to receptors on target cells in the body. The receptors may be located in the cell membrane (catecholamines, polypeptide hormones), the cytoplasm (steroids), or the nucleus (thyroid hormones and steroids). The binding of the hormone to the receptor leads to a series of changes in the cell that results in the metabolic action of the hormone. In the case of catecholamines and polypeptide hormones, there is activation of adenylyl cyclase, which stimulates intracellular production of cAMP. cAMP acts as an internal (second) messenger, effecting the specific biochemical change dictated by the hormone on the target cell. Other hormones such as cortico-steroids and thyroid hormone cause increased mRNA synthesis, leading to protein (enzyme) synthesis.

Endocrine diseases are frequently characterized by abnormal patterns of hormone secretion:
- Excessive secretion of hormones may be due to the presence of increased numbers of cells of the type that normally secrete the hormone. This may occur as primary hyperfunction, due to hyperplastic or neoplastic proliferation of the cells; or secondary hy-

perfunction, due to increased stimulation by increased levels of tropic hormones or decreased feedback inhibition. Excessive secretion may also be due to production of hormones by cells that do not normally secret the hormone, resulting in what we call ectopic hormone syndromes.

- Decreased secretion of hormones may be due to decreased numbers of hormones-secreting cells, which may in turn be due to primary hypofunction, from congenital absence or hypoplasia or from destruction of the gland by trauma, infection, ischemia, immunologic mechanisms, or neoplasms; or secondary hypofunction, from absence of stimulation by the tropic hormones on which the cells are dependent. Secondary hypofunction is characterized by atrophy of the hormone-secreting cells due to lack of stimulation. Diminished secretion may also be due to deficiency of enzymes required to synthesize the hormone. Decreased hormone activity may be caused by a defect in the target organ receptors, which is usually congenital. Because serum hormone levels are normal in such patients, the prefix *pseudo* -is attached to these hypofunctional states, e. g. pseudohypoparathyroidism.
- Secretion of abnormal hormones by endocrine glands is usually due to enzyme deficiency, e. g. in congenital adrenal hyperplasia.

DISEASES OF THE PITUITARY GLAND

NORMAL STRUCTURE AND FUNCTION

The pituitary (hypophysis) is a small gland (350-900 mg) located in the sella turcica, a bony compartment in the base of the skull. It is composed of an anterior lobe (adenohypophysis), which comprises about 75% of gland; a posterior lobe (neurohypophysis), which comprises about 25% of the gland; and a vestigial intermediate lobe (Figure 13-1).

Histologically, the anterior pituitary is composed of small round cells in nests and cords separated by a rich vascular network. The cells have variably staining cytoplasm on routine sections and were at one time called acidophils, basophils, and chromophobes based on their staining characteristics. They are now classified according to the specific hormones they produce (Table 13-1) as identified by immunohistochemical methods. About 15% - 20% of the cells in the anterior pituitary are nonreactive to immunohistochemical tests and are classified as nonsecretory cells.

The posterior lobe is composed of a mass of nerve fibers with supporting glial cells. These unmyelinated nerves are the axons of hypothalamic neurons. As shown by electron microscopy, they contain membrane-bound secretory granules (composed either of antidiuretic hormone [ADH] or of oxytocin). ADH and oxytocin are complexed with specific binding proteins (neurophysins).

The anterior and posterior lobes of the pituitary are under hypothalamic control. Control is direct in the case of the posterior lobe; neurons in the hypothalamic nuclei secrete ADH and oxytocin, which pass down the axons in the pituitary stalk for storage and eventually are released into the blood by the posterior pituitary. Hypothalamic control of the anterior pituitary is affected by releasing and inhibiting hormones produced in the hypothalamus and carried to the anterior lobe via the portal venous system (Table 13-2 and Figure 13-1).

Table 13-1 Cell types and hormones of the pituitary

Cell Type	Quantity	Hormone	Action
Anterior pituitary Somatotroph	40% - 50%	Growth hormone (somatotropin)	Growth of all body tissue; antagonist to insulin
Lactotroph	15% - 20%	Prolactin	Proliferation of ductal tissue in breast and initiation of milk secretion
Corticotroph[1]	15% - 20%	Corticotrophin (ACTH)	Stimulation of adrenocortical steroid synthesis and secretion
		Beta-lipotropic hormone	...
		Beta-endorphin	Endogenous opiate
		Alpha-melanocyte stimulating hormone	Dispersion of melanin in skin
Thyrotroph	5%	Thyrotropin (TSH)	Stimulation of thyroid hormone synthesis and secretion

(Continued)

Cell Type	Quantity	Hormone	Action
Gonadotroph[2]	5%	Follicle-stimulating hormone (FSH)	Preovulatory growth of graafian follicle and estrogen secretion; with LH, induces ovulation
		Luteinizing hormone (LH)	With FSH, induces ovulation, formation of corpus luteum, and progesterone secretion
Nonsecretory (null) cells	15%–20%	None	...
Posterior pituitary Hypothalamic nuclei		Antidiuretic hormone (ADH)	Water resorption in distal nephron; arteriolar constriction
		Oxytocin	Contraction of smooth muscle of uterus and breast ducts

[1] Beta-lipotropic hormone, beta-endorphin, and alpha-melanocyte stimulating hormone are peptides that are split off during corticotrophin synthesis.

[2] The same cell probably secretes both FSH and LH. Note that in the male, LH is identical to the interstitial cell-stimulating hormone (ICSH), which stimulates the testicular Leydig cells to secrete androgens.

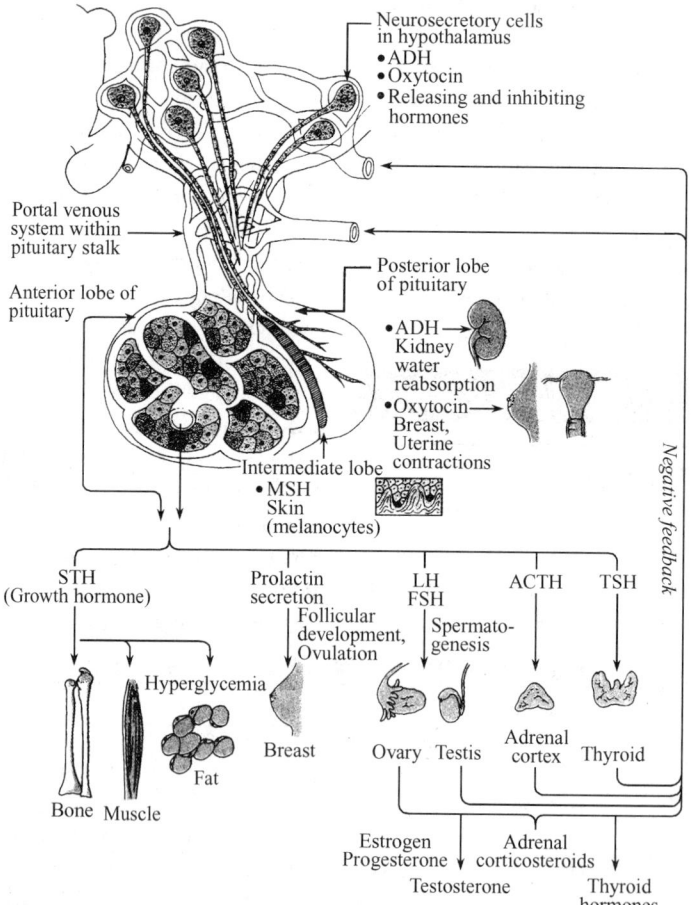

Figure 13-1 Principal hormones of the pituitary and hypothalamus, their target organs, and their effects. Hypothalamic neurosecretory cells secreting ADH and oxytocin have direct axonal connections with the posterior pituitary. Hypothalamic cells secreting releasing and inhibiting hormones that control pituicytes in the anterior lobe exert their controlling influence via the portal venous system in the pituitary stalk. (STH, somatotropic hormone; LH, luteinizing hormone; FSH, follicle-stimulating hormone; ACTH, adrenocorticotropic hormone (corticotropin); TSH, thyroid-stimulating hormone (thyrotropin); ADH, antidiuretic hormone.)

Table 13-2 Control mechanisms for pituitary hormones

Hormone	Control
Antidiuretic hormone (ADH)	Serum osmolality
Oxytocin	Neural
Grown hormone	Serum glucose; hypothalamic GHRH[1]
Prolactin	GHIH[1]
Thyrotropin	Hypothalamic PRH[1], PIH[1]
Gonadotropins	Serum thyroxine; hypothalamic TRH[1]
Corticotropin	Serum estrogen, progesterone, testosterone; hypothalamic GRH[1] (LHRH[1] and FRH[1]) Serum cortisol; hypothalamic CSH[1]

[1] These releasing and inhibiting hormones (factors) are produced by cells in the hypothalamus and transmitted to the anterior pituitary by a portal system (Figure 13-1).

Key: CRH = corticotropin-releasing hormone
FRH = FSH-releasing hormone
FSH = follicle-stimulating hormone
GHIH = growth hormone-inhibiting hormone (somatostatin)
GHRH = growth hormone-releasing hormone
GRH = gonadotropin-releasing hormone
LHRH = luteinizing hormone-releasing hormone
PIH = prolactin-inhibiting hormone
PRH = prolactin-releasing hormone
TRH = thyrotropin-releasing hormone

HYPOTHALAMUS-POSTERIOR PITUITARY DISEASE

Diabetes Insipidus

Diabetes insipidus is caused by failure of the hypothalamus and posterior pituitary to secrete antidiuretic hormone (ADH). Deficient water reabsorption in the renal collecting tubule then leads to the excretion of an increased amount of urine (polyuria) of very low specific gravity. Serum osmolality is increased, including thirst and polydipsia (excessive water intake). The superficial resemblance of the clinical features (polyuria, polydipsia) to diabetes mellitus, combined with the absence of a sweet (insipid) taste of the urine led historically to the term diabetes insipidus.

Diabetes insipidus may be caused by any condition that interferes with the hypothalamopituitary axis: (1) hypothalamic or pituitary neoplasms or (2) disruption of the pituitary stalk by trauma, meningeal disease (metastatic carcinoma, sarcoidosis, tuberculous meningitis), or bone disease (Hand-Schüller-Christian disease).

Diagnosis is based initially on the clinical features with confirmation by the water deprivation test. Deprivation of water fails to increase urine concentration in patients with diabetes insipidus due to the absence of ADH.

Precocious Puberty

Precocious puberty is due to gonadotropic hormone (GTH) that is secreted by the hypothalamus-pituitary in the premature stage, which is caused by the diseases of central nervous system (e.g. neoplasms, hydrocephalus) and inherited disorders. It is characterized by sex development before 6–8 years in girls and 8–10 years in boys.

HYPERSECRETION AND HYPOSECRETION OF ANTERIOR PITUITARY HORMONES

Hypersecretion of Anterior Pituitary Hormones

Nearly all cases of anterior pituitary hypersecretion are due to primary hyperfunction caused by benign neoplasms of a single cell type (pituitary adenoma). Hyperplasia of pituitary cells and pituitary carcinoma are extremely rare.

The clinical features of pituitary adenoma may be divided into effects resulting from local growth of the neoplasm and those resulting from hormone secretion (Table 13-3). The former depend on the size of the neoplasm and its invasive capability; the later depend on the type of hormone secreted.

Table 13-3 Clinical effects of pituitary adenoma

Mass Effects (Large Adenomas)	Excessive Hormone Secretion (Only Manifestation in Small Adenomas)
Enlargement of the pituitary gland, causing • Destruction of normal pituitary cells, → hypopituitarism diabetes insipidus • Expansion of sella turcica (visible on x-ray) • Suprasellar extension through diaphragma sella, causing (1) Compression of optic chiasm or nerves→visual field defects (2) Compression of hypothalamus→diabetes insipidus (3) interference with outflow of CSF from third ventricle→raised intracranial pressure and hydrocephalus (4) Compression of vessels→headache (5) Cranial nerve compression (rare) (6) Possible invasion of brain (invasive adenoma), paranasal sinuses, cavernous sinus	Absent in 30% of cases Prolactin in 30% →galactorrhes Growth hormone in 25% → gigantism in children and acromegaly in adults Corticotrophin in 10% →Cushing's syndrome Thyrotropin and gonadotropins in 5%

Systemic effects due to hormone excess:

A. Pituitary Gigantism and Acromegaly

Increased growth hormone levels cause increased growth of nearly every tissue in the body. The clinical effect depends on the age of patients. In the children, there is excessive uniform bone growth at the epiphyses, resulting in a massive but proportionate increase in height (gigantism). In adults, in whom adenomas occur much more commonly, the fused epiphyses do not permit increased height, but there is a generalized enlargement of bones that is most visible in the hands (spade-like hands), jaw, and skull (acromegaly). Tissues other than bone are also affected. Increased size of cartilages leads to enlargement of the nose and ears. Joint abnormalities occur, particularly in the vertebral column, causing osteoarthritis. Increased size of soft tissues produces coarsening of facial features and enlargement of all the viscera, notably the heart, liver, kidneys, adrenals, thyroid, and pancreas.

B. Hyperprolactinemia

The commonest hormone produced by a pituitary adenoma is prolactin. In women, prolactin causes amenorrhea, infertility, and galactorrhea (milk secretion in the absence of pregnancy). In men, it causes decreased libido, impotence, and galactorrhea.

These clinical features may be mimicked by other conditions, including hypothalamic diseases in which these is decreased production of prolactin inhibiting factor, and they may occur as a toxic response to drugs that block dopaminergic transmission (e. g. methyldopa and reserpine) to produce hyperprolactinemia. Since prolactin-secreting tumors may be microadenomas, the differential diagnosis is very difficult.

Hyposecretion of Anterior Pituitary Hormones

Hypopituitarism in adults (Simmonds' disease) is rare. The most common cause in the past was ischemic necrosis of a gland that had undergone hyperplasia during pregnancy (Sheehan's syndrome) (Table 13-4). This was duo to shock, usually precipitated by postpartum hemorrhage. With improved obstetric care, Sheehan's syndrome is now very uncommon in developed countries.

Table 13-4 Causes of hypopituitarism

Ischemic necrosis of the pituitary
Postpartum necrosis (Sheehan's syndrome)
Head injury
Vascular disease, commonly associated with diabetes mellitus
Neoplasms involving the sella turcica
Nonfunctional adenoma
Craniopharyngioma
Suprasellar chordoma
Histocytosis X (eosinophilic granuloma; Hand-Schüller-Christian disease)

	(Continued)
Intrasellar cysts	
Empty sella syndrome	
Chronic inflammatory lesions	
Tuberculosis, syphilis, sarcoidosis	
Infiltrative diseases	
Amyloidosis	
Hemochromatosis	
Mucopolysaccharidoses	
Defective end-organ growth hormone receptors (Laron dwarfism)	

Nonfunctioning neoplasms involving the sella now represent the most common cause of hypopituitarism in developed countries. Such tumors include nonfunctional pituitary adenoma and craniopharyngioma. Pituitary dwarfism occurs if hypopituitarism develops early in life due either to tumor or to other causes.

The clinical effects of hypopituitarism depend on whether the patient is a child or an adult.

Hypopituitarism in children results in a proportionate failure of growth due to absence of growth hormone (pituitary dwarfism). These children have normal intelligence and remain child-like, failing to develop sexually. A similar clinical picture of pituitary dwarfism occurs in children born with defective end-organ receptors to growth hormone (Laron dwarfism). These patients have normal levels of growth hormone in the serum.

In adults, hypopituitarism is characterized mainly by the effects of gonadotropin deficiency. In the female, there is amenorrhea and infertility; in the male, infertility and impotence. Thyrotropin and corticotropin deficiency may result in atrophy of the thyroid gland and adrenal cortex. However, decreased secretion of thyroxine and cortisol is rarely severe enough to cause clinical manifestations. Isolated growth hormone deficiency produces little abnormality in the adult.

PITUITARY NEOPLASMS -ADENOMA AND CARCINOMA

Introduction

Pituitary adenomas are uncommon, constituting about 10% of primary intracranial neoplasms. They occur at all ages but are most common in the age group of 20 to 50 years. They occur in men slightly more frequently than in women.

About 30% are nonfunctional, causing destruction of the normal gland. Patients present with general or selective hypopituitarism. About 30% secrete prolactin, 25% growth hormone, and 10% ACTH. The remainders secrete thyrotropin or gonadotropins (Table 13-3). Fifteen percent of adenomas secrete more than one hormone.

Occasionally, pituitary adenoma occurs as part of the multiple endocrine adenoma syndromes.

Pathologic Changes

Grossly, pituitary adenomas vary greatly in size from microscopic to very large. Microadenomas (diameter < 1 cm) are commonly found autopsy, but their significance is unclear. ACTH- and prolactin-secreting adenomas tend to be microadenomas at the time of presentation, whereas nonfunctional and growth hormone-secreting tend to reach a large size before they are discovered. Larger tumors expand the sella turcica and compress surrounding structures, especially the optic chiasm (Table 13-3).

Pituitary adenomas are circumscribed and often have a thin fibrous capsule. In a few cases-particularly when the adenoma recurs after surgical removal-the neoplasm is locally infiltrative with both upward extension to the base of the brain and downward extension into the sphenoid sinus. Such locally aggressive adenomas are called invasive adenomas; the diagnosis of carcinoma is made only when distant metastases are documented, which is extremely rare.

On cut section, pituitary adenomas are fleshy, gray to red masses that frequently show cystic degeneration, hemorrhage, and necrosis due to ischemia. Rarely, infarction of the entire tumor may occur.

Microscopically, the cells in a pituitary adenoma are mostly of one morphologic type and are arranged in nests and trabeculae separated by sinusoidal blood vessels. The cells are uniform, resembling normal pituitary cells in most cases. However, in a few tumors, particularly recurrent cases, there is cytologic pleomorphism and increased mitotic activity. These cytologic features correlate with locally aggressive tumor behavior.

Classification

The characterization of cell type requires either immunohistochemical or electron microscopic study (differences in granule types). The classification of pituitary adenomas into basophilic (ACTH, TSH), acidophilic (GH, prolactin), and chromophobic (nonfunctional) is inexact and should be discarded. Chromophobic adenomas can be shown immunohistochemically to produce hormones in many cases.

DISEASES OF THE THYROID GLAND

NORMAL STRUCTURE AND FUNCTION

The adult thyroid weight 20 - 25 g and is composed of two lateral lobes joined across the midline by an isthmus. A pyramidal lobe of varying size extends upward from the isthmus and represents the point of attachment of the thyroglossal duct. The pyramidal lobe cannot be palpated in a normal gland. The thyroid is firm, reddish-brown, and smooth. It is surrounded by a fibrous capsule that blends with the deep cervical fascia.

Histologically, the thyroid is composed of closely packed follicles separated by a rich vascular supply and little intervening stroma. The follicles are lined by cuboidal epithelial cells and contain colloid, a proteinaceous material composed mainly of thyroglobulin and stored thyroid hormones.

Dispersed between the thyroid follicles are the parafollicular or C cells, which secrete calcitonin.

DIFFUSE NONTOXIC AND MULTINODULAR GOITER

Introduction

Diffuse nontoxic and multinodular goiter represent the culmination of mild deficiency of thyroid hormone production followed by compensatory thyroid hyperplasia. Hyperplasia of the gland corrects the hormone deficiency and maintains the euthyroid (normal hormone levels) state at the expense of thyroid enlargement. The mechanism of thyroid hyperplasia is unknown. Serum TSH levels are normal. It is thought likely that there is an increased responsiveness of thyroid cells to TSH due to depletion of organic iodine in the cells resulting from impaired hormone synthesis. (Note that "goiter" means enlargement of the thyroid gland due to any cause.)

Etiology

The basic cause of diffuse nontoxic and multinodular goiter is failure of normal thyroid hormone synthesis.

A. Endemic Goiter

Endemic goiter is the result of chronic dietary deficiency of iodine. It occurs mainly in inland mountainous regions of the world such as the Alps, Andes, and Himalayas and inland regions of Asia and Africa. In these populations, up to 5% of individuals may have thyroid enlargement, sometimes massive. Endemic goiter is not common in coastal communities because of the high iodine content of seawater and seafood. Endemic goiter is more common in women because of increased iodine requirements in pregnancy and lactation.

The incidence of endemic goiter decreased greatly in countries such as the United States and Western Europe after iodization of common table salt was instituted.

Much less commonly, goitrogens are responsible for endemic goiter. Goitrogens are dietary factors that block thyroid hormone synthesis. They are found in plants such as cabbage and cassava and have been identified as a cause of goiter in South America, Netherlands, and Greece.

B. Sporadic Goiter

Sporadic goiter may occur anywhere and is usually due to increased physiologic demand for thyroxine at puberty or during pregnancy (also called physiologic goiter). Less commonly, sporadic goiter may result from mild deficiency of enzymes involved in thyroid hormone synthesis. Abnormalities relating to synthesis of thyroid-binding globulin may cause goiter because excess thyroxine-binding globulin (TBG) in plasma decreases delivery of free hormone to the periphery. In many patients with multinodular goiter, no cause can be identified.

Pathologic Changes

Changes in the thyroid gland progress through diffuse enlargement (diffuse nontoxic goiter) to multinodular goiter (Figure 13-2).

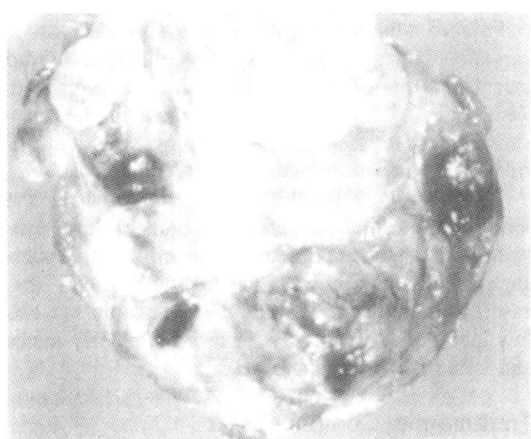

Figure 13-2 Multinodular goiter, showing part of a massively enlarged gland containing multiple nodules of varying size, some with hemorrhage

In the early stages, diffuse hyperplasia is characterized by small follicles lined by tall columnar cells, resembling the microscopic changes of Graves' disease. (The term diffuse nontoxic goiter is used for this stage because the patient is clinically euthyroid.) Involution follows, due probably to transient phases of adequate or excess hormone synthesis. The follicles become distended with colloid, and the lining epithelial cells become flattened or cuboidal. These changes are not uniform, and there may be a mixture of colloid-filled large follicles and small hyperplasitic follicles. At this stage, the thyroid is enlarged and nodular and its cut surface appears gelatinous and glistening owing to its colloid content.

Repeated episodes of hyperplasia and involution over a long period result in a markedly enlarged multinodular goiter. In endemic areas, it is not uncommon to see goiters so large that they hang to the chest. Multinodular goiter is characterized by nodules composed of colloid-filled enlarged follicles, areas of hyperplasia in which small follicles are lined by active epithelium, fibrosis, areas of hemorrhage, cystic degeneration, fibrosis, and calcification.

Clinical Features

Patients present with painless diffuse enlargement of the thyroid. As the disease progresses, the thyroid becomes larger and more nodular. Patients are euthyroid as a rule, and serum TSH by ultrasensitive assay is normal. The most common reason for surgical treatment is that the mass is cosmetically unacceptable. In a few patients, the presence of a dominant nodule may mimic a neoplastic process.

Individuals with congenital thyroid tissue in the mediastinum may present with a mediastinum mass (retrosternal goiter).

Abnormal thyroid hormone production may rarely occur in multinodular goiter. Hyperthyroidism is commoner than hypothyroidism and is due to the development of autonomous hyperplastic nodules in the gland (toxic nodular goiter). Hypothyroidism results in very rare cases when thyroid hyperplasia cannot compensate for severe deficiency of hormone synthesis.

The risk of development of carcinoma in a multinodular goiter is small.

DISORDERS OF THYROID SECRETION

Excessive Secretion of Thyroid Hormone (Diffuse Toxic Goiter; Graves' Disease; Hyperthyroidism)

A. Introduction

Graves' disease is responsible for the great majority of cases of hyperthyroidism. It is relatively common disease affecting females four to five times more commonly than males. It has its highest incidence in the 15- to 40-year age group. There is a familial tendency and an association in Caucasians with the histocompatibility antigens HLA-DR$_3$ and B$_8$. Patients with Graves' disease frequently suffer from other autoimmune disease such as pernicious anemia, and there is also an overlap with Hashimoto's disease.

B. Etiology

Graves' disease is an autoimmune disease characterized by the presence in serum of autoantibodies of the IgG class directed against the TSH receptor in the thyroid cell. The combination of the antibody with the receptor leads to stimulation of the cell to produce thyroid hormone.

Based on different in vitro system used to defect these autoantibodies, there are several different antibodies; (1) long-acting thyroid stimulator (LATS), (2) LATS protector, (3) thyroid-stimulating immunoglobulin (TSI), and (4) TSH-binding inhibitory immunoglobulin (TBII). TSI and TBII are most widely used in testing.

The precipitating cause is unknown. Serum levels of antibodies do not correlate precisely with severity of disease.

Because the stimulating antibodies are IgG, they cross the placenta in pregnancy and stimulate the female thyroid, causing neonatal hyperthyroidism; this condition spontaneously reverses after delivery as the maternal antibodies disappear from the body's blood, providing good evidence that the antibodies are responsible for the disease.

C. Pathologic Changes

The thyroid gland is diffusely and symmetrically enlarged and extremely vascular. Microscopically, thyroid follicular epithelial cells are increased in size and number. The follicles are closely packed and lined by tall columnar epithelium which is frequently thrown into papillary infoldings (Figure 13-3). Colloid is scanty, and its periphery is scalloped because of rapid thyroglobulin proteolysis. Lymphocytic infiltration of the interstitium is common, and lymphoid follicles with germinal centers may be present. Treatment with antithyroid drugs causes regression of these hyperplastic changes.

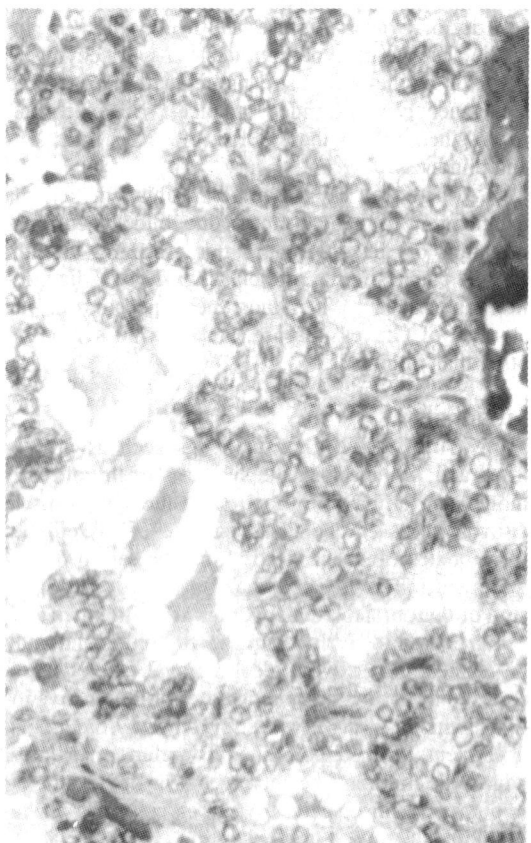

Figure 13-3 Graves' disease, showing small follicles with scanty colloid and enlarged follicle-lining epithelial cells

D. Clinical Features

The thyroid gland is diffusely enlarged and appears as a mass in the neck. A bruit resulting from the greatly increased blood flow is often present over the gland.

Eye changes are present in most patients with Graves' disease. These include exophthalmos, a staring gaze due to decreased blinking and impaired eye muscle function, eye changes help to distinguish Graves' disease from other causes of hyperthyroidism.

Laboratory evidence of hyperthyroidism-most reliably elevation of free thyroxine T_4 index-is present. Ten percent of patients show normal T_4 but elevated levels of free T_3 (T_3 toxicosis). Serum TSH is markedly decreased.

Thyroid scan shows increased uptake of radioiodine but is rarely needed for diagnosis. Most patients have autoantibodies directed the TSH receptor (most commonly TSI and TBII) in their blood, and this is of diagnostic value.

E. Associated Conditions

The following conditions may be associated with Graves' disease but are not always present.

1. Exophthalmos

Exophthalmos - protrusion of the eyeballs - occurs in 70% of patients with Graves' disease. Its presence is unrelated to the severity of Graves' disease, and its may rarely occur in the absence of hyperthyroidism. Lymphocytic infiltration of the orbital soft tissues with edema fluid and mucopolysaccharides produces the exophthalmos. When severe, there is risk of ocular infections and blindness.

2. Pretibial myxedema

Pretibial myxedema occurs in 5% of patients and is due to localized accumulation of mucopolysaccharide, forming circumscribed patches in the pretibial skin. It is of diagnostic of Graves' disease. It causes no symptoms other than itching.

Decreased Secretion of Thyroid Hormone (Hypothyroidism)

Decreased secretion of thyroid hormones results in cretinism if deficiency is present from birth and myxedema if it develops in an adult.

Hypothyroidism may be broadly classified as primary, due to a decrease in the thyroid hormone resulting from a disease process in the thyroid gland (common), or secondary, resulting from failure of pituitary TSH secretion (rare).

The diagnosis of hypothyroidism may be confirmed in the laboratory by decreased free thyroxine index. The T_3 level is of little value because it only falls in extreme hypothyroidism. The most sensitive diagnostic test in primary hypothyroidism is elevation of serum thyrotropin (TSH) concentration. This test is also useful in the differentiation of primary (increased serum TSH) and secondary (decreased serum TSH) hypothyroidism.

A. Cretinism

1. Etiology

Cretinism is an uncommon disease of childhood, but diagnosis is important because thyroxine administration soon after birth can prevent severe consequences in many cases.

The causes can be listed as follows: (1) Failure of development of the thyroid (thyroid agenesis). (2) Failure of hormone synthesis due to severe iodine deficiency in the diet of both the mother during pregnancy and the baby after birth. This condition is now rare in countries in which table salt is iodized but still occurs in some mountainous Third World countries (endemic cretinism). (3) Failure of hormone synthesis due to the presence of dietary substances (goitrogens) that block hormone synthesis. Thiocyanate in the cassava plant eaten in Central Africa is the best known of these substances. Goitrogens represent a very rare cause of endemic cretinism. (4) Failure of hormone synthesis due to autosomal recessive enzyme deficiency (sporadic cretinism). Many enzyme deficiencies have been identified, causing failure of iodide trapping, organification of iodide, coupling, and dehalogenation of monoiodotyrosine (MIT) and diiodotyrosine (DIT).

2. Pathologic changes

The appearance of the thyroid gland depends on the cause. In cretinism due to thyroid agenesis, the gland is absent. In cretinism caused by failure of thyroid hormone synthesis, the gland undergoes enlargement and hyperplasia because of increased secretion of pituitary thyrotropin resulting from decreased feedback inhibition (goitrous cretinism).

3. Clinical features

Babies with cretinism show lethargy, somnolence, hypothermia, feeding problems, and persistent neonatal jaundice. A hoarse cry, hypotonia of muscles, large protruding tongue, and umbilical hernia are common features. If the diagnosis is not made at birth, there is growth retardation (failure to thrive, delayed bone growth) and irreversible mental retardation. Replacement of thyroid hormones after diagnosis cretinism in the perinatal period prevents mental retardation to a large extent.

B. Myxedema

1. Etiology

Causes of hypothyroidism in the adult include the following: (1) Hashimoto's Autoimmune Thyroiditis: This disorder is responsible for most cases and is discussed below. (2) Pituitary Failure: Secondary hypothyroidism due to pituitary failure is uncommon but may be recognized by the markedly decreased thyrotropin level in the blood. (3) Iatrogenic Hypothyroidism: Hypothyroidism may result from administration of antithyroid drugs or ablation of the gland by surgery (total thyroidectomy) or by radiation. (4) Dietary Causes: Failure of thyroid hormone synthesis due to extreme dietary iodine deficiency very rarely results in adult hypothyroidism. In patients with iodine deficiency, decreased hormone production is usually compensated for by hyperplasia of the thyroid via the thyrotropin feedback mechanism, with the enlarged gland maintaining adequate hormone secretion. Certain dietary factors appear to induce similar effects by interfering with iodine metabolism (goitrogens).

2. Pathologic changes

The changes in the thyroid depend on the cause of hypothyroidism (see Hashimoto's thyroiditis and multinodular goiter).

3. Clinical features

Decreased levels of thyroid hormones cause a decreased rate of metabolism in all target cells, with the following results: (1) Lethargy, cold intolerance, weight gain, and constipation; (2) Loss of hair all over the body, but typically in the scalp and eyebrows; (3) Neurologic manifestations, including psychomotor retardation and slow thought processes and bodily movements. In many patients, overt psychotic features appear (myxedema madness). A useful physical finding is a prolonged relaxation phase in the deep tendon reflexes; (4) Anemia, usually normochromic normocytic, due to decreased erythropoiesis; (5) Pleural and pericardial effusions; and (6) Increased serum cholesterol and atherosclerosis.

The term myxedema is used for adult hypothyroidism because of the deposition of increased amounts of mucopolysaccharides in connective tissues. It is not known why this occurs. Mucopolysaccharides are deposited (1) in the skin, producing a peculiar kind of diffuse nonpitting doughy swelling; (2) in the larynx, causing hoarseness, an almost constant feature in severe hypothyroidism; and (3) in the heart, involving the interstitium between myocardial fiber degeneration also occurs. Hypothyroid patients may present with heart failure owing to the combined effect of this change and myocardial ischemia due to the associated atherosclerotic coronary artery disease. In treating hypothyroid patients with thyroid hormone replacement, care must be taken to ensure that the cardiac stimulation caused by administered thyroid hormone does not precipitate failure in the myxedematous heart.

INFLAMMATORY THYROID DISEASES

Subacute Thyroiditis

Subacute thyroiditis – also called granulomatous thyroiditis or DeQuervain's thyroiditis – is an uncommon inflammatory condition of the thyroid. It affects both sexes and all ages.

A. Etiology

A viral origin is considered most likely. Thyroid inflammation frequently follows upper respiratory infection. Viruses that have been implicated include adenoviruses, mumps virus, echovirus, influenza virus, Epstein-Barr virus, and-most consistently - coxsackieviruses. However, neither culture nor electron microscopy has demonstrated virus in affected thyroid tissue.

Autoimmunity has also been suggested as a possible mechanism but considered an unlikely one since antithyroid antibodies are present only transiently in a few patients. Subacute thyroiditis has no relationship to either Graves' disease or Hashimoto's thyroiditis.

B. Pathologic Changes

The thyroid is diffusely enlarged, firm, and often adherent to surrounding structures. Microscopically, there is extensive destruction and fibrosis of thyroid follicles with aggregates of macrophages and giant cells around fragments of colloid.

C. Clinical Features

There is acute onset of painful enlargement of the thyroid, often associated with fever, malaise, and muscle aches. Most patients are euthyroid but in a few cases there is transient hyperthyroidism, due probably to the sudden release of hormone from the damaged gland.

The disease is self-limited with recovery usually occurring within 3 months; it does not lead to hypothyroidism.

Chronic Thyroiditis

A. Chronic Lymphocytic Thyroiditis (Hashimoto's Thyroiditis)

Hashimoto's thyroiditis is responsible for most cases of primary hypothyroidism.

Hashimoto's thyroiditis affects middle-aged individuals – females 10 times more frequently than males. There is an association with histocompatibility antigen HLA-DR$_5$.

1. Etiology

Hashimoto's disease is believed to be the result of an autoimmune response against the thyroid. The most likely mechanism of thyroid cell destruction is by a cytotoxic T cell-mediated hypersensitivity reaction.

Most patients with Hashimoto's disease have in their serum several different IgG autoantibodies: (1) antithyroglobulin antibody; (2) antimicrosomal antibody; (3) antibody directed against a component of colloid other than thyroglobulin; and (4) antibodies against thyroid TSH receptors, including TSI and antibodies that stimulate cell growth (thyroid growth immunoglobulin, TGI). Serum levels of these antibodies do not correlate with severity of disease, and their exact relationship to thyroid cell destruction is uncertain. They are, however, of diagnostic value.

2. Pathologic changes

In the early stages, the thyroid is enlarged diffusely. The gland is firm and rubbery, with a coarsely nodular ("bosselated") appearance. As the disease progresses, the gland becomes smaller; the end result is a markedly atrophic, fibrosed thyroid.

Microscopically, there is evidence of destruction

of the thyroid follicles associated with severe lymphocytic infiltration of the gland (Figure 13-4). Large lymphoid follicles with germinal centers are commonly present. Surviving follicular epithelial cells are commonly transformed into large cells with abundant pink cytoplasm known as Hürthle cells. Hyperplastic nodules composed of Hürthle cells are sometimes present. Progressive fibrosis occurs.

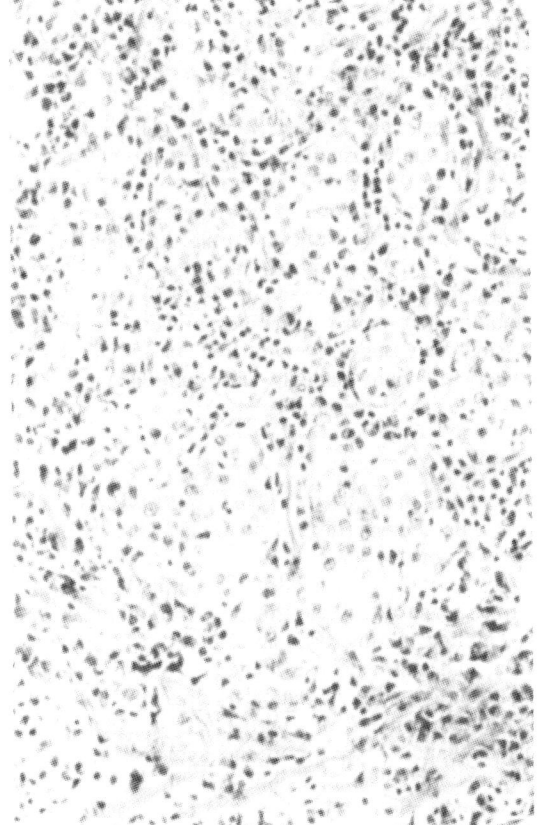

Figure 13-4 Hashimoto's autoimmune thyroiditis, showing marked lymphocytic infiltration and loss of thyroid follicles. Residual thyroid follicular epithelial cells are enlarged and have abundant cytoplasm (Hürthle cells)

The histologic changes are diagnostic of Hashimoto's disease only if the clinical background is consistent. Similar changes, usually of lesser degree and usually without the presence of Hürthle cells, occur commonly without Hashimoto's disease and are referred to as nonspecific lymphocytic thyroiditis.

3. Clinical features

Most patients with Hashimoto's thyroiditis present with gradual enlargement of the thyroid that may raise a suspicion of neoplasm.

Thyroid function at the time of presentation is variable. Patients are commonly either euthyroid or mildly hypothyroid. Rarely, there is mild hyperthyroidism in the early phase. In most cases, the disease progresses with increasing degrees of hypothyroidism.

Thyroid autoantibodies can be detected in the serum of almost all patients. High titers of these antibodies are diagnostic of Hashimoto's disease, multinodular goiter, and thyroid neoplasms, and low levels are seen in 50% or more of elderly males and 90% of elderly females.

B. Fibrous Thyroiditis (Riedel's Thyroiditis)

Riedel's thyroiditis is a rare chronic disorder occurring in older patients, with women affected more frequently than men.

Thyroid autoantibodies are usually not present. Riedel's thyroiditis is sometimes associated with similar fibrosing lesions in the retroperitoneum and mediastinum, suggesting that it may be a systemic disorder involving fibroblasts.

1. Pathologic changes

The gland is usually mildly enlarged and replaced wholly or in part by hard, grayish-white fibrous tissue (woody or ligneous thyroiditis), which extends beyond the capsule.

Microscopically, there is atrophy of thyroid follicles with replacement by dense, scar-like collagen. Scattered lymphocytes and plasma cells are present.

2. Clinical features

Both clinically and at surgery, Riedel's thyroiditis resembles a malignant neoplasm of the thyroid. It presents with painless rock-hard enlargement of the thyroid. The fibrosis may constrict the trachea, producing dyspnea and stridor; the esophagus, causing dysphagia; or the recurrent laryngeal nerve, causing hoarseness. Patients are usually euthyroid. In most cases the disorder causes slowly increasing fibrosis of the neck structures.

THYROID NEOPLASMS

Thyroid Follicular Adenoma

A. Introduction

Follicular adenoma of the thyroid is the commonest neoplasm of the thyroid, accounting for about 30% of all cases of solitary thyroid nodules. It may occur at any age; female are affected four times as frequently as males.

B. Pathologic Changes

Grossly, thyroid adenomas present as a solitary, firm gray or red nodular up to 5 cm in diameter (Figure 13-5); hemorrhage, fibrosis, calcification, and cystic degeneration may be present.

Microscopically, follicular adenomas are usually composed of follicles of varying size (microfollicular adenoma; macrofollicular adenoma). Less often, solid cords of thyroid epithelial cells form only rudimentary follicular structures (embryonal adenoma). Other adenomas are composed of cells with abundant pink granular cytoplasm (Hürthle cell adenoma). The cytologic features of adenomas are usually uniform; a few adenomas, however, show cellular pleomorphism and atypia (atypical adenoma).

Follicular adenomas are surrounded by a complete fibrous capsule of varying thickness, and the normal thyroid parenchyma around the adenoma is compressed (Figure 13-6). The capsule is intact, and

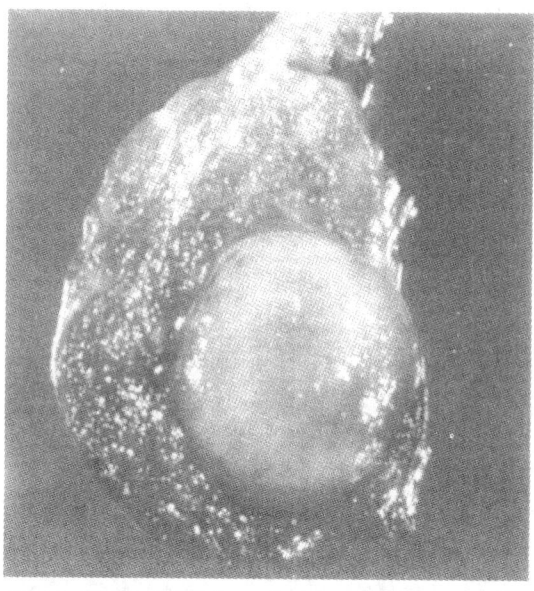

Figure 13-5 Follicular adenoma, showing a well-encapsulated solitary nodule in the thyroid. Microscopic evaluation is necessary to rule out carcinoma

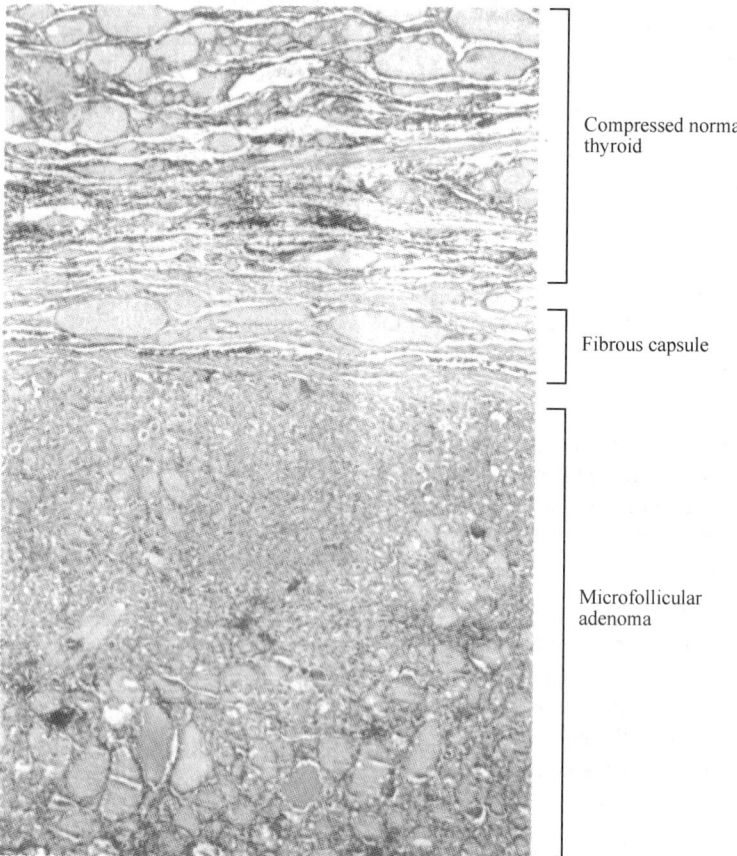

Figure 13-6 Follicular adenoma, showing microfollicular structure of the neoplasm, a thin fibrous capsule, and compressed normal thyroid

there is no vascular invasion. Absence of capsule and vascular invasion are the criteria used to differentiate follicular adenoma from follicular carcinoma.

C. Clinical Features

Patients are usually euthyroid. Thyroid scan shows the presence of a circumscribed cold nodule. Fineneedle aspiration usually shows a cellular smear with many microfollicles. Rare "toxic" adenomas produce sufficient hormone to cause hyperthyroidism.

Thyroid Carcinoma

A. Introduction

Thyroid cancer is uncommon, with an incidence in the United States of about 25 - 30 cases per million populations. It is responsible for about 7000 deaths per year in the United States. Thyroid cancer affects females about three times as frequently as males.

The incidence has increased greatly in the last 50 years, probably as a result of increased exposure to radiation. Radiation-induced thyroid carcinoma is most commonly of the papillary or follicular types.

B. Pathologic Changes

Thyroid carcinoma is classified on the basis of its microscopic appearance into four types (Figure 13-7). Three of these - papillary, follicular, and anaplastic - are derived from thyroid follicular epithelium. Medullary carcinoma is distinct and arises in the parafollicular calcitonin-secreting cells. Mixed papillary and follicular carcinomas also occur but behave exactly like pure papillary carcinoma.

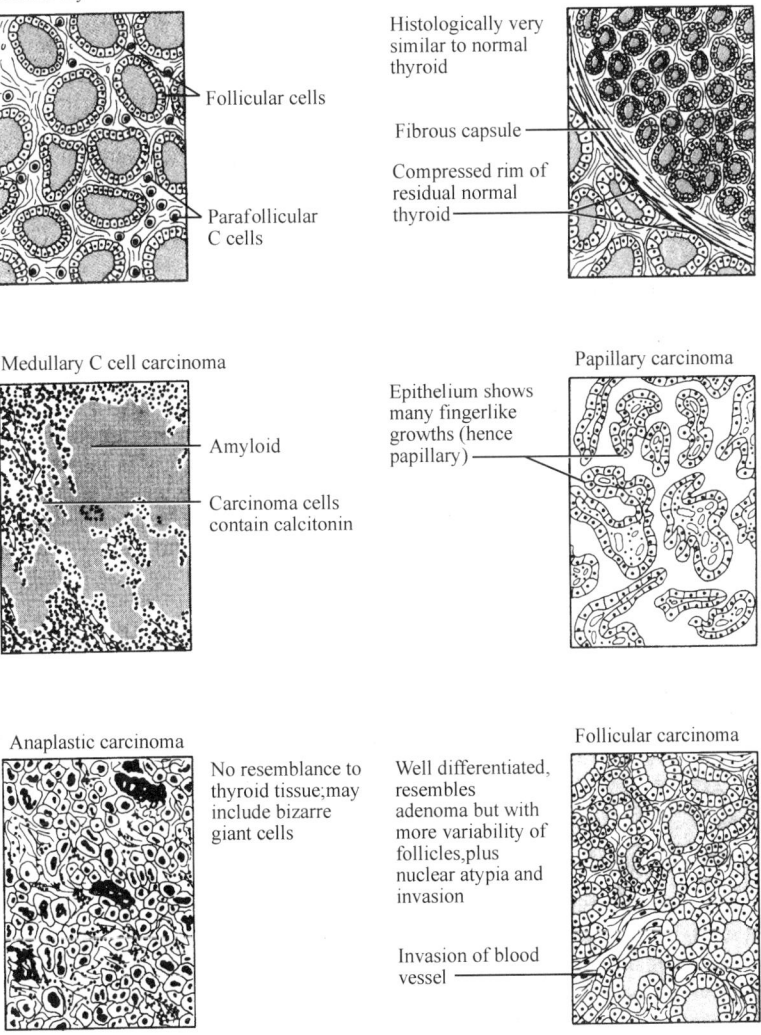

Figure 13-7 Common thyroid neoplasms, showing basic pathologic features

1. Papillary carcinoma

Papillary carcinoma is the most common type (Table 13-5). It affects females three times more commonly than males; younger individuals in the age range 15-35 years are predominantly affected.

Grossly, papillary carcinomas range from microscopic lesions to large masses over 10 cm in diameter. They are usually infiltrative lesions, but a small number appear as circumscribed nodules.

Microscopically, they are characterized by (1) an arrangement of cells in papillary structures (Figure 13-8); clear nuclei – resembling the eyes of the cartoon character Orphan Annie – which are virtually diagnostic of papillary carcinoma even though they represent an artifact produced by formalin fixation; (2) prominent nuclear grooves; (3) intranuclear inclusions caused by cytoplasmic invaginations into the nucleus; and (4) psammoma bodies, which are round, laminated, calcified bodies that are present in about 40% of papillary carcinomas. Papillary carcinoma is defined by its nuclear characteristics (clearing, grooves, and inclusions). Rare papillary carcinomas have an entirely follicular pattern (follicular variant of papillary carcinoma).

Papillary carcinomas grow very slowly. They commonly spread by local invasion, and many have invaded the thyroid capsule at the time of presentation.

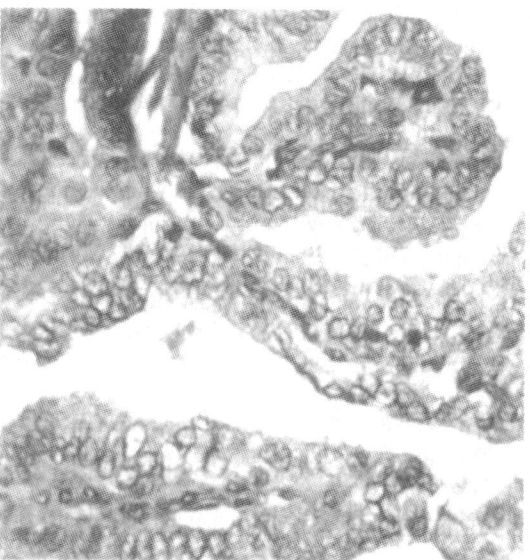

Figure 13-8 Papillary carcinoma, showing typical papillary structures composed of a fibrovascular core and lined by enlarged epithelial cells. Note that many of the cells have enlarged, clear nuclei

Lymphatic spread produces additional intraglandular foci of tumor are present in the opposite lobe. Cervical lymph node metastases – once mistakenly thought to be nodules of congenitally "aberrant" thyroid – are present in 40% of cases of papillary carcinoma at the time of presentation. Bloodstream dissemination is rare in papillary carcinoma.

Table 13-5 Differential features of thyroid carcinoma

	Papillary Carcinoma	Follicular Carcinoma	Anaplastic Carcinoma	Medullay Carcinoma
Cell of origin	Follicular epithelial cell	Follicular epithelial cell	Follicular epithelial cell	Parafollicular or C cell
Frequency[1]	70%	20%	5%	5%
Sex and age incidence	F > M = 3 : 1 ; 15 – 35 years	F > M all age; > 30 years	F > M; > 50 years	F = M ; 30 – 60 years
Local features	Infiltrative masses; Multifocal and bilateral; Lymph nodes often positive	May be grossly infiltrative or encapsulated; Angioinvasive	Massively infiltrating locally	Slowly growing mass; Infiltrative
Lymphatic metastasis	+ + +	+	+ + +	+
Blood-borne metastasis	Late, uncommon	+ + +	+ + +	+
Five-year survival rate	90%	65%	Nil	50%
Tumor markers	Thyroglobulin	Thyroglobulin	None	Calcitonin

[1] Percentages relate to frequency among thyroid carcinomas.

2. Follicular carcinoma

Follicular carcinomas comprise 20% of thyroid carcinomas. Again, females are affected more commonly than males. All ages are vulnerable, but the disease is more common in middle age.

Grossly, follicular carcinoma may be indistinguishable from adenoma (encapsulated follicular carcinoma), or it may form a large infiltrative mass. Microscopically, follicular carcinomas are composed of follicles of varying size lined by thyroid epithelial cells that resemble normal thyroid cells. Rarely, cells have clear cytoplasm (clear cell variant), are composed of Hürthle cells (Hürthle cell carcinoma), or have insular and trabecular rather than follicular architecture. Solid areas composed of cells showing cytologic atypia, pleomorphism, and increased mitotic activity are common. The diagnosis of carcinoma depends on the presence of invasion of the capsule or vascular structure (Figure 13-9).

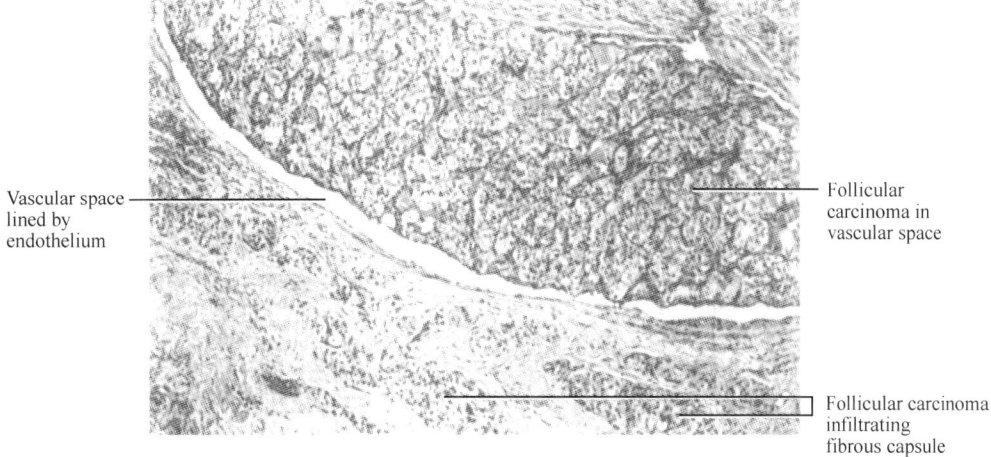

Figure 13-9 Follicular carcinoma, showing large vessel in the capsule of the neoplasm filled with tumor. Note also the irregular infiltration of the fibrous capsule by tumor

Follicular carcinoma is a slowly growing neoplasm that may, however, spread via bloodstream at an early stage, producing metastases in bone and lungs. Lymphatic metastasis to cervical nodes also occurs but to a lesser extent than in papillary carcinoma.

3. Anaplastic carcinoma

Anaplastic carcinoma is rare, comprising 5% of thyroid carcinomas. It occurs most commonly in patients over the age of 50 years.

Grossly, anaplastic carcinoma appears as a massive infiltrative lesion. It is hard, gritty, and grayish-white and frequently shows areas of necrosis and hemorrhage. Microscopically, it is composed of highly malignant-appearing spindle or giant cells, showing extreme pleomorphism and frequent mitotic figures.

Anaplastic carcinomas are aggressive, rapidly growing neoplasms that disseminate extensively. Death usually occurs within a year after diagnosis and is mainly due to local invasion of neck structures.

4. Medullary carcinoma

Medullary carcinoma is rare, accounting for about 5% of thyroid carcinomas. It is derived from the calcitonin-secreting parafollicular cells (C cells) of the thyroid. Ninety percent of medullary carcinomas occur as sporadic lesions; 10% are familial and may form part of the multiple endocrine adenomatosis (MEA type II) syndrome (concurrence of medullary carcinoma of the thyroid, pheochromocytoma of the adrenal medulla, and parathyroid adenoma). The familial form may be distinguished from the sporadic type by the occurrence in the former of C cell hyperplasia in the residual noncancerous thyroid.

Grossly, medullary carcinoma forms a hard, grayish-white infiltrative mass. Microscopically, it is composed of small spindle-shaped and polygonal cells arranged in nests, cords, and sheets. The cells stain positively for calcitonin by the immunoperoxidase technique (Figure 13-10). The stroma contains amyloid in most cases; the amyloid consists of calcitonin fragments. Electron microscopy shows the presence of membrane-bound dense-core neurosecretory granules in the neoplastic cells and fibrillar amyloid material in the stroma.

Medullary carcinomas have a slow but progressive growth pattern. Local invasion of neck structures is common, and both lymphatic and bloodstream metastasis occurs.

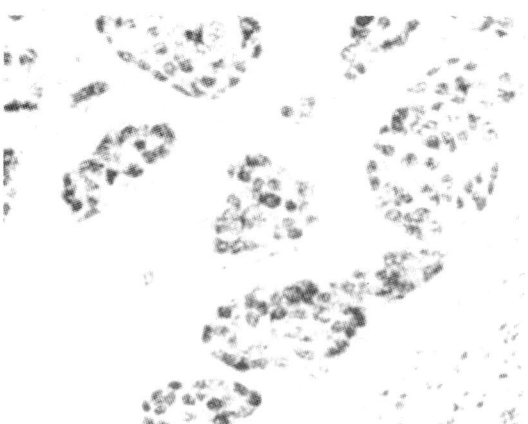

Figure 13-10 Medullary carcinoma of the thyroid. This is a section stained by immunoperoxidase for calcitonin, showing positive cytoplasmic staining in nests of neoplastic cells. The normal tissue comprising the stroma of the tumor is completely unstained

C. Clinical Features

Thyroid carcinomas commonly present with a painless solitary nodule in the thyroid. Thyroid scan commonly shows a lack of uptake (cold nodule). Fine-needle aspiration may be diagnostic of papillary carcinoma, medullary carcinoma, or anaplastic carcinoma, but the distinction of follicular carcinoma from follicular adenoma is rarely possible.

Patients with thyroid carcinoma are euthyroid as a rule. Very rarely, well-differentiated carcinomas secrete hormones and cause hyperthyroidism.

Important modes of presentation of thyroid carcinoma are with local invasion of neck structures or with distant metastases. In the case of papillary carcinoma, this is commonly in a cervical lymph node. In follicular carcinoma, the first manifestation of disease may be due to a metastasis in bone or lung.

D. Tumor Markers

Medullary carcinoma of the thyroid secretes calcitonin, which can be detected in the blood (by radioimmunoassay) and is useful in diagnosis and assessing response to treatment. Rarely, calcitonin production is sufficient to induce hypocalcemia. Identification of a thyroid carcinoma as medullary in type is facilitated by staining sections for calcitonin using immunoperoxidase methods.

Well-differentiated thyroid carcinomas (papillary and follicular types) form thyroglobulin, which can be demonstrated in tumor cells in histologic sections by immunoperoxidase techniques - useful in identifying a neoplasm as a thyroid carcinoma (Figure 13-11). Small amount of thyroglobulin, released by the tumor cells into the blood, can be detected by ultrasensitive assays for thyroglobulin. Thyroglobulin is also found in the blood after any form of damage to the thyroid. Serum thyroglobulin has no value in the initial diagnosis of thyroid carcinoma but is of value in assessing adequacy of treatment and in detecting disseminated disease or recurrence after treatment.

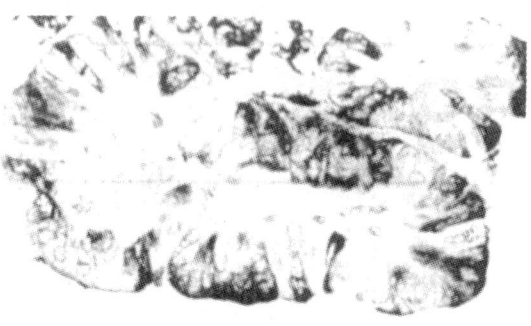

Figure 13-11 Papillary carcinoma of the thyroid stained for thyroglobulin by the immunoperoxidase technique, showing dark staining of the cytoplasm of most of the cells. Positive staining for thyroglobulin establishes the carcinoma as being of thyroid epithelial origin

Anaplastic carcinomas do not commonly stain for thyroglobulin and have no tumor markers in the blood.

E. Prognosis

The prognosis of papillary carcinoma is good, with 15-year survival rate of 90% and a 20-year survival rate of 85%. Even when metastases are present, patients survive for long periods after surgical excision of thyroid and metastatic tumor. Follicular carcinoma has a 5-year survival rate of about 65% and a 20-year survival rate of 30%. The presence of distant blood-borne metastases is a poor prognostic sign. Medullary carcinoma has a 5-year survival rate of 50%. Anaplastic carcinoma is a highly malignant neoplasm, and most patients die within a year after diagnosis; the 5-year survival rate is almost nil.

SUMMARY (FIGURE 13-7)

The solitary thyroid nodule is a common clinical problem that deserves special consideration before a discussion of thyroid neoplasia is undertaken.

In studies on autopsy material, it is found that 4%–12% of all patients have small thyroid nodules; clinical studies have shown that careful palpation of the thyroid reveals the presence of thyroid nodules in 4%–7% of all patients. Having detected a nodule clinically, the question is what to do about it.

A solitary thyroid nodule is malignant in less than 5% of cases. About 30% of solitary nodules are benign follicular neoplasms (adenomas). The remainder represent nonneoplastic lesions such as early nodular goiter (colloid nodular), Hashimoto's thyroiditis, and subacute thyroiditis. Over 60% of solitary nodules are benign colloid nodules. The physician's task is to identify those nodules that have a high likehood of being carcinoma.

DISEASES OF THE PARATHYROID GLAND

NORMAL STRUCTURE AND FUNCTION

Normally, there are four parathyroid glands, situated in two pairs with one above the other on the posterior aspect of the thyroid gland. Rarely, the parathyroids may be found inside the thyroid gland itself. In about 10% of individuals, the number exceeds four; on occasion, there are fewer than four glands. The inferior pair of parathyroids, which arise in the branchial arch that also gives rise to the thymus, may descend into the mediastinum.

Grossly, each parathyroid gland is an encapsulated ovoid structure with a distinctive yellowish-brown color. Its maximal diameter is 5 mm and its weight is 35–40 mg.

Microscopically, the normal parathyroid contains three types of cells: chief cells, water-clear cells, and oxyphil cells. All three are believed to produce hormone, and their relative numbers are of little significance. Variable amounts of adipose tissue are interspersed between parenchymal cells; the amount of adipose tissue increases with age.

The parathyroid glands secrete parathyroid hormone (PTH). PTH regulates the concentration of ionic calcium in plasma. Its main target cells are the renal tubular epithelial cells and bone osteoclasts. In the kidney, PTH increases reabsorption of calcium in the distal tubules and decreases reabsorption of phosphate in the proximal tubule. It also stimulates activation of vitamin D, which in turn increases intestinal absorption of calcium. PTH increases bone resorption (releasing calcium and phosphate) by stimulating osteoclastic activity. This function of PTH requires the synergistic action of active vitamin D. PTH also increases collagenase activity in bone, causing breakdown of the bony matrix.

The overall effect of PTH is an increase in total and ionized plasma calcium and a decrease in plasma inorganic phosphate.

The action of PTH is dependent on binding with cell membrane receptors to cause activation of intracellular adenylate cyclase. The result is increased synthesis of cAMP., which mediates the physiologic actions of PTH.

The rate of PTH synthesis and secretion are controlled by serum ionized calcium level.

EXCESSIVE SECRETION OF PTH (HYPERPARATHYROIDISM)

Hyperparathyroidism is defined as elevated serum PTH due to increased secretion. Primary hyperparathyroidism results from an intrinsic abnormality of one or more parathyroid glands. Secondary hyperparathyroidism is excessive secretion of PTH by the parathyroids in response to a lowered serum ionized calcium level.

Primary hyperparathyroidism is most commonly due to a solitary adenoma involving one gland; less often, diffuse hyperplasia of all four glands occurs (Table 13-6). In about 10% of cases, the gross findings at surgery are atypical, with two or three slightly enlarged glands found. These represent either irregular parathyroid hyperplasia or multiple adenomas. Adenomas and hyperplasia of the parathyroid usually occur sporadically. In a few cases, they are part of the multiple endocrine adenomatosis syndromes.

Secondary hyperparathyroidism is a compensatory hyperplasia of all four glands aimed at correcting a lowered serum calcium. In most cases, serum calcium levels are corrected toward normal but are not elevated. Rarely overcorrection occurs, and serum calcium levels exceed normal; the patient may then develop symptoms of hypercalcemia.

Table 13-6 Causes of hyperparathyroidism

Primary hyperparathyroidism
Single adenoma (80%–90%)
Multiple adenomas (1%–4%)
Diffuse hyperplasia (3%–15%)
Carcinoma (1%–2%)
Secondary hyperparathyroidism
Chronic renal failure
Malabsorption syndrome
Vitamin D deficiency
Medullary carcinoma of the thyroid
Ectopic parathyroid hormone (PTH) syndrome[1]
Squamous carcinoma of lung
Adenocarcinoma of kidney
Others

[1] Most malignant neoplasms secrete PTH-related peptide that is biologically active (activating PTH receptors on target cells) but does not cross-react with the immunologic testing reagents used in PTH assays.

Pathologic Changes

A. Parathyroid Adenoma

Parathyroid adenoma is a benign solitary neoplasm that involves one gland only; very rarely, multiple adenomas are present. Five to 10 percent of parathyroid adenomas are found in unusual locations such as the mediastinum (usually in relation to the thymus and rarely behind the pericardium or esophagus) or within the thyroid gland.

Grossly, parathyroid adenomas are usually small (commonly 1–2 cm in diameter and weighing 1–3 g) and may be difficult to locate at surgery. However, once located, they are well-encapsulated masses that are easily removed.

Microscopically, parathyroid adenomas are composed of a mixed population of chief, water-clear, and oxyphil cells, arranged in sheets, trabeculae, or glandular structures. The cells are usually small and uniform; rarely, there may be cytologic pleomorphism. Mitotic activity is very rare. There is no correlation between predominant cell type and hormone levels.

Parathyroid adenoma is differentiated from a normal gland by its increased size, the absence of fat in the gland, and the presence of a compressed rim of normal parathyroid tissue around the adenoma. In many parathyroid adenomas, there is no compressed rim of normal gland. In patients with a solitary adenoma, the other three parathyroid glands are normal in size and microscopic appearance.

B. Parathyroid Hyperplasia

1. Primary hyperplasia

Primary hyperplasia of the parathyroid is hyperplasia of all four glands in the absence of a known inciting cause. Hyperplasia usually affects all glands equally; rarely, one or two glands are disproportionately enlarged. The most accurate method of diagnosis of hyperplasia is to demonstrate increased weight of all four glands above 40 mg each. Gland weight can be assessed at surgery by estimating the volume by measurement and multiplying the result by the specific gravity of 1.06. In practice, a gland whose greatest diameter is over 5 mm is considered enlarged.

Microscopically, parathyroid hyperplasia is characterized by proliferation of all three cell types at the expense of the intraglandular fat. In some cases chief cells dominate and in others clear cells dominate, leading to the descriptive terms chief cell hyperplasia and clear cell hyperplasia. These histologic patterns have no clinical significance. In the majority of cases, the nature of the cells in hyperplasia is identical to that of an adenoma. Microscopic, examination of a single enlarged gland does not permit differentiation of parathyroid adenoma from hyperplasia except in cases where a rim of compressed normal gland is present in an adenoma. Differentiation of hyperplasia from adenoma requires biopsy of a second parathyroid gland; in hyperplasia, the second gland is microscopically abnormal, whereas in adenoma the second gland is normal.

2. Secondary hyperplasia

The pathologic findings in secondary parathyroid hyperplasia are histologically difficult to distinguish from those of primary hyperplasia. In most cases, chief cells dominate over water-clear and oxyphil cells.

C. Parathyroid Carcinoma

Carcinoma of the parathyroid is very rare. Patients with parathyroid carcinoma tend to have higher serum calcium and PTH levels. Carcinoma differs pathologically from adenoma in the following respects: (1) carcinoma tends to infiltrate outside the capsule, so that it is difficult to remove at surgery; (2) there is a high mitotic rate; and (3) broad bands of collagen frequently are present in the substance of a carcinoma. The pathologic differentiation of a parathyroid carcinoma from adenoma is difficult.

Parathyroid carcinoma tends to recur locally after excision. However, metastasis to regional lymph nodes or distant sites is the only proof of malignancy.

Clinical Features

A. Primary Hyperparathyroidism

Primary hyperparathyroidism is characterized by elevated serum PTH, elevated serum calcium, and decreased serum phosphate. In the early stages, patients are asymptomatic. The degree of elevation of serum calcium is usually not great, being in the 11 – 12 mg/dL range (normal, 9 – 11 mg/dL). In some patients, serum calcium is in the high normal range. However, when serum calcium and PTH levels are considered together, the PTH level is seen to be inappropriately increased. In rare patients with parathyroid carcinoma, serum calcium levels may be very high (15 – 20 mg/dL). One diagnostic pitfall is that there is reduced clearance of the inactive carboxyl terminal fragment of PTH in patients with renal failure, causing falsely elevated total serum PTH. Determination of amino terminal PTH or intact PTH is therefore recommended for assessment of parathyroid function, especially in patients with renal failure.

1. Urinary calculi

Urine calcium is increased owing to increased filtration of calcium, despite the fact that calcium reabsorption in the distant tubule is also increased. Phosphate excretion in urine is increased by direct PTH action. The result is an increased incidence of urinary calculi composed of calcium phosphate; 25% of patients with primary hyperthyroidism present with renal calculi.

2. Metastatic calcification

Calcification occurs as a result of elevated serum levels of ionized calcium. Calcium is deposited in the renal interstitium (nephrocalcinosis), causing renal failure, and in the walls of small blood vessels throughout the body. When extensive, this may result in widespread ischemic changes.

Increased calcium levels also interfere with cellular function (1) in the distal convoluted tubule, resulting in inability to concentrate urine and causing polyuria, nocturia, and thirst; (2) in the nervous system, causing disturbances in levels of consciousness, convulsions, and coma; and (3) in the heart, producing arrhythmias and electrocardiographic abnormalities.

3. Bone changes

Bone changes are characteristic and may be the presenting feature. Increased bone resorption leads to osteoporosis, fibrosis of the intertrabecular zone, and cyst formation (osteitis fibrosa cystica). Compensatory osteoblastic proliferation causes elevation of serum alkaline phosphatase. "Brown tumors"- solid masses of osteoclastic giant cells, fibroblasts, and collagen-resemble giant cell tumor of bone in histologic appearance, but they are nonneoplastic. The brown color is due to hemorrhage and hemosiderin deposition.

B. Secondary Hyperparathyroidism

Secondary hyperparathyroidism usually is accompanied by normal or slightly decreased serum calcium with high PTH and low serum phosphate levels. Bone changes caused by high PTH concentrations are similar to those seen in primary hyperparathyroidism. A few patients have high serum calcium levels and are liable to develop all the renal, vascular, and neurologic complications of hypercalcemia.

DECREASED SECRETION OF PTH (HYPOPARATHYROIDISM)

Etiology and Pathologic Changes

A. Hypoparathyroidism Complicating Neck Surgery

Accidental removal of parathyroid glands during neck surgery is the commonest cause of hypoparathyroidism. Two to 10 percent of patients undergoing total thyroidectomy, parathyroid surgery, and radical neck dissection for cancer develop hypoparathyroidism after surgery.

It is not uncommon to have transient hypocalcemia after thyroidectomy even when the parathyroids have not been removed; this is believed to be due to transient parathyroid edema or ischemia. Permanent hypoparathyroidism may result from accidental removal of the glands caused by interference with their arterial supply during surgery.

B. Idiopathic Hypoparathyroidism

Idiopathic hypoparathyroidism is rare disease with slight female predominance. It is believed to be the result of autoimmune destruction of the parathyroid cells. Parathyroid-specific autoantibodies are demonstrable in about 40% of patients, and there is an association with other autoimmune disease such as pernicious anemia, Addison's disease, and Hashimoto's thyroiditis. Microscopically, there is atrophy of parathyroid cells, lymphocytic infiltration, and fibrosis.

C. Congenital Absence of Parathyroids

Absence of parathyroids most commonly occurs when there is a generalized failure of development of the third and fourth branchial arches. It is then associated with thymic agenesis and marked deficiency of cellular immunity. Patients with congenital absence of parathyroids present with hypocalcemia and convulsions soon after birth.

D. Pseudohypoparathyroidism (Table 13-7)

This term denotes a group of rare inherited disorders characterized by lack of end-organ response to PTH caused by abnormal binding of PTH to PTH receptors on the target cell. The term pseudohypoparathyoidism is used because there is evidence of clinical hyoparathyroidism serum PTH levels in the face of normal. Examples of both autosomal and X-linked inheritance have reported.

Pseudohypoparathyroidism is commonly associated with Albright's osteodystrophy, characterized by short stature, short neck, abnormally developed metacarpal and metatarsal bones, and subcutaneous ossification. These features provide clues to diagnosis.

E. Hypomagnesemia

Several decrease in serum magnesium (to < 0.8 meq/L or 0.4 mmol/L) blocks PTH release by the parathyroid glands.

Table 13-7 Causes of hypoparathyroidism

Absence of PTH
Congenital absence of parathyroids (DiGeorge syndrome) (associated with thymic hypoplasia and T cell deficiency)
Hereditary hypoparathyroidisim (very rare; different patterns of inheritance)
Surgically induced (following thyroid and parathyroid surgery and radical neck dissection for cancer)
Idiopathic hypoparathyroidism (? autoimmune)

(Continued)

Defective release of PTH
Hypomagnesemia (when serum Mg^{2+} falls below 0.4 mmol/L)
PTH ineffective
Pseudohypoparathyroidism (end-organ resistance to PTH)

Clinical Features

Hypoparathyroidism is characterized by decreased serum levels of ionized calcium. This causes increased irritability of nerves, leading to numbness and tingling of the hands, feet, and lips and tetany. Tetany is manifested clinically as muscular spasms that affect the hands and feet (carpopedal spasms). Laryngeal spasm may occur, leading to respiratory obstruction. Muscular contraction is easily stimulated by such maneuvers as (1) inflating a blood pressure cuff (to above systolic pressure for at least 3 minutes) to produce transient ischemia, which precipitates carpal spasms; and (2) tapping the facial nerve at its exit at the stylomastoid foramen, which precipitates facial twitching. With severe hypocalcemia, particularly in children, there are generalized convulsions.

Serum phosphate is increased because of defective renal excretion of phosphate when PTH is deficient. High phosphate levels are associated with deposition of calcium phosphate in tissue (metastatic calcification). Increased bone density, calcification of the basal ganglia, and mineral deposition in the lens to form cataracts may be seen in patients with hypoparathyroidism.

DISEASES OF THE ADRENAL GLAND

NORMAL STRUCTURE AND FUNCTION

The paired adrenal glands are situated in the retroperitoneum above the kidneys. They are variably shaped and irregularly folded, flattened structures whose cut surface reveals an outer yellow cortex and an inner gray medulla. The normal adrenals have an aggregate weight of about 6 g (upper limit, 8 g).

The adrenal cortex is derived from the mesoderm of the urogenital ridge. Its origin is independent of that of the adrenal medulla, which is derived from the neural crest.

The cortex is composed of the subcapsular zona glomerulosa (10% - 15%), the zona fasciculate (80%), and the zona reticularis (5% - 10%). The zona glomerulosa secretes aldosterone and is controlled by the rennin-angiotensin mechanism, which is dependent of the pituitary. The zona fasciculate and reticularis secrete cortisol and androgenic hormones, respectively, and are under the regulatory control of the pituitary via corticotrophin (ACTH). ACTH secretion by the pituitary is under the control of (1) hypothalamic corticotrophin-releasing factor and (2) the feedback inhibitory effect of serum cortisol.

EXCESSIVE SECRETION OF ADRENOCORTICAL HORMONES

Cushing's Syndrome

Cushing's syndrome is a relatively common clinical abnormality of the adrenal cortex, usually affecting middle-aged individuals, women more often than men. It can be caused by several different disease processes.

A. Pathologic Changes

1. Adrenocortical adenoma
   See below.

2. Adrenocortical carcinoma
   See below.

3. Bilateral adrenal hyperplasia
   Once thought to be a primary disorder of the adrenal, bilateral adrenal hyperplasia is now believed to be almost invariably secondary to increased ACTH production, whether from a pituitary adenoma or a malignant nonpituitary neoplasm (usually small-cell undifferentiated carcinoma of lung). Both adrenal glands are enlarged to greater than their aggregate normal upper weight limit of 8 g. Careful weighting of the adrenal removed at surgery or autopsy after all periadrenal connective tissue has been dissected away is the most reliable means of making a diagnosis of adrenal hyperplasia. The enlarged glands may be nodular or diffuse. Microscopically, the zona fasciculate and reticularis are greatly widened.

4. Iatrogenic hypercortisolism
   In cases where hypercortisolism is the result of exogenous glucocorticoid administration, both adrenal cortices show diffuse atrophy due to inhibition of pituitary ACTH secretion by the exogenous steroids.

B. Clinical Features

Cortisol excess causes an extensive array of metabolic abnormalities. (1) Redistribution of body fat from the extremities to the trunk results in moon facies and truncal obesity with thin extremities. Hypercholesterolemia and accelerated atherosclerosis also occur. (2) The antagonistic effect of cortisol on the action of insulin produces diabetes mellitus. (3) Protein catabolism is increased. Gluconeogenesis is stimulated by cortisol, leading to muscle wasting. Growth retardation occurs in children. Other consequences of increased protein catabolism include thinning of the skin with development of striae, easy bruising, and delayed wound healing. Decrease in the amount of the protein matrix of bone leads to osteoporosis. (4) Cortisol has a significant mineralocorticoid action that results in retention of sodium in the distal renal tubule at the expense of potassium and hydrogen. Hypertension and hypokalemic alkalosis may occur as a result. (5) Cortisol has an inhibitory effect on lymphocyte, macrophage, and neutrophil function, resulting in increased susceptibility to infections. (6) Cortisol in excess has an effect on brain cells, and patients with Cushing's syndromes such as euphoria, mania, and psychosis (steroid encephalopathy). (7) Some degree of androgen excess coexists with cortisol excess in many patients, leading to hirsutism, acne, infertility, and menstrual disturbances in females.

Hyperaldosteronism

A. Etiology

1. Primary hyperaldosteronism (Conn's syndrome)
   This disorder is rare and is most commonly the result of an aldosterone-secreting adrenocortical adenoma (Figure 13-12). Less commonly, it may result from bilateral hyperplasia of the zona glomerulosa. Adrenal carcinomas only very rarely secrete aldosterone. In a few cases of hyperaldosteronism, no definite abnormality is detected in the gland.

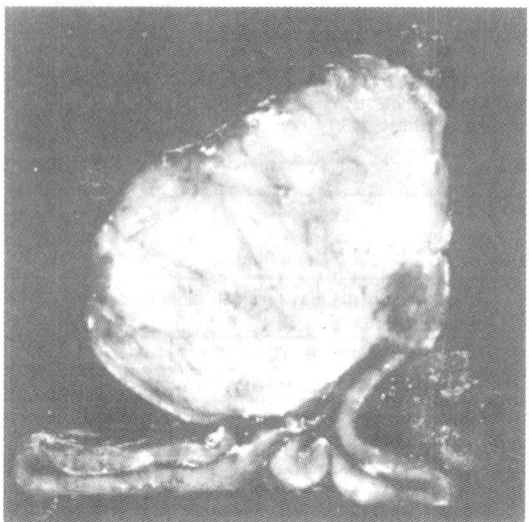

Figure 13-12 Cross section of adrenal gland, showing an adrenocortical adenoma. The gross and microscopic features do not permit differentiation of aldosterone- and cortisol-secreting adenomas

2. Secondary hyperaldosteronism

Secondary hyperaldosteronism is common. It is caused by a high rennin output from the juxtaglomerular cells of the kidney in response to (1) renal ischemia, such as occurs in renal artery stenosis and malignant hypertension; (2) reduced effective plasma volume, as occurs in cardiac failure and hypoproteinemic states; or (3) juxtaglomerular cell hyperplasia (Bartter's syndrome) or neoplasia.

B. Pathologic Changes

Most cases of primary aldosteronism are associated with an adrenocortical adenoma indistinguishable from an adenoma that produces cortisol except that it tends to be sma ller (usually < 2 cm in diameter) (Figure 13-12).

The adrenals appear grossly normal in patients with secondary hyperaldosteronism; microscopic demonstration of hyperplasia of the zona glomerulosa is difficult and subjective.

C. Clinical Features

Aldosterone causes sodium retention in the distal renal tubule in exchange for potassium and hydrogen ions, resulting in hypertension and hypokalemic alkalosis. Hypertension is the usual presenting feature. Less than 1% of patients with hypertention have primary hyperaldosteronism, but this cause is important to identify because it represents a surgically curable cause. Hypokalemic symptoms may occasionally dominate. They include muscle weakness, fatigue, paralyses, and paresthesias. Alkalosis may cause a decrease in serum ionized calcium, leading to tetany.

Secondary hyperaldosteronism occurs as a complication of a variety of diseases whose clinical manifestations usually dominate the clinical picture. In this situation, increased aldosterone secretion is a normal compensatory phenomenon and produces few symptoms except sodium retention, thereby contributing to the edema under these conditions. Hypokalemic alkalosis and its effects may also be present.

It is of interest that edema is rare in patients with primary hyperaldosteronism even though there is marked sodium and water retention. Lack of edema is due to the fact that increased atrial natriuretic factor secreted by cardiac tissue limits sodium retention.

Excess Sex Hormone Secretion

Excessive secretion of androgenic hormones by the adrenals is very rare. It may be due to adrenocortical neoplasms (particularly carcinomas) or congenital adrenal hyperplasia (adrenogenital syndrome). It may also occur as an associated phenomenon in patients with Cushing's syndrome.

Excessive estrogen secretion occurs very rarely with adrenocortical carcinomas.

DECREASED SECRETION OF ADRENOCORTICAL HORMONES

Etiology

Decreased secretion of adrenocortical hormones is uncommon.

A. Acute Insufficiency

Acute insufficiency may follow destruction of the adrenal cortices in severe bacteremias, most commonly meningococcal bacteremia (Waterhouse-Friderichsen syndrome). Clinically, this is a fulminant illness characterized by high fever, bacteremia, hemorrhagic skin rash, and shock, which progresses rapidly to death in most cases. Disseminated intravascular coagulation is believed to be responsible for petechial hemorrhagic throughout the body, including the adrenals.

Acute adrenocortical insufficiency (addisonian crisis) is most commonly seen today as an iatrogenic disease in patients being treated with synthetic glucocorticoids (e.g. prednisone) in high doses. These drugs suppress pituitary ACTH and result in atrophy of the adrenal cortex, destroying the patient's ability to secrete cortisol normally. If such a patient has a sudden increased demand for cortisol (as during stress or an infection) or if the exogenous steroids are withdrawn rapidly, acute adrenocortical insufficiency may occur.

B. Chronic Insufficiency (Addison's Disease)

Chronic insufficiency of adrenocortical hormone synthesis occurs in a variety of conditions associated with chronic destruction of the adrenal glands (Table 13-8).

Table 13-8 Causes of chronic adrenal insufficiency (Addison's disease)

Primary adrenal insufficiency (destruction of adrenals)
Autoimmune Addison's disease (idiopathic Addison's disease)
Infections: tuberculosis, histoplasmosis, HIV infection
Amyloidosis
Hemochromatosis
Surgical removal
Metastatic carcinoma, especially from lung
Failure of hormone synthesis
Congenital adrenal hyperplasia
Enzyme-inhibiting drugs: metyrapone, ketoconazole
Cytotoxic drugs: mitotane
Secondary adrenal insufficiency
Pituitary-hypothalamic disease
Suppression by exogenous steroids

With the declining incidence of tuberculosis and histoplasmosis, 90% of the adult cases in the USA are caused by autoimmune destruction of the adrenals. Fifty percent of patients with autoimmune Addison's disease have antiadrenal antibodies in the serum. The cell destruction is most likely mediated be sensitized cytotoxic T lymphocytes. Autoimmune Addison's disease is associated with other autoimmune disease such as Hashimoto's thyroiditis, Graves' disease, and pernicious anemia.

Pathologic Changes

When the adrenals are the site of a disease (tuberculosis, fungal infection, metastatic carcinoma, hemochromatosis, amyloidosis, etc), the gland shows the specific morphologic features associated with those disorders.

In autoimmune Addison's disease, the adrenals are markedly atrophic, with an aggregate weight less than 4 g. There is loss of normal architecture and lipid depletion of cells, resulting in a brown color. Microscopically, the cortex is greatly narrowed, with a diffuse lymphocytic infiltrate and fibrosis.

Clinical Features

The dominant clinical features of Addison's diseases are caused by decreased mineralocorticoid activity. There is increased weakness, fatigability, and weight loss (asthenia). Sodium excretion in the renal tubules is increased, with retention of potassium and hydrogen ions. Loss of sodium results in hyponatremia and contraction of plasma volume, leading to hypotension. Serum chloride is decreased, and there is a hyperkalemic acidosis. Hyperkalemia may cause muscular weakness and electrocardiographic abnormalities.

Patients are unable to respond to stresses such as infections, surgery, and trauma, which precipitate life-threatening circulatory collapse (addisonian crisis).

A compensatory increase in pituitary ACTH secretion occurs in all cases of adrenal insufficiency (except when caused by hypopituitarism). Plasma ACTH levels are increased. This causes increased skin pigmentation because of the melanocyte-stimulating property of ACTH.

In the early stages, patients have a normal plasma cortisol but a decreased adrenal reserve. This is best detected by ACTH stimulation tests, which fail to increase cortisol output by the adrenal. In later stages, plasma levels of cortisol and aldosterone are decreased.

Treatment is by glucocorticoid (cortisol) replacement. Fludrocortisone is usually necessary to correct the mineralocorticoid deficiency.

THE ADRENAL GLAND NEOPLASMS

Adrenocortical Adenoma

Grossly, adrenocortical adenomas appear as well-circumscribed nodular masses that are usually small (< 5 cm in greatest diameter and 5 – 10 g in weight; Figure 13-12). They usually have a bright yellow color and may show areas of cystic degeneration, fibrosis, and hemorrhage. The controlateral adrenal usually is atrophic.

Microscopically, adenomas are composed of uniform large cells arranged in nests and trabeculae. The cells have abundant lipid-filled cytoplasm and small uniform nuclei. Nuclear enlargement and pleomorphism are not uncommon, but mitotic figures are rare.

Not all adrenocortical adenomas produce hormones. Nonfunctional adrenocortical adenomas are present in about 5% of all autopsies and are being increasingly detected as incidental findings when abdominal CT scans are performed for other reasons. The diagnosis of a functional adrenocortical adenoma is best made by careful chemical assays for hormones in the serum before the adenoma is removed. Pathologic features of nonfunctional adenomas and those that secrete different hormones are similar and do not allow diagnosis of specific hormone-secreting adenomas.

Adrenocortical Carcinoma

Adrenocortical carcinomas usually appear as large (>6 cm and >50 g), poorly circumscribed masses that commonly show infiltration of perinephric fat and kidney. Gross, involvement of the adrenal and renal vein by the neoplasm may also occur.

Microscopically, adrenal carcinomas are composed of large, pleomorphic cells arranged in diffuse sheets. Mitotic figures are frequent and abnormal. Areas of necrosis, capsular invasion, and vascular invasion are common. The microscopic features permit accurate differentiation of adenoma and carcinoma.

Adrenal carcinoma behaves as a highly malignant neoplasm, metastasizing both to lymph nodes and via the bloodstream. Not all produce excess hormones; like adenomas, the pathologic features of nonfunctional carcinomas are similar to those that secrete hormones.

Adrenomedullary Neoplasm (Pheochromocytoma)

Pheochromocytomas are catecholamine-producing neoplasms of the adrenal medulla or extra-adrenal paraganglia. The term paraganglioma is commonly used for these tumors when they occur outside the adrenal gland itself.

Pheochromocytoma is an uncommon neoplasm. It usually occurs sporadically, but 5% of patients give a positive family history for the following diseases: (1) Familial occurrence of pheochromocytoma, with an autosomal dominant pattern of inheritance, which is very rare; (2) Generalized neurofibromatosis (von Recklinghausen's disease) is associated with an increased incidence of pheochromocytoma; (3) Multiple endocrine neoplasia types II a and II b (see below); (4) von Hippel-Lindau disease; and (5) Sturge-Weber disease.

A. Pathologic Changes

Pheochromocytoma is sometimes called "the 10% tumor" for the following reasons: (1) Its commonest location is in the adrenal medulla, but 10% of pheochromocytomas occur in extra-adrenal paraganglia - most often intra-abdominal, occasionally in the mediastinum, neck, or wall of the urinary bladder. (2) Ten percent of patients with pheochromocytoma have multiple tumors, most commonly involving both adrenal glands but also the extra-adrenal paraganglia. (3) Most pheochromocytomas behave as benign neoplasms, but 10% are malignant with local invasion and metastasis. In children, the 10% rule does not apply, as 25% are bilateral and 25% extra-adrenal.

Pheochromocytomas vary in size from very small (1 cm) to massive tumors, are well circumscribed, are frequently show areas of hemorrhage and necrosis (Figure 13-13). Fixation in a chromium salt fixative (such as Zenker's solution) imparts a brown color to the tumor - hence the older term chromaffin paraganglioma.

Microscopically, the tumor consists of large cells arranged in sheets and nests separated by a rich vascular stroma. Pleomorphism is common, but mitoses are rare. Invasion of capsule and vessels is common even in those neoplasms that behave in a generally benign fashion.

Electron microscopy shows the presence of membrane-bound, dense-core neurosecretory granules in the cytoplasm. Immunologic studies show the presence of markers for neuroendocrine cells such as neuron-specific enolase and chromogranin. Catecholamines can be demonstrated in the tumor if it a sample is assayed.

The biological behavior of a pheochromocytoma cannot be predicted by microscopic examination. Extra-adrenal paragangliomas are more frequently malignant than adrenal pheochromocytomas. The diagnosis of malignant pheochromocytoma is made only when metastasis demonstrated. Distinction must also be made between true metastases and multiple primary paragangliomas, which occur rarely and are usually benign. A diagnosis of metastatic pheochromocytoma is made only when a pheochromocytoma occurs in a site where paraganglia are not found (e.g. lung, bone, liver, brain).

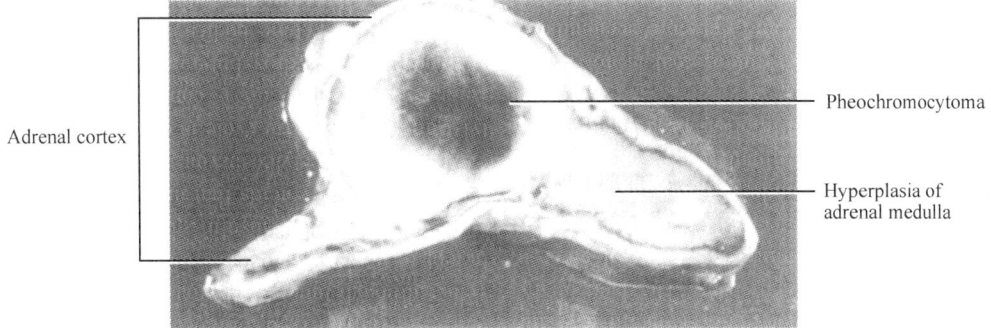

Figure 13-13   Cross section of adrenal gland, showing a pheochromocytoma associated with hyperplasia of the medulla in a patient with multiple endocrine neoplasia type II a. (He also had a medullary carcinoma of the thyroid and a large pheochromocytoma in the opposite adrenal)

B. Clinical Features

The clinical manifestations of pheochromocytoma are due to increased catecholamine secretion.

Hypertension is the most common presenting feature. Blood pressure elevation is the result of peripheral vasoconstriction and increased cardiac output caused by the alpha and beta effects of catecholamines. Hypertension is commonly persistent but may be paroxysmal, with return of the blood pressure to normal between paroxysms. Paraxysmal hypertension is caused by sudden release of hormone from the neoplasm and may be precipitated by bending, increased abdominal pressure (as during physical examination), meals, and - in those rare cases where the tumor is located in the urinary bladder wall - by micturition. During a hypertensive crisis, the systolic pressure can rise to 300 mmHg.

Hypertension, particularly when episodic, is accompanied by other manifestations of catecholamine excess such as palpitations, tachycardia, feelings of anxiety, and excessive sweating. Impaired glucose tolerance is common as the result of the insulin-antagonistic action of catecholamines.

Untreated, patients with pheochromocytomas die of cardiac failure or cerebral hemorrhage during a hypertensive crisis.

THE ENDOCRINE PANCREAS DISEASES

NORMAL STRUCTURE AND FUNCTION

The islets of Langerhans are microscopic structures 50 - 250 μm in diameter. They are scattered throughout the pancreas, with a maximum density in the tail. The islets appear to have a major problem even after 90% of the pancreas is removed in a distal pancreatectomy. The islets are not connected to the exocrine duct system; the hormonal products are secreted directly into the bloodstream.

Microscopically, the islets are composed of small uniform cells with round nuclei and scant cytoplasm. Routine microscopy does not permit differentiation of the various types of cells contained within the islets; this requires immunohistochemistry (Table 13-9 and Figure 13-14).

Table 13-9   Cell types in the islets of Langerhans

Cell Type	Frequency	Secretion
B (beta)	60% - 70%	Insulin
A (alpha)	10% - 20%	Glucagon
D (delta)	2% - 8%	Somatostatin
F	1% - 5%	Pancreatic polypeptide
D[1]	Rare	Vasoactive intestinal polypeptide
G	Rare	Gastrin

[1] Demonstrable by immunostaining methods using the appropriate antibody.

The most important hormone secreted by the pancreas is insulin. The B (beta) cells of the islets are the only source of insulin in the body, and failure of secretion of adequate amounts of insulin results in diabetes mellitus.

Glucagon, secreted by the A (alpha) cells, also plays a role in glucose metabolism. The role of glucagons is a less vital one, and absence of glucagons has not been shown to cause clinical disease. The physio-

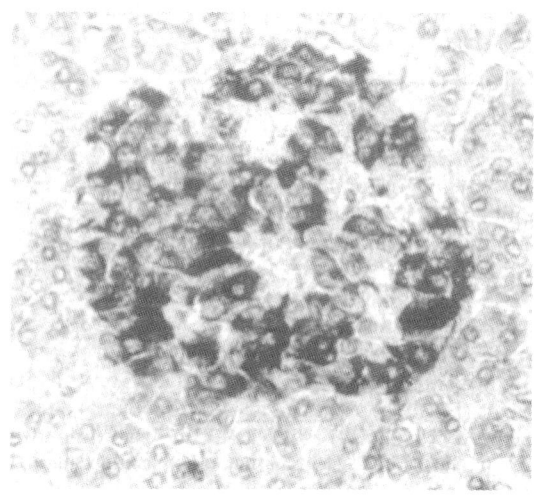

Figure 13-14 Pancreatic islet stained by immunoperoxidase technique with antibody against insulin, showing B cells in the islet, which stain darkly. The non-B cells of the islet and the pancreatic acini around the islet remain unstained

logic functions of pancreatic polypeptide (PP) and vasoactive intestinal polypeptide (VIP) have not been elucidated, and the amount of somatostatin and gastrin normally secreted by the pancreatic islets is thought to be too small to be of any physiologic significance. However, excessive secretion of any of these hormones by pathologic islets causes specific clinical syndromes.

Assessment of islets structure is very difficult because of their small size and scattered distribution in the pancreas. Only large islet cell neoplasms are distinguishable on computerized tomography. The main tests of islet function are serum assays of the various hormones secreted by the islets.

DIABETES MELLITUS

Introduction

Diabetes mellitus is a chronic disease characterized by relative or absolute deficiency of insulin, resulting in glucose intolerance. It occurs in 4-5 million persons in the Unites States (approximately 2% of the population).

Etiology (Table 13-10)

Diabetes mellitus is caused by a relative or absolute deficiency of insulin. In primary diabetes (95% of cases), there is no underlying disease process that might explain insulin deficiency. Primary diabetes is of two types: 1 and 2 (see below and Table 13-10). The remaining 5% of cases of secondary diabetes are due either to pancreatic destruction or to the presence of increased levels of hormones that antagonize the action of insulin.

There is an absolute deficiency of insulin in type I primary diabetes and in those cases of secondary diabetes associated with destruction of the pancreas. In type II primary diabetes - and in the presence of increased levels of antagonistic hormones - the insulin deficiency is relative, and serum insulin levels are usually normal and may even be elevated.

Table 13-10 Classification of diabetes mellitus

Primary diabetes mellitus (95%)
Type I: Insulin-dependent diabetes mellitus (IDDM)
Type II: Non-insulin-dependent diabetes mellitus (NIDDM)
Impaired glucose tolerance: IGT (latent diabetes)
Gestational diabetes mellitus[1]
Secondary diabetes mellitus (5%)
Destructive pancreatic disease
Chronic pancreatitis
Hemochromatosis (bronze diabetes)
Total pancreatectomy
Endocrine disease (high levels of insulin-antagonistic hormones)
Acromegaly (growth hormone)
Cushing's syndrome (cortisol)
Pheochromocytoma (catecholamines)
Glucocagonoma (glucagons)
Drug-induced diabetes (including diuretics such as thiazides, furosemide; propranolol; antidepressants; phenothiazines)
Stress disbetes[1]

[1] Gestation and stress diabetes probably represent patients with IGT or with a genetic predisposition to diabetes who are decompensated by the physiologic changes of pregnancy or stress. The "diabetes" is often reversible, but such patients show an increased incidence of true diabetes in succeeding years.

A. Type I Diabetes Mellitus

Type I diabetes mellitus (insulin-dependent diabetes mellitus, IDDM) is due to destruction of pancreatic B cells. Plasma insulin levels are very low, and ketoacidosis develops if the patients do not receive exogenous insulin. Rarely, in the early stage of type I diabetes, there may be enough insulin to prevent ketoacidosis, and the patients are not insulin-dependent (this is sometimes known as "type I diabetes in evolution"). The disease affects young patients (juvenile-onset diabetes mellitus), most commonly under 30 years of age, and there is a significant association with HLA-B8, -B15, -DR4. The HLA-D locus is closely associated with genes that confer increased susceptibility to type I diabetes. Ninety-five percent of patients with type I diabetes express DR3, DR4, or the heterozygous DR3/DR4 state. Increased susceptibility has also been linked with (1) the absence of aspartic acid in position 57 of the DQ_β chain and (2) the presence of the DQw8 allele. The genetic predisposition to type I diabetes is shown by the history of diabetes in about 20% of first-degree relatives - which is not as strong as in type II diabetes.

The cause of B cell destruction in type I diabetes is unknown. A few cases have followed viral infections, most commonly with coxsackievirus B or mumps virus, and several viruses have been shown to cause B cell damage when inoculated into mice. Despite these findings, the role of viruses in the etiology of human diabetes is thought to be that of an inciting factor for autoimmunity.

Autoimmunity is believed to be the major mechanism involved. Islet cell autoantibodies are present in the serum of 90% of newly diagnosed cases. Such antibodies are directed against several cell components, including cytoplasmic and membrane antigens or against insulin itself (IgG and IgE antibodies). Sensitized T lymphocytes with activity against B cells have also been demonstrated in some patients. Microscopic examination of the islets in patients with early type I diabetes shows the presence of a lymphocytic infiltrate in the islet ("insulitis"). One hypothesis is that a mild viral injury of B cells induces an autoimmune reaction against the injured cells. HLA-linked immune response genes may explain the genetic susceptibility; HLA-B8, -B15, -DR3, and -DR4, in addition to their association with diabetes, also occur at increased frequency in Graves' disease, Addison's disease, and pernicious anemia, all of which are characterized by the presence of autoantibodies.

Toxins such as nitrophenylureas (in rat poisons) and cyanide from spoiled food have been implicated in B cell destruction in rare cases.

B. Type II Diabetes Mellitus

The etiology of type II diabetes (non-insulin-dependent diabetes mellitus, NIDDM) is even less clearly understood. Two factors have been identified.

1. Impaired insulin release

Basal secretion of insulin is often normal, but the rapid release of insulin that follows a meal is greatly impaired, resulting in failure of normal handling of a carbohydrate load. The delayed phase of insulin secretion is also normal in the early stages but impaired in advanced disease. However, some level of insulin secretion is maintained in most patients, so that the abnormality of glucose metabolism is limited, and ketoacidosis is uncommon. In these patients, insulin secretion can be stimulated by drugs such as sulfonylureas. Exogenous insulin is therefore not essential in treatment. Most patients with type II diabetes first develop disease in adult life (adult-onset diabetes). A subgroup of type II diabetes develops disease at a young age (maturity-onset diabetes of the young, MODY). These patients have an autosomal dominant single-gene inheritance pattern.

It has been suggested that inheritance of a defective pattern of insulin secretion is responsible for the familial tendency of diabetes. The mechanism of inheritance is highly complex and probably involves multiple genes except in maturity-onset diabetes of the young. The genetic factor is very strong in type II diabetes, with a history of diabetes present in about 50% of first-degree relatives.

2. Insulin resistance (Table 13-11)

A defect in the tissue response to insulin is believed to play a major role. This phenomenon is called insulin resistance and is caused by defective insulin receptors on the target cells.

Insulin resistance occurs in association with obesity and pregnancy. In normal individuals who become obese or pregnant, The B cells secrete increased amounts of insulin to compensate. Patients who have a genetic susceptibility to diabetes cannot compensate because of their inherent defect in insulin secretion. Thus, type II diabetes is frequently precipitated by obesity and pregnancy.

In a few patients with extreme insulin resistance, antibodies against the receptors have been demonstrated in the plasma. These antibodies are mostly of the IgG class and may act in a manner analogous to the action of antiacetylcholine-receptor antibodies in myasthenia gravis. Decreased numbers of insulin receptors, defective binding of insulin to receptors, and abnormalities in the series of cellular events that follow insulin binding have also been postulated as causes of insulin resistance.

Table 13-11 Comparison of types of primary diabetes mellitus

	Type I	Type II
Incidence (% age of cases of primary diabetes)	15%	85%
Insulin necessary in treatment	Almost always	Sometimes
Age (commonly; Exceptions occur)	Under 30	Over 40
Association with obesity	No	Yes
Genetic predisposition	Weak, polygenic	Strong, polygenic
Association with HLA system	Yes, DR3, DR4	No
Glucose intolerance	Severe	Mild
Ketoacidosis	Common	Rare
Hyperosmolar coma	Rare	Common
B cell numbers in the islets	Reduced	Variable
Serum insulin level	Reduced	Normal or high
Classic symptoms of polyuria, polydipsia, thirst, weight loss	Common	Rare
Basic cause	? Viral or immune destruction of B cells	? Increased resistance to insulin

Pathologic Changes

The pathologic changes in the pancreatic islets in diabetes mellitus are variable from one patient to another and are not specific for diabetes. In type I diabetes, there is frequently a lymphocytic infiltration of the islets in the early phase, followed by a progressive loss of B cells.

The changes in type II diabetes are often minimal in the early stages. In advanced disease, there may be fibrosis and amyloid deposition in the islets; in diabetes, the amyloid appears to consist in part of precipitated insulin. Similar changes in the islets are sometimes present in elderly nondiabetic patients and are not considered diagnostic for diabetes.

Clinical Features

The classic symptoms of diabetes mellitus result from abnormal glucose metabolism. The lack of insulin activity results in failure of transfer of glucose from the plasma into the cells ("starvation in the midst of plenty"). The body responds as if it were in the fasting state, with stimulation of glycogenolysis, gluconeogenesis, and lipolysis producing ketone bodies

The glucose absorbed during a meal is not metabolized at the normal rate and therefore accumulates in the blood (hyperglycemia) to be excreted in the urine (glycosuria). Glucose in the urine causes osmotic diuresis, leading to increased urine production (polyuria). The fluid loss and hyperglycemia increase the osmolarity of the plasma, stimulating the thirst center (polydipsia). Stimulation of protein breakdown to provide amino acids for gluconeogenesis results in muscle wasting and weight loss. These classic symptoms occur only in patients with severe insulin deficiency, most commonly in type I diabetes.

Many patients with type II diabetes do not have these symptoms and present with one of the complications of diabetes.

A. Acute Complications

1. Diabetic ketoacidosis

Ketoacidosis occurs in severe diabetes, where insulin levels are greatly reduced and glucagons levels are increased. It is common in untreated type I diabetes but rare in type II diabetes, where insulin levels, although functionally inadequate, are still sufficient to prevent ketone body formation.

In the absence of insulin, lipolysis is stimulated releasing free fatty acids that are oxidized in the liver cell to form acetylcoenzyme A. The entry of acetyl-CoA into the citric cycle is defective in diabetes. As a result, acetyl-CoA is converted in the liver to acetoacetate, β-hydroxybutyrate, and acetone (collectively called ketone bodies). Glucagon excess is an important factor in the pathogenesis of ketoacidosis. While insulin lack mobilizes free fatty acids from adipose tissue, oxidation of fatty acids to ketone in the liver cell is induced by glucagons via its stimulatory effect on the hepatic carnitine-palmitoyl-transferase system. Glycagon also stimulates gluconeogenesis, aggravating the hyperglycemia. The ketone bodies enter the blood (ketonemia, ketosis) and represent an important source of energy for skeletal muscle that cannot utilize glucose effectively in diabetes. They also spill over to be excreted in the urine (ketonuria).

Ketone bodies are moderately strong acids and cause a metabolic acidosis with decreased blood pH and low serum bicarbonate. Respiration is stimulated, washing out carbon dioxide and leading to a decrease in Pco_2. An acid urine is excreted.

2. Hyperosmolar nonketotic coma

Patients who develop hyperosmolar coma are usually elderly, with severe uncontrolled diabetes. The disorder results from extremely high serum glucose levels that cause osmotic diuresis and marked fluid depletion, increasing plasma osmolarity. Hyperosmolar coma is treated with aggressive fluid replacement and insulin. It is associated with a high mortality rate.

3. Hypoglycemic coma

Hypoglycemic coma is not a direct complication of diabetes but rather a complication of therapy. In treating diabetes it is essential to balance the insulin dose and the dietary intake of carbohydrate ("glucose dose"). A fall in blood glucose may follow overdosage of insulin but is seen more often when the usually daily schedule of insulin injections is given and one or more meals is missed or lost by vomiting (i.e. when the "glucose dose" is reduced).

B. Chronic Complications

1. Diabetic microangiopathy (Small vessel disease)

Microangiopathy is one of the most characteristic and most important pathologic changes in diabetes. It is characterized by diffuse thickening of the basement membranes of capillaries throughout the body. The kidney (Figure 13-15), retina, skin, and skeletal muscles are commonly involved. A similar change involves other basement membranes in renal tubules, placenta, and peripheral nerves. Basement membrane thickening in capillaries is associated with increased permeability to fluid and protein macromolecules.

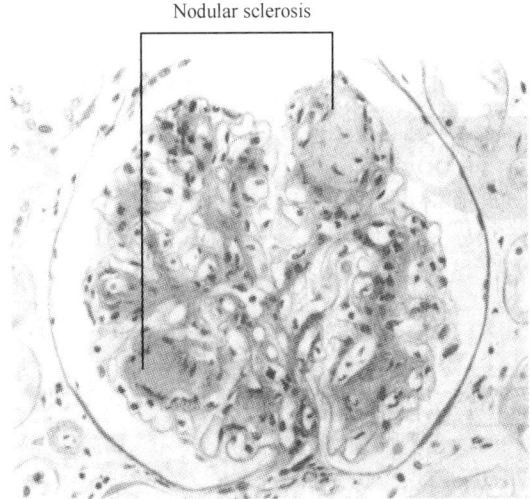

Figure 13-15 Diabetic nephropathy, showing nodular glomerulosclerosis (Kimmelstiel-Wilson disease)

The structure of the thick basement membrane in diabetics is abnormal. Increased amounts of collagen and laminin and decreased proteoglycans have been demonstrated. It has been suggested that prolonged elevation of serum glucose increases glycosylation of basement membrane proteins in a manner similar to glycosylation of hemoglobulin. This would explain why strict control of diabetes decreases the incidence and severity of microangiopathy. It is widely accepted - that tight control of diabetes decreases the risk of microangiopathy.

2. Large vessel disease

Diabetes mellitus is a major risk factor for development of atherosclerotic vascular disease; myocardial infarction and cerebral arterial occlusion (stroke) represent two of the most common causes of death in diabetics. The increased incidence of hyperlipidemia (both hypertriglyceridemia and hypercholesterolemia) in diabetes contributes to the development of atherosclerosis.

3. Neuropathy and cataract

Neuropathy and cataract in diabetic patients are believed to result from accumulation of sorbitol within nerve or lens tissue. The enzyme aldose reductase produces sorbitol in these tissues when glucose levels are high, and the accumulated sorbitol, which is osmotically active and nondiffusible, produces cellular swelling or death. It is postulated that nerve and lens tissue (and perhaps small vessels and kidney) may be particularly vulnerable to this effect because glucose can enter these cells even in low-insulin states – unlike other cells of the body, which require normal plasma levels of insulin for entry of glucose. Trials of drugs that inhibit aldose reductase are under way as a possible means of combating some of the chronic effects of diabetes.

4. Other complications

Other complications include a general increased susceptibility to infection and impaired wound healing. Chronic foot ulcers are common and difficult problem.

C. Clinical Course

The average life expectancy of diabetics is reduced by 9 years for males and 7 years for females when compared with nondiabetics. The reduction is greatest when the onset of disease is at a young age.

Quality of life is seriously affected for all diabetics because of the many disabling complications. In addition, the requirement for strict dietary control and continuous drug treatment for many patients calls for a continuous emotional struggle.

Causes of death in diabetes (in order of frequency) are myocardial infarction, renal failure, cerebrovascular accidents, infections, ketoacidosis, hyperosmolar coma, and hypoglycemia.

ISLET CELL NEOPLASMS

Adenomas derived from the islet cells are relatively common. In 10%-15% of cases, multiple adenomas are present. Islet cell carcinomas occur, but less frequently.

Grossly, islet cell neoplasms are firm nodules that typically have a yellowish-brown color. They vary in size from microscopic (microadenomas) to large masses that may weigh several kilograms. They may or may not show encapsulation.

Microscopically, islet cell neoplasms are composed of uniform small cells arranged in nests and trabeculae separated by endothelium-lined vascular spaces. The islet cell origin of a pancreatic neoplasm can be established (1) by the presence of membrane-bound, electron-dense neurosecretory granules in the cytoplasm on electron microscopy; and (2) by positive staining for neuron-specific enolase, chromogranin, or specific hormones by immunoperoxidase techniques.

Differentiation of adenomas from carcinomas of islet cells is difficult by light microscopic examination. Invasion of the capsule and cytologic atypia are common in neoplasms that show benign behavior and cannot be used as evidence of malignant change. Conversely, islet cell carcinomas may be well circumscribed and have little cytologic atypia. Features that favor a diagnosis of carcinoma are extensive invasion of the pancreatic stroma or perineural invasion. The only definite evidence of malignancy is the presence of metastatic lesions.

Islet cell adenomas are cured by surgical excision; carcinomas tend to grow slowly but are difficult to control if surgery fails. Even in the presence of metastatic disease, patients may survive several years because of the slow growth rate of islet cell carcinoma.

Most islet cell neoplasmas are composed of one cell type; less commonly, multiple cell types are involved. The diagnosis of the cell type is impossible by routine light microscopy and requires (1) electron microscopy, which demonstrates characteristic granules of the different cells; (2) serum assay for different pancreatic hormones; and (3) demonstration of hormone in the tumor cells by immunoperoxidase techniques. Some islet cell neoplasms do not produce sufficient hormone to be detectable in serum (nonfunctional islet cell neoplasms).

*SUPPLEMENT: MULTIPLE ENDOCRINE NEOPLASIA SYNDROMES

The multiple endocrine neoplasia (MEN) or multiple endocrine adenomatosis (MEA) syndromes are characterized by the familial occurrence of multiple endocrine neoplasms. They are rare and are inherited as an autosomal dominant trail with variable penetrance.

Three types of MEN syndromes are recognized:

MEN (MEA) Type I

MEN type I consists of pituitary adenoma, parathyroid hyperplasia or adenoma, and pancreatic islet cell neoplasms, including gastrinoma. Peptic ulcers also occur in these patients, probably related to gastrin production (Zollinger-Ellison syndrome). Adrenocortical adenomas rarely occur.

MEN Type II A (Sipple Syndrome)

MEN type II a consists of medullary carcinoma

and parafollicular cell hyperplasia of the thyroid and adrenal medullary hyperplasia or pheochromocytoma (Figure 13-13). Parathyroid hyperplasia or adenoma may also be present. These patients do not have pancreatic islet cell neoplasms or pituitary neoplasms and have no increased incidence of peptic ulcer.

MEN Type II B

A subgroup of MEN type II has been identified in which patients have mucocutaneous (tongue, eyelids, bronchus, intestine) neuromas in addition to the thyroid and adrenal neoplasms. This is sometimes also called MEN type III.

Chapter 14 Diseases of the Nervous System

Luo Dianzhong, Ma Yun

CHAPTER CONTENTS
- Structure of the Nervous System and Basic Pathologic Changes in Disorders of the Nervous System
    Structure of the Nervous System
      Basic Pathologic Changes in Disorders of the Nervous System
- The Cerebrospinal Fluid
    Hydrocephalus
    Cerebral Edema
    Increased Intracranial Pressure
- Infections of the Nervous System
    Meningeal Infections
    Infections of the Brain Parenchyma
- Degenerative Disease of the Nervous System
    Cerebrocortical Degenerations
    Basal Ganglia Degenerations
- Neoplasms of the Nervous System
    Neoplasms of the Central Nervous System
    Neoplasms of the Peripheral Nervous System

STRUCTURE OF THE NERVOUS SYSTEM AND BASIC PATHOLOGIC CHANGES IN DISORDERS OF THE NERVOUS SYSTEM

STRUCTURE OF THE NERVOUS SYSTEM

The Central Nervous System

The central nervous system is composed of the cerebral hemispheres, brain stem, cerebellum and spinal cord. Microscopically, the principal cell types are neurons and neuroglial cells (Table 14-1).

Neurons represent the basic function unit of the nervous system. Each neuron is composed of a cell body plus cytoplasmic processes, including dendrites, which synapse with processes from other neurons, and axons, which carry impulses away from the cell body. The neuron has a large nucleus with a prominent nucleolus and an abundant pale eosinophilic cytoplasm in which the ribosomes form clumped masses (Nissl substance). Neurons are postmitotic (permanent) cells that have no mitotic capability. Neurons are found in the cerebral cortex, the cerebellar cortex, the basal ganglia, and in the nuclei and gray matter of the brain stem and spinal cord.

Neuroglial cells form the supporting connective tissue of the brain that represents the white matter. Neuroglial cells include astrocytes, oligodendroglial cells, microglial cells and are capable of mitotic division and proliferate in a variety of conditions. **Astrocytes** are the major supporting cells in the brain and show some of the most common reactive changes. In cases of brain parenchymal injury, astrocytes respond by producing a dense network of processes, some what analogous to a fibrous scar occurring elsewhere in the body. In contrast to fibroblasts, astrocytes do not produce collagen. The glial scar is made up predominantly of cytoplasmic processes, with little or no extracellular protein. In routine sections, **oligodendroglia** cells are recognizable by their small, rounded, lymphocyte-like nuclei, often arranged in linear arrays. Despite their name, it is now generally accepted that **microglia** are derived from circulating monocytes rather than from the neural tube. The many functions of these ubiquitous cells are only now becom-

Table 14-1 Principal cell types in the central nervous system and the common pathologic changes they undergo

Cell Type	Basic Pathologic Change	Causes	Effects
Neuron (many subtypes)	Necrosis, usually liquefactive	Anoxia, commonly ischemic Hypoglycemia Toxins, including drugs Metabolites Infectious agents Neoplasm Trauma	Permanent loss of function subserved by neuron Neurons cannot divide by mitosis

	Chromatolysis: swelling with loss of Nissl substance
	Neurofibrillary tangles
	Cytoplasmic inclusions
	  Lipid
	  Mucopolysaccharide
	  Pick's bodies
	  Lewy bodies
	  Negri bodies
	Intranuclear inclusions
	  Viral inclusions
	  Axonal injury
		Axonal injury
		Alzheimer's disease
		
		Lipid storage diseases
		Mucopolysaccharidoses
		Pick's disease
		Parkinson's disease
		Rabies (viral inclusion)
		
		Cytomegalovirus
		Herpes simplex virus
		Papovavirus
			Associated with neuronal dysfuction

	Neoplasia	Central neurocytoma Gangliocytoma	
Astrocyte	Degeneration, loss	Toxic states. e.g. hepatic failure Infarction	No major known effect
	Proliferation (nonneoplastic)	Variety of injuries	Associated with gliosis (analogue of fibrosis in the brain)
	Neoplasia	Astrocytic tumors	Most common primary CNS neoplasm
Oligodendroglia	Degeneration, loss	Demyelinating diseases	Oligodendroglial cells are responsible for myelination in CNS
	Neoplasia	Oligodendroglial tumours	
Microglia	Proliferation and activation	Any cause of neuronal necrosis or demyelination	Analogue of macrophages in CNS Appear in activated state as swollen cells with foamy cytoplasm
Ependymal cells	Neoplasia	Ependymal tumours	

ing clear. Like their counterparts outside the central nervous system, microglia appear to serve as antigen-presenting cells in many inflammatory conditions. Virtually any form of central nervous system injury is associated with the presence of activated microglial cells; these then behave as active macrophages. **Ependymal cells** are specialized glial cells that line the ventricles and the central canal of the spinal cord.

The Peripheral Nervous System

The peripheral nervous system is composed of cranial and spinal nerves that originate in the brain stem or spinal cord and end in the periphery. The autonomic nervous system, with sympathetic and parasympathetic components, may be regarded as a specialized part of the peripheral nervous system with regulatory functions. Periphe-ral nerves are usually mixed motor and sensory nerves and are composed of bundles of nerve fibers that have their cell bodies in the motor nuclei (the anterior horn of the spinal cord or cranial nerve nuclei), the sensory nerve root ganglis, or the autonimmic ganglia.

BASIC PATHOLOGIC CHANGES IN DISORDERS OF THE NERVOUS SYSTEM

There are the following basic pathologic changes in disorders of the nervous system.

A. Coagulation Necrosis

A change occurs most frequently in association with hypoxic-ischemic injury. Morphologically, neuronal necrosis is characterized by a loss of cytoplasmic ribonucleoproteins and denaturation of cytoskeletal proteins, resulting in the development of intense cytoplasmic eosinophilia (**Red neurons**) in hematoxylin and eosin stained section.

B. Chromatolysis

Chromatolysis is a common reaction to axonal injury and is characterized by dispersion of the Nissl substance and swelling of the neuronal cell body.

C. Inclusion Bodies

A number of infectious agents may produce characteristic nuclear or cytoplasmic inclusion bodies within neurons. Examples include the intracytopasmic Negri bodies of rabies and the intranuclear inclusion of cytomegalovirus. Inclusion bodies also can form in the other conditions, for example, Lewy body formation in Parkinson disease.

D. Neurofibrillary Tangles

Neurofibrillary tangles appear as coarse, filamentous aggregates within the cytoplasm of neurons and are composed of insoluble, protein-rich paired helical filaments. Neurofibrillary tangles can be found in Alzheimer disease.

E. Wallerian Degeneration

When a proximal segment of an axon is injured, the axon distal to the site of injury rapidly degenerates and ultimately disappears, a process termed Wallerian degeneration.

F. Microglial Nodues

Microglia may aggregate in compact clusters in response to various insults (e.g. viral infections) to form microglial nodules.

G. Neuronophagia

A process, Microglia or macrophage may engulf injured neurons, is known as Neuronophagia.

H. Gitter Cells

In a setting of tissue necrosis and demyelinating diseases, activated macrophages and microglia may accumulate abundant intracellular lipid to form cells with foamy cytoplasm, termed gitter cells.

I. Astrogliosis and Glial Scar

Astrogliosis or simply gliosis is a process that astrocytes multiply both in and about the localized sites of tissue injury, such as in contusions, penetrating wounds, abscesses, granulomas, infarcts, and cerebral hemorrhages. Astrocytes finally form a "**glial scar**", which is composed predominantly of cell processes rather than collagen.

THE CEREBROSPINAL FLUID

The cerebrospinal fluid (CSF) fills the ventricular system of the brain, the central canal of the spinal cord, and the subarachnoid space.

CSF is secreted by the choroids plexuses, which are situated in the lateral ventricles. From the lateral ventricles, CSF passes through the foramen of Monro into the third ventricle and then through the cerebral aqueduct (aqueduct of Sylvius) in the midbrain into the fourth ventricle (Figure 14-1). The fourth ventricle houses the foramina of Luschka and Magendie, which permit the passage of CSF into the subarachnoid space. CSF then passes over the convexity of the brain to the region of the superior sagittal sinus, where it is absorbed into the venous system by the arachnoid villi.

HYDROCEPHALUS

Hydrocephalus is defined as abnormal dilation of the ventricles (Figure 14-2). It is readily diagnosed by computerized tomography. Hydrocephalus may result from (1) increased secretion of CSF, as occurs very rarely with neoplasms of the choroids plexus; (2) obstruction to the flow of CSF, either in the ventricular system or in the subarachnoid space; (3) failure of absorption of CSF (Table 14-2).

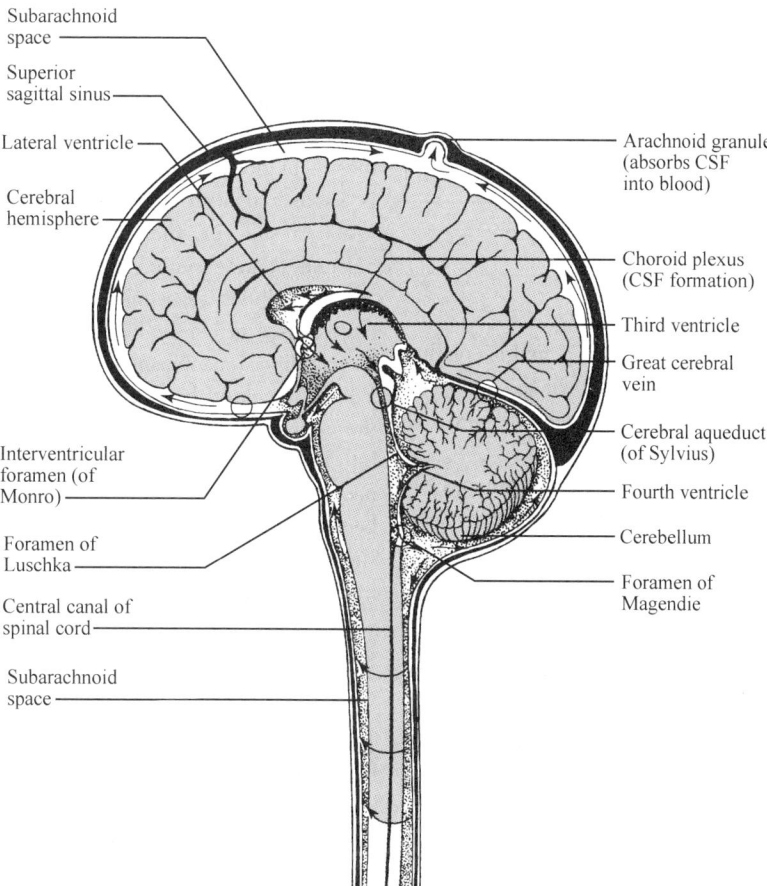

Figure 14-1 Production, circulation, and absorption of cerebrospinal fluid

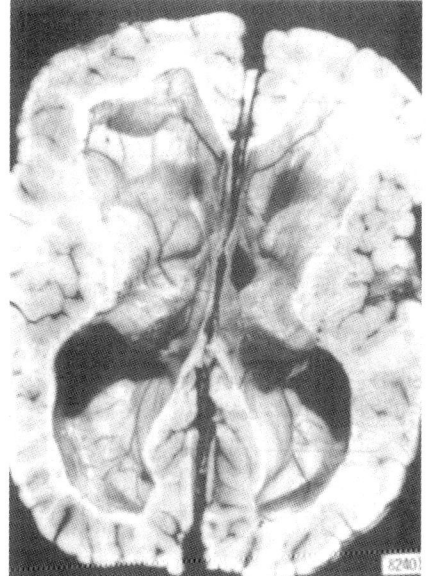

Figure 14-2 Congenital hydrocephalus. Section of whole brain, showing a markedly dilated ventricular system

Table 14-2 Causes of hydrocephalus

Noncommunicating hydrocephalus
Congenital
Aqueductal stenosis and atresia
Dandy-Walker syndrome
Acquired
Neoplasms and cytsts obstructing cerebral aqueduct and third ventricle
Gliosis and chronic inflammation involving aqueduct
Obstruction of fourth ventricle openings
Organized subarachnoid hemorrhage, obstructing flow at base of brain
Communicating hydrocephalus
Choroids plexus papilloma (increased secretion)
Arnold-Chiari malformation
Deficient absorption of cerebrospinal fluid

(Continued)
Communicating Dural sinus thrombosis
Organized subarachnoid hemorrhage
Organized meningitis
Deficiency of arachnoid villi

Classification

A. Anatomic Classification

- Noncommunicating (obstructive) hydrocephalus occurs where there is an obstruction in the ventricular system that prevents CSF from passing into the subarachnoid space.
- Communicating hydrocephalus occurs when CSF passes normally out of the ventricular system but either flow is obstructed in the subarachnoid space or reabsorption is reduced.

B. Functional Classification

- High-pressure hydrocephalus is due to obstruction to CSF flow. If obstruction occurs after fusion of skull sutures, it causes an increase in intracranial pressure. When it occurs in the fetus or infant before fusion of the sutures, it causes the skull to expand.
- Low-pressure (or normal pressure) hydrocephalus is uncommon. There is slow dilation of the ventricles associated with free flow of CSF, cerebral atrophy, and dementia. The cause is unknown in most cases.

CEREBRAL EDEMA

Cerebral edema or brain parenchymal edema indicates the presence of increased water content within the brain parenchyma. It may be categorized as vasogenic edema or cytotoxic edema.

- Intracellular cytotoxic cerebral edema is an early manifestation of cell injury resulting from failure of normal energy production and implies an increase in intracellular fluid secondary to cellular injury. It is most commonly seen in hypoxic-ischemic states. In these situations, energy failure at the cellular level is associated with abnormalities of ion transport, which result in the accumulation of increased amounts of water within the cell.
- Extracellular vasogenic edema is responsible for most causes of cerebral edema, occurring in infections, trauma, neoplasms, and metabolic disorders. Edema is caused by capillary damage, disruption of the normal blood-brain barrier, and leakage of fluid into the interstitium. New blood vessel formation in neoplasms or in the walls of abscesses causes edema because the new vessels are poorly developed and show increased permeability with lesser degrees of injury than do normal vessels.

Pathology

The edematous brain is softer than normal brain. The gyri are flattened, the intervening sulci narrowed, and the ventricular cavities compressed.

INCREASED INTRACRANIAL PRESSURE

Increased intracranial pressure is defined as elevation of the mean CSF pressure above 200 mm water (15 mmHg) when measured with the patient in the lateral decubitus position. Raised intracranial pressure is a common and important pathologic state; it is a frequent cause of neurologic symptoms and, when severe, can cause death.

Etiology (Table 14-3)

Table 14-3 Causes of increased intracranial pressure

Hydrocephalus	(See Table 14-2)
Space-occupying lesions	
Hemorrhage or hematoma	Extradural, subdural, subarachnoid, or intracerebral
Infarction	With local edema or hemorrhage
Neoplasm	Primary or secondary (mass effect and local edema)
Infection	Abscess (mass effect and local edema)
Cerebral edema	
Cytotoxic	Anoxia of any cause; hypoglycemia

(Continued)

Vasogenic	Hypertensive encephalopathy; associated with altered capillaries of tumors, abscesses; toxins (e.g. lead poisoning); uremia
Infection	Meningitis, encephalitis
Trauma	
Hypercapnia in chronic obstructive lung disease	
Benign intracranial hypertension (pseudotumor cerebri)	Mainly in young women, in pregnancy, or with drugs (tetracycline, oral contraceptives)

A. Due To Obstructive Hydrocephalus

See above.

B. Due to a Space-occupying Mass Lesion in the Cranial Cavity

In general, the degree of elevation of intracranial pressure is proportionate to the size of the mass and the rate of expansion. For example, a slowly expanding subdural hematoma is associated with a lesser increase in intracranial pressure than a rapidly expanding extradural hematoma.

C. Due to Cerebral Edema

Cerebral edema is accumulation of water in the brain (see above).

Pathology

Raised pressure occurring within the fixed volume of the bony cranial cavity causes displacement of the brain (Figure 14-3).

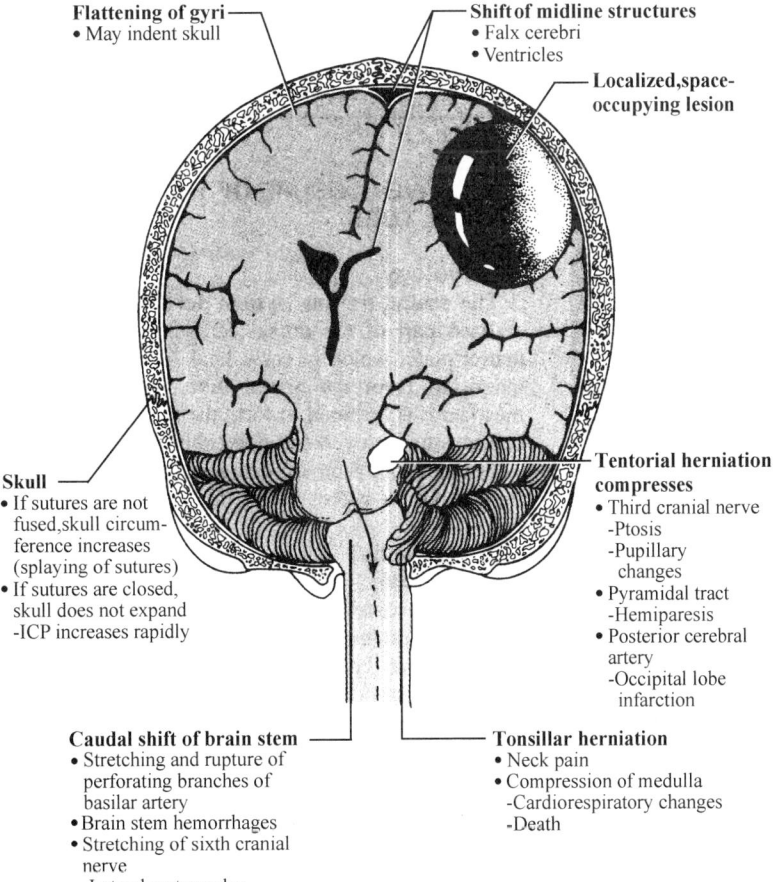

Figure 14-3 Possible consequences of increased intracranial pressure (ICP) resulting from a mass lesion in the right supratentorial compartment

A. Supratentorial Lesions

• **Caudal displacement of the entire brain stem** may stretch the sixth cranial nerve (causing paralysis of the lateral rectus muscle) and may rupture vessels passing from the basilar artery to the brain stem. The resulting brain stem hemorrhages interfere with vital centers and are a common cause of death.

• **Herniation of the uncinate gyrus of the temporal lobe** through the tentorial opening (tentorial herniation) stretches the third nerve, causing eye muscle paralysis, ptosis, and papillary changes. Compression of the pyramidal tract in the crus cerebri may also occur, causing motor paralysis in the contralateral side of the body.

B. Posterior Fossa Lesions

Posterior fossa lesions cause herniation of the cerebellar tonsils through the foramen magnum; late supratentorial lesions have a similar effect. Resulting compression of the medulla affects the cardiorespiratory centers. Leading to death. Tonsillar herniation is particularly likely to occur if lumbar puncture is performed in patients with markedly raised intracranial pressure.

Clinical Features

Increased intracranial pressure presents with headache, vomiting, and papilledema. The headache is typically described as bursting, is present on waking in the morning, and is increased by coughing and straining, maneuvers that further increase the intracranial pressure. Vomiting is typically effortless, unaccompanied by nausea, and often projectile. Papilledema is edema of the optic disk as shown by ophthalmoscopic (funduscopic) examination of the retina. Prolonged papilledema leads to atrophy of the optic disk (secondary optic atrophy) and blindness.

Raised intracranial pressure also produces false localizing signs, caused by displacement of the brain. As noted above, sixth and third nerve palsies, pyramidal tract compression, and brain stem dysfunction are the commonest of these. Hemorrhage into the brain stem may cause unconsciousness and death.

The diagnosis of increased intractanial pressure is made by clinical examination. If increased intracranial pressure is suspected, lumbar puncture should not be performed because of the danger of precipitating fonsillar herniation.

INFECTIONS OF THE NERVOUS SYSTEM

Infections of the nervous system are classified according to the infected tissue into (1) meningeal infections (meningitis), which may involve the dura primarily (pachymeningitis) or the pia-arachnoid (leptomeningitis); and (2) infection of the cerebral and spinal parenchyma (encephalitis or myelitis). In many cases, both the meninges and the brain parenchyma are affected to varying degrees (meningoencephalitis). Infectious agents may gain access to the nervous system by one of several routes. These include hematogenous spread, direct implantation in the setting of trauma or congenital CNS malformations (e.g. neural tube defects) local extension of infection in a contiguous structure (e.g. the middle ear and sinuses), and invasion via the peripheral nerves, as in the case of rabies.

MENINGEAL INFECTIONS

Leptomeningitis, or meningitis refers to inflammation of the leptomeninges and subarachnoid space. When the term meningitis is used without qualification, it means leptomeningitis. Most cases result from infection. Infectious meningitis can be divided into acute purulent meningitis, usually caused by bacteria; acute lymphocytic meningitis, usually caused by viruses; and chronic meningitis, caused by a number of different infectious agents.

Acute Leptomeningitis

Acute leptomeningitis is an acute inflammation of the pia mater and arachnoid, and is an important cause of morbidity and mortality at all ages. Most cases are caused by infectious agents; rarely, release of keratinaceous contents from an intradural epidermoid cyst or teratoma causes a chemical meningitis.

A. Classification

Acute meningitis may be classified according to the etiology.

1. Acute bacterial meningitis

The bacterium involved varies with the age of the patient and other factors (Table 14-4). About 70% of all cases occur in children under 5 years of age. Neonatal meningitis is acquired during passage of the fetus through the birth canal. Organisms found in the maternal vagina, commonly *Escherichia coli* and *Streptococcus agalactiae* (a group B streptococcus) are responsible.

In children up to 5 years of age, the most common pathogen causing meningitis is *Haemophilus influenzae*. In adolescents, Neisseria meningitidis (meningococcus) is the most common cause. *Streptococcus pneumoniae* (pneumococcus) causes meningitis in all age groups. *Listeria monocytogenes* and Gram-negative bacilli are important causes in older, debilitated, and immunosuppressed patients.

Table 14-4 Etiologic agents in bacterial meningitis.

Organism	Patients Profile
Streptococcus pneumoniae	Most common agent in patients over age 40 years 30%–50% of cases in adults 10%–20% of cases in children 5% of cases in infants
Neisseria meningitidis	Most common agent in patients aged 5–40 years 25%–49% of cases in children aged 5–15 years 10%–35% of cases in adults
Haemophilus influenzae	Most common agent in patients aged 1–5 years 40%–60% of cases in children aged 1–5 years 2% of cases in adults
Listeria monocytogenes	1% of all cases of bacterial meningitis. Common in infants, elderly, or immunosuppressed patients
Streptococcus agalactiae (group B)	40% of cases in neonates
Escherichia coli	40% of cases in neonates
Gram-negative bacilli (other than *E coli*)	Posttraumatic Postneurosurgical; 20% of cases in patients over age 50 years and in debilitated patients
Staphylococcus aureus	Postneurosurgical, posttraumatic
Staphylococcus epidermidis	75% of cases of meningitis complicating shunts

2. Acute viral meningitis

Most of viral meningitis (90%) occurs in patients under 30 years of age. This is a mild, benign illness, which rarely causes death. It is caused most commonly by enteriviruses, mumps virus, and lymphocytic choriomeningitis (LCM) virus. An acute meningitis occurs in 10% of patients with HIV infection, most commonly at the time of seroconversion.

3. Tuberculous meningitis

Tuberculous meningitis is typically chronic; however, in the early stages there may be an exudative phase that resembles acute meningitis.

4. Other causes

The fungi *Cryptococcus neoformans*, *Histoplasma*, *Blastomyces*, and *Candida albicans* may cause meningitis in immunocompromised patients. Free-living amebas belonging to the genera *Naegleria* and *Acanthamoeba* are rare causes of pyogenic meningitis.

B. Routes of Infection of the Meninges

Bloodstream spread accounts for the majority of cases; the primary entry site of the organism may be the respiratory tract (*N. meningitides*, *H. influenzae*, *S. pneumoniae*, *C. neoformans*, many viruses), skin (bacteria causing neonatal meningitis), or intestine (enteroviruses).

Meningitis may also result from direct spread of organisms from an infected middle ear or paranasal sinus, especially in childhood. Meningitis may be associated with skull fractures, especially those at the base of the skull causing free communication between the subarachnoid space and the upper respiratory tract; brain surgery; or lumbar puncture. Organisms may also gain entry through the intact nasal cribriform plate (e.g. free-living soil amebas in stagnant swimming pools).

Tuberculous meningitis may occur during severe tuberculous bacteremia (miliary tuberculosis) or as a result of reactivation of a meningeal focus, in which case the patient may have no evidence of tuberculosis elsewhere.

C. Pathology

Grossly, the leptomeninges are congested and opaque and contain an exudate. Microscopically, acute meningitis is characterized by hyperemia, fibrin formation, and inflammatory cells. In bacterial meningitis, neutrophils dominate (Figure 14-4A and 14-5); in acute viral meningitis, neutrophils are rare and lymphocytes dominate (Figure 14-4B). In acute tuberculous meningitis, there is an inflammatory exudate that contains increased numbers of both neutrophils and lymphocytes.

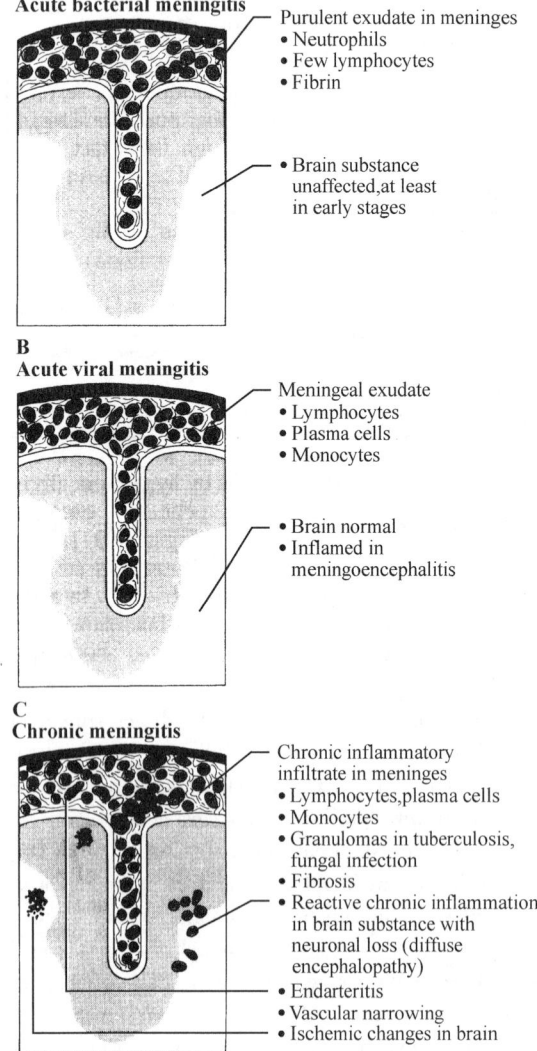

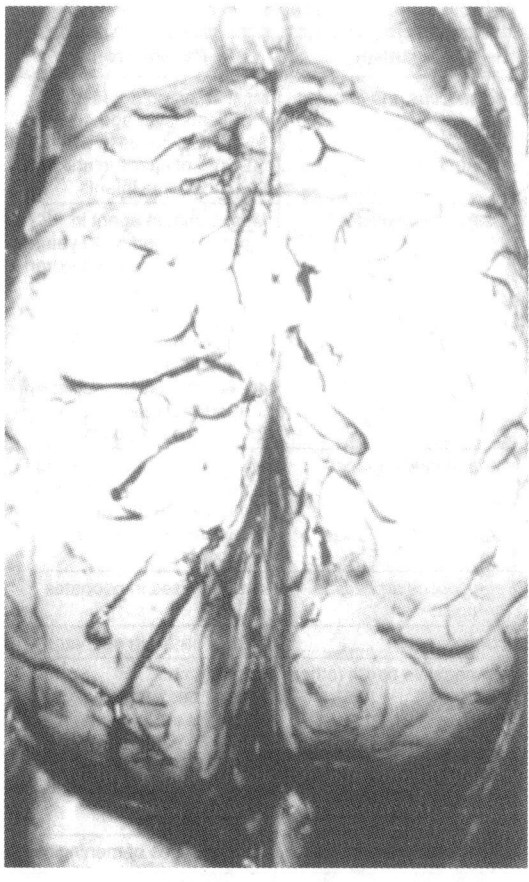

Figure 14-5 Pyogenic meningitis, showing obliteration of the gyri of the brain surface by the purulent exudate

D. Clinical Features

Acute meningitis presents with fever and symptoms of meningeal irritation, which include headache, neck pain, and vomiting. Physical examination reveals neck stiffness and a positive Kernig sign (inability to straighten the raised leg because of pain), both of which are due to reflex spasm of spinal muscles, a consequence of irritation of nerves passing across the inflamed meninges.

In general, bacterial meningitis is a serious disease with considerable risk of death while viral meningitis is usually a mild, self-limited infection. Tuberculous meningitis has an insidious onset and a slow rate of progression but is frequently a severe illness with a fatal outcome if not treated.

Chronic Meningitis

Chronic meningitis is caused by facultative intracellular organisms such as *Mycobacterium tuberculo-*

Figure 14-4 Contrasting histologic features in different types of meningitis

sis, fungi, and *Treponema pallidum*. It is now relatively uncommon in the western countries but more prevalent in parts of Africa, India, South America, and Southeast Asia.

Pathology and Clinical Features

Chronic tuberculous and fungal meningitis are characterized by caseous granulomatous inflammation with fibrosis (Figure 14-4C). Marked fibrous thickening of the meninges is the dominant pathologic feature. The entire brain surface is involved, with the basal meninges more severely affected in cases of tuberculoses. The causative agent may be identified in tissue sections specially stained for acid-fast bacilli and fungi.

The meningovascular phase of syphilis also causes a basal chronic inflammation with marked fibrosis and obliterative vasculitis, with large numbers of plasma cells infiltrating the meninges; granulomas are not present.

Complications of chronic meningitis include (1) obliterative vasculitis (endarteritis obliterans) which may produce focal ischemia with microinfarcts in the brain and brain stem; (2) entrapment of cranial nerves in the fibrosis as they traverse the meninges, resulting in cranial nerve palsies; and (3) fibrosis around the fourth ventricular foramina, causing obstructive hydrocephalus.

Clinically, chronic meningitis is characterized by an insidious onset with symptoms of diffuse neurologic involvement, including apathy, somnolence, personality change, and poor concentration. These symptoms are thought to stem from a concomitant diffuse encephalopathy (Figure 14-4C). Headache and vomiting are less severe than in acute meningitis, and fever is often low-grade. Focal neurologic signs and epileptic seizures result from ischemia, cranial nerve palsies, or hydrocephalus.

INFECTIONS OF THE BRAIN PARENCHYMA

Cerebral Abscess

Cerebral abscess is a localized area of suppurative inflammation in the brain substance. The cavity contains thick pus formed from necrotic, liquefied brain tissue and large numbers of neutrophils and is surrounded by a fibrogliotic wall.

A. Etiology

Cerebral abscesses are caused by a large variety of

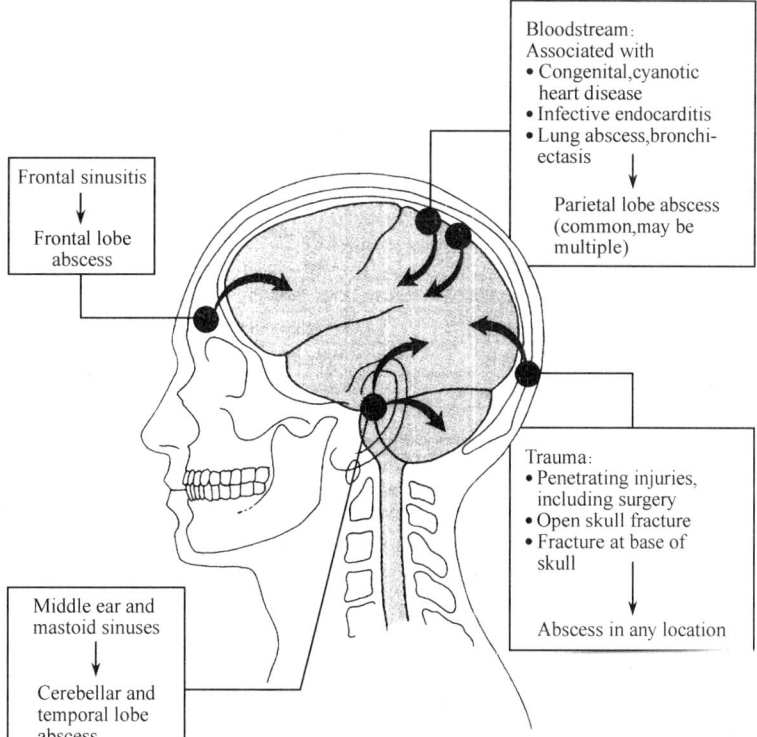

Figure 14-6 Cerebral abscess - common sites and routes of infection

bacteria; several organisms may occur in a single abscess, and anaerobic bacteria such as *Bacteroides* and anaerobic streptococci are common. *Nocardia*, *Staphylococcus aureus*, and Gram-negative enteric bacteria may also be isolated.

Cerebral abscesses occur as complications of other diseases (Figure 14-6).

- **Chronic suppurative infections of the middle ear and mastoid air spaces and of the paranasal sinuses.** The middle ear is separated from the middle and posterior cranial fossas by thin bony plates that may be eroded by infection. The temporal lobe and the cerebellum are usually involved. Infections of the paranasal sinuses are occasionally associated with frontal lobe abscesses.
- **Infective endocarditis** with embolization to brain. These patients commonly develop parietal lobe abscesses, which are often small and multiple.
- **Right-to-left shunts** (e.g. in patients with congenital cyanotic heart disease) may divert infected systemic emboli to the brain.
- **Suppurative lung diseases** such as chronic lung abscess and bronchiectasis are rarely complicated by embolization of infected material to the brain, leading to parietal lobe abscesses.

B. Pathology

Grossly, a cerebral abscess appears as a mass lesion in the brain. It has a liquefied center filled with pus and a fibrogliotic wall whose thickness depends on the duration of the abscess (Figure 14-7). The surrounding brain tissue frequently shows vasogenic edema.

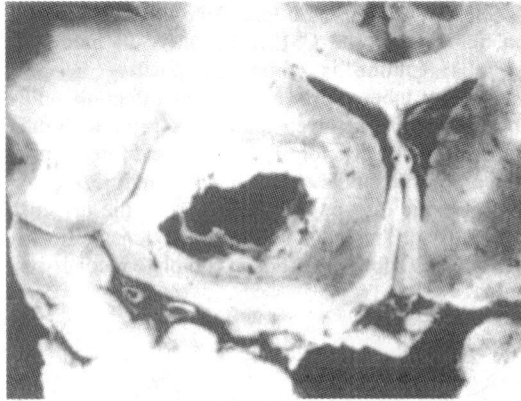

Figure 14-7 Cerebral abscess, showing a cavity in the region of the basal ganglia lined by inflammatory exudate. The cavity was filled with pus that drained when the brain was cut

C. Clinical Features and Diagnosis

Cerebral abscess presents with (1) features of a space-occupying lesion, including evidence of increased intracranial pressure (headache, vomiting, papilledema) and focal neurologic signs, depending on the location of the abscess; (2) features relating to the source of infection, such as chronic otitis media, supperative lung disease, and endocarditis; and (3) general evidence of infection, such as fever, rapid (elevated) erythrocyte sedimentation rate, and weight loss in chronic cases.

In untreated cases, the abscess progressively enlarges and may cause death from increased intracranial pressure or rupture into the ventricular system.

The diagnosis of cerebral abscess is made clinically and confirmed by CT scan or MRI. Lumbar puncture is dangerous because of the risk of precipitating tonsillar herniation. The CSF may be normal or may show mild increases in protein, neutrophils, and lymphocytes. CSF culture may or may not be positive.

Viral Encephalitis

Encephalitis means inflammation of brain tissue secondary to viral infection. The frequency of viral encephalitis is difficult to estimate. Most of viral encephalitis are presumptive diagnoses - the etiologic virus is identified in only about 30% of cases. Worldwide, many cases of acute cerebral dysfunction in which no attempt is made to identify a virus probably go unreported.

Epidemics of encephalitis are most commonly the result of arthropod-borne viruses (arboviruses), mainly togavituses and bunyaviruses (Table 14-5). Arboviruses have animal hosts, are transmitted to humans by arthropod bites, and have a distinctive geographic distribution. Sporadic cases of encephalitis may be caused by a large number of other viruses, most commonly herpes simplex virus.

Table 14-5 Causes of viral encephalitis

Diffuse encephalitis
Epidemic (arbovirus) encephalitis
Eastern equine encephalitis
Western equine encephalitis
Venezuelan equine encephalitis
St. Louis encephalitis

Chapter 14 Diseases of the Nervous System

(Continued)
California encephalitis
Japanese B encephalitis
Sporadic encephalitis
Herpes simplex encephalitis
Enterovirus encephalitis
Measles encephalitis
Varicella (chichenpox) encephalitis
Encephalitis in the immunocompromised patient
Herpes simplex encephalitis
Progessive multifocal leukoencephalopathy (PML)
Cytomegalovirus
HIV (AIDS) encephalitis
Specific types of encephalitis
Poliomyelitis
Rabies
Subacute sclerosing panencephalitis (SSPE)
Prion (slow virus) infections

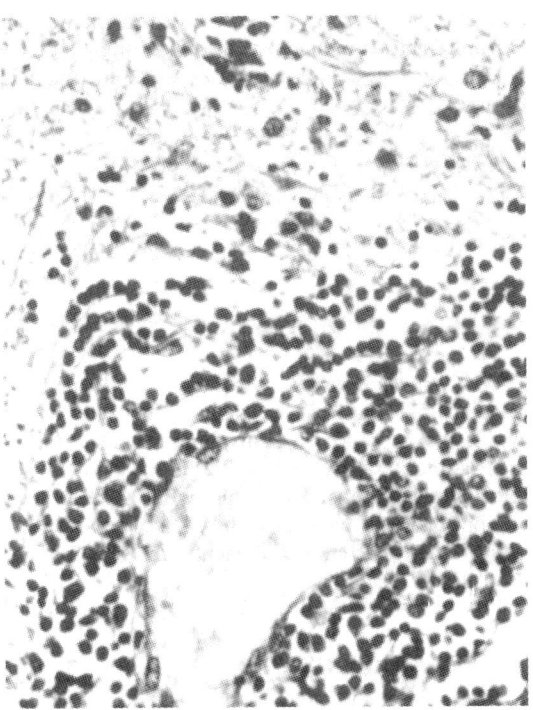

Figure 14-8 **Viral encephalitis, showing perivascular lymphocytic cuffing**

1. Pathology

The virus usually reaches the brain via the bloodstream. It infects brain cells, causing neuronal necrosis and marked cerebral edema, which in turn leads to acute cerebral dysfunction and increased intracranial pressure. **Perivascular lymphocytic infiltration (perivascular cuffing)** is characteristic (Figure 14-8) and consists of mononuclear cells, including lymphocytes and macrophages. **Microglial nodules** are usually present and sometimes associated with phagocytosis of neurons by microgia and macrophages (**neurophagia**). In some cases, **inclusion bodies** appear within the nuclei or cytoplasm of viral infected cells. In severe cases, hemorrhages occur.

2. Clinical features

Viral encephalitis has an acute onset with fever, headache, and signs of brain dysfunction, the nature of which depend on the areas of brain involved. Convulsions may occur. There may be papilledema if cerebral edema is severe. In many cases of viral encephalitis, there is concomitant meningeal inflammation causing neck stiffness and CSF abnormalities typical of viral meningitis. The diagnosis is based on the clinical picture. Lumbar puncture with examination and culture of CSF may provide an etiologic diagnosis.

A. Japanese B Encephalitis (Epidemic Encephalitis B)

1. Epidemiology and incidence

Japanese B encephalitis, as an epidemic forms, first appeared in Japan in 1924, affected thousands of people and killed many of them. It is widespread throughout temperate and tropical Asia. Japanese encephalitis keeps the leading cause of viral encephalitis in Asia with 30 - 50,000 cases reported annually. In China, the disease is prevalent in almost all provinces except few west-northern provinces such as Xinjiang, Qinghai, and Tibet. In 2004, 5420 new cases are reported in China, which indicates a great of decrease of incidence compared to over 10,000 cases reported annually in the end of last century. The mosquito plays an important role in the transmission of the disease, which explains the disease epidemic in summer and autumn, and in rural areas of China. Children are more frequently affected especial those who are under 10 years old.

2. Transmission

The JE virus belongs to the family Flaviviridae and is in the genus *Flavivirus*. It can be transmitted between small birds by Culex mosquitoes, and domestic pigs and wild birds are carriers and amplifying hosts of the virus. Human being also gets infected by Culex mosquitoes coincidentally, but there is not person-to person transmission pattern.

3. Pathology

The gross appearance of the brain is not characteristic. Congestion is marked, and small hemorrhages and necroses may be scattered within the parenchyma in severe cases. Microscopically, the chief lesion is the familiar perivascular cuffing, usually accompanying with neurophagia and Microglial nodules. In some severe cases, liquefaction necroses occur to form so-called "soften foci", which is well-circumscribed and pale stained incompleted necrotic area. It was presumed that both immunologic and circulated factors contributed to the lesion formation. Unfortunately, none of any above lesion is characteristic for diagnosis.

4. Clinical features

The clinical picture of the acute stage of this disease is similar to that of other kinds of encephalitis. Most infected people develop only mild symptoms or no symptoms at all. In more severe cases symptoms include fever, chills, nausea and vomiting, and lethargy. Although signs of general nervous system involvement are present at the beginning of the disease, the patient who recovers after treatment makes a complete recovery.

5. Sequelae

Case-fatality ratio range from 0.3% to 60%, and about 30% cases present serious neurologic sequela.

B. Herpes Simplex Encephalitis

1. Incidence and Etiology

Herpes simplex encephalitis occurs in 3 classes of patients:

Neonates are infected during delivery to a woman with active genital herpes. The presence of herpes genitalis in the mother is an absolute indication for cesarian section. Herpes simplex type 2 is responsible for most cases.

Adults are infected through the bloodstream from a minor focus of viral replication, usually in the mouth. Herpes simplex type 1 is commonly involved.

Immunocopromised persons, particularly patients undergoing chemotherapy for the treatment of cancer, have an increased susceptibility not only to become infected by herpes simplex virus but also to develop viremia and encephalitis.

2. Pathology

Herpes simplex encephalitis affects the temporal and inferior frontal lobes selectively, producing a necrotizing, hemorrhagic acute encephalitis that may rapidly cause death. Patients who survive frequently suffer permanent neuologic defects, the nature of which depends on the neuronal loss.

3. Diagnosis

The diagnosis may be made by brain biopsy, which shows cerebral edema, necrosis, lymphocytic infiltration, and presence of intranuclear Cowdry A inclusions in infected cells. Electron microscopy or, preferably, immunohistochemical or in situ hybridization tests demonstrate the virus in the majority of cases (Figure 14-9).

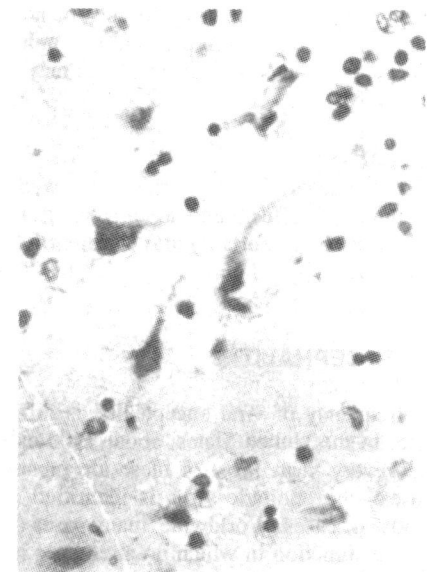

Figure 14-9 Herpes simplex encephalitis. This section has been stained for herpes simplex viral antigens by the immunoperoxidase technique. The darkly staining (positive) cells are infected with the virus

C. HIV Encephalitis

HIV is a neurotrophic virus that cause subacute encephalitis characterized pathologically by small nodules composed of demyelination, reactive astroglial proliferation, and infiltration by lymphocytes and microglial cells. These microglial nodules occur in about 30% of patients with AIDS. Their relationship to the occurrence of dementia in AIDS patients is uncertain.

D. Rabies

Rabies is rare in humans but occurs in a variety of wild animals and domestic pets, including doges and cats, in whom it causes a fatal illness called hydrophobia characterized by abnormal behavior, difficulty in swallowing, and convulsions. Humans are infected when bitten by an infected animal. The rabies virus enters the cutaneous nerve radicles at the site of inoculation and passes proximally to the central nervous system. The incubation period is 1 – 3 months and is shortest in facial bites.

Rabies virus causes a severe necrotizing encephalitis that maximally affects the basal ganglia, hippocampus, and brain stem. Infected neurons show diagnostic eosinophilic intracytoplasmic inclusion bodies (Negri bodies). The virus can also be identified in the infected cells by electron microscopy and immunoperoxidase techniques.

Clinically, rabies presents with fever and generalized convulsions that are precipitated by the slightest of sensory stimulation such as a gust of wind, a faint noise or the sight of water. Death is inevitable.

Because there is no treatment, prevention is essential and consists of controlling the disease in wild animals, rabies immunization of domestic pets, and administration of antirabies vaccine to humans immediately after viral exposure.

Spongiform Encephalopathies

The spongiform encephalopathies represent a group of uncommon, transmissible disorders that includes classic and new variant Creutzfeldt-Jakob disease, kuru, and fatal familial insomnia. Creutzfeldt-Jakob disease and kuru are infections of the human brain that are characterized by a long latent period after infection followed by a slowly progressive disease ending in death. Scrapie, an encephalopathy in sheep and goats, and bovine spongiform encephalopathy (BSE, or mad cow disease) in cattle are apparently animal counterparts. All of these diseases were once thought to be caused by slow-acting viruses because material remained infectious after passage through a filter sufficiently fine to exclude all bacteria. In the early 1980s evidence began to accumulate that these diseases might be caused by an agent consisting solely of protein, a prion (for *proteinaceous infectious* particle). The mode of transmission and whether or not activation of host genes is involved in pathogenesis remain unclear. About 10% of cases of Creutzfeldt-Jackob disease may be inherited as a dominant trait; a gene responsible for production of prion proteins has been located in chromosome 20.

Creutzfeldt-Jakob disease has occurred in patients who had received transplants of infected tissue (e.g. corneal and dural transplants). It is also important medically because the infectious agent is resistant to inactivation by formalin; this imposes a great risk of infection on pathologists and other medical personnel who handle infected tissues. Historically, Creutzfeldt-Jakob disease mainly affects persons 50 – 75 years old and occurs worldwide. The recent correlation of cases in younger persons in Great Britain with an outbreak of BSE in cattle that has been given feed containing protein derived from sheep carcasses has caused investigators to focus on possible transmission between species. Kuru has occurred mainly among cannibalistic tribes in Papua New Guinea, where the disease is believed to be transmitted by the ritualistic practice of eating brain tissue from deceased persons. The incidence of kuru is rapidly decreasing.

Clinically, patients present with confusion and dementia followed by ataxia. Symptoms progress slowly but relentlessly to a fatal outcome. There is no treatment.

Pathologically, both Creutzfeldt-Jakob disease and kuru are characterized by slowly progressive degeneration of the brain, with neuronal loss, demyelination, and spongiform change in the cerebral white matter. There is no inflammatory cell infiltration. Kuru tends to affect the cerebellum and is characterized microscopically by the presence of kuru plaques, which are amyloid bodies with radially arranged spicules. The plaques appear to consist of filaments of prion protein.

DEGENERATIVE DISEASE OF THE NERVOUS SYSTEM

CEREBROCORTICAL DEGENERATIONS

Alzheimer's Disease

Alzheimer's disease is extremely common – responsible for more than 50% of all cases of dementia (Table 14-6). It is characterized by progressive loss of neurons in the entire cerebral cortex. The frontal lobe is involved preferentially. Neuronal loss leads to dementia, which is the characteristic clinical presentation.

Table 14-6 Principal causes of dementia

Primary dementia with no other features
Alzheimer's disease (over 50% of cases)
Pick's disease
Secondary dementia with other neurologic features
Huntington's disease
Parkinson's disease
Chronic subdural hematoma
Hydrocephalus, low-pressure
Ischemic conditions
Multiple small infarcts (multi-infarct dementia)
Chronic arterial disease causing subcortical encephalopathy (Binswanger's disease)
Vasculitis (SLE, polyarteritis nodosa)
Chronic infections
AIDS dementia
Syphilis
Progressive multifocal leukoencephalopathy (JC virus)
Subacute sclerosing panencephalitis
Creutzfeld-Jakob disease
Chronic meningitis (tuberculous, fungal, sarcoidosis)
Endocrine and metabolic disorders
Hypothyroidism (myxedema madness)
Pellagra (niacin deficiency)
Thiamin (vitamin B_1) deficiency (beriberi)

(Continued)

Vitamin B_{12} deficiency
Cushing's syndrome (hypercortisolism)
Chronic hypoglycemia
Toxic disorders
Chronic alcoholism (alcoholic dementia)
Dialysis dementia (aluminum toxicity)
Drug and narcotic abuse
Heavy metal poisoning (lead)
Dementia following diffuse brain damage
Postencephalitic dementia
Pugilistic dementia

The term Alzheimer's disease was initially applied to patients who developed dementia under 65 years of age (presenile dementia), whereas dementia occurring after age 65 was called senile dementia. It has now become clear that the changes seen in most patients with senile dementia are identical to those of Alzheimer's disease. Alzheimer's disease occurs in 20% of person over 80 years old.

A. Etiology

The cause remains unknown. However, abnormalities of chromosomes 14, 19, or 21 have been identified in affected families, providing some clues to possible pathologic mechanisms. Patients with Down syndrome (trisomy 21) frequently develop lesions of Alzheimer's disease in the third or fourth decade of life. The gene encoding the β-amyloid protein of Alzheimer's disease has been localized to chromosome 21, leading to the suggestion that the presence of an additional or defective copy of the gene may be instrumental in causing the deposition of β-amyloid in plaques. In addition, the formation of neurofibrillary tangles has been attributed to the presence in Alzheimer's patients of apoprotein E4 (ApoE4), which is less effective in stabilizing microtubules than ApoE2, the form present in most individuals. The gene for ApoE is on chromosome 19. Levels of the enzyme choline acetyltransferase, an essential catalyst of acetylcholine synthesis, also are consistently reduced in the cerebral cortex of patients with Alzheimer's disease.

B. Pathology

Grossly, there is atrophy of the cerebral cortex, with thinning of the gyri and widening of the sulci affecting the frontal parietal sad medial temporal lobes. The cortical gray matter is greatly thinned and poorly demarcated. The lateral ventricles show compensatory dilatation.

Microscopically, there is neuronal loss and disorganization of the cerebrocortical layers. Alzheimer's disease is characterized by the presence of **neurofibrillary tangles** in the cytoplasm of affected neurons (best seen in silver stains). These are complexly interwoven masses of paired helical filaments 10 nm in diameter consisting of various proteins, including an abnormally phosphorylated form of the microtubule protein tau, and ubiquitin. Also characteristic of Alzheimer's disease - and best seen on silver stains - are **neuritic plaques**, which are large (150 μm) extracellular collections of degenerated cellular processes disposed around a central mass of β-amyloid protein material (Figure 14-10). The degenerated neuritic material contains paired helical filaments identical to those found in neurofibrillary tangles in affected neurons.

Amyloid protein similar to that seen in neuritic plaques is also present in the walls of small meningeal and cortical arteries (cerebral amyloid angiopathy) in patients with Alzheimer's disease.

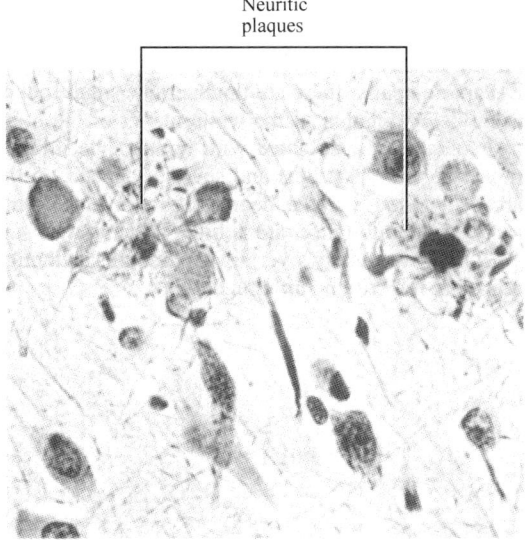

Figure 14-10 Neuritic plaques in cerebral cortex in Alzheimer's disease, showing cellular processes disposed around a central mass of β-amyloid

C. Clinical Features

Alzheimer's disease usually occurs in patients over 50 years of age. The clinical symptoms are subtle at first, manifested as a loss of higher cortical functions. The loss of ability to solve problems, decreased agility of thought processes, and mild emotional lability are common early features. The dementia progresses inexorably over the next 5 - 10 years to an extent that the patient becomes unable to carry out daily activities. There is no effective treatment.

BASAL GANGLIA DEGENERATIONS

A. Idiopathic Parkinson's Disease

Idiopathic Parkinson's disease is a common disease, affecting 5% of persons over 70 years of age. The exact cause is unknown. There is degeneration of the pigmented nuclei of the brain stem, particularly the substantia nigra, producing dysfunction of the extrapyramidal system. Patients with Parkinson's disease have depletion of dopamine in the affected areas. Because dopamine is an important neurotransmitter in the extrapyramidal system, it has been postulated that failure of normal dopamine synthesis is responsible for the disease.

1. Pathology

Grossly, patients with Parkinson's disease have depigmentation of the substantia nigra and locus ceruleus. Microscopically, loss of pigmented neurons is accompanied by gliosis in the substantia nigra and other basal ganglia. Lewy bodies - rounded eosinophilic cytoplasmic inclusions - may be present in the remaining neurons; they are characteristic of Parkinson's disease.

2. Clinical features

Onset is usually after the age of 50 years, and the disease is slowly progressive. It is characterized by extrapyramidal dysfunction, which causes increased rigidity of muscles, resting tremors, and slowness of movements (bradykinesia). Patients have a typical gait, walking stooped forward with short, quick shuffling steps (festinating gait). Up to 20% of patients with parkinsonism develop dementia. Slow, difficult speech is due to motor retardation.

Treatment with levodopa produces a good clinical response in most cases. However, the disease is progressive, and over time, control becomes difficult. Transplantation of autologous adrenal medulla or fetal tissue containing substantia nigra neurons into the basal ganglia by stereotactic surgery is under trial. The overall prognosis is poor.

B. Other Causes of Paekinson's Syndrome

Identical clinical features may be caused by several diseases that affect the extrapyramidal system.
- postencephalitic parkinsoninsm, which occurred in association with the influenza epidemic of 1914 – 1918, tended to occur in younger individuals and is uncommon today.
- Ischemic damage to the basal ganglia is associated with atherosclerosis.
- Wilson's disease is due to deposition of copper in the basal ganglia.
- Damage to the basal ganglia may result from exposure to toxic agents such as carbon monoxide and manganese.
- Several drugs in therapeutic doses, notably the phenothiazines and reserpine, produce reversible Parkinson's syndrome.
- Shy-Drager syndrome is intractable hypotension with various autonomic defects and Parkinson's syndrome.

NEOPLASMS OF THE NERVOUS SYSTEM

NEOPLASMS OF THE CENTRAL NERVOUS SYSTEM

Intracranial and spinal neoplasms may be primary or metastatic; in most autopsy series, metastatic tumors are more common. Primary intracranial neoplasms number about 13,000 new cases per year in the United States and represent about 2% of deaths from malignant neoplasms. They are the second most common group of neoplasms in children, after leukemia and lymphoma if considered as one group. Taken overall, 65% of primary intracranial neoplasms are of glial origin (gliomas), 10% meningiomas, 10% acoustic schwannomas, 5% medulloblastomas and 10% others. Primary malignant lymphomas of the central nervous system have recently increased in frequency because they are common in patients with AIDS. Tumors of neurons per se are extremely uncommon except in childhood (e.g. medulloblastoma). Primary neoplasms in the central nervous system are somewhat different from neoplasms arising in other sites, in the sense that even histologically benign lesions may result in death, owing to compression of vital structures. Furthermore, even histologically malignant primary tumors of the brain rarely disseminate to other parts of the body.

A. Classification

1. Histogenetic classification

Classification on a histogenetic basis has great theoretical value and provides a means of logically remembering all the different kinds of intracranial neoplasms (Table 14-1).

2. Topographic classification

When a patient presents with an intracranial neoplasm, its location can usually be ascertained by clinical examination and radiologic studies. According to their location, intracranial neoplasms may be classified as supratentorial or infratentorial. Further subdivisions in these main compartments are recognized, leading to a topographic classification. When the location of the neoplasm is combined with the patient's age, a clinically useful differential diagnosis of the histologic type of the neoplasm can be derived. For example, if a child presents with a neoplasm in a cerebellar hemisphere, it is most likely a juvenile pilocytic astrocytoma.

3. Classification according to biologic potential

The criteria used to determine malignancy in neoplasms are somewhat different from those used elsewhere in the body:
- Even highly malignant intracranial neoplasms generally do not metastasize outside the craniospinal axis. Metastasis within the craniospinal axis via the cerebrospinal fluid does occur, most commonly with medulloblastoma, pineoblastoma, malignant ependymoma, pineal germinoma, and glioblastoma.
- Destructive infiltration of the brain is the major criterion of malignancy for intracranial neoplasms, and infiltration of brain substance usually prevents complete removal at surgery. Actually all glial neoplasms invade brain, and all must be considered malignant. Neurologic deficits resulting from destructive invasion by malignant neoplasms are irreversible. Benign neoplasms, on the other hand, cause neurologic deficits due to compression; these often reverse when the neoplasm is removed.
- The rate of growth of neoplasms also correlates well with malignant behavior. Rapidly growing neoplasms such as glioblastoma and medulloblastoma are highly malignant. Low-grade malignant neoplasms such as

well-differentiated astrocytoma and oligodendroglioma grow slowly. Benign neoplasms usually grow very slowly, enlarging over several years.
- Recurrence after treatment is almost invariable with malignant intracranial neoplasms. Recurrence also occurs with many benign neoplasms such as meningioma and craniopharyngioma, and therefore recurrence of itself is not a criterion of malignancy.
- The term benign for any intracranial neoplasm is probably inappropriate. Benign intracranial neoplasms frequently produce extremely serious clinical disease and may cause severe neurologic deficits and death unless treated. The term thus does not mean that these neoplasms are harmless but implies rather that they are slow growing and do not infiltrate the brain substance.

B. Pathology and Clinical Features (Figure 14-11)

The specific clinicopathologic features of intracranial neoplasms will be considered with the individual neoplasms. In general, intracranial neoplasms cause the following clinical and pathologic changes:

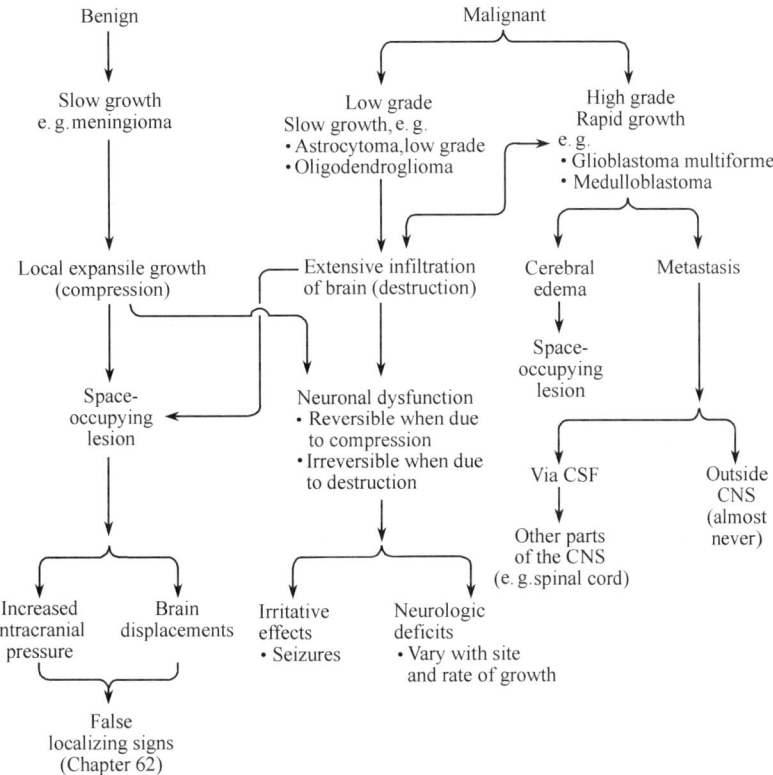

Figure 14-11 Clinical effects related to the biologic behavior of intracranial neoplasms

1. Compression

Compression of adjacent neural tissues occurs with all expanding neoplasms. When the rate of growth is slow, compression leads to atrophy, which may cause symptoms of dysfunction. e.g. atrophy of the motor cortex adjacent to a meningioma causes upper motor neuron paralysis; compression of a cranial nerve may cause cranial nerve palsy. In general, relief of compression is followed by significant recovery of function. With long-standing compression, there may be a permanent deficit.

2. Destruction

Destruction of neural tissues by direct infiltration with a malignant neoplasm produces an irreversible deficit.

3. Cerebral edema

Cerebral edema is commonly present around infiltrative neoplasms and may be severe. It is believed to result from the neovascularization that accompanies malignant neoplasms. The new vessels have a poorly developed blood brain barrier that permits exit of proteins and fluids more easily than from normal vessels. Cerebral edema tends to be most marked in highly malignant neoplasms. Cerebral edema causes elevation of intracranial pressure that is additive to the mass effect of the tumor.

4. Irritative effects

Irritation of neural tissues may occur with both compressing and infiltrating neoplasms. Abnormal stimulation is usually manifested as either simple or complex partial focal epilepsy. A neoplasm near the motor cortex may generate an abnormal electrical potential that causes motor stimulation of the entire contralateral half of the body (jacksonian epilepsy). Up to 5% of individuals with intracranial neoplasms experience one or more seizures. Note that although only a minority of cases of epilepsy are due to tumors, seizures should be fully investigated for cause due to tumor or other treatable disease, particularly when the onset is in adult life or when the seizure is focal rather than generalized.

5. Hydrocephalus

Neoplasms in the region of the third ventricle or in the posterior fossa may cause obstructive hydrocephalus. This causes marked elevation of intracranial pressure.

6. Increased intracranial pressure

Intracranial neoplasms cause increased intracranial pressure due to (1) the mass effect of the neoplasm itself, (2) cerebral edema, or (3) hydrocephalus. Many patients with intracranial neoplasms present with the effects of increased intracranial pressure - headache, vomiting, papilledema, and false localizing signs due to displacement of the brain and to herniations. Shift of structures can often be detected radiographically and provides a clue to the site of intracranial neoplasms.

C. Diagnosis

Clinical examination and radiologic imaging provide excellent localization of mass lesions of the nervous system. Specific diagnosis, however, is based on microscopic examination of a sample from the tumor. Stereotactic biopsy and open resection are the methods available for obtaining tissue samples. Examination of cerebrospinal fluid is rarely useful because (1) lumbar puncture is not usually performed in the presence of mass lesions, and (2) the yield of neoplastic cells in cerebrospinal fluid is low even with highly malignant neoplasms.

Astrocytomas

A. Cerebral Hemisphere Astrocytoma

Astrocytoma in the cerebral hemisphere is the most common primary neoplasm of the brain and occurs chiefly in adults.

1. Well-differentiated astrocytomas (Grade I)

Well-differentiated (grade I) astrocytomas are infiltrative, slowly growing neoplasms that form firm, white, ill-defined masses (Figure 14-12). Microscopically, they show slightly increased cellularity and astrocytes with cytologic features that deviate very slightly form normal Neurofibrillary processes are present and, often, abundant (fibrillary astrocytoma). Well-differentiated astrocytomas, although low-grade malignant neoplasms, are practically impossible to excise surgically because of irregular extension beyond the apparent margin. They progress slowly to cause death approximately 5 - 10 years after presentation.

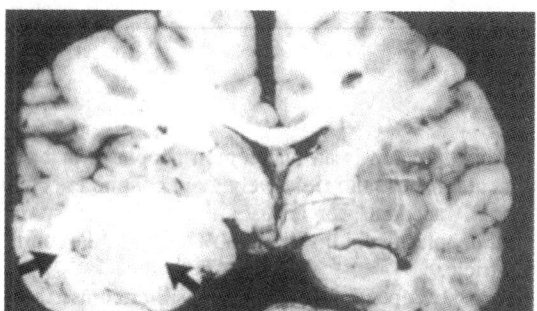

Figure 14-12 Well-differentiated (low-grade) astrocytoma of the left temporal lobe (arrow), characterized by poorly circumscribed homogeneous expansion of the white matter that has obliterated normal markings

2. Anaplastic astrocytomas (Grade II and Grade III)

Anaplastic astrocytoma is a more rapidly growing neoplasm that forms a white infiltrative mass in the cerebral hemisphere. Microscopically, it is composed of astrocytes that show greater cellularity, more pleomorphism, neovascularization with prolife-ration of endothelial cells, and an increased mitotic rate. Anaplastic astrocytomas show a higher rate of cell proliferation than well-differentiated astrocytoma. The proliferative rate may be measured by (1) the percentage of cells in the S phase of the cell cycle and (2) the ercentage of cells expressing proliferation-associated antigens such as Ki67. They commonly cause death after 1 - 5 years.

3. Glioblastoma (Grade IV Astrocytoma)

Glioblastoma is the most common type of astrocytoma. It is also one of the most malignant and rapidly growing neoplasms of the brain. Grossly, glioblastomas appear as large infiltrative masses that typically extend across the midline as the so-called "butterfly" tumor. The cut surface commonly shows hemorrhage and necrosis (Figure 14-13). Microscopically, they are composed of highly pleomorphic astrocytic cells with frequent mitotic figures. Necrosis is an important indicator of aggressive behavior (Figure 14-14). Prominent neovascularization is common. Glioblastoma is highly malignant, with a median survival of one year after diagnosis.

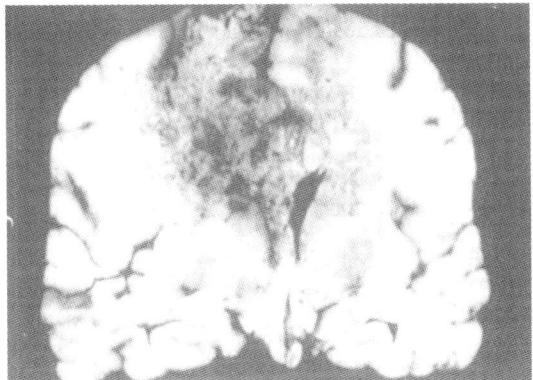

Figure 14-13 Glioblastoma of deep cerebral white matter, showing an extensively destructive and infiltrative mass extending across the midline to involve both hemispheres (butterfly lesion). Necrosis was present on microscopic examination

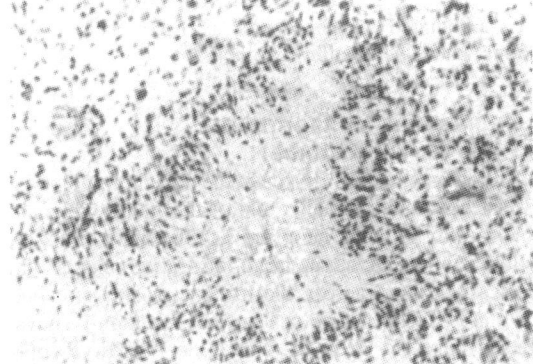

Figure 14-14 Glioblastoma, showing areas of necrosis surrounded by palisading neoplastic astrocytes

B. Juvenile Pilocytic Astrocytoma

Juvenile pilocytic astrocytoma is a neoplasm of children and adolescents found most commonly in the cerebellar hemispheres. It accounts for 25% of intracranial neoplasms in children under age 10 years. Grossly, it is well circumscribed and often cystic. Microscopically, it shows hypercellularity and is composed of cytologically uniform fibrillary astrocytes. Microcystic change and the presence of enlarged astrocytic fibers (Rosenthal fibers) are characteristic features.

Juvenile cerebellar pilocytic astrocytoma is a very slowly growing tumor that is extremely well circumscribed. It is almost benign in its biologic behavior. Surgical removal results in permanent cure in most cases.

Juvenile pilocytic astrocytoma may also occur in the region of the hypothalamus. Though slowly growing and circumscribed, it is rarely possible to completely remove a hypothalamic pilocytic astrocytoma, and it frequently causes death.

Oligodendroglioma

Oligodendroglima occurs in the cerebral hemisphere in adults 30 - 50 years of age. It is uncommon in pure form but more often is part of a mixed glial neoplasm with astrocytic and oligodendroglial components.

Grossly, oligodendrogliomas are well-circumscribed solid neoplasms. Seventy-five percent of oligodendrogliomas have speckled calcification that is visible on x-ray. Microscopically, the neoplasm is composed of numerous small uniform oligodendroglial cells. Mitotic activity is scarce.

Clinically, oligodendroglioma is a slowly growing neoplasm. The prognosis after surgical removal is good, although recurrence is common.

Ependymal Neoplasms

Ependymoma

Ependymoma is an uncommon neoplasm that occurs at all ages but is relatively more common in children. It accounts for 60% of intramedullary spinal cord neoplasms; in the brain, 60% occur in the fourth ventricle.

Grossly, ependymomas form well-circumscribed, reddish-brown nodular masses that occur in relation to the ventricular system. They grow slowly but have the ability to spread via the cerebrospinal fluid and should be considered as low-grade malignant neoplasms.

Microscopically, ependymomas are highly cellular, with small polygonal cells that form ependymal tubules and perivascular pseudorosettes. Well-differentiated ependymomos tend to grow slowly and may be cured by complete surgical removal. Less differentiated ependymomas infiltrate, grow rapidly, and have a poor prognosis.

A specific type of ependymoma called myxopapillary ependymoma occurs in the filum terminale and presents as a cauda equina tumor in young adults.

Medulloblastoma

Medulloblastoma is derived from primitive neuroectodermal cells. It occurs mainly in children, accounting for 25% of all intracranial neoplasms in children under age 10 years. Its most common location is the midline cerebellar vermis in the posterior fossa.

Grossly, medulloblastoma appears as a grayish-white fleshy mass with infiltrative margins. Microscopically, the tumor is highly cellular and composed of sheets of small primitive cells with hyperchromatic nuclei and scant cytoplasm. Mitotic figures are frequently present.

Medulloblastoma is highly malignant and frequently seeds the cerebrospinal fluid to produce metastases around the spinal cord. The prognosis is poor, but recent aggressive chemotherapeutic regimens have improved the outlook somewhat.

Pineal Neoplasms

The pineal gland is situated in the midline, dorsal to the midbrain and the posterior part of the third ventricle. It is composed of pinealocytes, which are modified neuroectodermal cells.

A. Pinealocyte Neoplasms

Pineocytoma is a benign or low-grade malignant neoplasm composed of well-differentiated pinealocytes. It occurs mainly in adults.

Pineoblastoma resembles medulloblastoma. It occurs in childhood and is highly malignant.

B. Germ Cell Neoplasms

Neoplasms arising from primitive germ cells in the nervous system occur most commonly in the pineal region. Germinoma, which resembles the testicular seminoma microscopically, is most common and typically forms a well-circumscribed mass that compressed the midbrain, causing abnormalities in ocular movement and hydrocephalus. Germinomas are malignant and tend to spread along CSF pathways. Germinomas are extremely radiosensitive neoplasms, and cures have been recorded following radiation therapy.

Other germ cell neoplasms occurring in the region of the pineal gland include teratoma, embryonal carcinoma, yolk sac carcinoma, and choriocarcinoma. All are very uncommon.

Meningioma

Meningioma can occur at any age but is rare in childhood. Meningiomas occur most frequently in middle-aged women - the predominance in women is probably related to the presence of progesterone receptors on the tumor cells. As the second commonest intracranial tumours, most maningiomas are benign and with the best prognosis among tumous of central nervus system.

A. Pathology

Meningiomas usually arise outside of the brain substance and have an attachment to the dura. They present grossly as a firm encapsulated mass that compresses adjacent neural structures (Figure 14-15). In filtration of the dura is usual and does not indicate malignancy. Meningiomas are frequently associated with hypertrophy of the overlying bone (hyperostosis); this may be so pronounced as to cause a palpable mass in the skull. Meningiomas may also infiltrate bone and extend into the scalp, a locally aggressive behavior pattern that still dose not necessarily indicate malignancy. The term malignant meningioma is used only when the neoplasm infiltrates the underlying brain.

Microscopically, meningioma is composed of sheets or whorls of meningothelial cells, which are plump spindle cells with oval nuclei and scant cytoplasm (syncytial or meningothelial meningioma). In some cases, the meningothelial cells are more elongated, resembling fibroblasts (fibroblastic meningioma). Psammoma bodies (round, laminated calcifications) occur in many meningiomas. Mitoses are rare. When there is necrosis, cellular pleomorphism, or a high mitotic rate, the term atypical meningioma may be used.

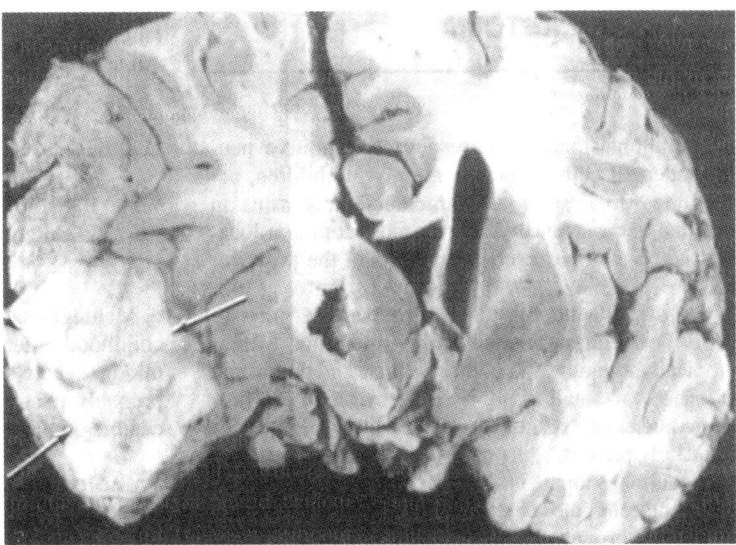

Figure 14-15 Meningioma of the convexity, causing marked compression of the underlying brain and shift of midline structures. Note the excellent demarcation between the cerebral cortex and the noninfiltrative neoplasm

B. Biologic Behavior

Meningioma is a benign neoplasm. However, because of infiltration of dura and bone, complete surgical removal may be difficult in some cases, and there is a 10% recurrence rate. The recurrence rate increases in (1) atypical meningiomas (20%-30% recurrence rate) and (2) malignant meningiomas (90% without radiotherapy).

C. Clinical Features

Meningiomas occur throughout the craniospinal axis, producing specific clinical features that depend on their location (Figure 14-16). Sites of predilection are (1) the parasagittal region and falx cerebri, giving rise to motor deficits; (2) the surface of the cerebral hemispheres, causing focal epilepsy and cortical dysfunction depending on exact location; (3) the olfactory bulb, compressing the optic nerve and causing blindness; (4) the sphenoidal ridge, compressing the cranial nerves passing into the orbit; (5) the posterior fossa, with features of a cerebellopontine angle tumor; and (6) the spinal cord, causing spinal compression.

Metastatic Neoplasms

Neoplasms metastatic to the brain are common and may be derived from melanomas or from primary tumors in almost any organ, most commonly the lung, breast, kidney, stomach, and colon. The brain metastasis may be the first manifestation of a previously occult malignant neoplasm, in which case differentiation from a primary intracranial neoplasm is difficult without biopsy. More frequently, metastasis to the brain occurs during the terminal phase in a patient with disseminated cancer. Meningeal involvement by metastatic neoplasms occurs frequently in patients with acute leukemia. This presents a problem because the blood-brain barrier prevents chemotherapeutic agents from reaching the meningeal leukemic cells. The diagnosis of meningeal involvement can be made by identifying leukemic cells in cerebrospinal fluid. These patients can then be treated either with intrathecal chemotherapy or craniospinal irradiation.

NEOPLASMS OF THE PERIPHERAL NERVOUS SYSTEM

Neoplasms of peripheral nerves are common. They may occur in any nerve and may be classified anatomically as (1) neoplasms within the skull or spinal canal; (2) neoplasms that involve both the spinal canal and the paraspinal soft tissue (termed dumbbell tumors because of their shape - 2 large masses connected by a narrow mass within the intervertebral foramen); (3) neoplasms arising in large nerve trunks in extraspinal or extracranial soft tissues.

In all of these anatomic sites, neural tumors fall

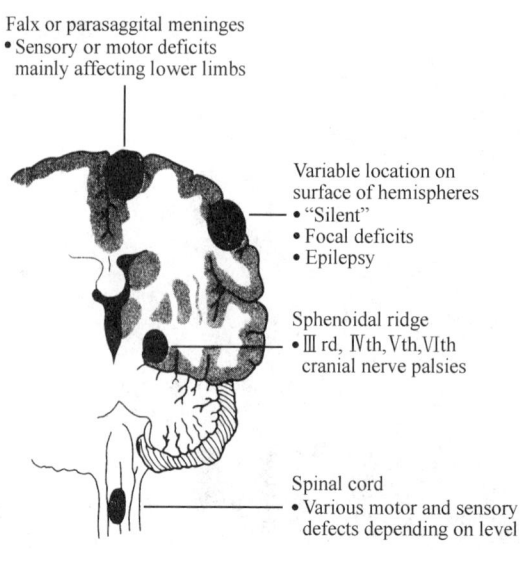
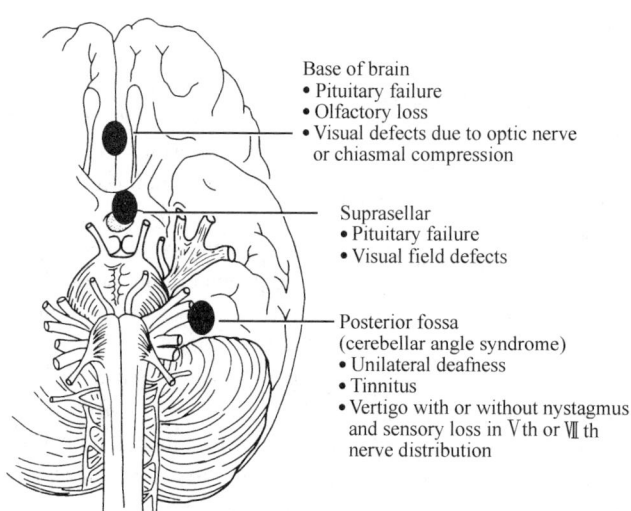

Figure 14-16 Intracranial meningiomas - common sites and symptomatology

into 3 groups: (1) schwannoma, (2) neurofibroma, and (3) malignant peripheral nerve sheath tumor - a type of sarcoma also called malignant schwannoma or neurofibrosarcoma (Figure 14-17). Most neural neoplasms occur as sporadic lesions. In a small number of cases, multiple neural neoplasms occur as part of the familial generalized neurofibromatosis syndrome of von Recklinghausen.

Schwannoma (Neurilemmoma)

Schwannoma is a slowly growing benign neoplasm that commonly occurs in relation to large nerve trunks. Sensory cranial nerves (eighth and fifth nerve schwannoma) and the sensory root of spinal nerves are common locations. In the extra-axial soft tissues, they most commonly occur in the posterior mediastinum, the retroperitoneum, the head and neck, and the extremities. Schwannomas are usually solitary; multiple schwannomas may be associated with von Recklinghausen's neurofibromatosis.

Clinically, schwannomas present as a mass lesion, usually causing compression of surrounding structures. Compression of the nerve of origin causes irritative and paralytic symptoms - e.g. acoustic schwannoma results in tinnitus followed by nerve

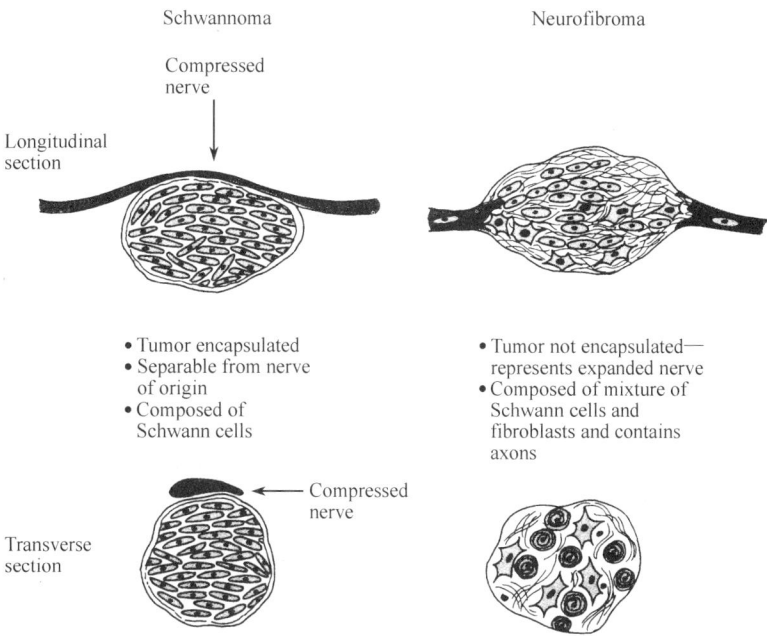

Figure 14-17 Differences between schwannoma (left) and neurofibroma (right). A schwannoma is a true encapsulated neoplasm, composed of Schwann cells, that compresses the nerve of origin. A neurofibroma is a hamartomatous proliferation of several cell types that expand the involved nerve

deafness. Pain in the distribution of affected sensory nerves is a common finding.

On gross examination, schwannomas appear as encapsulated masses that compress the nerve of origin, which is frequently splayed out on one side of the mass. There is usually a plane of cleavage separating the nerve from the mass that may permit the tumor to be removed surgically without sacrificing the nerve. Areas of hemorrhage and cystic change are seen commonly in schwannomas; rarely, the neoplasm is composed predominantly of a cyst.

Histologic examination shows the tumor to be composed of Schwann cells arranged in one or both of two distinct patterns (Figure 14-18). The Antoni A pattern is characterized by highly cellular, compact, spindle-shaped cells arranged in short bundles or fascicles. Palisade arrangement of nuclei (nuclei of a fascicle of cells arranged one below the other) and Verocay bodies (structures formed by two rows of palisaded nuclei separated by an oval mass of pink cytoplasm) are characteristic histologic features. The Antoni B pattern is a loose, haphazard arrangement of Schwann cells in a richly myxomatous stroma. Large vascular spaces with hyalinized walls are a common feature. Nuclear pleomorphism and atypia, sometimes marked may be present. Mitotic figures may also be present. Neither cytologic atypia nor mitotic activity indicates malignancy. Immunohistochemical studies show the presence of S100 protein in the Schwann cells.

The malignant potential of schwannomas is very low.

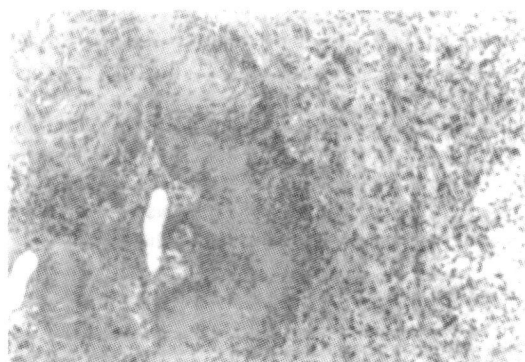

Figure 14-18 Schwannoma, showing compactly arranged Antoni A type of tissue with nuclear palisading (left half of photograph) and the loosely arranged Antoni B type of tissue (right half)

Neurofibroma

Neurofibroma is a slowly growing benign neoplasm that occurs (1) in relation to large nerve trunks and (2) in peripheral tissues such as skin, where it arises from very small nerves. Neurofibroma most commonly occurs as a solitary neoplasm. In patients with von Recklinghausen's disease, there are multiple neurofibromas in the skin and viscera.

Clinically, neurofibroma presents as a soft tissue mass. It is commonly associated with pain.

On gross examination, neurofibromas of large nerves appear as an expansion of the affected nerve. The mass is firm and rubbery, not demarcated from the nerve, and cannot be removed surgically without sacrificing the nerve. Cystic degeneration is common.

Histologic examination shows a varied spindle cell population composed of Schwann cells and fibroblasts. Cellularity is variable, and myxomatous change is commonly present in the stroma. Nuclear atypia and pleomorphism may be observed without indicating that the neoplasm is malignant. The presence of mitotic activity in a neurofibroma indicates a strong likelihood of malignant biologic potential. Immunohistochemical studies show the presence of S100 protein; this is a reliable method of confirming the histologic diagnosis of both schwannoma and neurofibroma. Neurofibroma carries a low but significant risk of malignant transformation. Risk of malignancy is greatest in patients with von Recklinghausen's disease.

Malignant Peripheral-nerve-sheath Tumor

The term malignant peripheral-nerve-sheath tumor is applied to all malignant neural neoplasms and is synonymous with malignant schwannoma and neurofibrosarcoma. Most such tumors occur de novo; a few complicate preexisting neurofibromas, particularly in patients with von Rcklinghausen's disease.

Malignant peripheral-nerve-sheath tumors appear clinically as soft tissue neoplasms. Any location may be affected; most common are the extremities and retroperitoneum. The rate of growth varies, being slow in low-grade neoplasms and rapid in high-grade ones. The tumors are diffusely infiltrative, frequently invading surrounding structures. Many patients have evidence of metastatic disease at the time of presentation. The most common site of metastasis is the lung.

Grossly, malignant peripheral-nerve-sheath tumors are fleshy masses, frequently large and showing extensive infiltration. Areas of necrosis and hemorrhage are common. Microscopically, they are highly cellular spindle cell sarcomas with marked cytologic atypia and pleomorphism and a high mitotic rate. The diagnosis of malignant peripheral-nerve-sheath tumor may be made when (1) a sarcoma has its origin from a large peripheral nerve, (2) a sarcoma of appropriate histologic type occurs in a patient with von Recklinghausen's disease, (3) S100 protein is demonstrated in the tumor cells, or (4) electron microscopy demonstrate features typical of Schwann cells. Less than 50% of malignant peripheral-nerve-sheath tumors stain positively for S100 protein.

Chapter 15　Infectious Deseases

Shen Hong

CHAPTER CONTENTS
- Tuberculosis
    - Pulmonary Tuberculosis
    - Extrapulmonary Tuberculosis
- Typhoid fever
- Bacillary dysentery
- Leprosy
- Leptospirosis
- Epidemic hemorrhagic fever
- Sexually transmitted disease
    - Gonorrhea
    - Condyloma Acuminata
    - Syphilis

Infectious diseases are a group of diseases caused by infectious agents that can be transmitted from one host (person or animal) to another directly or indirectly. Infectious diseases are also known as communicable disease. Transmission means that an infectious agent is moved through the environment from an infected host or reservoir to a susceptible host. The chain of transmission must include infectious agent, host, and environment.

Infectious agent denotes a microorganism, capable of infecting a host, whose presence is necessary for disease to occur. The host is an individual or population of persons or animals that provides a habitat and subsistence for an infectious agent. Environment is the universe external to the human host. Environmental factors include: geography/geology, climate, season, biologic environment, socioeconomic environment, and sociocultural influences. Agent, host, and environment are the epidemiologic triad, which are necessary for the production of communicable disease (Figure 15-1).

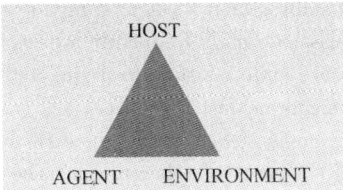

Figure 15-1　The epidemiologic triad of communicable disease

Although there has been continuing progress in controlling some vaccine-preventable childhood diseases such as polio, neonatal tetanus, and measles, infectious disease remains the most common cause of death globally. Based on the report of National Intelligence Council of U. S., "The Global Infectious Disease Threat and Its Implications for the United States", of the estimated 54 million deaths worldwide in 1998, about one-fourth to one-third were due to infectious diseases, most of them in developing countries and among children. Infectious diseases accounted for 41 percent of the global disease burden, as compared to 43 percent for noninfectious diseases and 16 percent for injuries. Even in the U. S., during the period 1980 – 1992, infectious diseases became the third leading cause of death (after CV disease and malignancy). At least 29 previously unknown diseases (exclusive of SARS) have appeared globally since 1973, many of them incurable, including HIV/AIDS, Ebola hemorrhagic fever, and hepatitis C. Most recently, SARS (Severe Acute Respiratory Syndrome) was identified. Twenty well-known diseases such as malaria, TB, cholera, and dengue have rebounded after a period of decline or spread to new regions, often in deadlier forms.

If this trends continues, developing countries will continue to experience the greatest impact from infectious diseases, because of malnutrition, poor sanitation, poor water quality, and inadequate health care. The developed countries also will be affected. HIV/AIDS and TB are likely to account for the overwhelming majority of deaths from infectious diseases in developing countries by 2020. Acute lower respiratory infections, including pneumonia and influenza, as well as diarrheal diseases and measles, appear to have peaked at high incidence levels. Asia and the Pacific, where multidrug resistant TB, malaria, and cholera are rampant, are likely to witness a dramatic increase in infectious disease deaths, largely driven by the spread of HIV/AIDS in South and Southeast Asia and its likely spread to East Asia. By 2010, the region could surpass Africa in the number of HIV infections.

In this chapter, TB, typhoid fever, bacillary dysentery, leprosy, leptospirosis, epidemic hemorrhagic fever, and sexually transmitted diseases (STD) are discussed. Hepatitis is discussed in chapter 8, epidemic cerebrospinal meningitis and epidemic encephalitis B in chapter 14, HIV/AIDS in chapter 10, and parasitosis in chapter 16.

TUBERCULOSIS

Tuberculosis (TB) is an infectious disease caused by several different species of mycobacteria. Once, it was one of the most common and lethal infectious diseases throughout the world. The incidence was 200 deaths per 100,000 per year in the USA at the beginning of the twentieth century. The rate decreased sharply to 4.1 per 100,000 per year in 1965, decrease sharply. More recently emergence of multi-drug-resistant organisms in developed countries and the appearance of the acquired immunodeficiency syndrome (AIDS) have lead to a resurgence of the disease. WHO declared TB a global emergency in 1993 and the threat continues to grow. Several million new cases occur annually. The disease is prevalent especially in Russia, India, Southeast Asia, Sub-Saharan Africa, and parts of Latin America. There were up to 7.4 million new cases in 1998 and more than 1.5million people died, excluding those infected with HIV/AIDS. TB caused 1 million deaths in the Asia and Pacific region in 1998, more than any other single disease, with India and China accounting for two-thirds of the total. Some high-risk populations such as and those with HIV/AIDS have experienced death rates from TB as high as 70 to 90percent. One-quarter of the increase in TB incidence involves co-infection with HIV. TB probably will rank second only to HIV/AIDS as a cause of infectious disease deaths by 2020.

Clinically, symptoms may vary from insidious weight loss with night sweats and a mild chronic cough, to rampant bronchopneumonia with fever, dyspnea and respiratory distress (galloping consumption). Most early cases of primary tuberculosis are clinically silent.

Etiology, Transmission and Pathogenesis

A. Etiology

Tuberculosis is caused by *mycobacterium tuberculosis*, which is a slender slightly curved rod-shaped aerobic bacterium. Its length varies from 1 to 4 μm. Staining characteristics include resistance to decolourization by acid and alcohol (acid-fast) associated with long-chain fatty acids in the capsule. The organism stains red with a Ziehl-Neelsen stain and can be stained with auramine resulting yellow fluorescence under UV light. The organism grows slowly and the colonies may only be visible after 4 weeks on the egg-based Lowenstein-Jensen medium or the agar-based Middlebrook 7H10 and 7H11. Direct examination of smeared material, e. g. sputum, gives a sensitivity of detection of 55% (22%-80%). It is stressed, however, that there is no way of identifying microscopically which species of mycobacterium has caused the disease. Newer DNA based detection methods have reduced the time and increased the sensitivity of tests compared to conventional staining.

Originally only mycobacterium tuberculosis *var. horninis* and *var. boris* were identified as pathogenic for human being. In recent years, the unclassified mycobacteria, anonymous, have become important.

B. Transmission

The main routes of tuberculous infection are (1) pulmonary, (2) intestinal, (3) tonsillar, (4) cutaneous, and (5) placental (congenital). The disease usually is spread by droplets from a patient with a cavitary lesion that opens into a bronchus. Coughing, sneezing, and spitting emit a potent spray to which members of the same family frequently are exposed. The organisms are quite resistant to drying and persist as infective agents in dust.

In some areas of the world, infected milk causes up to 10% of cases of tuberculosis. The organisms swallowed from outside the body (usually the bovine variety) may infect the tonsils and cervical lymph nodes. The tonsillbar disease may pass unnoticed, whereas the cervical node enlargement is prominent. Similarly, the first intestinal lesion is mucosal ulceration, which tends to heal readily, leaving the impression that disease commenced in the mesenteric lymph nodes. The investigation established that primary tuberculosis in the lung is not caused by alimentary tract infection.

Inoculation of tubercle bacilli into the skin is among the lesser dangers faced by pathologists and rarely leads to infection of the internal organs. Butchers may be infected when handling contaminated meats.

Rare congenital tuberculosis is caused by transplacental infection when pregnant women suffering from TB given birth.

Pathogenesis

Five strains of mycobacterium tuberculosis are recognized (human, bovine, murine, avian and reptilian) and infection can occur by inhalation, ingestion (rare following testing of cattle and pasteurization) and inoculation. A single organism is potentially infective, but there must be one million bacilli or clumps of bacilli per milliliter of bacterial suspension before microscopic examination can reveal more than one organism per ten oil immersion fields. The tissue damage associated with tuberculosis is due to the specific reactivity of the immune system occurring as a result of the presence of the bacterium. This expresses itself in two ways:
- Enhanced resistance to infection and more effective clearing of the bacterium.
- Appearance of hypersensitivity causing most of the damage.

As for the virulence of mycobacterium tuberculosis: No exotoxin is secreted. Different strains exhibit differences in their power to cause disease. Increased virulence is associated with components that protect the organism from intracellular killing. These components are:

'Cord' factor: a surface glycolipid, when present causes the organism to grow in cords. This is associated with the ability to induce granuloma formation and inhibits neutrophil chemotaxis.

Sulfatides-surface glycoproteins: it can inhibit fusion between lysosomes and phagosomes.

Lipoarabinomannan (LAM): a lipopolysaccharide resembling endotoxin, which can inhibit up regulation of macrophage killing by interferon, increases output of TNF, which associated with fever, weight loss and tissue destruction, and increases in IL-10 secretion which inhibits induced T cell proliferation.

Tuberculous granuloma is the main feature of the tuberculosis pathological changes. How does it evolve and form? It progresses as the following: First, local tissues show initial mild and transient acute inflammatory reaction. After this, mycobacteria are engulfed by local macrophages with the antigen being presented to T-helper cells which are transported to regional lymph nodes and stimulate them to enlarge and develop into caseous necrosis. This interaction leads to a proliferation of specifically coded T cells and the release of cytokines. Next, there is infiltration by macrophages, which accumulate at the site of infect-ion and undergo epithelioid change, and some fuse to form multi-nucleate giant cells, the Langhans giant cell. So, the nodule containing tuberculous granulomas is formed. Within 10 - 14 days evidence of coagulative necrosis begins to appear, characterized by 'cheesy' material (caseation).

The chief factor in the modulation of the degree of tissue destruction in tuberculosis is hypersensitivity to some antigenic components of the bacillus. This causes caseation necrosis. Liquefactive necrosis may occur with active local proliferation of baceria. This liquefied tissue contains a lot of bacteria and may rupture or get into bronchi, lymphatics and blood vessels.

How about the tissue response to mycobacterium tuberculosis? Different tissues and different individuals may react differently to the presence of mycobacterium tuberculosis. These differences are probably related to virulence of the organism, dose of bacterium, degree of local and general resistance, type and degree of hypersensitivity, age and innate immunity. The more virulent the strain and the more vulnerable the organ, the greater the extent of the immediate reaction is. A higher dose of this bacterium, leads to a greater probability of invasion. Also, the wicker the degree of local and general resistance, the heavier the degree of hypersensitivity, and the more susceptible to invasion. Some races appear inherently more susceptible to tuberculosis because of a lack of innate immunity, e.g. North American Indians and black races appear more susceptible to tuberculosis. The very young age (under 5 years) and elderly appear more at risk of developing tuberculosis. Immunosuppression resulting from AIDS, or treatments associated with prolonged high-dose corticosteroids increases the risk of tuberculosis. Figure 15-2 shows the main courses of pathogenesis and pathological progression of pulmonary tuberculosis.

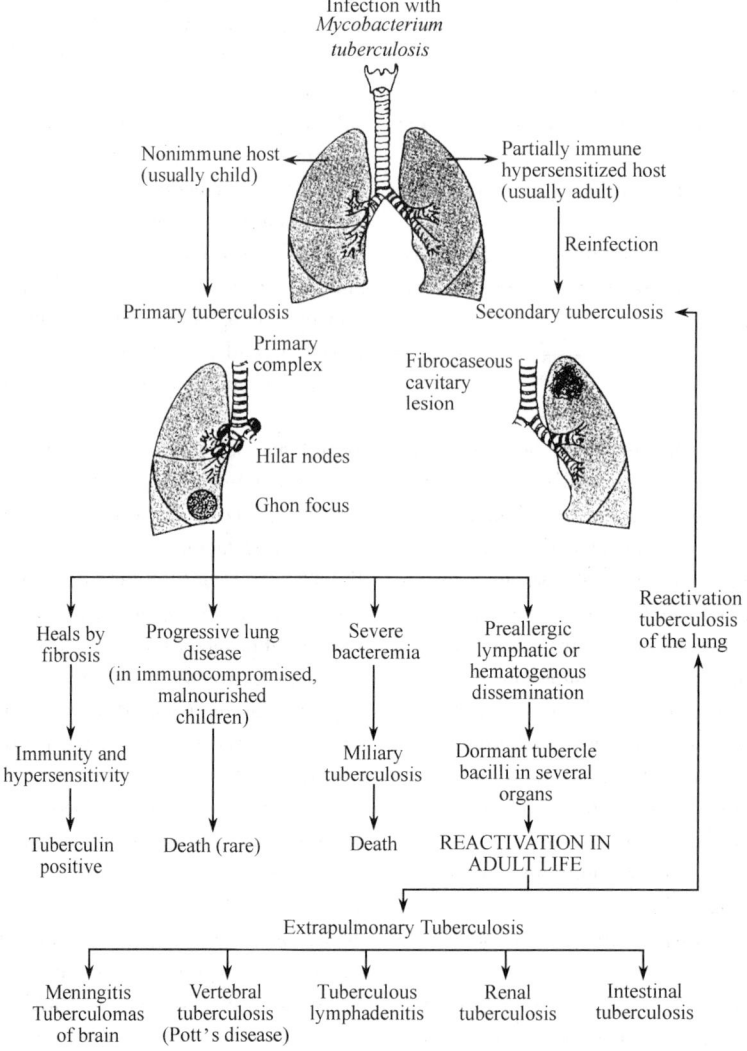

Figure 15-2 Pathogenesis and pathological progression on pulmonary tuberculosis

Basic Pathological Changes and Sequences

Susceptive tissue: Tissue susceptibility is as noticeable in this disease. In children, the lymph nodes are particularly heavily attacked, and the meninges, lungs, and spleen often are involved. Among adults, the lungs bear most of the disease. The second place is roughly the adrenal glands, kidneys, epididymides, meninges and serous membranes. The liver, spleen, bone, red bone marrow, and lymphoid tissue come next. The mucosae of the upper respiratory tract and intestine of adults are rather resistant unless the dose is massive. Rarely infected are cardiac and skeletal muscle, stomach, thyroid gland, pancreas, testis, and breast.

1. Basic pathological changes

The features of the pathological changes of tuberculosis is the formation of tuberculous granuloma or tubercle, which is showed typically by: (1) Caseous necrosis; (2) Epitheliod cells; (3) Langhans' giant cells; (4) lymphocytes; (5) Fibrosis. There are three forms of pathological changes, i.e. exudation, proliferation and alteration. The feature in most is the formation of tubercle and caseous necrosis.

• Exudative changes. The exudative reaction is an expression of poorer host resistance as compared met with in the proliferative reaction and is most often seen in the lungs in rapidly progressive tuberculosis. Reactions of tissues to infection show as: edema, hyperemia, and neutrophilic infiltration. There is exudation of fibrinous fluid into the alveoli, with outpouring of neutrophils and mononuclear phagocytes. It may progress to massive caseation. Numerous organisms are present in acute exudative tuberculosis. However, if the lesion becomes caseous, few organisms can be found in the cheesy matter. If it later becomes semiliquid, the organisms usually multiply at a great rate.

• Proliferative changes. The end of the proliferative reaction is the hard tubercle, which signifies merely that there is no necrosis. Tubercle bacilli are much fewer than in the exudative phase.

The tubercle contains a lot of a score of a special form of mononuclear phagocyte, which have a plentiful, palely eosinophilic cytoplasm and an oval vesicular nucleus. These cells have only the faintest resemblance to epithelial cells, So they were long ago called "epithelioid cells." Among the cells or at their periphery, there is often a giant cell with a plentiful pink cytoplasm and as many as about twenty to forty round or oval nuclei in 2-dimensional sections. The nuclei are arranged in a complete or partial marginal ring. This kind of the cell is described as a Langhans' giant cell (Figure 15-3).

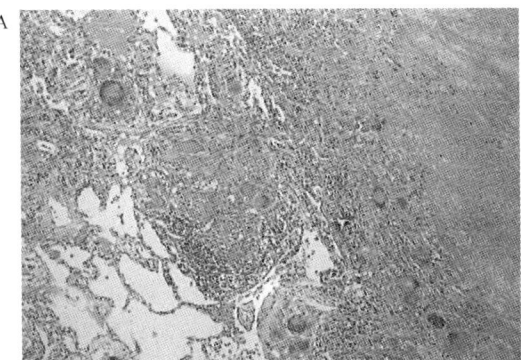
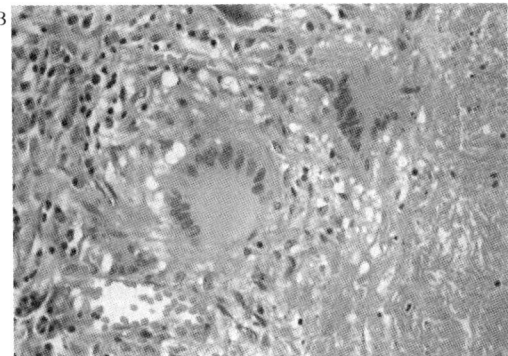

Figure 15-3 A: **Pulmonary tuberculosis, showing multiple granulomas with caseous necrosis.** B: **Granuloma of tuberculosis with epithelioid cells, giant cells and caseation**

• Alterative changes. Starting in the center of the tubercles, the tissue and the epithelioid cells become necrotic and are then replaced by an eosinophilic substance which at first in coarsely granular and dotted. Once it becomes homogeneous and quite structureless, it is termed caseous (cheesy), having the naked-eye appearance of a thick, pasty, pale yellow-white substance in the 1 or 2 mm miliary tubercle. Few organisms are present in it. The term "miliary" implies a resemblance to the millet seed, an object seen by few occidental pathologists. This total obliteration of structure is what distinguishes caseation from coagulation necrosis because even the interstitial fibrous tissue has gone. The dead tissue is rich in lipids, and it may persist for a very long time, apparently because the lipids inhibit proteolytic enzymes.

2. Advance changes in development

What happens next is either further spread of the disease or healing, depending on the host-bacillus relationship (Figure 15-2).

• Healing. Healing in tuberculosis means the focus is lysed and absorbed, with increasing fibrosis spreading into the diseased area, creating a scar with calcium deposition, i.e.: calcification.

a. Lysis and absorb: These denote that the focus is lysed by enzyme and absorbed by capillary and lymph vessels, and the focus is eliminated.

b. Fibrosis and Calcification: Calcification is very common. It is in no sense a protective process. Calcium carried in blood plasma to caseous areas is deposited as relatively insoluble compounds, possibly influenced by the high concentration of lipids.

Reportedly, calcification can appear in primary lesions after two months. Calcium must accumulate for about a year to be seen radiologically. After about three years, the lesion attains a chalky character. Stony foci are at least five years old and may be ossified. At first, the calcium is seen in routine sections as irregular pale blue clouds. With time, the color intensifies, particularly at the periphery. Viable bacilli may still be present in non-calcified areas.

Calcification in tuberculosis, therefore, merely indicates that caseous necrosis has taken place but is

not evidence of cure or sterilization. Identical pulmonary calcification can be produced by histoplasmosis.
• Depravation. In the progression of tuberculosis to depravation, the focus becomes invasive and spreads.
a. Invasion: Under this circumstance, the focus shows exudation changes, including edema, hyperemia, and neutrophil and mononuclear phagocytes infiltration. It may progress to massive caseation necrosis.
b. Spread: If the number of organisms in the circulation is large and the host resistance low, spread may be via the bloodstream, lymph vessels and by natural anatomical pathways such as through the bronchial system, up into the larynx and subsequently into the bowel. Spread by bloodstream can result in military tuberculosis, which is featured by numerous small granulomas of almost equal size in many organs. Lesions are commonly found in the lungs, meninges, kidneys, bone marrow and liver, but no organ is exempt. It can be the consequence of either the primary or secondary tuberculosis. This type of spread may also be seen in the elderly receiving immunosuppressive therapy and in patients with AIDS. Childhood miliary tuberculosis can heal without trace, but the adult variety rarely does. This is an acute medical emergency necessitating prompt treatment with antituberculous therapy.

Acute systemic military tuberculosis: Tubercle bacilli can spill into the blood, directly or via lymphatic vessels. Penetration of a pulmonary vein is likely to infect all of the body, whereas entrance of bacilli into a pulmonary artery is likely to restrict them to its territory within the lung. Entering major lymphatic vessel, mycobacteria will be returned by the right ventricle to both lungs. A small tubercle is formed. A harmless infection leaves a residue of tiny calcified dots in the liver, spleen, apices of the lungs, mening-es, or skeletal system. For a while, it is possible for one of these to light up as active disease. If so, the condition of miliary tuberculosis is set up.

Infection may come from a primary focus or from a later stage of tuberculosis, in which the miliary disease may be merely a terminal event. In the adult, miliary tuberculosis is more likely to be of extrapulmonary origin. The lung is seen to be infected the most heavily even though it contains chronic lesions that initiated extrapulmonary disease.

In children, miliary tuberculosis may be more or less confined to the lung. More often, in addition, liver, spleen, and kidneys bear a great number of tubercles, followed by meninges, bone marrow, lymph nodes, and thyroid gland. Only muscle tissue is spared.

The pleura generally show little reaction. The cut surface of the lung is studded with firm white tubercles 1 mm in diameter or caseating tubercles several millimeters in diameter. Tubercles in the upper lobes are the largest, but the distribution of tubercles is even throughout. The heavier the infection, the closer and more numerous they will be (Figure 15-4).

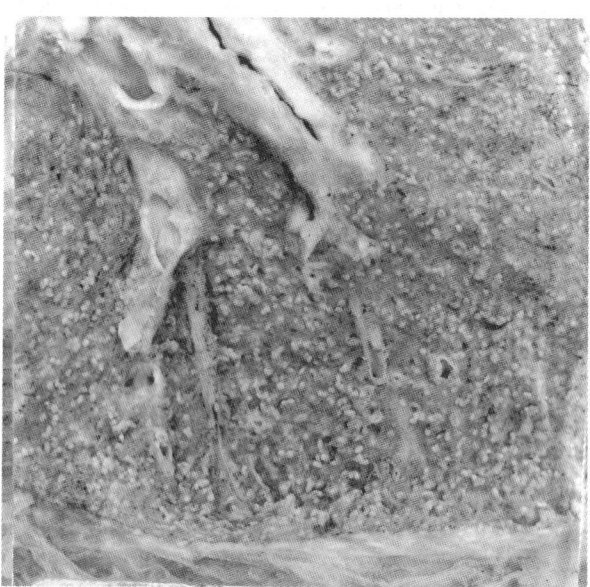

Figure 15-4 Acute military pulmonary tuberculosis. The cut surface of the lung is studded with numerous firm gray-white tubercles 1 mm in diameter

Sub acute military tuberculosis: The military tuberculosis that is between the acute and chronic military tuberculosis in term can be called sub acute military tuberculosis. The size of military nodule in sub acute military tuberculosis is usually bigger than that in acute, and the number of military nodules in sub acute is small than in acute.

Chronic military tuberberculosis: Chronic and recurrent types of pulmonary miliary tuberculosis occasionally are found in adults. The lungs are heavy, and the pleurae are fibroic. On the cut surface, tubercles are seen to have coalesced into small nodules with central caseation and eventual cavitation. In other patients, there is extensive fibrosis around the nodules. Chronic disseminated tuberculosis can also involve several other organs.

PULMONARY TUBERCULOSIS

Pulmonary tuberculosis is caused by Mycobacterium tuberculosis. It is a major cause of death in the world, and it is the principal cause of HIV-related death in, for example, Africa and Far East. It still takes a heavy toll in underdeveloped countries or among malnourished people anywhere living in overcrowded conditions. The common human strain infects only humans and not animals. Patients with pulmonary tuberculosis who cough up bacilli in the sputum are the main source of transmitted infections.

Pulmonary tuberculosis could be divided as two types. One is primary pulmonary tuberculosis, also called as childhood tuberculosis, or first infection type. Another is secondary pulmonary tuberculosis, also named as adult-type pulmonary tuberculosis.

Primary Pulmonary Tuberculosis

A. Definition

Primary pulmonary tuberculosis occurs when a child who has not been previously exposed to tubercle bacilli inhales the organism. The organism enters the alveoli and leads to the formation of the primary complex, or Ghon complex (Figure 15-2), which is composed of a focal tuberculosis lesion (the Ghon focus), inflammatory lymphatic vessels and the enlarged regional lymph nodes. The Ghon focus is an epithelioid-cell granulomatous inflammation at the site of parenchymal infection. This lesion is almost always situated just below the pleura either in the basal segment of the upper lobe or the apical segment of the lower lobe.

Most early cases of primary tuberculosis are clinically silent. In almost all cases, a primary lesion will form a fibrocalcific nodule in the lung, and there will be no clinical sequelae. However, tubercle bacilli may still be present within such scarred foci and may persist as viable organisms for years.

B. Pathology

The combination of the rather inconspicuous parenchymal lesion and the prominent lymphadenopathy for primary infection is known as the primary or Ghon complex. The Ghon focus is an epithelioid-cell granulomatous inflammation at the site of parenchymai infection. The pulmonary lesion consists of a central zone of caseous necrosis surrounded by palisaded epithelioid histiocytes, the occasional Langhans' giant cell, and lymphocytes. Similar granulomas are seen in lymph nodes at the portion of the lung. It is usually small and sub pleural but may be large and located anywhere in the lung. It occurs with equal frequency on either side and tends to be subpleural in the midportion of a lobe rather than apical. Rare multiple primary complexes may be the result of exposure to a source of heavy infection. One lesion can be in the lung and the other extrapulmonary. The lymphatic vessel component may not be seen at all in some lungs. The lymph nodes have massive enlargement. Before immunity is established, tubercle bacilli survive in the macrophages that phagocytose them and are transported via lymphatics and the blood stream throughout the body.

Most primary lesions both in the lung parenchyma and in the lymph nodes heal with complete replacement of the caseous necrosis by fibrous tissue or (more often) by walling off of the necrotic area by scar tissue followed by dystrophic calcification in the caseous material. In the latter cases organisms can survive in the calcified foci for many years. If high grades hypersensitivity develops there may be an outpouring of fibrin-rich exudate. Spreading may take place via the bronchi or bloodstream, usually after softening of the necrotic material.

The development of an immune response against the tubercle bacillus results in (1) macrophage activation by the lymphokine macrophage activating factor, leading to destruction of tubercle bacilli; (2) inhibition of macrophage migration by the lymphokine macrophage migration-inhibiting factor, which reduces further spread of bacilli in the body;

and (3) delayed hypersensitivity (type IV), which leads to caseous necrosis of granulomas in the Ghon focus and elsewhere in the body. Hypersensitivity is responsible for tuberculin conversion: The infected individual gives a positive reaction to intradermal injection of tuberculin (purified protein derivative of tubercle bacilli, or PPD).

In 95% of cases, immunity stops disease progression and healing occurs. The lesions heal by fibrosis and may calcify. There may or may not be radiologic evidence of healed primary infection. Complications occur in 5% of cases of primary pulmonary tuberculosis. Rapidly progressive pulmonary disease, causing extensive caseous consolidation of the lung (caseous pneumonia), usually occurs only in malnourished or immunodeficient children. Erosion of a caseous granuloma into a bronchus may result in tuberculous bronchopneumonia; erosion into a blood vessel may cause severe bacteremia in which numerous small tuberculous granulomas are found all over the body (miliary tuberculosis).

C. Effects of Primary Tuberculosis

An individual who has recovered from primary tuberculosis shows the following evidence of infection:
- Tuberculin Positivity: A positive skin test to tuberculoprotein may remain for a long period, often for several years.
- Partial Immunity to Tuberculosis: An individual who is tuberculin-positive requires a higher dose to be reinfected by tubercle bacilli.
- Presence of Dormant Tubercle Bacilli: Tubercle bacilli may remain dormant in the lungs, brain, meninges, bone, kidneys, lymph nodes, intestines, etc (Figure 15-2). Organisms are present in these tissues as a result of preallergic lymphohe matogenous dissemination of bacilli. Not all of the bacilli in these foci are killed by the immune response, and some remain dormant for long periods within inactive caseous granulomas. When becoming reactivated many years later, it will lead to secondary pulmonary and extrapulmonary tuberculosis (Figure 15-2). Rarely, dormant granulomas are visible radiologically due to the presence of calcification. Chemoprophylaxis with isoniazid is indicated in tuberculin-positive patients to eradicate these dormant bacilli.

Secondary Pulmonary Tuberculosis

Secondary tuberculosis in adult is almost always symptomatic. The most common symptom is chronic cough, frequently with hemoptysis due to erosion of a blood vessel in the wall of the cavity. Marked weight loss, low-grade fever, and night sweats are common.

Physical examination and chest x-ray show the changes of apical fibrosis and cavitation. The normal lung is replaced by an opacity caused by fibrosis and granulomatous inflammation. The occurrence of central cavitation is typical. Bronchopneumonia due to spread of bacilli in the bronchial tree may occur in elderly, debilitated, and immunodeficient patients.

A. Definition and Etiology

Secondary tuberculosis occurs in patients who have had a prior primary infection. It usually occurs in an adult as a result either of reinfection or reactivation, with the latter more common.
- **Reinfection**: Because of partial immunity, the number of organisms that must be inhaled to reinfect such an individual is large; the source of infection is usually a patient with active pulmonary tuberculosis who is discharging large numbers of organisms in sputum.
- **Reactivation**: The mechanism that keeps dormant bacilli in check is uncertain, as are the reasons why they become reactivated. Reactivation represents some breakdown of immunity and commonly occurs when an individual harboring tubercle bacilli, i.e. a tuberculin-positive individual, is given immunosuppressive drugs such as corticosteroids. Such patients should be treated with antituberculous drugs.

In the adult, the parenchymal lesions usually start in the sub-apical region of the upper lobe (Assman foci). No prominant lymph node involvement is seen although microscopic involvement may be present.

B. Pathology

Multiplication of tubercle bacilli occurs in the presence of a rapidly developing secondary immune response, characterized by rapid lymphokine production by specifically activated T lymphocytes that limit dissemination of infected macrophages and localize the tubercle bacilli to the area of reactivation or reinfection. Enhanced delayed hypersensitivity produces a heightened local response with extensive caseous necrosis. The exact mechanism by which caseous necrosis is produced is unknown.

Secondary pulmonary tuberculosis may occur in any tissue reactivation. The most common site is the lung apex, due probably to the greater availability of oxygen in this better ventilated zone of lung that favors multiplication of the aerobic tubercle bacilli.

Secondary pulmonary tuberculosis may also result from reinfection in adult life. The pathologic features of reinfection and reactivation types of secondary pulmonary tuberculosis are identical. Note that extrapulmonary tuberculosis may occur in a patient without overt lung involvement.

The earliest lesions are small epithelioid cell granulomas characterized by caseous necrosis and fibrosis. These coalesce to form a large solid mass of fibrocaseous granulomatous inflammation called a tuberculoma. The caseous material is at first solid, but with continued multiplication of bacilli it undergoes liquefaction. The liquefied granuloma may open into a bronchus, leading to the following consequences: (1) Infected sputum, with coughing up of large numbers of tubercle bacilli. The patient is now highly infective. (2) Cavitation of the tuberculoma. The tuberculous cavity is lined by caseous granulomatous inflammatory tissue and associated with marked fibrosis. This is called cavitary fibrocaseous tuberculosis. It is the typical lesion of secondary tuberculosis. (3) Dissemination via the bronchial tree, lymphatics, or bloodstream usually occurs late in the disease. With hematogenous spread, secondary granulomas may develop in any location in the body. Dissemination occurs early in the course of disease only in debilitated or immunodeficient patients.

C. Natural History of Adult-Type Pulmonary Tuberculosis

1. Healing

If there is a high degree of immunity lesions may heal with scarring and calcification.

2. Softening and cavitation

Softening with caseous necrosis may occur and if this is associated with erosion into a bronchus there may be cavitation. Communication with an airway increases oxygen tension and favours bacterial multiplication. The patient will cough up potentially infectious material. Blood vessels in the wall of the cavity may show thrombotic occlusion or may be eroded with resultant massive haemorrhage. Involvement of overlying pleura may be associated with a serous pleural effusion, a persistent fibrinous exudate or tuberculous empyema, which is the pleural space containing partly liquefied caseous material.

3. Spread

Spread may be via the bloodstream, lymph vessels or by natural anatomical pathways, such as through the bronchial system, up into the larynx and subsequently into the bowel.

D. Pathological Type of Secondary Pulmonary Tuberculosis

1. Focal pulmonary tuberculosis

It is the early change of the secondary pulmonary tuberculosis. The lesions is usually located at the apex of the lungs and is approximate 0.5 to 1 cm in diameter. The color of the lesions is gray-white or yellow which is caseation. The edges of the lesions are sharp with surrounding fibroses (Figure 15-5). There may be single or multiple lesions. So, one or more shadows of nodulus can be seen by radiograph of the chest. Microscopically, it appears mainly as proliferation and the caseous necrosis may occur in the center of the lesions. This kind of tuberculosis is inactive. The patients are clinical asymptomatic.

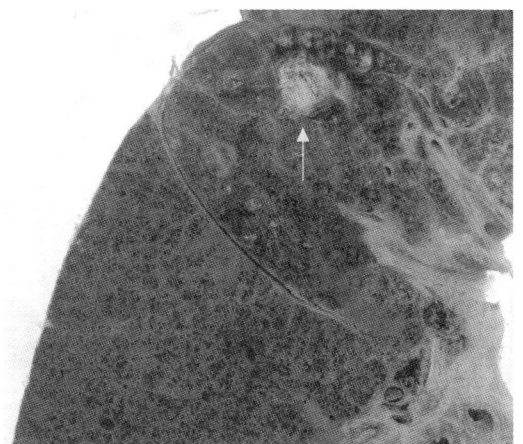

Figure 15-5 **Focal pulmonary tuberculosis**

2. Infiltrating pulmonary tuberculosis

It is the most common type of the secondary pulmonary tuberculosis. Usually, it results from the depravation of focal fulmonary tuberculosis. At this circumstance, the focus becomes invasion and fuzzy. It appears as cloudy-like shadows and indistinct edges in radiograph of the chest (Figure 15-6). There is an evident exudation with edema, hyperemia and infiltration of neutrophil and mononuclear phagocytes, and caseation in the lesions. The lesion enlarges and the area of the caseation expands with the tuberculosis progressing. If the necrosis erodes the bronchus, the central caseous material will spread from the lesions into the bronchus, result in the formation of an acute cavity, which is lined by caseous material. So, the tubercle bacilli are disseminated by bronchus and cause caseous pneumonia.

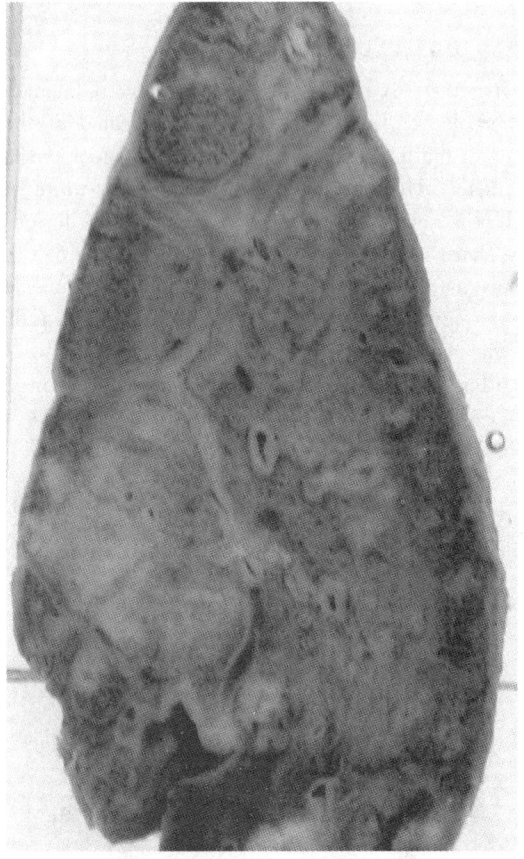

Figure 15-6 Infiltrating pulmonary tuberculosis, the focus becomes invasion and fuzzy. The edge is indistinct

Patients often have low grade fever, feel weary, cough, and emptysis, etc. With prompt adequate treatment, the process can be stopped. The lesion with hyperplasia or necrosis can heal by fibrosis and calcification. And, the acute cavity can heal by hyperplasia of wall granulation tissue, and eventually be closed by formation of scar tissue. It can also be healed by cavity collapse and formation of band scar. The acute cavity, if it is not healed for a long time, can progress to chronic fibrotic cavitary tuberculosis.

3. Chronic fibrotic cavitary tuberculosis

A newly formed chronic cavity has necrotic, ragged walls, with adherent, pale yellow, cheesy material. The cavities have thick walls and communicate with larger bronchi by wide openings. There is large area of caseation with attempts at fibrous encapsulation (Figure 15-7). There is also extensive tuberculous bronchitis. No odor is present. The wall of the active cavities has three definite linings. Innermost is the caseous tissue with debris, many bacilli, and, in places, epithelioid cells and some fibro blasts. Beyond this is a red zone of tuberculous granulation tissue composed of many dilated capillaries, epithelioid and Langhans' cells, and fibroblasts. The external layer is a thin gray zone of loose connective tissue, which has arisen from organization of the perifocal zone. This merges indefinitely into consoli dated or normal lung. The opening into the bronchus may be very small.

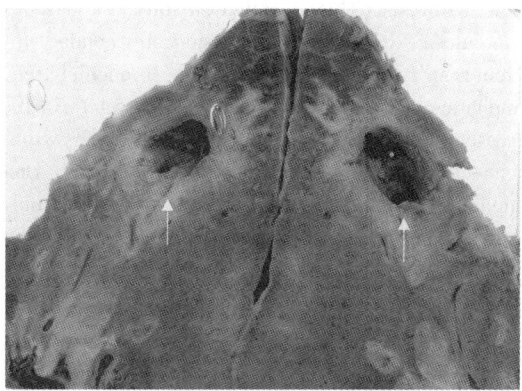

Figure 15-7 Chronic fibrotic cavitary tuberculosis

Chronicity is indicated by a fibrous outer wall, which forms from organization of the perifocal reaction and is 1 or 2 mm thick. The outline tends to be markedly irregular because of uneven breakdown of the tissues. Several cavities may intercommunicate, and the bronchus of each may be identified.

The lining of older cavities is gray or pink and shaggy. A smooth fibrous lining replaces this granulation tissue when the infection is overcome. Around it are foci of tuberculous bronchopneumonia, caseation, fibrosis, and bronchiectasis. The overlying pleura is fibrotic.

The cavities can lead to the danger of bronchogenic dissemination of bacilli. An upper lobe cavity tends to infect other parts of that lobe and the apex of the lower lobe, less often its post erobasal region. Infection also can spread to the opposite lung, usually its lower lobe. Tubercle bacilli in sputum may set up ulcerative tracheal or laryngeal tuberculosis or, in late stages of the disease, infect the tongue and mucosal lymphoid tissue of the small and large intestines. Hematogenous miliary dissemination can also occur.

4. Caseous pneumonia

Tuberculous caseous pneumonia is a rapidly progressive secondary pulmonary tuberculosis. It occurs when a caseous hilar node erodes a bronchial wall and when there is perforation of a tuberculous cavity into a bronchus. A great amount of infected material is spilled over, the affected area at first includes one or two lobules, which are solid, dry, gray, and granular.

Large quantities of tuberculoprotein reach uninfected tissue of an already hypersensitive individual, provoking a vigorous exudative response in the alveoli, with many bacilli. Tissue necrosis follows rapidly, and adjacent foci enlarge and coalesce. Microscopic tubercles are uncommon. Soon the gray turns to yellow or gray-red, and the whole lobe is felt to be firm. A whole lung, or most of both lungs, can be affected, and those parts not massively consolidated may show bronchopneumonia around caseous bronchi. The peripheral zones may be moist, translucent, shiny, smooth, and somewhat gelatinous pneumonia, which show microscopically as filling of intact thick-walled alveoli by much fluid and fibrin with many macrophages. Other inflammatory cells are much fewer.

The larger the disease area, the more likely is it that caseation and cavitation will occur in the center of the older areas. The cut surface show as firm, dry, opaque, yellow-white color. Tubercles are found in and around the bronchi, which are ulcerated and may be destroyed. Tuberculous pleurisy and caseous hilar nodes are very frequently present. Eventually, an opening will be forced into a large bronchus. Miliary dissemination is common. The most severe cases used to be called "galloping consumption." If such widespread disease can be arrested, the eventual fibrosis is most extensive (Figure 15-8).

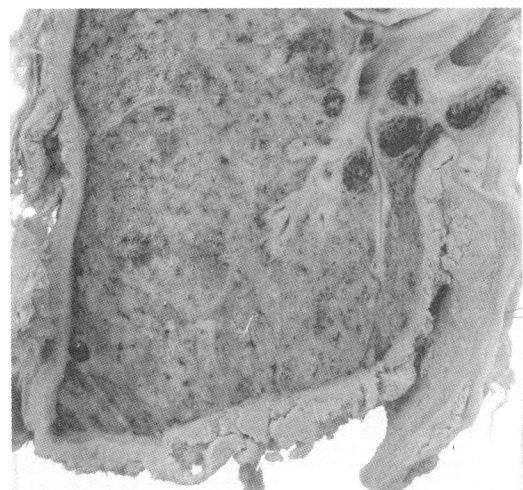

Figure 15-8 Caseous pneumonia and siccus tuberculous pleuritis

5. Tuberculoma

A tuberculoma is a nodular, conglomerate area of caseous necrosis with a well formed fibrous capsule. It occurs in adults with reinfection tuberculosis. Usually, the diameters of the tuberculomas vary from 0.5 to 4 cm. Most are solitary and occur in an upper lobe. The cut surface shows a uniform or lamellate, dry, caseous matter with areas of calcification. The capsule is 1 to 3 mm thick, and the surrounding lung is normal or has minimal tuberculosis. Although tuberculomas are thought as inactive, they may break down and discharge their contents into the bronchial tree, indicating reactivation (Figure 15-9).

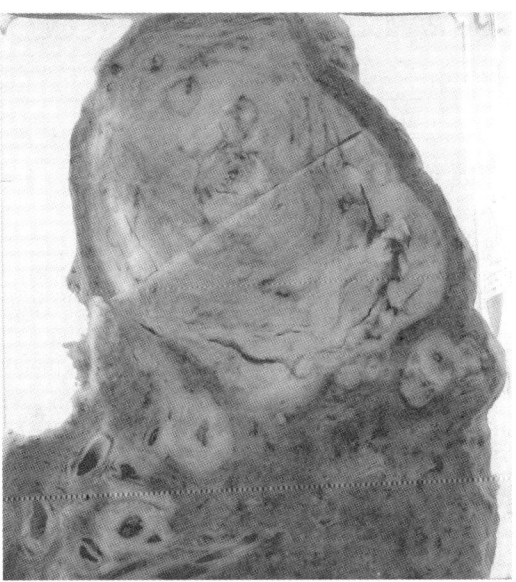

Figure 15-9 Tuberculoma

6. Tuberculous pleuritis

With the progressions of pulmonary tuberculosis, the tuberculous pleuritis may develop with serous pleural effusions and pleural fibrous. Based on the morphological characteristics of tuberculous pleuritis, it can be classified as humectous tuberculous pleuritis and siccus tuberculous pleuritis.

Humectous tuberculous pleuritis, also be called exudative tuberculous pleuritis, is featured by serous fibrinous inflammation. It may accompany hematodes. If the effusion is large, it is difficult to absorb and can result in the pleural thickening and adhering.

Siccus tuberculous pleuritis, also called hyperplastic tuberculous pleuritis, is featured by localized hyperlasia and the pleural effusion is extremely minute. It mostly locates at the apex of lungs and heals by fibrosis.

E. Diagnosis

The diagnosis of tuberculosis must always be confirmed by microbiologic techniques.
- Demonstration of tubercle bacilli in smears of sputum or in tissue sections.
- Culture of *M. tuberculosis* from sputum or tissue: Culture of the slowly growing organism takes 4 – 6 weeks but represents the most accurate method of diagnosis.
- Find tuberculosis granulomas or tubercle with caseous necrosis in paraffin section.

EXTRAPULMONARY TUBERCULOSIS

Intestinal Tuberculosis

A. Aetiology

Mycobacterium tuberculosis and *Mycobacterium bovis* are the main causes of intestinal tuberculosis. It is primarily from drinking infected milk (*M. bovis*); A secondary source is the swallowing of infected sputum from patients with pulmonary tuberculosis.

In the past, the bovine strain of *M. tuberculosis* infected dairy herds, causing human infection via contaminated milk. Bovine tuberculosis has now been almost eradicated from dairy herds in most developed countries, and pasteurization of milk has further decreased the risk of human infection. Bovine tuberculosis typically involved the oropharynx or intestine because the organism was ingested in milk and not inhaled. The primary focus would thus be found in the gastrointestinal tract.

B. Pathomorphology

Intestinal tuberculosis occurs most commonly in the jejunum and ileum, and it may also occur in the following sites (in order of frequency): appendix, colon, rectum and duodenum. It is very rare in the anus.

The morphological feature of intestinal tuberculosis is the formation of circumferential ulcers, which is often perpendicular to the long axis of the intestine. And there may be an inflammatory process extending through the thickness of the bowel forming a mass of inflamed fibrous tissue. The intestine proximal to the ulcers and mass is dilated secondary to intestinal obstruction (Figures 15-10, 15-11).

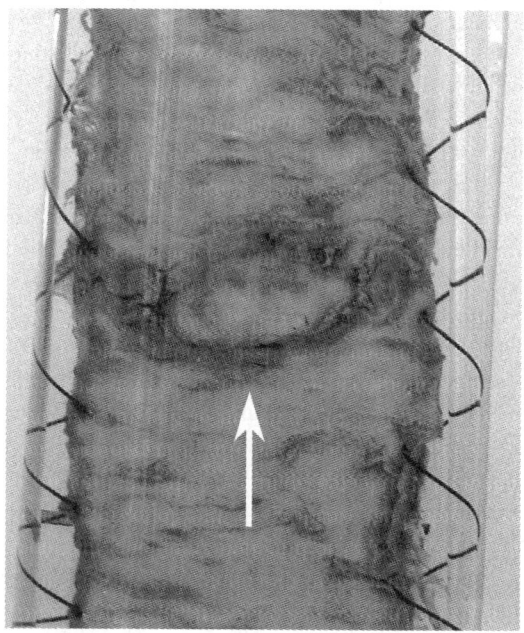

Figure 15-10 Showing transverse ulcer of intestinal tuberculosis

- Primary Intestinal Tuberculosis. Primary tuberculous infection of the intestine has become rare as a result of pasteurization of milk and eradication of bovine tuberculosis in dairy herds. It is characterized by a small focus in the intestine and large mesenteric lymph nodes, analogous to the primary complex in the lung.

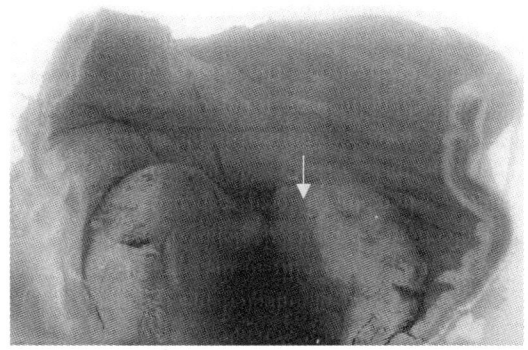

Figure 15-11 Hyperplastic cecal tuberculosis. The intestine proximal to the mass is dilated secondary to the intestinal obstruction by that mass

• Secondary Intestinal Tuberculosis. This form of tuberculosis still occurs as a result of swallowing of infected sputum by patients with active pulmonary disease or reactivation of a dormant intestinal focus, usually in the terminal ileum or cecum. Typical caseous granulomas form. The organisms spread locally in the intestinal lymphatics, resulting in ulcers that are transverse (Figure 15-10) because the intestinal lymphatics pass circumferentially. Involvement of the serosa results in fibrous adhesions between loops of intestine. Fistula formation may occur.

Clinically, intestinal tuberculosis is a chronic illness characterized by lower grade fever and diarrhea, which may be tinged with blood. A mass may be palpable in a few cases (hyperplastic cecal tuberculosis, Figure 15-11). The clinical diagnosis is made by cultured tubercle bacilli from the stools.

Complications of intestinal tuberculosis include intestinal obstruction and dilation, caused by mass, strictures, fistulas, and tuberculous peritonitis.

Tuberculous Meningitis

Tuberculous meningitis most often affects infants and children. It has an insidious onset with nonspecific prodrome including anorexia, malaise and episodes of vomiting lasting 2 - 3 weeks. This is followed by signs of meningeal irritation, which are less severe than that in acute bacterial meningitis.

Morphology: The base of brain is most severely affected. The tuberculosis granulomas can be seen by microscope in the focus. However, in the early stage, there may be an exudative phase.

Renal Tuberculosis

Renal tuberculosis still occurs frequently in parts of the world where tuberculosis is endemic. It is most common in patients 20 - 50 years of age. The kidneys are initially infected in the primary pulmonary stage by hematogenous dissemination. The bacilli remain dormant and become reactivated much later. Approximately half of the patients with renal tuberculosis have a normal chest x-ray because the original infection has long since healed.

The lesion usually begins in the corticomedullary region as a caseous granuloma (tuberculoma). Multiple granulomas are common. The kidney is grossly enlarged, and cut section shows several yellow crumbling foci. With progression, the granulomas open into the pelvicaliceal system, leading to discharge of the caseous material in the urine and cavitation of the lesion (Figure 15-12). Microscopically, there is central caseous necrosis surrounded by epithelioid cells, lymphocytes, and fibroblasts. Marked fibrosis is usually present. Acid-fast bacilli can be demonstrated in most cases.

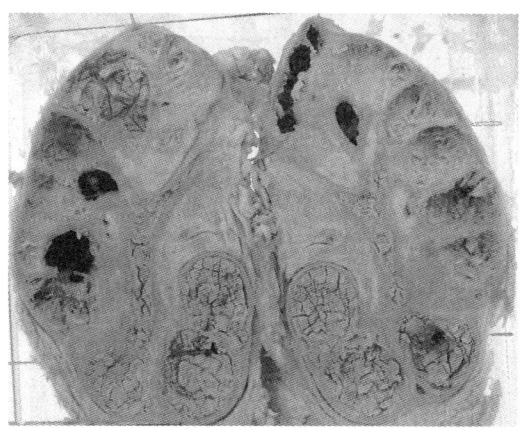

Figure 15-12 Renal tuberculosis with caseous necrosis and cavitation

Clinically, patients have a combination of chronic inflammatory and urinary symptoms: low-grade fever, weight loss, hematuria, frequency, and mild lumbar pain. The urine shows numerous neutrophils. Ordinary urine culture is sterile (leading to the misnomer "sterile pyuria"). However, the examination for mycobacteria is positive.

Tuberculosis of Bone

Tuberculosis of bone shows as tuberculous osteomyelitis. It has become rare in the areas where the pulmonary and intestinal tuberculosis has been good controlled. It is still common in some developing countries. The vertebral column, mainly the thoracic and lumbar vertebrae, is the commonest site. The bones of hip, knee, ankle, elbow and wrist can be also involved. It is usually due to blood infection. For the tuberculosis of spine it is also called Pott's disease. This disease starts in vertebral body and extends into the disc space causing collapse. Area of bone destruction associated with granulomatous inflammation with caseation (Figure 15-13). When the tuberculosis is invaded to the muscles, the liquefied caseous emerge as "abscess". These "abscesses" are "cold". They lack heat and redness of acute pyogenic abscesses. So they are called as cold abscess.

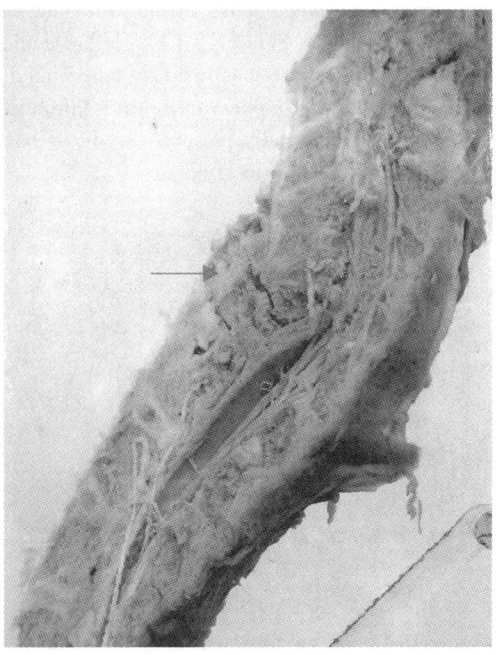

Figure 15-13　Pott's disease with vertebra collapse

Lymph Node Tuberculosis

The lymph nodes involved tuberculosis are most frequently pulmonary hilar nodes associated with a lung primary complex. It may be seen in cervical nodes associated with ingested organisms that pass to the nodes from the pharynx (scrofula).

The nodes are enlarged and matted together. The cut surface reveals cheesy material (caseation). In the section, numerous granulomas composed of chiefly the epithelioid cells can be seen by microscopy. The centres of granulomas undergo caseation necrosis resulting in featureless areas of eosinophilic material. Langhans' Giant cells are almost always present. The granulomas are surrounded by lymphocytes. Organisms may or may not be identified when special stains.

Testis Tuberculosis

The testis is relatively resistant to tuberculous involvement. It usually occurs when tuberculosis spread by haematogenous way. The epididymis is the primary target. Under the microscope, in the epididymis the features are the same as seen in other organs. Caseation necrosis is usually severe.

Tuberculosis continues to be a major cause of disease and death in endemic areas. In addition, the emergence of multi-drug resistant strains is an increasing problem in treating tuberculosis.

TYPHOID FEVER

Typhoid fever is an acute intestinal infectious disease, still prevalent in Third World countries. In as much as the principal lesions are those of lymphoid tissue of intestine, the ileum is most affected, although the jejunum, appendix, and colon also may be involved. According to the World Health Organization 1994 census, approximately 17 million cases occur per year worldwide. Among these cases, 7 million distribute in Asia, 4 million in Africa, and 0.5 million in Latin America, with 600,000 fatalities. The global incidence is about 0.5%, but incidence rates as high as 2% have been reported in hot spots, such as Indonesia and Papua New Guinea, where typhoid fever ranks among the 5 most common causes of death.

Etiology and Pathogenesis

Typhoid fever is caused by *Salmonella typhi*; *Salmonella paratyphi* may produce a similar illness. *S. typhy* is a motile, gramnegative bacillus. The organism infects only humans, and the minimal infective dose is less than 10,000 bacteria. The infection results from contamination of food and water with feces from a symptomatic case or asymptomatic carrier of typhoid. The incubation period of typhoid fever averages 10–20 (range 3-56) days. In paratyphoid fever, the incubation period ranges from 1-10 days. The duration of illness in an untreated individual is usually 4 weeks.

The ingested bacillus invades the small intestinal mucosa, where it is taken up by macrophages and transported to regional lymph nodes. S. typhi is a facultative intracellular organism and multiplies in the intestinal lymphoid tissue during the 1 to 3 week incubation period (Figure 15-14).

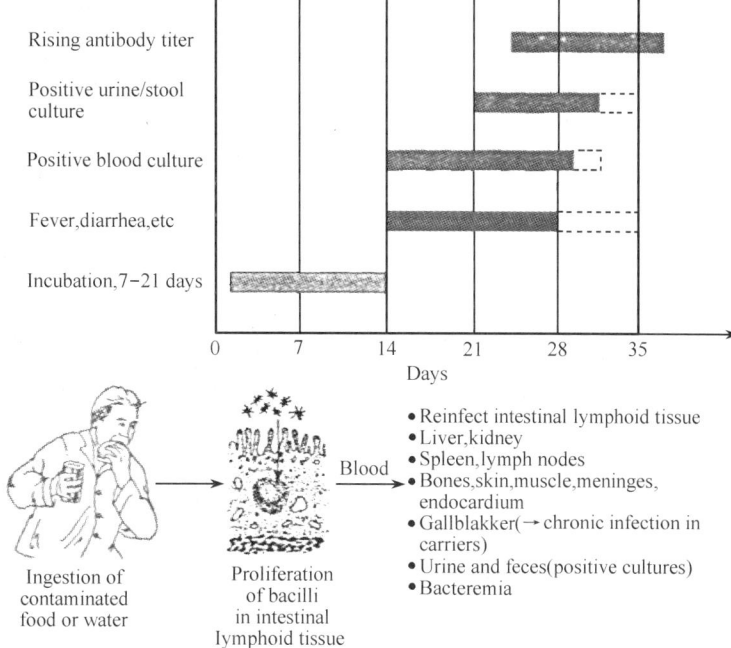

Figure 15-14 Typhoid fever, showing the course and diagnostic tests. In the example above, the incubation period is 14 days (range, 7-21 days)

At the end of the incubation period, the bacilli enter the bloodstream (bacteremic phase), resulting in fever, headache, and muscle aches. Many tissues, including liver, heart, kidney, lungs, meninges, and bone, may be infected during this phase.

In the second week of illness, S. typhi reenters the intestinal lumen by way of biliary excretion (intestinal phase). The organism reinfects lymphoid tissue in the small intestine and colon in large numbers, causing acute inflammation, necrosis, and ulceration. Necrosis is the result of direct invasion plus endotoxin released by the bacillus, together with delayed hypersensitivity, which has developed by this time. The mucosal ulcers tend to take the shape of the underlying lymphoid follicles and typically occur as longitudinal ulcers overlying the Peyer's patches in the ileum.

Pathological Changes

The hallmark histologic finding in typhoid fever is the infiltration of tissues by typhoid cells, which is a characteristic large macrophages containing phagocytized erythrocytes or lymphocytes, bacteria, and necrotic cellular debris. This kind of cells is called typhoid cell, and this kind of lesion, aggregates of these macrophages, is known as typhoid granuloma or typhoid nodule (Figure 15-15), and are commonly found in the intestine, mesenteric lymph nodes, spleen, liver, and bone marrow. A striking feature of typhoid lesions is the virtual absence of polymorphonuclear leukocytes.

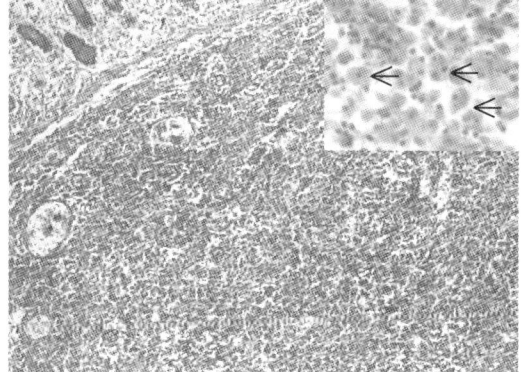

Figure 15-15 Showing typhoid granuloma (low power), and typhoid cells (high power) which contain phagocytized lymphocytes

The early changes in intestine are degeneration and proliferation of Peyer's patches and of the solitary lymphoid follicles of the intestine. Large numbers of typhoid cells constitute the most conspicuous histological feature of the disease.

The longitudinal ulcer, which takes the shape of Peyer's patch (Figures 15-16, 15-17), is typical of typhoid fever macroscopically. Other changes observed by microscopic examination show edema and acute inflammation. The cellular infiltrate in typhoid is deficient in neutrophils. Lymphocytes and plasma cells could be seen. Necrosis and ulceration follow. The change in the terminal small intestine have been divided into 4 classic stages.

phoid granuloma with a large number of typhoid cells can obviously be seen.

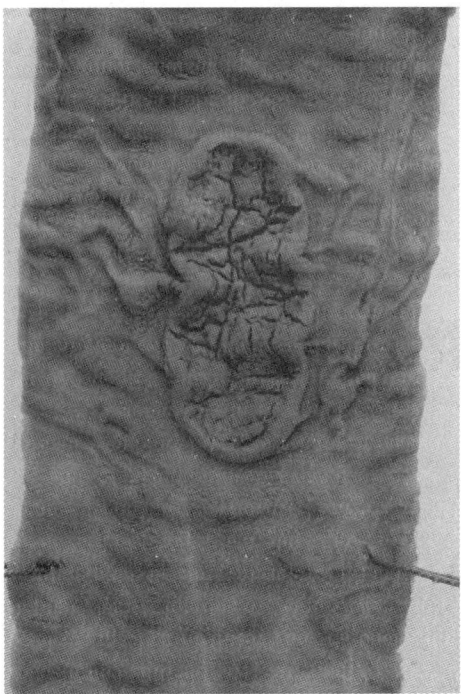

Figure 15-17 Typhoid fever, showing the necrosis of Peyer's patches, which is fuzzy

B. Necrosis Stage

In the second week about, the focus in the intestine is complicated by necrosis, i.e.: necrosis take place within the Peyer's patches of the ileum and the solitary lymph follicles. The structure of enlarged Peyer's patches becomes fuzzy. The surface on the necrosis may covered with greenish yellow exudate. The typhoid granuloma can be seen at the margin of necrosis (Figure 15-17).

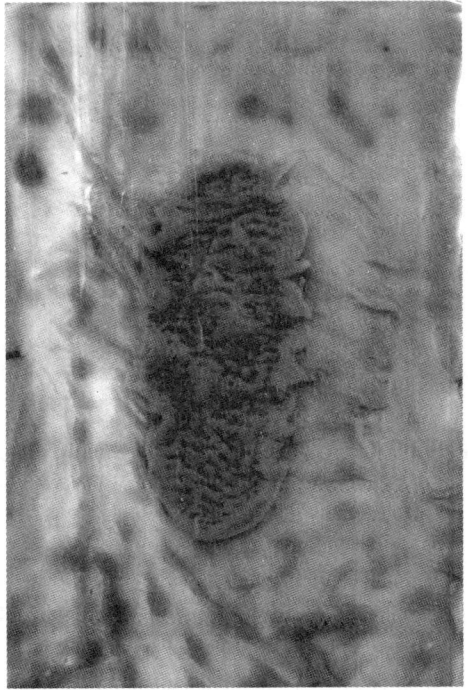

Figure 15-16 Typhoid fever, showing the hyperplasia of Peyer's patches of ileum, which is button-like elevation

A. Stage of Hyperplasia of Peyer's Pathes

During the first week, the lymphoid tissue of the intestinal tract, The Peyer's patches of the ileum and the solitary lymph follicles in the region of the cecum, show proliferation and hyperplasia, and appear as button - like protrusions. The mesenteric lymph nodes become markedly hyperplasia too, as a result of infection via lymphatics (Figure 15-16). Ty-

C. Ulceration Stage

In the third week about, those necrosis tissues progress to exuviations from the focus areas and result in the ulceration formation in intestine (Figure 15-18). The shape of ulcerations is elongated generally with the long axis in line with that of the intestine in the terminal ileum and more or less rounded or oval. Hemorrhage may often occur and the ulcer can extend down to the submucosa, muscularis and serosa, which leads to perforation (Figure 15-19). Peripheral remnants of preserved hyperplastic lymphoid tissue usually elevate their margins.

tocytes are replaced by a phagocytic mononuclear aggregate (typhoid nodule). Kupffer cell is hyperplasia and proliferation. These distinctive nodules also occur in the bone marrow and lymph nodes. Gallbladder colonization, may causes a chronic carrier state. Typhoid fever differs from bacillary dysentery in being essentially systemic rather than limited to the gastrointestinal tract.

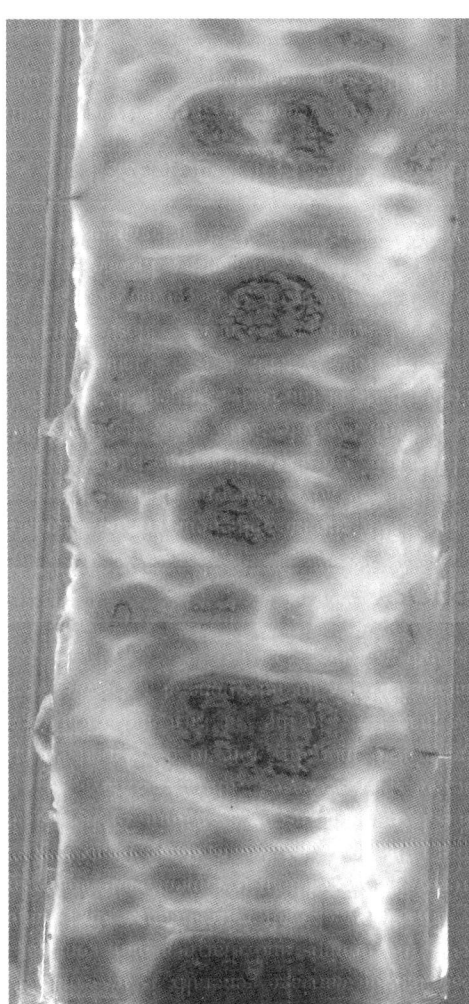

Figure 15-18　Typhoid fever, showing the multi ulceration of intestine

D. Healing Stage

In the fourth week about, ulceration show followed by granulation tissue formation, and ultimately epithelial regeneration takes place.

Along with this, the reticuloendothelial system as a whole is responding to tile septicemia, which causes proliferation of phagocytes with enlargement of reticuloendothelial and lymphoid tissues throughout the body. The typhoid nodules, usually in focal collections and associated with loci of necrosis, are also conspicuous in the spleen, liver, bone marrow, and lymph nodes etc. The spleen is enlarged, with obliterated follicular markings, and prominent sinus histiocytosis. The liver shows small, randomly scattered foci of parenchymal necrosis in which the hepa-

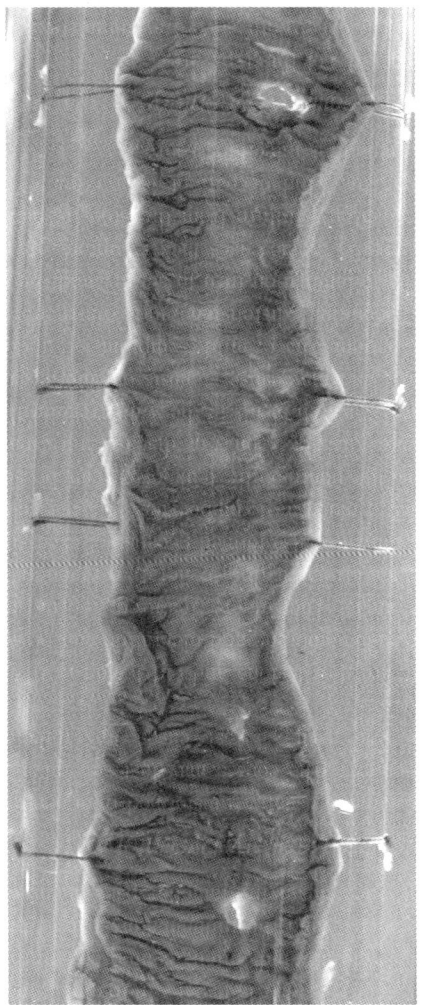

Figure 15-19　Typhoid fever, showing the perforation of intestine

Clinical Feature, Complications and Prognosis

A. Clinical Feature and Complications

Clinically, the intestinal phase is characterized by diarrhea and continued fever. Leukopenia is an important characteristic and clinical sign, since very few bacterial infections are associated with a low white blood cell count. The diagnosis can be established by stool and urine culture, which is positive at this stage. Blood culture is positive in 95% of cases in the first week. And it is still positive in about 60% of patients in the second week of illness.

Bacteremia is common and often fatal if the patient is not treated. Toxemia of typhoid fever is often extreme, especially early in the disease. A toxic confusional state, characterized by disorientation, delirium, and restlessness, is characteristic of late-stage typhoid.

The two common and most serious complications are intestinal bleeding and perforation, occurs in about 5% of patients, which may be life-threatening. Bleeding usually is noted after the second week of the disease, but perforation and the resultant peritonitis may occur unexpectedly after the patient has begun to improve.

Maculopa pular rash (rose spots) lasting a few days can be seen in skin during the second week. Skeletal muscle may characteristically shows widespread focal necrosis (Zenker's degeneration), particularly affecting the abdominal wall and thigh muscles.

Toxic myocarditis is about 1%-5%, which occurs in patients who are severely ill and toxemic and is characterized by tachycardia, weak pulse and heart sounds, hypotension, and electrocardiographic abnormalities.

Subclinical disseminated intravascular coagulation occurs commonly in persons with typhoid fever.

Nephritic syndrome may complicate chronic S. typhi bacteremia associated with urinary schistosomiasis.

Other complications include pneumonia, acute cholecystitis, and acute meningitis. Pancreatitis and simultaneous acute renal failure and hepatitis with hepatomegaly have also been reported. Jaundice may occur in persons with enteric fever and may be due to hepatitis, cholangitis, cholecystitis, or hemolysis. Occasionally, meningitis, arthritis, endocarditis, chondritis, osteomyelitis and endophthalmitis can occur. Spontaneous splenic rupture and multiple brain abscesses also have been reported.

Typhoid fever differs from bacillary dysentery in being essentially systemic rather than limited to the gastrointestinal tract.

B. Prognosis

Before 1909, the preantibiotic era, the mortality rate in patients with intestinal perforation in typhoid fever was 66%-90% but now is significantly lower. Toxic myocarditis occurs in 1%-5% of persons with typhoid and is a significant cause of death in disease-endemic countries. Altered mental status has been associated with a high case-fatality rate.

Today survival rates exceed 96% in developed countries but remain less than 90% in parts of the developing world despite antibiotic availability.

Studies show that 1%-5% of patients become chronic carriers, who harbor S typhi in their gall bladders. The risk of carrier status is correlated to underlying biliary pathology and co-infection with schistosomiasis. This carrier state is believed to be due to persistent low-grade infection in the kidney and gall bladder. They continue to excrete bacilli in urine or feces. Carriers represent a public health hazard, particularly if they are involved in handling food.

Relapse occurs in as many as 10% of patients, while 1%-3% of patients become long-term carriers following recovery.

BACILLARY DYSENTERY

Bacillary dysentery is an acute infectious inflammatory disease of the colon, occasionally involving the ileum as well, caused by microorganisms of the *genus Shigella*. It is also known as SHIGELLA COLITIS. The infection is the result of contamination of food or water supplies with the feces of individuals who either have the disease or, less often, are symptomatic carriers of the organism.

The epidemiology of bacillary dysentery and the severity of the individual case vary greatly with the species of Shigella involved, as well as with the character of the population at risk. Thus, the disease is particularly severe in infants and young children, as well as in the case of Shigella dysenteriae (shiga) infections in the tropics.

Etiology and Pathogenesis

Bacillary dysentery is caused by Shigella species, including Shigella dysenteriae, *S. flexneri*, *S. boydii* and *S. sonnei*. These kinds of bacterial are slender bacilli with Gram-negative. Then natural habitat is the primate gut. It is spread through fecal-oral transmission. The minimal infective dose is less than 1000 organisms. All the 4 kinds of Shigella species can produce endotoxin (lipopolysaccha ride) derived from the cell wall, which result in the lesion of intestine. The *Shigella dysenteriae* can produce exotoxin that affects the bowel and CNS. *Shigella sonnei* and *Shigella flexneri* are the common species and cause a relatively mild illness. *Shigella boydii* is uncommon. *Shigella dysenteriae* type I (Shiga's bacillus) can produce a severe illness and is endemic in parts of Asia.

It is postulated that the lesion is caused by the action of a bacterial endotoxin upon the deeper cells lining the intestinal crypts. Invasion of the mucosal epithelium is followed by the formation of small abscesses in the wall of the colon and terminal ileum. Diagnosis is made by stool based on the etiology detection, such as bacillary culture.

Pathological Changes and Clinical Types

Shigella species affect the colon, producing an acute inflammation with diffuse hyperemia, edema, and multiple superficial ulcers. Neutrophils are the dominant inflammation cells. Bacteremia is rare, occurring only in severe cases, particularly with *S. dysenteriae* type I.

The anatomic changes are characterized by the formation of a pseudomembrane and ulcers (Figure 15-20). The pseudomembrane consists of fibrin cell debris, necrotic mucosa, acute inflammatory cells and bacteria (Figure 15-21). Ulcers are usually shallow but deep ulcers may occur. In contrast to amebic colitis, the ulcers are not undermined. The lesion is of an acute, pyogenic inflammation that may progress from edema and leukocytic infiltration of the mucous membrane to necrosis, bleeding, and ulceration. Healing is with granulation tissue formation, but in the usual case there is little scarring.

The disease is usually self-limited and resolves completely. However, on occasion the acute infection may evolve into chronic recurrent disease with episodes of diarrhea or dysentery or, rarely, into the asymptomatic carrier state.

Following three types could be divided based on the clinical and pathological changes.

A. Acute Bacillary Dysentery

This type is of the above typical pathological changes and it also makes a feature of following:
● It is shown as an acute intestine inflammation, accompanied by hyperemia, and nentrophil infiltration. The course lasts 1-2 week and patients recover with adequate treatment.

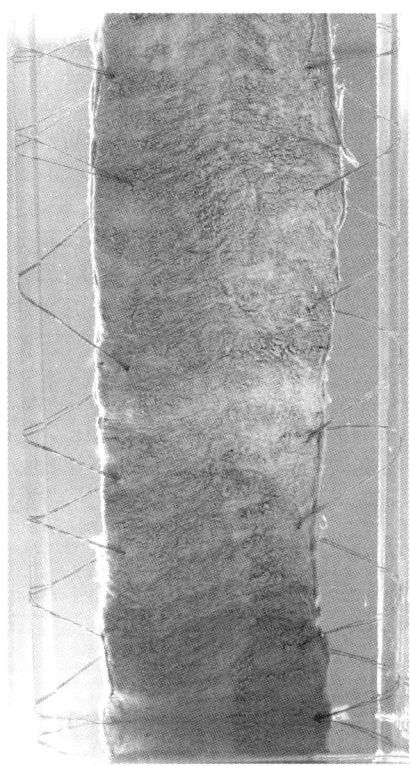

Figure 15-20 Bacillary dysentery, showing the pseudomembrane and irregular ulcers

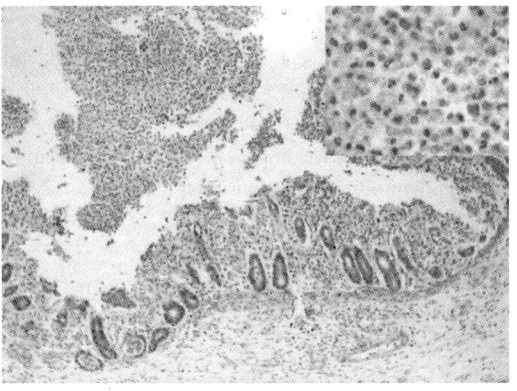

Figure 15-21 Bacillary dysentery, showing pseudomembrane (low power) and its compositions (high power)

● Gross pathological changes are mucosal edema, erythema, superficial ulceration, and focal mucosal hemorrhage involving the rectosigmoid junction primarily. Microscopic pathological changes consist of epithelial cell necrosis, polymorphonuclear infiltrates and mononuclear infiltrates in lamina propria, and crypt abscess formation. It features distinctive pseudomembranous and ulceration, and eventually resolves with healing. The pseudomembrane, which showing as gray-white, consists of fibrin, necrotic tissue, nentrophil cells, erythrocyte and bacilli. Ulceration following the shedding of presudmembrane is showing different size and shape, like map. Hemorrhages can occur.

● Clinically, it is characterized by sudden onset high fever, abdominal pain, severe diarrhea, tenesmus, and neutrophilic leukocytosis. The diarrhea is watery, and within a few days it becomes more solid with mucus and blood in the stool. Passage of 10-40 stools per day is usual. Individual stools are of small volume and often composed entirely of blood, mucus, and the inflammatory exudation, occasionally accompanying lamellar pseudmembrane.

B. Chronical Bacillary Dysentery

● This status is usually transformed from acute bacillary dysentery. The course may last several months, even several years. Most cases are infected by *S. flexneri*.

● There are new lesions and old lesion in the intestine. Pseudomembrane and ulceration can be seen in disease area. The ulcers featured by its edges, which show irregular due to iterative regeneration to repair. Polypi is also formed because of excessive hyperplasia in mucosa. Lymphocytes, plasma cells and sometime the neutrophilic leukocytes can be seen in the disease district. Some of disease intestinal wall are fibrosis, which result in the wall irregular thicken and hard, and may cause stenosis of enteric cavity.

● The patients have mild symptom of abdominal pain, abdominal distension and diarrhea. Some time, the inflammation turn to acute, and the symptoms intensify. Some cases lack symptoms or signs, but the bacillary culture from the stool is persistent positive. This kind of patient is a chronic carrier and an important infectious source.

C. Toxic Bacillary Dysentery

The features of this type are:
● It sudden onset with severe systemic toxic symptom and mild symptom of intestine. Toxic shock or respiratory failure will occur in several hours after onset and can lead to death.
● Children at the age of 2-7 years old are sensible to this type.
● Most cases are result from the *Shigella* species of *S. sonnei* and *S. flexneri*.

Complications and Prognosis

A. Complications

Infection with *Shigella* species may be associated with extragastrointestinal complications.
● Bacteremia and septicemia occurs primarily in malnourished children and carries a mortality rate of 20% as a result of renal failure, hemolysis, thrombocytopenia, gastrointestinal hemorrhage, and shock.
● Hemolytic uremic syndrome (associated with strains that produce Shiga toxin, e. g. *S dysenteriae*) may complicate infections with *Shigella* species and *Escherichia coli*, and it carries a mortality rate greater than 50%. Hemolytic uremic syndrome is characterized by acute hemolysis, renal failure, uremia, and disseminated intravascular coagulation.
● Central nervous system lesions.
● Myocarditis.

B. Prognosis

Postinfection carriage generally is less than 3-4 weeks. Mild cramps and diarrhea may continue for many days to weeks after treatment. Most patients can recover even without treatment, although illness is more prolonged and severe if not treated. Usually, the fever defervescences within 24 hours. Frequency of stool deceases within 2-3 days.

The overall mortality rate in developed countries is less than 1%. In the Far East and Middle East, the mortality rates for infections of *S dysenteriae* may be as high as 20%-25%.

LEPROSY

Leprosy is a chronic infectious granulomatous disease caused by Mycobacterium leprae. It is also called Hansen's disease. It is transmitted by person to person with low infectivity rates. It affects chiefly the cooler parts of the body, principally the skin and peripheral nervous system. It is a common disease in tropical and subtropic countries. Most patients are found in Asia. Worldwide, 80% of the cases are found in 5 countries: India, Myanmar, Indonesia, Brazil, and Nigeria. It is rare in Western communities.

Etiology and Pathogenesis

Mycobacterium leprae is an acid-fast bacillus, which has the same morphological characteristics as other mycobacteria, such as Mycobacterium tuberculosis, but more easily decolourized by acid necessitating, Wade-Fite stain, a modification of the Ziehl-Neelsen stain for identification. The organism is an obligate intracellular parasite and cannot be cultured but can proliferate in the footpad of the mouse and nine-banded armadillo.

There are two basic extremes of leprosy, tuberculoid leprosy and lepromatous Leprosy. Different kinds of leprosy are of different pathogenesis. And the body response to infection by Mycobacterium leprae is variable depending on the degree of T cell mediated response.

Tuberculoid leprosy occurs in patients who build up a good T cell response to the bacillus, which is localized to the area of entry. So the bacteremia spread is rare and the number of lesions is small. Involvement of large peripheral nerves (ulnar, common peroneal, greater auricular) produces palpable thickening and nerve palsies. Tuberculoid leprosy has a slowly progressive course naturally. It can be successfully treated now.

Lepromatous leprosy occurs in patients who have a low level of cellular immunity. In the absence of an effective T cell response, the bacillus multiplies unchecked in skin macrophages, forming large foamy lepra cells where many acid-fast bacilli are found. Aggregation of macrophages causes thickening and nodularity of the skin. The bacillus can also spreads via the blood stream, result in widespread lesions in the skin, eye, upper respiratory tract, and testis. Leprosy bacilli prefer to grow at temperatures less than 37℃, so the internal viscera such as the spleen and liver are rarely involved. Mycobacterium leprae can causes extensive destruction of tissue, such as fingers, nose, and ears, and produces marked disfigurement. Therapy is unsatisfactory.

Intermediate forms of tissue response exist with those more closely resembling the lepromatous form containing more bacteria.

Morphological Changes

The sites that the *mycobacterium leprae* invaded are principally the skin, nasal mucosa, peripheral nerves and testis. Based on the characteristics of pathology, leprosy can be divided as three main types, tuberculous leprosy, Lepromatous leprosy and Borderline Leprosy.

A. Tuberculous Leprosy

The characteristics of tuberculous leprosy is that the production of epithelioid cell granulomas, which usually are arranged in clusters or cords and may or may not contain giant cells of Langhans' type. Tuberculoid leprosy of the skin histopathologically resembles Boeck's sarcoid, tuberculosis without caseation, and other diseases in which the host reaction is that of epithelioid granulomas with Langhans' giant cells. In contrast to lepromatous lesions, there is no "clear zone" between the infiltrate and the overlying epidermis.

The skin lesion is characterized histologically by epithelioid cell granulomas, numerous lymphocytes, and small numbers of leprosy bacilli. Scantier lesions but peripheral nerve involvement is common. Histologically there are tightly packed organized granulomas without caseation. Lymphocytes are numerous. Bacteria are very difficult to identify. Cutaneous hypersensitivity can be demonstrated showing that there is some cell-mediated immunity.

In this form of the disease, small dermal nerves generally show severe histopathologic involvement. The infiltrate of the small nerves may consist of epithelioid cells or cells indistinguishable from lymphocytes. In tuberculoid lesions of the skin, nerve destruction occurs early. Therefore, in more advanced lesions, no nerves may be seen in the histopathologic sections. The absence of nerves in a granulomatous skin lesion should cause a pathologist to suspect leprosy. In the chronic tuberculoid lesion, bacilli, if present, are usually within small nerves, and only two or three bacilli may be found in an entire section. In reactive tuberculoid leprosy, however, a fairly large number of bacilli may be observed in the edematous epithelioid cell infiltrate as well as in the nerves.

B. Lepromatous Leprosy

In the type of leprosy widespread lesions are present in the skin and mucous membranes. These lesions contain large numbers of foamy macrophages, some lymphocytes, plasma cells and mast cells, which consist of nodules. The nodules in skin may break, resulting in ulceration. Enormous numbers of bacilli are present in the macrophages. Macrophages on "aging" contain many bacilli and exhibit lipid vacuolization. The name Virchow lepra cell is commonly applied to these old, foamy macrophages (Figures 15-22, 15-23). Acid-fast-stained slides, in the moderately advanced and advanced lesions demonstrate numerous bacilli within the macrophages, which are called lepra cells, or Virchow lepra. Characteristically, bacilli are frequently arranged in parallel or cigarette packs, and in the older lesions it can be seen in compact globular masses (globi). When the cell walls are destroyed, the freed bacilli may coalesce to form large compact rounded masses that frequently are found in foreign " body giant cells. The bacilli generally are present in large numbers within the small skin nerves. The infected nerves may show very little histopathologic change other than the increased number of macrophages and Schwann cells in which the bacilli are found. Bacilli may be seen in macrophages, in the endothelial cells of blood vessels, and in the epithelial cells of hair follicles, but are rarely observed within the cells of sweat and sebaceous glands.

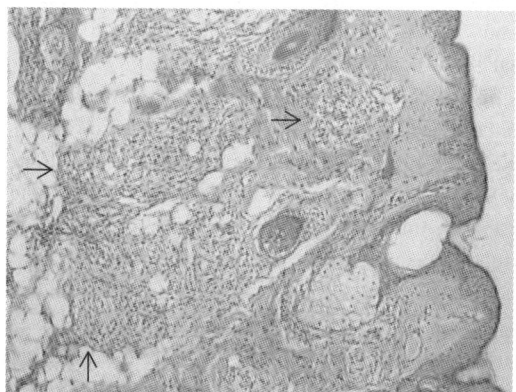

Figure 15-22 Lepromatous leprosy, showing nodules of lepromatous leprosy (low power)

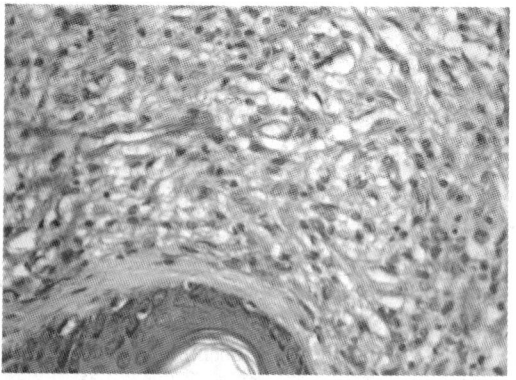

Figure 15-23 Lepromatous leprosy, showing Virchow lepra cell, the foamy macrophages (high power)

Other special changes of lepromatous leprosy:
- Erythema nodosum leprosum: In some lepromatous leprosy, the immune reaction may result in immune complexes being deposited in small subcutaneous blood vessel walls causing inflammation of the subcutaneous fat, the panniculitis, which are painful nodules in skin show as tender erythematous, with large numbers of macrophages (containing numerous leprosy bacilli), neutrophils infiltration, and an acute vasculitis involving dermal and subcutaneous arterioles.
- Lucio's phenomenon: A flare-up vasculitis that occurs in some patients with lepromatous leprosy. It is thought that the immune complex deposition due to type III hypersensitivity in small to medium sized arteries run it. It is characterized by the presence of numerous bacilli in the vessel wall, marked intimal fibrosis, and narrowing of the lumen. Ischemic changes may occur due to that the arteries are involved.

C. Borderline Leprosy

Borderline leprosy has features intermediate between lepromatous and tuberculoid leprosy. A single slide of borderline may contain infiltrates of lepra cells containing many bacilli and focal aggregates of epithelioid cells with few bacilli. The nerves may reveal varying degrees of cellular involvement and usually contain bacilli.

Clinical Feature, Complication and Prognosis

A. Clinical Features (Table 15-1)

The clinicopathologic features of leprosy are dependent on the immunologic reactivity of the host to the leprosy bacillus. There is a spectrum of disease pattern ranging from tuberculoid to lepromatous, with borderline an intermediate pattern. In the table, the lepromin test consists of an intradermal injection of Mycobacterium leprae antigens. A positive response (e.g. induration) indicates the presence of type IV hypersensitivity against leprosy antigens.

Except above, other clinical features are that: (1) In advanced lesions, the epidermis is thinned over nodular lesions, fete pegs are absent, and papillae are flattened; (2) Because the large peripheral nerves is involvement, leading to nerve palsies, wrist drop and foot drop are common presenting features.

Table 15-1 Clinicopathologic types of leprosy (from concise pathology)

Items	Lepromatous	Borderline	Tuberculoid
Cell-mediated immunity	Deficient	Intermediate	Present
Lepromin test	Negative	Positive or negative	Positive
Number of lesions	Numerous	Many	Few
Visceral lesions	Common	Uncommon	Absent
Skin lesion appearance	Nodular	Variable	Macular
Hypoesthesia of lesions	Rare	Rare	Common
Number of lymphocytes	Few	Intermediate	Numerous
Number of organisms	Numerous	Many	Few
Lepra cells	Numerous	Present	Absent
Distribution of macrophages	Diffuse	Aggregates	Granulomas
Erythema nodosum leprosum	Common	Common	Rare

B. Complications

- Deformities: These complications are most due to neuropathy. The effects include crippling deformities of the hand, contractures due to paralysis, and recurrent injuries to the hands, feet, and eyes due to insensitivity, separately leading to progressive absorption of the extremities, to the blindness, and to the formation of lagophthalmos, ectropion, and entropion. These commonly show as ulcerations on the plantar surfaces and sides of the feet and toes and on the hands. Shortening of digits on feet and hands may occur as a result of destructive osteomyelitis. Contractures can develop and result in fixation.
- Lucio phenomenon: It is characterized by thrombosis of the deep subcutaneous arteries resulting in necrosis of the skin and subcutaneous fat. The underlying tendons and muscles may be exposed. The outcome is often fatal.
- Secondary amyloidosis.

C. Prognosis

If severe and left untreated, leprosy can cause significant debilitating deformity. So, the prognosis depends on the stage of disease. In borderline cases, the disease has the potential to be down-graded to LL; these patients may have nerve damage. Even with corticosteroid treatment, neuritis may not be curable.

The prognosis also depends on the patient's access to therapy, the patient's compliance, and the early initiation of treatment. Since 1943, when sulfone was introduced as the first effective treatment for leprosy, antibiotic treatment has dramatically improved patients' outcomes. Early diagnosis and effective antimicrobial treatment can arrest and even cure the disease.

Progression of tissue and nerve damage can be limited, but recovery of lost sensory and motor function is variable and generally incomplete. Hyperpigmentation, hypopigmentation, and loss of skin organs persist.

LEPTOSPIROSIS

Leptospirosis is an infectious disease caused by the genus Leptospira. It affects both humans and animals, and is considered the most common zoonotic disease in the world. Leptospirosis is often referred to as swineherd's disease, swamp fever, or mud fever. The important disease of humans caused by the group of Leptospira is Weirs disease, while canicola fever, swineherd's disease, mud fever, Fort Bragg fever, rice field fever and cane field fever are less common. The infection is usually transmitted by contaminated water with urine and feces from patients or ill animals suffered from the Leptospirosis. It causes a systemic illness that often leads to renal and hepatic dysfunction. Some of the leptospiroses have a worldwide distribution, but others are limited to Australia, South America, and Japan. Leptospirosis may be spread epidemically in large populations in conditions of widespread flooding during the summer months when heavy rains and floods occur. The majorities of cases occur in the warm season and in rural areas because leptospires can persist in water for many months.

Etiology

Leptospirosis is caused by pathogenic spiral bacteria, which belonging to the genus *Leptospira*, the family *Leptospiraceae* and the order Spirochaetales. These spirochetes are finely coiled, thin, motile, obligate, slow-growing anaerobes. They differ from the other spirochetes morphologically in that they are generally smaller and slimmer and their spirals are very fine and close. They can be readily cultivated and produce high titers of agglutinating complement-fixing antibodies. Their flagella allow them to burrow into tissue. The genus *Leptospira* was originally thought to comprise only 2 species, *L interrogans*, which is pathogenic, and *L biflexa*, which is saprophytic. More recent work has identified 7 distinct species of pathogenic leptospires, which appear as more than 250 serologic variants (serovars). They survive best in fresh water, damp alkaline soil, vegetation, and mud with temperatures higher than 22℃.

Chain of Infection

A. Sources of Infection

Natural hosts are usually various domestic and wild animals, such as the dog, horse, pig, skunk, raccoon, and various rodents. Urinary shedding of organisms from these infected animals is the most important infectious source of these pathogens. Contact with the organism via infected urine or urine-contaminated media results in human infection. Such media include animal bedding, soil, mud, and aborted tissue.

B. Routes of Infection

The organism enters the body via abraded skin or mucous membranes, such as the conjunctiva or alimentary tract. In some status, the organism may even enter the body through intact skin. Infection has occurred after animal and rodent bites, after contact with abortion products of infected animals, after ingestion of contaminated food and water, and after contact with contaminated environmental sources.

C. Susceptibility Herd

Occupational exposure probably accounts for 30%–50% of human cases. The main occupational groups at risk include farm workers, veterinarians, pet shop owners, field agricultural workers, abattoir workers, plumbers, meat handlers and slaughterhouse workers, coal miners, workers in the fishing industry, military troops, milkers, livestock workers and sewer workers.

Infected rats may contaminate sewer water. Partial or total immersion in mud and water plays a role in facilitating infection in sewer workers and rice-field workers.

Pathogenesis and Pathological Changes

After the organism gains entry via skin or mucosa, the organism multiplies in blood and tissue, which result in leptospiremia and spread to the body, particularly to the kidney and liver.

When the organism get into the kidney, it migrates to the interstitium, renal tubules, and tubular lumen and causes acute interstitial nephritis and marked tubular degeneration and necrosis accompanied by glomerular and interstitial hemorrhages. The kidneys are enlarged and edematous. For renal failure develop, it usually is due to tubular damage, but hypovolemia from dehydration and from altered capillary permeability also can contribute to renal failure.

The most important organ affected is the liver, which is enlarged and of deep greenish yellow color. Severe liver cell degeneration, with centrilobular necrosis, bile stasis, and parenchymal hemorrhages, proliferation of Kupffer cells can be observed. Jaundice may occur as a result of hepatocellular dysfunction.

Leptospires also may invade voluntary muscles, as well as the heart muscle, causing inflammation, vacuolization of myofibrils, and focal necrosis. And there is a heavy infiltrate of both lymphocytes and plasma cells. Muscular microcirculation is impaired and capillary permeability is increased, with resultant fluid leakage showing as edema and circulatory hypovolemia.

In severe disease, a disseminated vasculitic syndrome may result from damage to the capillary endothelium.

The central nervous system shows perivascular infiltration of lymphocytes and chromatolysis with neuronophagia of the neurons. There may be a mild leptomeningitis of the lymphocytic type.

Leptospires may invade the aqueous humor of the eye, where they may persist for many months, occasionally leading to chronic or recurrent uveitis.

Despite the possibility of severe complications,

the disease is most often self-limited and nonfatal. Over time, a systemic immune response may eliminate the organism from the body, but it also may lead to a symptomatic inflammatory reaction that can produce secondary end-organ injury.

It should be stressed that the organisms of spirochetes can be demonstrated by the silver impregnation technique in various organs, particularly in the kidney. Spirochetes can also be found in abundance in the blood during the first stage and in the urine during the second stage.

Clinical and Prognosis

A. Clinical Features

The incubation period of leptospirosis is usually 7 – 12 days, with a range of 2 – 20 days. The patient is characterized by fever, chills, weakness, bleeding, myalgias, petechiae, purpura, ecchymosis, splenomegaly, abdominal tenderness, subconjunctival suffusion, pharyngeal injection, splenomegaly, hepatomegaly, mild jaundice, muscle tendernes, maculopapular, erythematous, urticarial, or hemorrhagic rash. Other symptoms are sore throat, cough, chest pain, hemoptysis, rash, dyspnea, respiratory distress, frontal headache, photophobia, mental confusion, and the symptoms of meningitis, etc. Many patients (77%) experience headache, which is intense and poorly controlled by analgesics. Aseptic meningitis is the most important clinical syndrome.

Some patients show as Weil syndrome. This severe form of leptospirosis primarily manifests as profound jaundice, renal dysfunction, hepatic necrosis, pulmonary dysfunction, and hemorrhagic diathesis. Patient's condition can deteriorate suddenly at any time.

B. Prognosis

Most patients suffer from leptospirosis can recover. For elderly patients and pregnant women, the mortality rates are high. Patients with hepatic dysfunction and renal failure have a good chance of recovering renal and hepatic dysfunction. Weil syndrome carries a mortality rate of 5% – 10%. The most severe cases of Weil syndrome, with hepatorenal involvement and jaundice, carry a case-fatality rate of 20% – 40%.

EPIDEMIC HEMORRHAGIC FEVER

Epidemic hemorrhagic fever (EHF) is an infectious disease featured by fever, hemorrhagic and renal failure and caused by the genus *Hantavirus*. Hemorrhagic fever with renal failure syndrome (HFRS) occurs mainly in Europe and Asia. Airborne contact with secretions from rodent hosts infected with the genus Hantavirus can cause EHF. It was initially recognized between 1913 and 1930 by Soviet scientists and came to the attention of the western world in 1950 when American soldiers in Korea developed a febrile illness associated with shock, hemorrhage, and renal failure. In 1993, an outbreak of respiratory illness in the southwestern United States caused by the *Sin Nombre* virus belonging to the Hantavirus genus occurred and is described as the *Hantavirus* pulmonary syndrome (HPS). The severe HFRS is in China, Japan, and Singapore, but the milder HFRS is in Sweden, Finland, Norway and Denmark. The number of cases reported in China is approximately 100,000 – 250,000 per year. The disease is observed throughout the year. The mortality and morbidity rates vary from 5% – 15%.

Etiology

A group of viruses belonged to the genus *Hantavirus* of the family Bunyaviridae cause different forms of HFRS. The severity of the illness depends on the infected virus type.

Korean hemorrhagic fever, a severe type of HFRS observed in Asia, is caused by the Hantavirus and is transmitted by the infected *Apodemus agrarius* (striped field mouse).

Balkan hemorrhagic fever, a severe type of HFRS observed in Balkan countries, is caused by the Dobrava virus and is transmitted by the infected *Apodemus flavicollis* (yellow-necked field mouse).

A mild-to-moderate form of HFRS is caused by the Seoul virus and is transmitted by the infected *Rattus rattus* (black rat) or the *Rattus novergicus* (urban rat).

Nephropathia epidemica (NE), a mild form of HFRS observed in Europe, is caused by the Puumala virus and is transmitted by the infected *Clethrionomys glariolus* (European bank vole).

Pathogeneses and Pathological Changes

The pathogenesis is in study and it is still largely unknown, but some studies suggest that immune reaction play a significant role. It is found that the marked cytokine production, kallikrein-kinin activation, complement pathway activation, and an increasing in circulating immune complexes occur following the infection. These components play an important role to the febrile and hypotension of the disease. It was reported that the nitric oxide production increased during the acute phase of the illness, and the level of nitric oxide are correlated with the disease.

Damage to the vascular endothelium, capillary dilatation, and leakage are significant features of the disease. That result in the hemorrhage. So the hemorrhage can be observed in different organs, especially in renal, lung, heart (intraventricular and the right atrium), pancreas, brain, adrenal glands, and elsewhere. Larger extravasates of blood are sometimes found in the pituitary gland and in the right auricle. The hemorrhage in skin shows as petechia like.

Except the widely hemorrhage, the kidneys show first to marked subcortical congestion, with variable degrees of stasis of blood, and then in HFRS exhibited as alterations, which are featured by acute interstitial nephritis, including acute tubular necrosis and damage of glomerular and endothelia. Hemorrhagic necrosis can be identified in renal medulla (Figure 15-24).

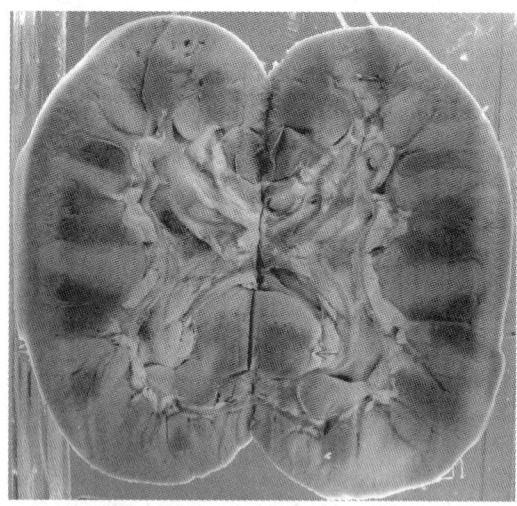

Figure 15-24 Epidemic hemorrhagic fevers, showing hemorrhage in renal medulla

Pulmonary infiltrates may be observed, and, occasionally, pulmonary edema is present.

The pituitary lesion was associated with necrosis, particularly in the anterior portion. There was generalized, intense capillary congestion.

Infiltration of large atypical mononuclear cells in the spleen, lymph node, and hepatic portal triad has been reported.

Clinical and Prognosis

A. Clinical Features

The patients progress the follow 5 stage. First, the febrile stage, which lasts about 4 - 6 days, an abrupt onset of fever of 40℃ occurs. Patients may complain of headache, chills, abdominal pain, and malaise. Flushing of the face, neck and chest, and petechia in the axilla and soft palate, subconjunctival hemorrhage and absolute bradycardia may be observed. Leucocytosis with thrombocytopenia usually occurs. Proteinuria may be onset. Following the hypotensive stage lasts approximately a few hours to 2 days. It coincides with defervescence. Patients may have tachycardia, acute abdomen caused by a paralytic ileus or convulsions or purposeless movements. The coagulation profile may include prolonged bleeding time, elevated prothrombin time, and activated thromboplastin time. The oliguric stage followed lasts about 3 - 6 days, featured by oliguria, hypertension, bleeding tendency caused by uremia, edema, and sometime pulmonary edema. After the followed diuretic stage, which lasts 2 - 3 weeks, and the Diuresis range between 3 to 6 L/d, which lead to rapid signs of dehydration and may be severe shock, it progress to the convalescent stage, patients recover gradually, which may be 3 to 6 months.

B. Complications

The complications are rare. During the oliguric or early diuretic phase, renal rupture may occur in some patients. Pulmonary edema and intraventricular hemorrhage can also occur. Pituitary hormonal can lead to delayed diuresis and late appearance of Sheehan syndrome.

C. Prognosis

The mortality and morbidity rates vary from 5% - 15%, mainly depending on the strain of the virus. HFRS is a self-limiting disease, and most patients can recover without any sequelae. Clinical recovery usually begins in the middle of the second week, with gradual resolution of symptoms and azotemia. In few residual patients, neurological and renal tubular defects may persist. Some of the patients are of increased sodium excretion because defective sodium reabsorption occurs. The renal tubular concentrating capacity recovers over many months. Chronic renal insufficiency and hypertensive renal disease have been reported. Approximately 10% of adult patients with end-stage renal disease (ESRD) have shown to have hantaviral-specific antibodies.

SEXUALLY TRANSMITTED DISEASE

Sexually transmitted diseases (STDs) is a group infectious disease which is transmitted by sex intersection or its related contact action. Traditionally, it mainly include gonorrhea, non-gonococcal urethritis, condyloma acuminatum, syphilis, herpes genitalis, chancroid, lymphogranuloma venereum, and granuloma inguinale, which are called veneral diseases. More recently, HIV, hepatitis B, and human papillomavirus infection have been included in this group. The increasing in the incidence of sexually transmitted diseases has now resulted in major public health problems. In this section, only the very common traditional sexually transmitted diseases, include gonorrhea, condyloma acuminatum and, syphilis, will discussed.

GONORRHEA

Gonorrhea is a purulent inflammation of mucous membrane surfaces caused by a sexually transmitted microorganism, *Neisseria gonorrhoeae*. It causes urethritis, cervicitis, epididymitis, pharyngitis, proctitis, and pelvic inflammatory disease. Virtually any mucous membrane can be infected and it can spread throughout the body to cause both localized and disseminated disease. It is one of the most common and widespread STD and can be observed in all parts of the world. Approximately 200 million new cases of gonorrhea appear each year in the world. Gonorrhea has a high prevalence in teenagers in large cities, in nonwhites, in drug abusers, and among lower socioeconomic groups.

The common presentation in men is with dysuria and purulent urethral discharge. Cervicitis may produce a vaginal discharge in women. In both sexes', gonorrhea may be asymptomatic, constituting a source of apparently healthy carriers, who is the main reason why the disease is difficult to control. The risk of infection during a single act of unprotected intercourse with an infected partner is estimated to be 20%–30%.

Etiology and Pathogenesis

Etiology: Gonorrhea is caused by *Neisseria gonorrhoeae* belonging to the genus *Neisseria*. It was detected by Neisser in 1879 in the exudate from gonorrheal lesions. Under the microscope, the organism appears as a Gram-negative diplococcus with the adjacent sides flattened and with the long axis vertical to the plane of junction. In infected men, the organism usually can be detected from the purulent discharge of the acute urethritis, and in the chronic stage of the disease it can be found in the secretion obtained from prostatic massage. In infected women, it is usually contained in the discharge from the urethra or cervix. In acute cases, gonococci may be found both extracellularly and intracellularly, but they are often obscured by the presence of other organisms, particularly the very similar *Mimea herellea*. Failure to detect gonococci is often due to inadequate methods of obtaining smears, and fresh material always must be examined. In case of doubt, culture methods should be used, which make it possible to increase up to 50% the number of cases in which gonococci can be successfully demonstrated. A distinct diagnostic advance is the use of the immunofluorescent method for the detection of gonococci. Not only is it more rapid than culture methods, but it also possesses a greater sensitivity. Indeed, by this method it was possible to detect gonococci in 80% of female contacts with known gonorrhea.

Pathological Changes

In men, the organism infects chiefly the urethra, producing acute urethritis. The prostate, seminal vesicles, and epididymis are commonly involved, causing suppurative acute inflammation followed by fibrosis and sometimes sterility. In women, the cervix is the main site of infection. The urethra, Bartholin's and Skene's glands, and the uterine tubes are commonly involved. Salpingitis, a kind of pelvic inflammatory disease, leads to fibrosis of the uterine tube, causing infertility and an increased risk of ectopic pregnancy.

The histopathology of an acute gonorrheal infection consists of a nonspecific purulent inflammatory process that is usually limited to the superficial layers of the affected mucous membrane. Extensive ulcerations are usually absent. The histopathology of chronic gonorrhea consists in the development of a nonspecific pyogenic granulation tissue that later leads to extensive fibrosis and the formation of strictures or adhesions. Purulent processes observed in the epididymis and the fallopian tube is often either sterile or contaminated with secondary invaders – mainly *staphylococci* or *Escherichia coil*.

The infection can occurs also at other sites in the genital tract. And with varied sexual methods, gonococcal pharyngitis and anal gonorrhea may occur. Gonococcal proctitis is frequent in sexually active male homosexuals.

Entry of gonococci into the pelvic peritoneum in the female via the uterine tubes may cause peritonitis. Perihepatitis, manifested by right upper quadrant pain and a hepatic friction rub (Fitz-Hugh and Curtis syndrome) is recognized. Entry of gonococci into the bloodstream may cause (1) bacteremia, with fever and a skin rash; (2) gonococcal endocarditis, which tends to affect both the right- and left-sided valves of the heart; and (3) gonococcal arthritis, frequently moarticular, affecting large joints, most commonly the knee joint.

In addition, gonocoecal infection may be transmitted to the fetus during delivery through the birth canal, producing neonatal ophthalmitis, the end result of which is often blindness.

Pathological Development and Clinical Related Feature

Pathologic lesions. The incubation period of gonorrhea varies with the virulence of the organism. But, as a rule, symptoms appear two to ten days after contact. In men, there is usually a burning sensation in the urethra, aggravated by urination and accompanied by the appearance of a purulent exudation at the urethral orifice. The inflammatory process is often limited to the mucous membrane of the anterior portion of the urethra but may extend beyond its usual confines and involve the posterior portion, leading to prostatitis and vesiculitis. Finally, the infection may spread along the vas deferens, causing very painful epididymitis. The infection in the prostate and seminal vesicles may become chronic and lead to abscess formation. Destruction of the epididymis by the inflammatory process may lead to sterility. One of the more common complications of gonorrhea is a deep infiltration of the urethra followed by scarring and the development of a stricture.

The first symptom of acute gonorrhea in women is usually the appearance of an irritating discharge, with a burning sensation on urination and swelling of the infected Bartholin glands. More often, however, the acute infected woman has very little discomfort, so that she may be unaware of the disease. In uncomplicated cases, the infection usually remains limited to the superficial layers of the urethral and cervical mucosae, and the purulent discharge may gradually subside. During pregnancy or immediately after delivery, the gonorrheal infection may invade the endometrium and from there spread to the fallopian tubes, where it produces an acute purulent salpingitis. This may lead to unilateral or bilateral tubo-ovarian abscesses, followed by pelvic or generalized peritonitis that may prove fatal. In chronic cases, there will be severe pelvic and back pain and destruction of the tubal mucosa, which will lead to pyosalpinx and the formation of tubo-ovarian abscesses. If the pelvic peritoneum is involved, pus may accumulate in the space of Douglas, and the inflammatory process may lead to the formation of a mass of adhesions involving all pelvic organs, a condition known as chronic pelvic inflammatory disease. Eventually the patient becomes a chronic invalid, suffering from severe pain, menstrual disturbances, premature cessation of ovarian function, and sterility.

Invasion of the bloodstream by the gonococci takes place during the acute or chronic stage of the disease. A frequently observed extragenital manifestation is gonorrheal arthritis, which often appears in the form of a monarthritis affecting a single large joint such as the knee joint. The organisms can be detected in the purulent exudation. Less commonly observed systemic manifestations of gonorrhea include the appearance of skin lesions, bacterial endocarditis, and general peritonitis.

Young infants may be infected by contact with the infectious discharge from the mother during the birth process, or they may be contaminated by infected hands, towels, etc. The two most important manifestations are a severe purulent conjunctivitis, which may lead to the formation of corneal ulcers and blindness, and acute purulent vulvovaginitis and proctitis.

Diagnosis

Identification of asymptomatic carriers by tracing sexual contacts of newly infected symptomatic patients is crucial. The diagnosis of gonorrhea is made by direct smear of the urethral or vaginal discharge. Gram staining reveals gram-negative diplococci both extracellularly and inside neutrophils. The diagnosis should be confirmed by culture, which is essential because *Neisseria* species other than gonococci may be present as commensals in the vagina.

Complication and Prognosis

A. Complication

- Scarring of the upper reproductive tract in women with PID possibly leading to infertility, chronic pelvic pain, and ectopic pregnancy. Ectopic pregnancy is a life-threatening complication.
- Urethral scarring in men possibly leading to decreased fertility or to bladder-outlet obstruction.
- Disseminated infection may lead to meningitis or endocarditis, which may result in permanent neurologic sequelae or destruction of cardiac valves, which can leading to congestive heart failure and death.
- In pregnant women, it is possible to result in prematurity, neonatal infection, and miscarriage.
- It is possible to lead to corneal scarring and permanent vision impairment or blindness resulting.
- It is possible to lead to sepsis in infants following neonatal exposure to maternal gonorrhea.
- Destruction of joint articular surfaces.

B. Prognosis

Most gonococcal infections respond quickly to antibiotic therapy. Prognosis is excellent if the diagnosis is made and treatment is started and completed before progression or complications occur.

The prognosis for patients with gonorrhea is excellent if the diagnosis is made and treatment is started before progression or complications occur.

CONDYLOMA ACUMINATA

Condyloma acuminata, also called venereal warts or genital warts, is a kind of STD caused by human papillomavirus (HPV), mainly the HPV 6 and HPV 11. Local infections appear as warty papillary condylomatous lesions. Approximately two thirds of individuals who have sexual contact with an infected partner develop genital warts. A 4 fold or more increase in prevalence has been reported in the last 2 decades. An estimated 500,000 to 1 million new cases of genital warts are diagnosed each year. In adolescents and young adults, HPV may be the most common STD. Data from STD clinics indicates a prevalence rate of 4%–13%.

Etiology and Pathogenesis

A. Etiology

It is considered that several of the epidermotropic HPVs cause condyloma acuminata. This kind of virus was first recognized in 1907. With the development of molecular, it is found that HPV is a group of double-stranded DNA viruses. The genome encodes 6 early open reading frames (E1, E2, E4, E5, E6, and E7) and 2 late open reading frames (L1, L2). Today, more than 120 distinct HPV subtypes have been identified. Among them, about 60 different types of HPV can potentially infect the anogenital tract. HPV infections in the genital area are sexually transmitted. This group of viruses is linked to the development of cervical dysplasia, cervical cancer, and vulvar dysplasia.

B. Pathogenesis

This group of viruses can infect many different sites, including the perianal region, vulva, vagina, cervix, larynx, skin, mouth, esophagus, and the anogenital tract. As for the incubation time, most investigators believe that it is 3 months.

HPVs associated with genital tract lesions can be divided into low risk, moderate risk and high risk based on each genotype's association with benign or malignant lesions. Most genital condylomata are due to infection by HPV-6 or HPV-11, which are most commonly types isolated, and belong to low risk because these 2 types replicate as an episome and rarely incorporate their genetic material into the host DNA. Approximately 90% of condyloma acuminata are related to HPV types 6 and 11. Types 33, 35, 39, 40, 43, 45, 51-56 and 58 belong to moderate. Types 16 and 18 belong to high risk, which can be recovered in approximately 70% of squamous cell carcinomas of the cervix. These high-risk HPV types, along with types 31, 33, 45, 51, 52, 56, 58, and 59 incorporate a portion of their genetic material into the host DNA. The E6 and E7 genes can produce oncoproteins that alter cell growth regulation. Specifically, E6 oncoprotein inactivates the tumor suppressor gene p53, and the oncoprotein produced by E7 inactivates pRB (retinoblastoma). Male sexual partners of women with cervical intraepithelial neoplasia often have infections with the same viral type.

Cells of the basal layer of the epidermis are invaded by HPV. These viruses penetrate through skin and cause mucosal microabrasions. A latent viral phase begins with no signs or symptoms and can last from a month to several years. Following latency, production of viral DNA, capsids, and particles begins. Host cells become infected and develop the morphologic atypical koilocytosis of condyloma acuminata.

Consider sexual abuse as a possible underlying problem in pediatric patients; however, keep in mind that infection by direct manual contact or indirectly by fomites rarely may occur. Finally, passage through an infected vaginal canal at birth may cause respiratory lesions in infants.

Pathological Changes

A. Site

The most commonly affected areas are the penis, vulva, vagina, cervix, perineum, and perianal area. Uncommon mucosal lesions in the oropharynx, larynx, and trachea have been reported. HPV-6 even has been reported in other uncommon areas (e.g. extremities). Multiple simultaneous lesions are common and may involve subclinical states as well-differentiated anatomic sites.

B. Macroscopy

- On gross inspection, condyloma acuminatum is raspberry-shaped or cauliflower-shaped, usually located on the sulcus. The neoplasm may be a single or multiple or conglomerated papular eruptions. The eruptions may appear pearly, filiform, fungating, cauliflower, or plaquelike. They can be quite smooth, particularly on penile shaft, verrucous, or lobulated (Figure 15-25). Eruptions' color may be the same as the skin, or they may exhibit erythema or hyperpigmentation. Typical condyloma is usually a discrete papillary growth that arises from a single stalk. Condyloma acuminata can involve a large area in a sessile fashion.
- Subclinical infection is another common presentation of condyloma. Tiny, slightly raised areas can be felt or visualized on the vagina or cervix.
- These flat warts can be well visualized using 3%- 5% acetic acid and a colposcope. Areas infected with HPV appear acetowhite.

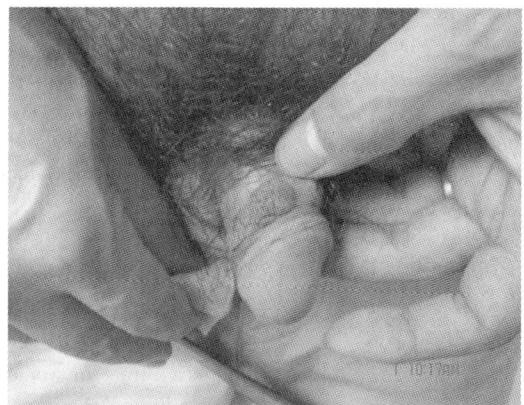

Figure 15-25 Condyloma acuminate, showing cauliflower-shaped in penis

C. Histopathological Findings

Microscopically, biopsy of the condyloma acuminatum show that it is essentially squamous papilloma-like characterized by marked hyperkeratosis, acanthosis and hyperplasia of the prickle cell layer. The papillae extend much deeper. Parakeratosis is present but normal. Koilocytosis, which is perinuclear cytoplasmic halos, is commonly observed in the superficial epithelial cells. The rete ridges are elongated and may be branching, but they all extend to about the same level (Figure 15-26). Mitoses, if exist, are limited to the basal layers. A chronic inflammatory infiltrate is often observed within the dermis. The growth is usually characteristically upward toward the surface and not downward into the tissue. Sometimes, the neoplasm is quite extensive. Clinically, they behave as cancer, and recurrence is the rule, but histologically they are benign.

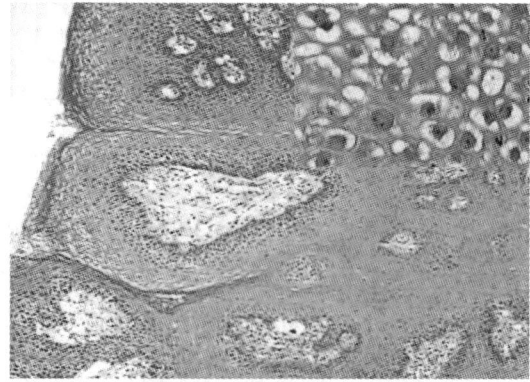

Figure 15-26 Condyloma acuminate, showing squamous papilloma-like structure (low power), koilocytes and koilocytosis (high power)

Clinical

Condyloma acuminatum is often asymptomatic. Pruritus or occasional bleeding may lead the patient to seek medical care. On gross inspection, it shows as above detailed on macroscopy.

Many investigators report that women in pregnant have higher rates of HPV infections. For pregnant patients of condyloma acuminata, the lesions may become activated with rapid growth, and the lesions often increase or tend to bleed easily, and may make vaginal delivery difficult if in cervix, vagina, or vulva. The responsible factors for these are considered to be the suppression of immunity and the hormonal changes during pregnancy. These lesions often spontaneously regress after delivery.

Pregnant women with genital warts can transmit the virus to the neonate. And the incidence of perinatal transmission to the infant pharynx can be as high as 50% and which occurs most frequently with HPV types 6 and 11. Incidence of genital infection in the neonate is 4%. The infants can develop laryngeal papillomatosis in the first 5 years. Approximately 60% of mothers with infants having laryngeal papillomatosis be reported suffering from genital warts.

Complication and Prognosis

A. Complication
- Disfigurement. Lesions can lead to local disfigurement of involved area(s).
- Transformation to malignancies. It is an important complication to the patients exposed HIV develop to dysplasia or squamous cell cancer. Most research indicates that HPV infection is strongly associated with the development of cervical dysplasia and cervical carcinoma. Approximately 90% of the risk for the development of cervical dysplasia attribute to HPV. Exposure to HPV is also associated with vaginal dysplasia.
- Transmission to neonate or partners.

B. Prognosis

In patients with immunologic deficiencies, HPV infection appears to be worse. Recurrence rates, size, discomfort, and risk of developing dysplasia or cancer of the vulva, vagina, cervix or penis are highest among those patients.

During pregnancy, the illness often becomes active and worse. Bleeding has been reported in large lesions. Cervical, vaginal, or vulvar condyloma acuminata may interfere with parturition.

Many patients fail to respond to treatment, or recur after adequate response to condyloma acuminata. Recurrence rates exceed 50% after 1 year.

Mortality is secondary to malignant transformation to carcinoma. Patients who are exposed to high-risk HPV types, such as HPV-16 and 18, are at high risk for developing high-grade dysplasias or carcinomas.

SYPHILIS

Syphilis is a common sexually transmitted infectious disease caused by *Treponema pallidum*, a spirochete. The attack rate of syphilis among sexual contacts of an infective person is around 50%. The organism can also be transmitted via placenta and blood to infect the unborn child.

Syphilis remains prevalent in many developing countries and in some areas of North America, Asia, and Europe, especially Eastern Europe. In some regions of Siberia, as of 1999, prevalence was 1300 cases per 100,000 population. The common age for contracting syphilis is shifting from the mid 20s to the teen years. Between 1977 and 1982, over 50% of all new cases were in homosexual males. The incidence in this population has declined sharply, largely because of changing sexual practices in response to the AIDS epidemic. Currently, syphilis has the highest incidence in heterosexuals in large cities, with most reported cases involving nonwhites from low socioeconomic groups. Routine testing of transfused blood and pregnant women for syphilis has resulted in a dramatic decline of transfusion syphilis and congenital syphilis.

Etiology and Pathogenesis

A. Etiology

The spirochaete *Treponema pallidum* is a delicate corkscrew-shaped bacillus (Figure 15-27), approximately 0.15 μm long and 6–50 μm in diameter. It can survive only briefly outside of the body; thus transmission almost always requires direct contact with the infectious lesion(s). The organism is sensitive to heat and cannot survive drying or exposure to disinfectants. Thus, fomite transmission, e.g. from toilet seats, is virtually impossible. And it cannot be cultured but can be maintained in the tissues of living animals such as rabbit testis. The organism can cross the placenta leading to the transplacental infection. It is solely a human pathogen and does not naturally occur in other species. The organism can be visualized in fluid taken from ulcerated lesions either by silver impregnation techniques or by using dark-field microscopy. There is an anti-phagocytic mucopolysaccharide capsule and the organism can down-regulate the T cell response.

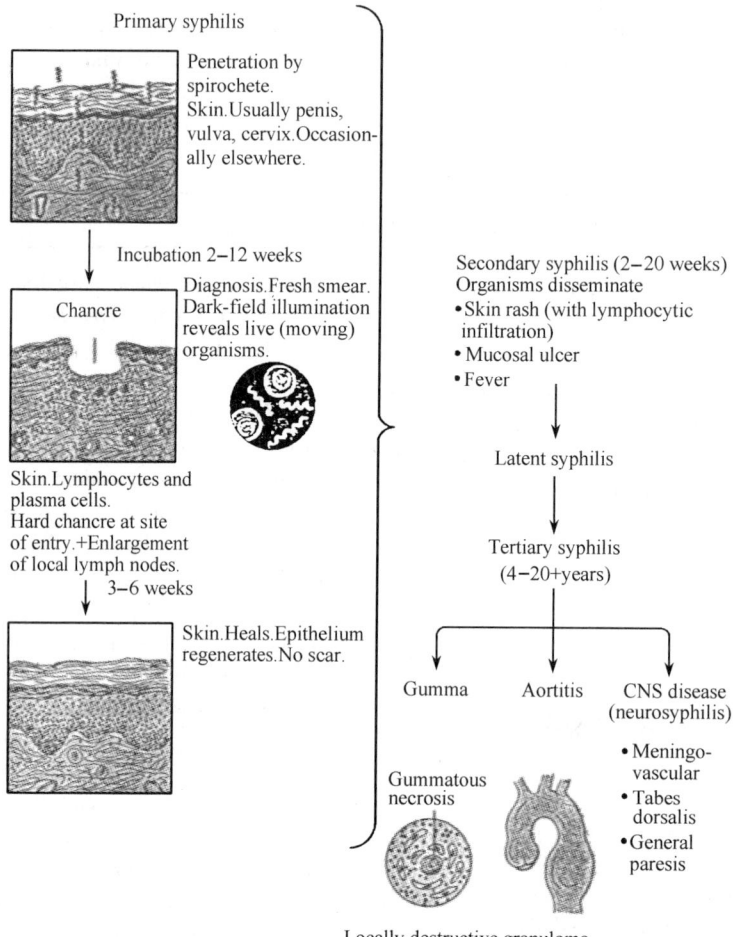

Figure 15-27   Course and pathologic features of syphilis

B. Pathogenesis

Based on the pathogenesis and development, syphilis can be classified as acquired syphilis and congenital syphilis. On acquired syphilis, it is transmitted in 3 ways. the first one is from intimate sexually contacting with infectious lesions, which is the most common way; the second is from blood transfusions; the third is transplacental from an infected mother to her fetus.

Transmission occurs by penetration of the spirochetes *T. pallidum* through mucosal membranes and abrasions on epithelial surfaces, although asymptomatically, via the blood vessels and lymphatics (Figure 15-27). Syphilis transmitted sexually requiring direct intimate contact because mucous membranes are the optimal sites of infection. Entry of the organism is facilitated by the presence of minute abrasions in the skin and mucous membranes. It cannot penetrate intact skin. It is heat and drying sensitive, so transmission on inanimate objects (e.g. tea cups) is unlikely.

Incubation time from exposure to development of primary lesions averages 3 weeks but can range from 9 - 90 days. During this time, the *T. pallidum* multiply locally and spread to lymph nodes and blood.

Within 1 - 3 weeks of the first lesion, the antibodies can be detected. Two groups of antibodies have been identified, one of which forms the basis of diagnostic tests: the VDRL (Venereal Disease Research Laboratory) and Wassermann reactions.

Wassermann reaction is an immune reaction by Wassermann antibodies (anti-cardiolipin), which is an IgM molecule reacting to cardiolipin. Not specific for syphilis and may be seen in association with malaria, leprosy, glandular fever, trypanosomiasis, other treponemal infections (yaws, pinta, bejel), mycoplasma pneumonia, some autoimmune haemolyic anaemias, sytemic lupus erythematosus, and after *Coxsackie B* infection. Cardiolipin has been shown to be present in *Treponema* which may act as the antigen but the antibodies do not react with the intact organism.

As for congenital syphilis, it is the transplacentally transmitted result from an infected mother to her fetus.

Pathological Changes

There are two basic tissue responses, which are small blood vessel changes and Gummatous necrosis

A. Gumma

Gumma is a localized destructive granuloma. It is also called syphiloma. It may occur anywhere in the body with predilection for the skin, liver, bone, testis, subcutaneous tissue and oral cavity. Grossly, it produces a large mass that may be mistaken for a neoplasm (Figure 15-28). It is an area of rubbery coagulative necrosis (Figure 15-29). Microscopically a gumma is composed of a central area of gummatous (rubbery) necrosis, surrounded by epithelioid cells, lymphocytes, numerous plasma cells, and plump fibrosis. Spirochetes cannot usually be demonstrated in gummas. Blood vessels in the periphery show narrowing of the lumen (Figure 15-30). *Treponemas* are very scanty. It is considered that type IV immunologic hypersensitivity is probably involved in the pathogenesis of the granuloma.

B. Small Blood Vessel Disease

These include obliterative endarteritis and periangiitis. The prominent histologic features of the human response to the presence of *T. pallidum* are vascular changes with associated endarteritis and periarteritis. There is periadventitial cuffing by lymphocytes and plasma cells. Endothelial cells swell and may proliferate and can lead to obliteration of the lumen (Figure 15-30). In the cardiovascular system the ascending and thoracic parts of the aorta are the chief targets. Involvement of the vasa vasorum and their extensions into the aortic wall leads to destruction of the elastic laminae and smooth muscle of the media and thus to aneurysm formation. The intimal surface shows a wrinkled appearance likened to tree-bark. But neither of these changes is specific for syphilis.

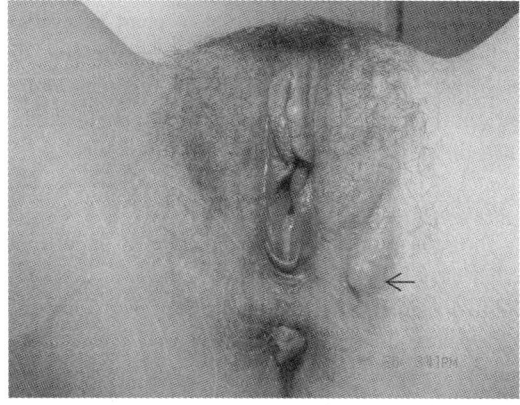

Figure 15-28 Syphilis, showing syphiloma or gumma

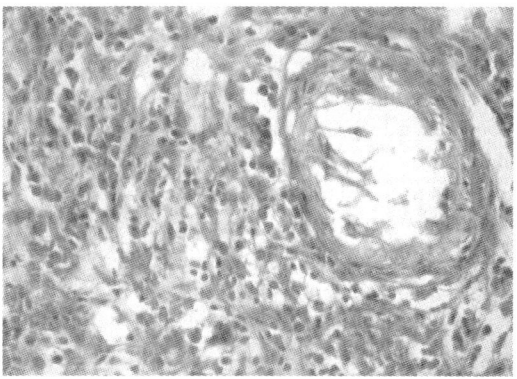

Figure 15-29 Syphilis, showing epithelioid cells, lymphocytes, plasma cells, and plump fibroblasts in gumma (high power)

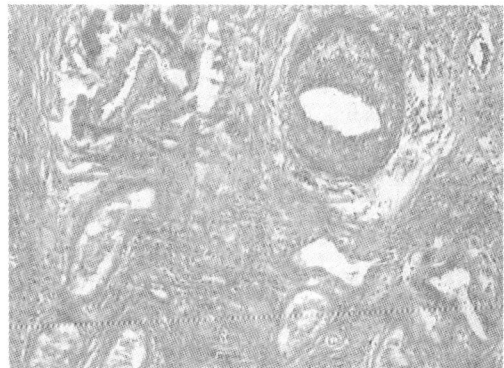

Figure 15-30 Syphilis, showing obliterative endarteritis and periangiitis (low power)

Pathological Development and Clinical Related Features

Untreated syphilis progresses through 3 stages: primary, secondary and tertiary stages. Early syphilis (primary and secondary) responds to penicillin. Late syphilis (tertiary) does not respond to antibiotic therapy and represent a chronic progressive disease that frequently causes considerable morbidity and, ultimately, death. So it is important to distinguish different stages.

1. Primary syphilis

The primary syphilis develops after an incubation period of 10 - 90 days, with the average 21 - 28 days. The first visible lesion is termed the primary chancre. The chancre appears at the site of initial invasion—usually the penis (glans or shaft) in the male and the vulva in the female. Other sites include the cervix, scrotum, anus, rectum, and oral cavity.

The primary chancre is a painless, indurated papule and often ulcerates (hard chancre) consisting of chronic inflammatory tissue. It occurs usually within a month of infection. Its surface exudes a serous fluid containing large numbers of treponemes. Painless enlargement of the inguinal lymph nodes may be present, but there are no systemic symptoms and the patient feels well.

Microscopically there is an inflammatory infiltrate in perivascular, chiefly be plasma cells, lymphocytes and macrophages. Endothelial cells lining blood vessels in the lesions proliferate, swell and may subsequently occlude the lumen of the small blood vessels. The draining lymph nodes may be enlarged. Organisms are usually plentiful and may be found in the fluid that oozes from the areas of ulcerated chancre. The chancres heal spontaneously. In about 50% the disease progesses no further but in the other half widespread dissemination of the treponema occurs leading to the secondary stage.

The diagnosis of syphilis is best made at this stage by identifying spirochetes in the serous exudate from the chancre by dark-field microscopy. Serologic tests for syphilis may be negative in the early primary stage, and the organism can not be cultured. The primary chancre heals spontaneously in 3 - 6 weeks.

2. Secondary syphilis

Secondary syphilis usually follows the primary stage after 2 - 20 weeks but may begin before the primary chancre heals. It is noted by fever, malaise, myalgia, and arthralgias, generalized enlargement of lymph node, and there is a generalized maculopapular skin rash, particularly in face, palms and soles, usually with red or coppercolour (Figure 15-31). Orogenital mucosal lesions are common. The mucous membranes of the mouth show white patches that break down to form lesions known as 'snail-track ulcers'. Flat papules (condylomata lata) occur at moist cutaneous/mucocutaneous areas, e. g. anus, vulva and perineum, which contain large numbers of treponemas and are very infectious. Hepatitis, meningitis, nephritis (immune complex type), and osteochondritis may also occur. Immune complexes may cause lesions in the kidney.

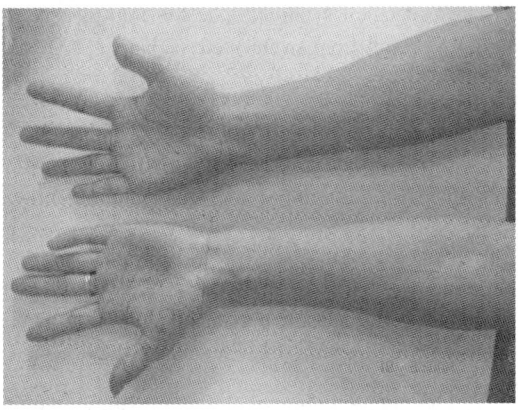

Figure 15-31 Secondary syphilis, showing maculopapular skin rash with red color

Microscopically, these lesions are characterized by a nonspecific chronic inflammatory response with numerous plasma cells. Spirochetes are present in large numbers and can be demonstrated in tissue sections with Dieterle's silver stain. Skin lesions reveal hyperkeratosis of the epidermis, capillary proliferation with endothelial swelling in the superficial corium, and transmigration of polymorphonuclear neutrophils. In the deeper dermis, perivascular infiltration by monocytes, plasma cells, and lymphocytes occurs.

The symptoms and the lesions disappear spontaneously over a few months and the patients are then no longer infectious. Complete clearance of the organism is rare and the treponemas appear to enter a latent phase.

Diagnosis is by demonstration of the living organism in smears made from lesions and examined by dark-field microscopy, special stains of tissue section from a lesion such as a condyloma latum, or positive serologic tests.

3. Tertiary syphilis

Manifestations of tertiary syphilis or late syphilis occur 1-4 or more years from the date of primary infection. Even without treatment, only 30% of cases of early syphilis ever develop tertiary syphilis. Primary and secondary stages may have been so subtle (subclinical) that patients with tertiary syphilis frequently give no history of symptoms of early syphilis.

The lesions in this stage are mainly obliterative endarteritis, periangiitis, and Gummatous necrosis, and they are very destructive. The clinical features will depend on the location. The Gummatous necrosis consist of granulomatous inflammation with a center of coagulated necrotic material and margins composed of plump or palisaded macrophages and fibroblasts surrounded by large numbers of mononuclear leukocytes, chiefly be plasma cells. Treponemes are scant in these gummas and are difficult to demonstrate. Healing occurs with criss-crossing fibrous bands and coarse scarring. Besides, aortitis reveals inflammatory scarring of the tunica media, secondary to obliterative endarteritis of the vasa vasorum. A patchy uneven loss of the medial elastic fibers and muscle cells is evident. The lesions of central nerves system and cardiovascular system are often involved in this stage, leading to neurosyphilis and cardiovascular syphilis.

a. Neurosyphilis. Forty percent of patients with early syphilis develop cerebrospinal fluid infection. Asymptomatic neurosyphilis is diagnosed in patients who have an abnormal cerebrospinal fluid featured by elevated protein and cells with a positive serologic test for syphilis. Twenty percent of patients with untreated asymptomatic neurosyphilis progress to clinical neurosyphilis, which is manifested as chronic meningovascular syphilis, tabes dorsalis, or general paresis. Tertiary syphilis in the central nervous system falls into two groups.

- **Meningovascular syphilis.** It involves either the leptomeninges, which are more frequently, or pachymeninges. Leptomeningitis occurs mainly at the base of the brain with swelling and thickening. Gummatous necrosis may occasionally be seen. Cranial nerve involvement is not uncommon and there may be obstruction of the 4th ventricle causing hydrocephalus. Pachymeningitis may occur over the surface and in relation to the spinal cord.

- **Parenchymatous Neurosyphilis**

Tabes dorsalis

It is characterized by degeneration of certain sensory fibres in the posterior nerve roots and posterior columns of the spinal cord. The posterior columns atrophy and become grey. This is associated with fibre loss and demyelination. The degeneration leads to loss of function especially in respect to deep pressure sensation, vibration and position sense and co-ordination leading to a stamping gait. There may be severe shooting pains in the limbs with lightning pains. The lack of sensation may lead to disorganization of joints, which is called Charcot's joints.

General paresis of the insane

In this state the brain becomes shrunken and the cerebral cortex is disorganized with degeneration of nerve cells and fibres especially in the grey matter which is associated with proliferation of astrocytes. Intracerebral blood vessels show perivascular plasma cells cuffing and endothelial swelling. Treponemas are relatively easy to find. Clinically there is deterioration in personality and changes in mental function which may express themselves in bizarre and grandiose delusions. If untreated there is dementia.

b. Cardiovascular syphilis. Involvement of the aorta is common in tertiary syphilis, usually occurring 10-40 years after the primary infection. Symptomatic cardiovascular syphilis occurs in 10% of patients with untreated late syphilis. The incidence at autopsy is as high as 50%. Cardiovascular syphilis is characterized by aneurysms in the ascending thoracic aorta, aortic valve incompetence, and myocardial ischemia secondary to coronary ostial narrowing due to aortic fibrosis.

In many patients the disease will pursue a course lasting many years if untreated and falls into three clear defined stages. And some of the infected persons are clinically symptomatic, i.e. latent syphilis.

c. Latent syphilis. This conception denotes that a diagnosis of latent syphilis is made when a specific treponemal antibody test is positive in a person with no clinical features of syphilis and normal cerebrospinal fluid. Over 70% of patients never develop late stages of syphilis. A minority do. However, patients with latent syphilis can intermittently seed the blood with treponemes and are capable of causing transfusion and transplacental infections.

d. Congenital syphilis (Figure 15-32). Transplacental infection and spread of the fetus usually occurs in the fifth month of pregnancy if the mother has untreated early (first 4 years) syphilis. The risk of fetal infection if the mother has early untreated syphilis is over 75%. Routine serologic testing and treatment of women in early pregnancy prevents congenital syphilis, which now occurs only when there is deficient prenatal care. Intrauterine infection may lead to abortion, stillbirth, and development of congenital syphilis in the neonatal period or latent infection.

Abortion and intrauterine death of the fetus occurs in 40% of infections. If the infection causes lesions in the perinatal period these are dominated by skin and mucous membrane involvement, i. e. desquamative skin rashes and ulcerating patches on mucous membranes. These lesions are highly infective and contain numerous spirochetes. Congenital infection with a prolonged latent period shows similar manifestations to the tertiary stage of acquired infection. Osteochondritis and perichondritis have severe effects on growing bone and cartilage, especially the nose, causing nasal bridge collapse (saddle nose), and formation of new bone over the surface of the tibia giving a sabre-like appearance (sabre shins). The Liver involvement may leads to diffuse hepatic fibrosis. There may be interstitial fibrosis and inflammation in the lung (pneumonia alba). The cornea may characterized by keratitis, leading to blindness. The teeth can show characteristic changes with screw-driver or peg-shaped incisors, which is called Hutchinson's teeth or Moon's molars (Figure 15-7-8). Nerve deafness can occur due to meningovascular inflammation. Gummas and neurosyphilis may occur in all forms of congenital syphilis; syphilitic aortitis is extremely uncommon.

Congenital syphilis with a prolonged latent period shows similar manifestation to the tertiary stage of acquired syphilis.

The diagnosis of congenital syphilis is based on clinical manifestations, dark-field microscopy, and serologic tests. Serologic tests are difficult to interpret because of transplacental transfer of maternal IgG antibodies to the fetus. An IgM FTA-ABS test that measures only fetal IgM treponemal antibodies has been used to the diagnosis of congenital syphilis.

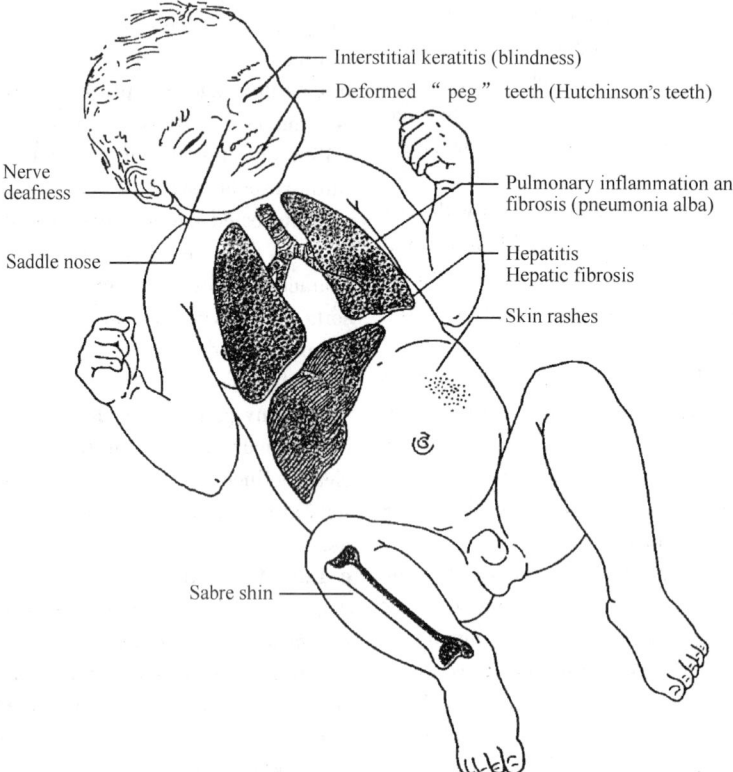

Figure 15-32 Clinical and pathologic features of congenital syphilis

Lab Diagnosis

Direct visualization of the organism by darkfield microscopy, immunofluorescent stain, or serologic test is necessary for diagnosis of syphilis because that *T. pallidum* cannot be cultivated in vitro and can not be seen under the light microscope. Darkfield microscopic diagnosis of oral lesions should be avoided because of the difficulty in distinguishing *T. pallidum* morphologically from *Treponema macrodentium* and *Treponema microdentium*, both are nonpathologic treponemes which can be found in the mouths of healthy individuals. A positive result of darkfield examination is the only means of making an absolute diagnosis of syphilis. A negative result of darkfield examination does not eliminate the diagnosis, and the lesion should be reexamined. The sensitivities of nontreponemal tests, VDRL and rapid plasma reagent (RPR), to diagnose syphilis are approaching 80% in patients with symptomatic primary syphilis and virtually 100% in patients with secondary syphilis. So it is valuable to screen syphilis. Patients with a positive VDRL or RPR should have to confirmed by specific treponemal testing, such as the fluorescent treponemal antibody absorption (FTA-ABS) and the microhemagglutination assay for *T. pallidum* (MHA-TP).

Complications and Prognosis

A. Complication

Virtually any organ in the body can be involved. The mainly complication include cardiovascular disease, CNS disease, Membranous glomerulonephritis, paroxysmal cold hemoglobinemia, irreversible end-organ damage, and Jarisch-Herxheimer reaction.

B. Prognosis

For patients with tertiary syphilis, overall prognosis depends on the duration and extent of disease activity, along with prior attempts to treat the disease.

The prognosis in primary and secondary syphilis is good following appropriate treatment. *T. pallidum* is sensitive to the penicillins and cure is likely in the early stages. Primary syphilis can heals spontaneously in 3-7 weeks. Symptom of secondary syphilis usually resolves without treatment.

Tertiary syphilis is associated with serious illness and disability; death may result in approximately 20% of untreated patients, with most of those deaths resulting from cardiovascular syphilis and neurosyphilis. In patients with neurosyphilis complicated by optic atrophy and blindness, the ability to regain vision remains poor despite attempts with high-dose penicillin. So, the prognosis in tertiary syphilis is less sanguine, although a significant number of patients demonstrate cure with antibiotic therapy.

Congenital syphilis is the most serious outcome of syphilis in women. It has been shown that a higher proportion of infants are affected if the mother has untreated secondary syphilis, compared to untreated early latent syphilis. For patients who are pregnant and have early syphilis, it is likely that the mother will deliver a child not infected by syphilis (assuming the mother was treated appropriately). Since *T. pallidum* does not invade the placental tissue or the fetus until the fifth month of gestation, syphilis causes late abortion, stillbirth, or death soon after delivery in more than 40% of untreated maternal infections. Neonatal mortality usually results from pulmonary hemorrhage, bacterial superinfection, or fulminant hepatitis.

Chapter 16 Parasitosis

Dong Jianguo

CHAPTER CONTENTS
- Amebiasis
    - Intestinal Amebiasis
    - Extraintestinal Amebiasis
- Schistosomiasis
- Clonorchiasis
- Paragonimiasis
- Hydatid Disease
    - Echinococcosis Granulosus Disease
    - Echinococcosis Multilocularis Disease

Parasitoses are common diseases worldwide and are diseases caused by parasites regarded as pathogens. The disease is initiated when the infectious stage of a parasite is transmitted to a susceptible host. Many factors such as physical and biologic factors can influence the probability of successful transmission. Physical factors include geographic locale, climate, humidity, altitude, season and so on. Biologic factors are such parameters as the abundance and distribution of appropriate host and vectors as well as the biotic habitat of a given locale. The levels of sanitation and hygiene present among the population of the region are also important for successful transmission of parasite to host.

Parasitic lesions can be acute but most of them are chronic. The lesions vary depending on parasitic virulence, physical size, phase of their life cycle, location within or on the host's body, abundance within the host, and the host's response to parasitic infection. In addition, the movements of parasites through their hosts provide portals of entry and sites for other pathogens to initiate secondary infection. Some of cases can be asymptomatic carriers.

Parasitoses are common diseases worldwide but more prevalent in underdeveloped countries.

AMEBIASIS

Amebiasis is the infection caused by the *Entameba histolytica*, a protozoan whose life cycle involves several changes in structure. From the medical standpoint, the cystic and the trophozoite or motile forms are more important. Infection occurs by ingestion of cysts in food and water contaminated with feces. The protozoan inhabits the bowel but may penetrate the mucosa and possibly invade locally or by hematogenous spread to other organs such as liver, lung, brain or skin and cause the organs of **amebic abscesses.**

E. histolytica is a common pathogen throughout the world and is maintained in the population by carriers. It is more prevalent in the tropics and subtropics than in the cooler climates. However, in unsanitary conditions in temperate and colder climates, infection rates have been found to be the same to that seen in the tropics. In China it occurs mainly in southern countryside but also has been found in northern areas during summer.

INTESTINAL AMEBIASIS

Intestinal amebiasis is a disease caused by *E. histolytica* that inhabits the intestinal tract. Clinically, patients present with bloody and mucous diarrhea accompanied by low-grade fever, therefore, intestinal amebiasis is often called **amebic dysentery.**

Etiology and Pathogenesis

Several protozoan species in the genus *Entameba* infect humans, but not all of them are associated with disease. *E. histolytica* is well recognized as a pathogenic ameba, associated with intestinal and extraintestinal infections. All species have a simple life cycle that usually consists of an infective cyst stage and a multiplying trophozoite stage. The trophozoite stage exists only in the host and in fresh feces and is responsible for tissue damage. Cysts are stage in the life cycle of protozoan parasites that are spherical and have a refractile wall that protects them against the hazards of the environment outside of the host's body and are capable of surviving days to weeks outside the host in water and soils and on foods, especially under moist conditions. The cyst is infectious, and E. histolytica is transmitted when humans swallow mature cysts in food, water, or hands contaminated by feces.

After cyst ingestion by humans, no changes occur in an acid environment because the cyst wall is resistant to destruction by the acid content of the stomach; however, it is destroyed by the alkaline intestinal medium, the encysted organism becomes active, with the outcome being four separate small trophozoites. These organisms develop into the adult trophozoites, which vary in size from about 20 to 40 μm. The adult trophozoite or motile form moves downstream and colonizes the large intestine, particularly the cecum. Once in the colon, E. histolytica can behave either as a commensal or as a highly invasive pathogen. Organisms recovered from diarrheic or dysenteric stools are generally larger than those in a formed stool from an asymptomatic individual. The cytoplasm is differentiated into a clear outer ectoplasm with a more granular inner endoplasm. The nucleus is characterized by having evenly arranged chromatin on the nuclear membrane and the presence of a small, compact, centrally located karyosome. The cytoplasm is usually described as finely granular with glycogen masses and few ingested bacteria or debris in vacuoles. In a patient with dysentery, red blood cells may be visible in the cytoplasm, and this feature is usually diagnostic for E. histolytica.

Although the exact mode of mucosal penetration is not know, microscopy studies suggest ameba have enzymes that lyse host tissue, possibly from lysosomes on the surface of the ameba or from ruptured organisms.

Pathologic Changes and Clinical Manifestations

Ingested cysts release active amebas (trophozoites) that invade the large intestinal mucosa and enter the submucosa, which is the site of maximal involvement. The amebas cause multiple areas of enzymatic necrosis of tissue and acute inflammation, leading to mucosal ulcer throughout the colon.

Ulcers are usually raised with a small opening on the mucosal surface and a larger area of destruction below the surface, leading to "flask-shaped" submucosal abscesses (Figure 16-1). The mucosal surface show multiple ulcers separated by healthy-appearing mucosa, which is, however, undermined by the submucosal abscesses. Confluence of mucosal ulcers results in large areas of denuded mucosa covered by a necrotic base. Amebas are found in the walls of the ulcers (Figure 16-2). The trophozoites typically contain phagocytosed erythrocytes in their cytoplasm.

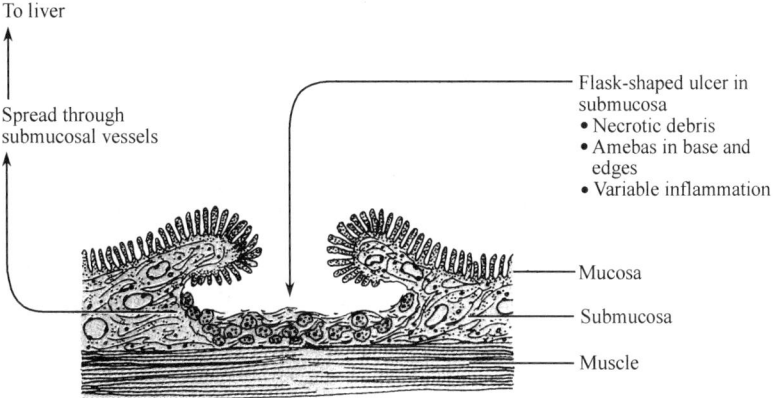

Figure 16-1 Amebic colitis, showing typical flask-shaped ulcers with maximal involvement of the submucosa

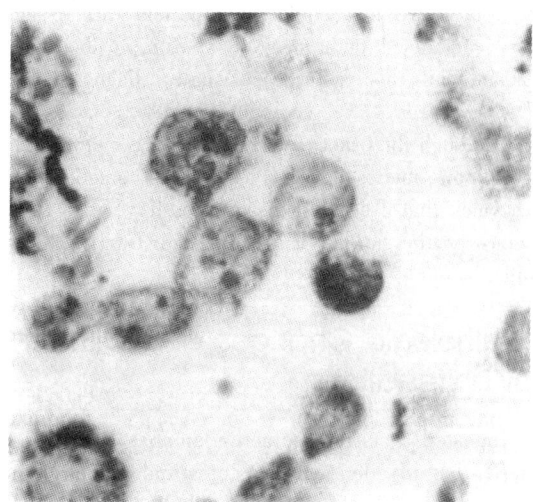

Figure 16-2 Amebic colitis. High-magnification photograph of the edge of an ulcer, showing trophozoites of *Entamoeba histolytica*. Note the presence of ingested erythrocytes that characterize tissue forms

Infection is usually localized to the submucosa and mucosa. Rarely, necrosis involves the muscle, leading to intestinal perforation. Hemorrhage and toxic megacolon may also occur with severe infection Venous spread to the liver may also occur. Microscopic examination of an ulcer reveals necrosis caused by parasites' proteolytic enzymes. The ulcers are often flask shaped because of destruction of the submucosa and overgrowth by epithelial cells in longitudinally sectioned tissue. Inflammation usually does not occur unless there has been secondary bacterial invasion. Occasionally, parasites that have ingested red blood cells can be observed and this is pathognomonic for *E. histolytica*. **Amebomas, granulomatous formations**, are observed infrequently in patients suffering from chronic intestinal amebiasis. Although amebomas respond to appropriate chemotherapy but they resemble carcinomas clinically, the differential diagnosis between ameboma and cancer is difficult to make, and as a result most amebomas are not discovered until after surgery.

EXTRAINTESTINAL AMEBIASIS

Amebic Liver Abscess

Hepatic amebiasis is the most common complication of intestinal infection by *E. histolytica*. The disease may be acute or chronic and ordinarily occurs several months or even years after intestinal infection. Hepatic amebiasis is caused by the entry of amebic trophozoites into portal venous radicles in the colonic submucosa, whence they are carried to the liver. Hepatic infection usually occurs in patients with subclinical or chronic intestinal amebic infection and very rarely during an attack of acute amebic colitis. About half the patients with hepatic amebiasis give no history suggestive of preceding amebic colitis.

When they reach the liver, the amebas cause focal enzymatic necrosis of hepatocytes and usually a single abscess forms in the right lobe of the liver. In the early stage of the disease, there are **multiple microabscesses** throughout the liver. Although the term "abscess" is used, amebic liver abscesses are not true abscesses because they contain few neutrophils and are composed of liquefied necrotic hepatic tissue. The patient presents at this stage with high fever, right upper abdominal pain, and tender hepatomegaly. With progression, the microabscesses coalesce to form larger abscesses.

Grossly, **amebic abscesses** are large, lined by an irregular wall, and contain amebic "pus," which has the typical reddish-brown hue (likened to anchovy paste) of liquefied liver (Figure 16-3). Abscesses compress the liver parenchyma around them, and a **pseudocapsule** of pale fibrous tissue is formed. Trophozoites of *E. histolytica* may be found in the abscess wall but are rarely demonstrable in the necrotic material.

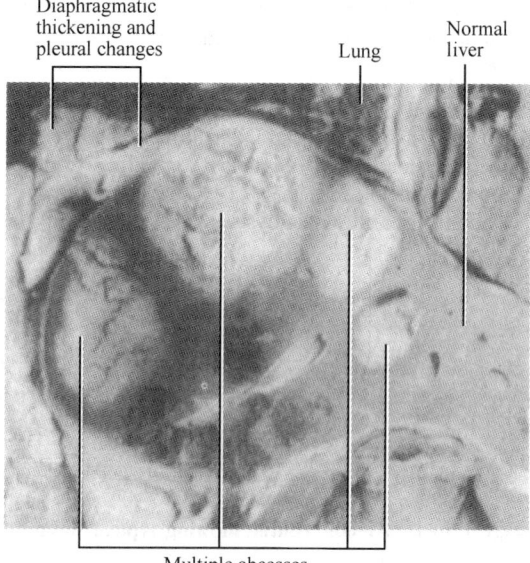

Figure 16-3 Amebic liver abscesses

Typical complaints in clinic include: right upper quadrant pain, fever, weight loss, and night sweats. Signs include liver tenderness and hepatomegaly. Without treatment, amebic liver abscess has a high mortality rate. Deaths are due to (1) rupture into the free peritoneal cavity; (2) rupture into the pleural cavity and lung; (3) rupture into the pericardial sac (in left lobe abscesses), causing acute pericardial tamponade; and (4) systemic spread of trophozoites, resulting in amebic abscesses in the brain and lung.

Amebic Lung Abscesses

The most frequent mechanism in the formation of lung abscesses is direct extension of hepatic abscesses through the diaphragm into the right lobe of the lung. Hematogenous pulmonary abscesses may develop as a result of amebic emboli transported in the bloodstream. These emboli originate in the branches of the hepatic vein or in the colonic blood vessels.

Amebic Brain Abscesses

Amebic abscesses of the brain are usually solitary and located in either cerebral hemisphere but the cerebellum is rarely involved. The amebas can reach the meninges and the cerebral substance, where they produce **encephalomalacia.**

SCHISTOSOMIASIS

Schistosomiasis refers to infection by dioecious trematodes of the genus *Schistosoma*. Man acquires the disease when cercaria successfully penetrates the skin. The adult worms live in the intestinal venous plexuses and produce eggs that are carried via the portal vein to the liver, where they are deposited in the portal areas. They produce granulomas in the acute phase followed by **pipestem fibrosis** of the portal areas in the chronic phase.

The major *schistosome* species that infect humans are: *Schistosoma haematobium*, which occurs in Northen Africa, *Schistosoma japonicum*, which is indigenous to Asia, and *Schistosoma mansoni*, which causes intestinal infection in Africa, the Middle East, South America, and some Caribbean countries. *S. japonicum* is the only species involved in China.

S. japonicum is mainly distributed in drainage area of Yangtse River and the southern areas of the river. Schistosomiasis was in infestation more than two thousands years ago, which were found in Han dynasty bodies excavated in tomb no. 1 at Mawangdui in the city of Changsha in Hunan province in 1972 and in tomb no. 168 at Fenghuangshan in Jiangling county in Hubei province in 1975. Schistosomiasis was controlled after establishment of People's Republic of China and it was disappeared in most endemic areas. However, it deserves attention to that the disease recurs in some areas recently.

Etiology and Infection

The life cycle of *S. japonicum* include stages of egg, miracidium, sporocyst, cercariaeum, schistosomulum and adult worm (Figure 16-4). In addition to humans, numerous animals such as cats, cattle, dogs, pigs, horses and mice are naturally infected and become reservoir hosts in many endemic areas. Development of schistosoma from miracidium to cercariaeum is in *Oncomelania* snails, which are operculated, amphibious, and able to survive prolonged periods of desiccation with the infection.

The infection is singularity because humans become transmitted by penetration of cercaiae through intact skin. Cercariae consist of a body containing glands whose material is used to penetrate skin and a bifurcated tail that is lost when the cercariae penetrate the skin. Once the cercariae have successfully entered the host, it is termed a schistosomulum. The schistosomulum migrates through the tissues and finally invades a blood vessel. On entry into the blood vessels, the schistosomulum is carried to all of the body. Only those able to pass from the arterial to the venous side survive and this takes place for the most part in the abdominal organs drained by the portal system, where each schistosomulum develops into an adult male or female worm. The adult worms migrate against the mesenteric circulation, where they copulate and where the females deposit their ova in the small venules of the liver and the submucosa of the intestine. The eggs are immature when first laid and take about 11 days to develop a mature miracidium. Eggs deposit intravascularly and then the eggs work their way through the tissues into the intestine to be released from the body in the feces. Egg migration through the tissues is facilitated by the miracidium's release of enzymes through the eggshell and these enzymes help digest the tissue. Eggs containing a mature miracidium that is released when the egg is in contact with water. The actively swimming miracidium seeks a suitable snail host, which it penetrates. Within the snail, the miracidium develops into a mother sporocyst, which in turn produces daughter sporocysts. The daughter sporocysts develop in the snail's hepatopancreas and produce cercariae. The cercariae are released from the snail into water, where they may infect humans by penetrating the skin. The typical incubation period takes four to six weeks to complete, and chronic infections lasting 25 to 30 years are common. The lifespan of the typical female schistosome is thought to range from five to ten years.

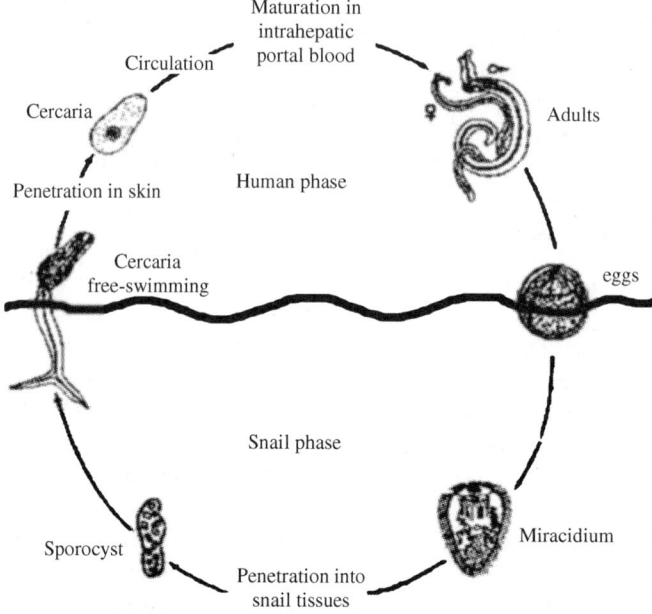

Figure 16-4　The life cycle of *S. japonicum*

Basic Morphology and Pathogenesis

Cercariae, schistosomulum, adult worm, egg in the life cycle of schistosomes all can be pathogen but it is the most severe that eggs cause the damage of the body in all of them.

A. Lesions Caused by Cercariae

The onset of acute schistosomiasis often begins shortly after cercarial penetration and it is signaled by **petechial hemorrhages** with edema and pruritus and maculopapular eruptions at the sites of skin penetration. That is so-called "**cercarial dermatitis.**" Cercarial dermatitis lasts for two to five days then disappear naturally. Cutaneous sign is a feature of human infection with cercariae in the subcutaneous tissues and immediate hypersensitivity reactions at the invasion sites.

B. Lesions Caused by Schistosomulum

After infection and the transformation of cercariaeum to schistosomulum, the schistosomulum expresses antigens on its surface that evokes a host immune response providing some degree of resistance to reinfection. The eosinophil is the major component of the host immune response against the schistosomula. Eosinophils adhere to the surface of the schistosomulum in the presence of antibody or complement. This is followed by degranulation and the release of granule contents, which include lysosomal hydrolytic enzymes, peroxidase, and major basic protein. In addition to the lesion of host caused by eosinophil-mediated effectors the schistosomulum migration through the tissues can cause mechanistic damage.

C. Lesions Caused by Adult Worms

Adult worms become less antigenic because the worms are able to incorporate host antigen onto their surface, thus preventing the host from recognizing these parasites as foreign material. Therefore the adult worms do not appear to cause severe damage to the host, nor do they evoke much of an immune response.

D. Lesions Caused by Eggs

1. Acute egg nodule

Granuloma aggregation in the intestinal wall is the major cause of pathological change. With the production of eggs by the adult worms, the eggs become trapped in the fine venules and are able to pass through the tissues, escaping into the intestine or other organs of body. Eggs remain viable from three weeks to a year or more, and at the same time release enzymes and a soluble egg antigen (SEA). Experimental studies have shown that SEA gives rise to a delayed hypersensitivity response and evokes **minute abscesses**, which facilitate their passage into the lumen of the intestine. As eggs are deposited in the tissues, the antigenic substances secreted by the eggs invoke a host immune response that causes the formation of granulomas around the eggs trapped in the tissues. Cellular infiltrates include lymphocytes, eosinophils, macrophages, and fibroblasts.

2. Chronic egg nodule

After death of the embryo in the acute egg nodule the egg granulomas can induce collagen formation accompanied by sporadic foreign body giant cell and filtration of lymph cells. The chronic egg nodule with centrally located ova is classic **bilharzial pseudotubercle**, which is evident in biopsy specimens obtained 80 days after infection. At the end the egg nodule becomes fibrosis and hyaline and consequentially the organs involved extensive fibrosis and deformed. The reparative fibrosis that follows the destruction caused by the egg granulomas is not sufficient to explain the extensive fibrosis. It seems that the egg granulomas can induce collagen formation through a mechanism other than necrosis followed by reparative fibrosis, for example, the collagen metabolism induced by SEA.

E. Lesions Caused by Circulating Antigens and Immune Complex

Circulating antigens and immune complex appear to be correlated with the worm burden of the host. These antigens and immune complex may be deposited on the basement membrane and glomerular capillaries, causing nephrosclerosis and kidney failure. The majority of cases have histopathologic findings consistent with a diffuse membranoproliferative glomerulonephritis in which immune complexes are detected by both immunoliuorescence and electron microscopy.

Pathologic Changes of Some Organs and Their Consequences

S. japonicum adults are mainly found in the radicles of the portal venous system and also have a tendency to be found in ectopic sites. Because of the higher egg production and the smaller egg size, an infection with just a few worm pairs can be very serious. The reason is that the eggs can be free in the general circulation to be filtered out in the liver, lung, and even the central nervous system.

A. Colonic Schistosomiasis

S. japonicum mainly inhabit the mesenteric veins and it's eggs are deposited in capillaries and venules of the large intestine and rectum. So the distal parts of the colon are more frequently and severely affected in intestinal schistosomiasis. The eggs cause acute egg nodules then turning to chronic egg nodule. The wall of the intestine becomes inflamed, thickened and polyps may form that protrude into the lumen. These **inflammatory polyps** may reach 1 cm and may produce bleeding from their ulcerated surfaces from where eggs are released to the lumen and passed with feces. During heavy infection the wall of the colon becomes densely fibrotic and very rigid, reducing in size of the intestinal lumen and leading to **mechanical obstruction**. Association between schistosomiasis and colonic carcinoma has been reported by investigators in China.

B. Hepatosplenic Schistosomiasis

Those eggs that do not enter the intestinal lumen or are not trapped in the mucosa will be carried to the liver via the hepatic portal system. Eggs deposited in the portal triads of the liver stimulate a granulomatous response, leading to continuous fibrosis of the periportal tissue. The fibrotic tissue is white and hard and has been referred to as **"pipestem" fibrosis** in the gross descriptive term because of the prominent vascular and fibrotic changes in the portal areas, the latter are moderately broadened and lengthened and stand out in cross section. The liver increases in size as a result of the lesions induced by the eggs at early stage and may decrease in size as a result of the extensive fibrosis in the liver portal spaces at the end. Contrary to the findings in classic liver cirrhosis, findings in the adjacent liver parenchyma and the majority of the liver function tests in uncomplicated schistosomiasis are negative. The most frequently encountered vascular lesion is that in which the intrahepatic portal radical is totally replaced by a granuloma that occludes the lumen. Occasionally an acute endophlebitis of the intrahepatic radicles is encountered, which is probably most important in the final causation of the intrahepatic vascular block. Inflammation and destruction of the coats of the vessels lead to thrombosis and the thrombi are organized. Portal blood is significantly diminished because of periportal fibrosis and vascular destruction, which leads to **portal hypertension, splenomegaly**, and the development of **collateral circulation**, such as esophageal varices. **Ascites** may be evident, depending on the degree of liver obstruction. The spleen becomes congested and increases greatly in size with subsequent fibrosis of the parenchyma and formation of brown siderotic nodule.

C. Schistosomiasis in other organs

Inhabitation of an adult worm or deposition of eggs found in tissues out of portal system such as lung, brain, spinal cord and pancreas is called **ectopic parasitism.** Pulmonary schistosomiasis is more common. Eggs and even worms may reach the lung via portasystemic anastomoses, leading to arteritis, granuloma formation and fibrosis of the pulmonary bed. The subsequent development of pulmonary hypertension leads to cor pulmonale. Clinical signs of the disease include fatigue, cough with possible hemoptysis, palpitations, dyspnea, right ventricular hypertrophy and pulmonary artery dilation. Because of anastomoses of the mesenteric, pelvic, and spinal veins, both the worms and eggs may reach the central nervous system more readily and evoke inflammatory reaction with focal lesions and generalized epileptiform seizures. Eggs trapped in the brain have caused cerebral atrophy and falling sickness. Neurologic symptoms and signs may include lethargy or coma, decreased mental ability, or spastic paralysis of one or more limbs. The severity of kidney disease is associated with the worm burden and the degree and duration of hepatic fibrosis.

CLONORCHIASIS

Clonorchiasis is caused by the trematode *Clonorchis sinensis*. Adult worm inhabits the intrahepatic distal portion of the bile duct, hence the name **liver fluke**, although flukes have been found throughout the biliary passages, gall bladder, and even the pancreatic duct of heavily infected hosts. The worm is endemic to Asia and can be found in most of areas except the northwestern in China.

Etiology and Infection

The life cycle of *C. sinensis* begins when contaminated feces containing viable eggs reach water. If susceptible snail species ingest the eggs, the miracidia hatch in the digestive tract of the snail, penetrate the visceral wall, and metamorphose into the sporocyst stage. The sporocyst stage contains germinal tissue that gives rise to a number of rediae. After another period development, the rediae produce thousands of organisms known as cercariae. Cercariae infect the freshwater fish that serve as the second intermediate host and encyst in their muscle tissue, at which point the larval fluke is called a metacercaria. Infection occurs after man ingests raw or inadequately cooked fish that contain metacercariae. Metacercariae excyst in the duodenum or intestine, enter the common bile duct then migrate to the distal bile capillaries, where they develop into adult worms.

Pathologic Changes and Complications

The extent and intensity of pathological changes is related to intensity and duration of infection. Lesions are mainly confined to the biliary system and are the result of mechanical irritation and toxic products produced by the worms. Flukes and ova may be found (Figure 16-5). In light infections there appears to be little or no change in liver parenchyma, while in heavy infections there is thickening and localized dilations of the bile ducts with hyperplasia of the mucinous glands. As a result, the biliary tract may become obstructed, causing bile retention, periductal inflammatory infiltration of lymphocytes, plasma cells, and eosinophils. Severe portal fibrosis ensues, followed by cirrhosis with portal hypertension. The

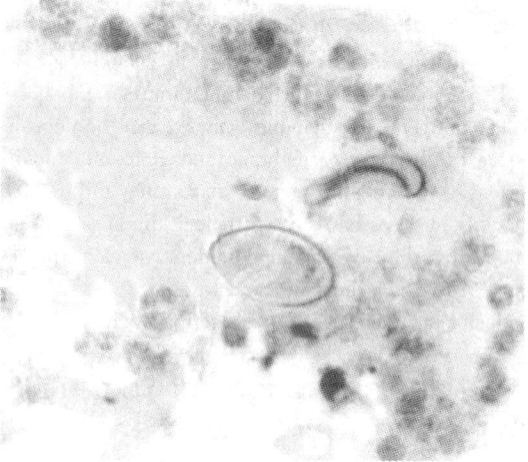

Figure 16-5 Aspirate of bile in oriental cholangiohepatitis, showing ova of *Clonorchis sinensis*

adenomatous hyperplasia of biliary duct epithelium is common and there are documents that *C. sinensis* has been linked to carcinoma of the bile duct.

PARAGONIMIASIS

Paragonimiasis is a disease of human or other mammals with flukes of *Paragonimus westermani* mainly found in the lung. Within the lungs the parasites become surrounded by fibrous, inflammatory capsule which eventually ruptures liberating ova and debris into the bronchioles. The disease is distributed throughout China.

Etiology and Infection

Reservoir hosts include dogs, cats and pigs besides human beings in areas of endemic infection. Eggs escape from the encapsulated tissue through the bronchioles and expectorated in the vicinity of water where they hatch in 2 to 3 weeks, releasing a miracidium to infect a susceptible snail host. Cercariae are released after a sporocyst and rediae generation. Cercariae infect crabs or crayfish and encyst in the gill vessels and muscles. Humans are infected by ingesting raw or pickled crustacea containing infectious metacercariae. The metacercariae excyst in the duodenum and migrate through the intestinal wall into the abdominal cavity. After migrating through the diaphragm, the larvae enter the lung parenchyma and reach maturity where they discharge their eggs into the bronchial secretions.

Pathogenesis and Pathologic Changes

Migration through the tissue produces localized hemorrhage and leukocytic infiltrates. When the worms finally reach the lungs and mature, a pronounced tissue reaction occurs with infiltration of eosinophils and neutrophils and a dense fibrotic capsule forms around the worm. The cysts produced by the presence of the worms contain brownish purulent fluid that is rather viscid and resembles anchovy sauce. The fluid is composed of the inflammatory exudates, erythrocytes, eosinophils necrotic debris, metabolic by-products, and numerous ova. Many of the cysts perforate into the bronchioles and release their contents into the respiratory tract. The eggs may also enter the pulmonary tissue or they may be carried by the circulatory system to other body sites, where they cause a **granulomatous reaction.** The patient may experience mild fever, and a cough with increased production of viscous blood-tinged sputum and increasing chest pain. Eventually chronic bronchitis develops with increasing dyspnea. Cachexia may develop in heavy infections and there may be secondary pulmonary infections.

Occasionally the worms may lodge in ectopic sites other than the lungs. Cysts have been detected in the liver, intestinal wall, muscles, the peritoneum, brain, or spinal cord.

HYDATID DISEASE

Hydatidosis, or Echinococcosis, is a zoonose in which man is really the intermediate host of the etiologic agent *Echinococcus* that is a species of tapeworm. There are mainly *Echinococcus granulosus* and *Echinococcus multilocularis* founding in human body. *Echinococcus granulosus* is more than *Echinococcus multilocularis* in China. Hydatidosis has endemic foci in sheep and cattle raising areas of the northwestern in China. Man is infected when he ingests ova.

ECHINOCOCCOSIS GRANULOSUS DISEASE

Etiology and Infection

Adult *E. granulosus* are small tapeworms (2 – 7 mm long) inhabiting in intestines of canids such as domestic dogs or wolves and possessing a scolex and three proglottids. Ova are passed in canine feces and ingested by herbivores such as sheep, cattle, or camel, which are intermediate host when they graze. The ova hatch in the duodenum, liberating the embryos, known as oncospheres or hexacanthes, which using their hooklets, find their way through the intestinal mucosa into the lumen of blood vessels and gain entrance into the hepatic portal system. Once in the circulation most embryos are filtered out of the blood within the liver. Only few of the embryos are pass through the liver or lymphatic system to infect the lungs, brain, spinal column, bones, or other visceral organs. After several months unilocular hydatid cysts appear in the liver or other tissue. Canidssuch as dogs act as definitive host when they eat the viscera of sheep or cattle with hydatid cysts. Larval tapeworms called protoscoleces are liberated in the small intestine of the dog and then become adult *E. granulosus* in about two months. Transmission of the parasite occurs when man contaminates his hands or food with ova and subsequently ingests them.

Pathogenesis and Basic Morphology

Although most of the oncospheres invaded into tissue are killed by macrophages, those that do begin to grow and develop into **hydatid cysts** containing numerous scolices provided with hooklets. Usually by the fifth month, the wall of the hydatid cyst has become differentiated into an outer friable, laminated, non-nucleated layer and an inner nucleated germinal layer. The cysts may reach a diameter of 10 to 20 cm and contain abundant clear fluid. A great deal of **daughter cysts** bud off from the inner germinal layer and may remain attached or float free interior of the fluid-filled cyst. The individual scolices bud of from the inner wall of the daughter cyst. Some of the cysts may collapse and undergo fibrosis and, not infrequently, calcification.

Pathologic Changes and Their Consequences

Hydatid disease in humans is potentially dangerous but size and organ location will greatly influence the outcome. In general hydatid cysts will remain undetectable for many years until they grow large enough to crowd the tissue around or other organs. The most common site of *E. granulosus* in humans is liver (about 70%) and they often infect the right lobe of the liver. Then there may be hepatomegaly, right upper quadrant pain, and possibly eosinophilia. Cysts in the lungs are usually asymptomatic until there is cough, shortness of breath, or chest pain.

There may be small fluid leaks into the systemic circulation that sensitize the patient during the life of the cyst. Later on if the cyst should burst or there is a large fluid leak, serious allergic response may occur, including anaphylactic shock.

ECHINOCOCCOSIS MULTILOCULARIS DISEASE

Etiology and Infection

The morphology of adult worms (1.4 - 3.4 mm) is similar to *E. granulosus* but smaller than it. The life cycle of *E. multilocularis* is essentially identical to that of *E. granulosus* with the following exceptions: the definitive hosts tend to be dogs, foxes, wolves and cats, while the intermediate hosts have been identified as field mice, ground squirrels, and shrews. Occasionally human may also be infected as an intermediate host by swallowing eggs.

Pathologic Changes

To be different to *E. granulosus*, the cyst of *E. multilocularis* is composed of many irregular cavities with little or no fluid, rare or no free scolices, and often central necrosis and cavitation of the lesion.

The alveolar form of hydatid disease has been mainly found in the liver although occasionally found in other tissues such as lung and brain. The disease may resemble a slow growing carcinoma and may present symptoms of hepatomegaly and splenomegaly. In full-developed disease, the liver may be destroyed severely and cause hepatic fibrosis, portal hyertension, jaundice, ascites and cachexia.